BSAVA Manual of
Canine and Feline
Radiography and Radiology
A Foundation Manual

Editors:

Andrew Holloway
BVSc CertSAM DVDI DipECVDI MRCVS
RCVS and European Specialist in Veterinary Diagnostic Imaging
Centre for Small Animal Studies, Animal Health Trust,
Kentford, Newmarket, Suffolk CB8 7UU

J. Fraser McConnell
BVM&S DVR DipECVDI CertSAM MRCVS
RCVS and European Specialist in Veterinary Diagnostic Imaging
Small Animal Teaching Hospital, University of Liverpool,
Leahurst, Chester High Road, Neston, Wirral CH64 7TE

Published by:

British Small Animal Veterinary Association
Woodrow House, 1 Telford Way,
Waterwells Business Park, Quedgeley,
Gloucester GL2 2AB

A Company Limited by Guarantee in England.
Registered Company No. 2837793.
Registered as a Charity.

A catalogue record for this book is available from the British Library.

ISBN 978-1-905319-44-2

The publishers, editors and contributors cannot take responsibility for
information provided on dosages and methods of application of drugs
mentioned or referred to in this publication. Details of this kind must be verified
in each case by individual users from up to date literature published by the
manufacturers or suppliers of those drugs. Veterinary surgeons are reminded
that in each case they must follow all appropriate national legislation and
regulations (for example, in the United Kingdom, the prescribing cascade)
from time to time in force.

Printed in the UK by Severn, Gloucester GL2 5EU – a carbon neutral printer
Printed on ECF paper made from sustainable forests

17176PUBS21

Titles in the BSAVA Manuals series:

For further information on these and all BSAVA publications, please visit our website: **www.bsava.com/shop**

Contents

To enable readers to view the radiographs in this manual on a larger scale, access to the online version is included. Go to **bsavalibrary.com/radiography-manual** and then to the 'Figures & Tables' tab for each chapter to view the images.

Contributors

Avi Avner BSc BVSc CVR DVDI MRCVS
RCVS Recognized Specialist in Veterinary Diagnostic Imaging
Chavat Daat Veterinary Specialist Referral Center, Beit Berl 44905, Israel

Elizabeth A. Baines MA VetMB DVR DipECVDI FHEA MRCVS
RCVS and European Specialist in Veterinary Diagnostic Imaging
Willows Referral Service, Highlands Road, Shirley, Solihull, West Midlands B90 4NH

Esther Barrett MA VetMB DVDI DipECVDI MRCVS
RCVS and European Specialist in Veterinary Diagnostic Imaging
Wales and West Imaging, Jubilee Villas, Tutshill, Chepstow, Gwent NP16 7DE

Kate J. Bradley MA VetMB PhD DVR DipECVDI MRCVS
European Specialist in Veterinary Diagnostic Imaging
School of Veterinary Services, University of Bristol, Langford House,
Langford, Bristol BS40 5DU

Abby Caine MA VetMB CertVDI DipECVDI MRCVS
European Specialist in Veterinary Diagnostic Imaging
Dick White Referrals, Station Farm, London Road, Six Mile Bottom, Suffolk CB8 0UH

Ruth Dennis MA VetMB DVR DipECVDI MRCVS
RCVS and European Specialist in Veterinary Diagnostic Imaging
Centre for Small Animal Studies, Animal Health Trust, Kentford, Newmarket, Suffolk CB8 7UU

Gawain Hammond MA VetMB MVM CertVDI DipECVDI FHEA MRCVS
European Specialist in Veterinary Diagnostic Imaging
School of Veterinary Medicine, University of Glasgow, Bearsden Road, Glasgow G61 1QH

Andrew Holloway BVSc CertSAM DVDI DipECVDI MRCVS
RCVS and European Specialist in Veterinary Diagnostic Imaging
Centre for Small Animal Studies, Animal Health Trust, Kentford, Newmarket, Suffolk CB8 7UU

J. Fraser McConnell BVM&S DVR DipECVDI CertSAM MRCVS
RCVS and European Specialist in Veterinary Diagnostic Imaging
Small Animal Teaching Hospital, University of Liverpool, Leahurst,
Chester High Road, Neston, Wirral CH64 7TE

Tobias Schwarz MA Dr.med.vet. DipECVDI DACVR DVR MRCVS
RCVS and European Specialist in Veterinary Diagnostic Imaging
Department of Veterinary Clinical Studies, Royal (Dick) School of Veterinary Studies,
The University of Edinburgh, Roslin EH25 9RG

Foreword

You know that you have reached a certain stage in your career when you are asked to write a Foreword for a Textbook or Manual. I was, however, delighted to be asked by the editors to write the Foreword for this *BSAVA Manual of Canine and Feline Radiography and Radiology*.

I was fortunate enough to be involved with the first publication on veterinary radiography that the BSAVA produced for practitioners. Called '*A Guide to Diagnostic Radiography in Small Animal Practice*' (edited by Peter Webbon) it was a thin A5 booklet with thick cardboard covers, which disguised the fact that there were not too many pages of text when it was published in 1981. The spiral binding was designed so that the book would lie flat on the X-ray table and it provided the practitioner with nuggets of information that were then only available in larger and more expensive textbooks. Simple line drawings augmented the text.

It is quite staggering how the depth and extent of knowledge relating to diagnostic imaging has increased over my professional life. The first edition of the *BSAVA Manual of Small Animal Diagnostic Imaging* (edited by Robin Lee), published in 1989, was a much larger publication than the original A5 booklet and also included an introduction to diagnostic ultrasonography. This Manual still relied upon line diagrams to demonstrate radiological signs, as radiographic reproductions were just not adequate in portraying these changes in enough detail. By the second edition, published in 1995, it was becoming clear that with the advances in diagnostic imaging it would no longer be possible to capture the depth of information that was emerging with newer imaging techniques, such as computed tomography or magnetic resonance imaging, in one book. This spawned the truly excellent and comprehensive BSAVA Manual series that includes thoracic imaging, abdominal imaging and musculoskeletal imaging as separate volumes. Indeed, each volume is bigger than the *Manual of Small Animal Diagnostic Imaging*, which they replaced.

This proliferation of imaging techniques, however, does not suit everyone and radiography still remains the lifeblood of diagnostic imaging in many veterinary practices due to its availability and, now with digital imaging, its immediacy. Digital images can be reviewed and manipulated almost immediately and, if necessary, sent electronically to an expert for further interpretation. So, it is in this context that the BSAVA have decided to return to the original concept to produce an informative and practical *Manual of Canine and Feline Radiography and Radiology*.

The editors have produced an excellent and exciting Manual. They have encouraged some of the best diagnostic imagers to contribute to this new Foundation Manual, which helps and supports busy practitioners with up-to-date information. The Manual includes both line drawings and radiographic reproductions to demonstrate the important radiological signs, which provides quick and accessible clinical information.

This is an excellent Manual. I just wonder where veterinary diagnostic imaging will go in the next 30 years.

Michael E. Herrtage MA BVSc DVSc DVR DVD DSAM DipECVDI DipECVIM-CA MRCVS
Professor of Small Animal Medicine
University of Cambridge

Preface

The original edition of the *BSAVA Manual of Small Animal Diagnostic Imaging*, edited by Robin Lee, was first published nearly 25 years ago. Since then, advances in veterinary diagnostic imaging have progressed rapidly with the widespread introduction and access to diagnostic ultrasonography, digital radiography and the cross-sectional imaging techniques of magnetic resonance imaging (MRI) and computed tomography (CT). The BSAVA now publishes separate titles on thoracic, abdominal and musculoskeletal imaging, as well as ultrasonography.

The purpose of the *BSAVA Manual of Canine and Feline Radiography and Radiology: A Foundation Manual* is to return to the fundamental principles of image interpretation for all body systems, as confident radiographic interpretation remains a considerable challenge for many, presenting, arguably, a more difficult skill to master than that of advanced cross-sectional imaging techniques.

Our own understanding of radiographic interpretation was greatly facilitated and developed by the film reading sessions held at Cambridge Veterinary School during the early 1990s, led by Mike Herrtage and Heike Rudorf. These sessions introduced us to a structured approach to radiographic interpretation (necessitating a rigorous examination of the entire radiograph), the value of consistent descriptive terminology using Röntgen signs, the construction of a list of relevant differential diagnoses and the need to consider appropriate and focused further investigations. This instruction instilled an appreciation of the significance and importance of individual Röntgen signs and a realistic understanding of the value of radiographic studies.

This Manual is not intended to illustrate the radiological appearance of a long list of diseases, as these are covered more exhaustively in other Manuals. Instead, the *BSAVA Manual of Canine and Feline Radiography and Radiology* aims to describe an approach to radiological interpretation, the range of variants and the key fundamental principles and their application to common diseases. In addition, throughout this Foundation Manual, the approach has been to highlight the importance of understanding the expectations and limitations of radiographic studies, as well as the errors which may lead to misinterpretation.

The publication of this Manual would not have been possible without access to the radiographic archives of the Animal Health Trust and the University of Liverpool (see below). In particular, we would like to thank Kate Bradley (University of Bristol), the Queen's Veterinary School Hospital at the University of Cambridge and Amy Pemberton for their assistance in tracking down additional images.

We would especially like to thank Katie McConnell for her invaluable assistance and guidance during the editing process. The editorial team at the BSAVA must be thanked for their patience and tolerance during the preparation of the manuscript and thanks also go to the illustrator, Samantha Elmhurst, for the schematics. We wish to thank all the contributing authors for their cooperation and patience during the period it has taken to compile this Manual.

We wish to thank our families for their understanding and support.

Andrew Holloway
Fraser McConnell
May 2013

Figure acknowledgements
The Animal Health Trust is thanked for providing Figures 2.9a, 2.14, 2.15, 5.37, 5.42, 5.94, 5.98, 5.99, 5.100, 5.102, 5.104, 5.105, 5.106, 6.12b, 6.13, 6.17, 6.18, 6.20, 6.23, 6.26, 6.34, 6.40, 6.45, 6.51, 6.66, 6.78, 6.97 and 9.9.
The University of Liverpool is thanked for providing Figures 2.9b, 2.32, 4.15, 5.38, 5.40, 5.47, 5.59, 5.65, 5.68, 5.73, 5.97, 5.103, 6.7, 6.11, 6.15, 6.21, 6.25, 6.29a, 6.31, 6.32, 6.33, 6.36, 6.37, 6.41, 6.43, 6.44, 6.53, 6.55, 6.64, 6.68, 6.79, 6.80, 6.83, 6.84, 6.86, 6.91, 6.93, 6.96, 6.99, 6.101, 6.103, 8.26, 8.27a, 8.32cd, 8.35, 8.36, 8.65, 8.80, 8.83, 8.84a, 8.89 and 9.51.

Physics and equipment

Ruth Dennis

Basic principles of radiography

X-rays are produced by X-ray machines when electricity from the mains is transformed into a high voltage current, following which some of the energy in the current is converted to X-ray energy. X-ray energy has some physical features of particles and some of wave-like energy, but can be thought of as tiny packets of energy, known as photons or quanta. The intensity and penetrating power of the emergent X-ray beam varies with the size and complexity of the apparatus and the exposure settings used. Portable X-ray machines are capable only of a relatively low output, whereas larger machines are far more powerful.

X-ray photons travel in straight lines and can be focused into an area called the primary beam, which is directed at the patient. Some of the photons are absorbed or scattered within the tissues of the patient; others pass through the tissues and are detected either by photographic X-ray film or by a digital recording system. Subsequent conversion to a permanent, visible radiographic image occurs with chemical processing of conventional X-ray film or with computer manipulation of the data in the case of digital radiography.

Properties of X-rays

X-rays form part of the electromagnetic spectrum, which defines different types of radiation by wavelength and frequency (Figure 1.1). The energy in a given type of radiation is directly proportional to the frequency and indirectly proportional to the wavelength. X-rays and gamma rays are similar types of electromagnetic radiation, which have very high frequencies, very short wavelengths and therefore high energies. X-rays are created by X-ray machines and gamma rays by the decay of radioactive materials; the latter are used in nuclear imaging (scintigraphy). The properties of the electromagnetic spectrum are that radiation:

- Does not require a medium for transmission and can pass through a vacuum
- Travels in straight lines
- Travels at the same speed (3×10^8 m/s) in a vacuum
- Interacts with matter by being absorbed or scattered.

X-rays have some additional properties which mean that they can be used to create images of the internal structures of biological material. These properties include:

- Penetration – because of their high energy, X-rays can penetrate substances that are opaque to visible ('white') light. The X-ray photons are absorbed to varying degrees, depending on the nature of the substance penetrated and the energy of the photons themselves, but the most energetic pass right through the patient, emerging at the other side. The shorter the wavelength, the higher the energy of the X-ray photon and the greater the penetrating ability
- Effect on photographic film – X-rays have the ability to create a latent image on photographic film, which is rendered visible by processing (hence, photographic film in a camera is damaged by exposure to X-rays)
- Fluorescence – X-rays cause crystals of certain substances to fluoresce (emit visible light) and this property is utilized in the composition of radiographic intensifying screens and digital radiography systems.

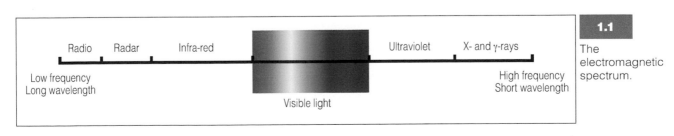

1.1 The electromagnetic spectrum.

Radio   Radar   Infra-red   Ultraviolet   X- and γ-rays

Low frequency
Long wavelength

High frequency
Short wavelength

Visible light

X-rays also produce biological changes in living tissues by altering the structure of atoms or molecules, or by causing chemical reactions due to ionization of atoms and the generation of free radicals. Some of these effects can be beneficial for the radiotherapy of tumours, but are harmful to normal tissues and constitute a safety hazard.

Properties of atoms

Electrons are present in the atoms of all elements and are small, negatively charged particles that orbit around the atomic nucleus (which comprises larger, positively charged protons and neutrons that have no electrical charge) in different planes or 'shells'. The innermost shells are known as the K, L and M shells; K being closest to the nucleus. The number of electrons is normally equivalent to the number of protons, so the atom as a whole is electrically neutral. The number of protons within the nucleus is unique to the atoms of each element and is known as the atomic number. Thus, with increasing atomic number, the number of electrons within the atom also increases. If an atom loses one or more electrons, it becomes positively charged and may be denoted as X^+ (where X is the symbol for the element). If an atom gains electrons, it becomes negatively charged and may be denoted as X^-. Atoms with a charge are called ions or are said to be ionized: a positively charged ion is known as a cation and a negatively charged ion is known as an anion. Compounds are a combination of two or more elements and usually consist of positive ions of one or more elements combined with negative ions of others (e.g. silver bromide in X-ray film emulsion consists of silver (Ag^+) and bromide (Br^-) ions).

Production of X-rays

X-ray photons are created when rapidly moving electrons are slowed down or stopped. In an X-ray tube head, X-ray photons are produced by collisions between fast-moving electrons (i.e. an electric current) and the atoms of the 'target' element. A small percentage of electrons are completely halted by, and give up all their energy to, the target atoms, forming X-ray photons with the most energy in the X-ray beam. Those electrons that merely decelerate give up smaller and variable amounts of energy to the target atoms, resulting in lower energy X-ray photons. Thus, the X-ray beam contains photons with a range of energies and is said to be polychromatic. If the number of incident electrons is increased, more X-ray photons are produced, and the intensity of the X-ray beam is increased. If the speed of the incident electrons is faster, they have more energy to lose, and so the X-ray photons produced are more energetic. This results in an increase in the quality of the X-ray beam and a greater penetrating power. The intensity and quality of the X-ray beam can be altered by adjusting the settings on the X-ray machine.

X-ray tube head

The X-ray tube head is part of the part of the machine where the X-ray photons are generated. The simplest type of X-ray tube, a stationary or fixed anode tube, is shown in Figure 1.2.

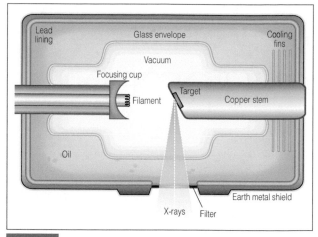

1.2   A stationary or fixed anode X-ray tube.

Production of electrons: The X-ray tube head contains two electrodes: the negatively charged cathode and the positively charged anode. Electrons are produced at the cathode, which is a coiled wire filament. When a small electrical current is passed through the filament, it is heated and releases a cloud of electrons by a process called thermionic emission. Tungsten is used as the filament material because:

- It has a high atomic number (74) and therefore many electrons
- It has a very high melting point (3380°C) and so can be safely heated
- It has appropriate mechanical properties, which mean that fine, coiled filaments can be constructed.

The electrical current required to heat the filament is small, so the mains current to the filament is reduced by a step-down or filament transformer, which is wired into the X-ray machine (a transformer is a device for increasing or decreasing an electric current).

Movement of electrons: The cloud of electrons must be accelerated at high speed across the short distance from the filament to the target (the anode). This is achieved by applying a high electrical potential difference between the filament and the target, so that the filament becomes negative (and therefore repels the electrons) and the target becomes positive (and therefore attracts the electrons). Thus, the filament becomes the cathode and the target becomes the anode.

The mains electrical supply is an alternating current (AC), which means that its two poles alternate from positive to negative at a high frequency (50 Hz). Since the target must always remain positive relative to the cathode, the high voltage supply needs to be corrected so that the polarity does not change. The process of converting alternating current to direct current is known as rectification. The electrons are formed into a narrow beam by the fact that the filament sits in a nickel or molybdenum focusing cup, which is also negatively charged and so repels the electrons. The electron beam constitutes a weak electric current across the tube (the tube current), which is measured in thousandths of an ampere or milliamperes (mA). Multiplying the mA by the duration (in seconds) of the exposure reflects the total quantity of X-ray photons emitted, known as milliampere seconds or mAs; although it should be noted that this is not a direct measurement of the number of X-ray photons which are produced only at the target.

The potential difference applied between the filament and the target needs to be very high (measured in thousands of volts or kilovolts, kV) and many times the voltage of the mains supply (240 volts in the UK). The large potential difference in the X-ray tube is created from the mains current in a second electrical circuit using a step-up or high-tension transformer, which is wired into the X-ray machine.

X-ray generation: The stream of electrons strikes the target (anode) at very high speed. Tungsten or rhenium–tungsten alloy is used as the target material because its high atomic number renders it a relatively efficient producer of X-rays. Despite this >99% of the energy lost by the electrons is converted to heat, so the anode must be able to withstand extremely high temperatures without melting or cracking. The high melting point of tungsten is therefore useful in the target as well as in the filament.

Two processes occur in the tungsten target to give rise to X-ray photons, and result in a continuous spectrum of X-ray energy and characteristic radiation of specific energies (Figure 1.3a).

- The continuous spectrum occurs when electrons pass close to the positively charged nuclei of target atoms and in doing so are decelerated and deflected. As a result, some of their kinetic energy is lost and converted to X-ray energy. The energy of the photon emitted depends on the degree of deceleration. A few incident electrons collide with the nuclei and come to a complete halt, losing all their kinetic energy. This results in the generation of an X-ray photon with maximum energy, known as E_{max}. The continuous spectrum is also known as 'braking' or 'white' radiation or *Bremsstrahlung*.
- Characteristic radiation arises when incident electrons collide with electrons orbiting within the inner atomic shells (K and L shells) and eject them, creating a vacancy in the shell. This is an unstable situation, so an electron from a shell further out falls into the vacant place, emitting an X-ray photon as it does so. The energy of these photons is characteristic of the difference in energy between the two shells, with the maximum energy produced when electrons fall into the innermost K shell. K and L peaks of characteristic radiation are superimposed over the continuous spectrum.

The appearance of the X-ray spectrum is altered by several factors, including:

- The voltage across the X-ray tube (Figure 1.3b). As the potential difference across the X-ray tube is increased, the maximum energy of any X-ray photon produced is proportionally increased, shifting the maximum energy of the curve to the right-hand side. It also results in an X-ray spectrum with a higher peak as more X-ray photons are produced. In addition, the peak is shifted to the right-hand side as the average energy of the beam is increased

- Tube current (Figure 1.3c). As the current applied to the filament increases, more electrons are produced and accelerated across the tube. More X-ray photons are created at the anode and the X-ray spectrum produced has a higher peak, but the maximum energy of the X-ray photons remains unchanged

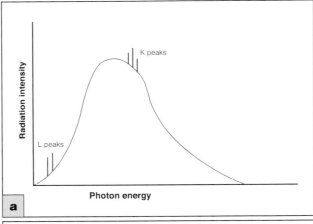

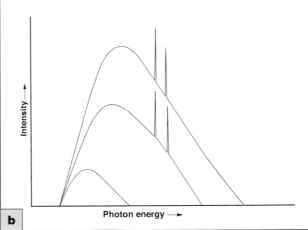

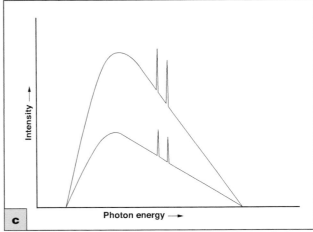

1.3 **(a)** The X-ray spectrum representing radiation emission at the target. The K and L peaks of characteristic radiation for tungsten are superimposed over the continuous spectrum. **(b)** Effect of increased tube voltage on the X-ray spectrum. The quality of the beam is increased (peak of the curve has shifted to the right), the intensity is increased (area under the curve) and the maximum energy of the beam is increased (maximum velocity on the right-hand side of the curve). **(c)** Effect of increased tube current on the X-ray spectrum. The intensity is increased (area under the curve) but the quality of the beam and characteristic radiation remain unchanged.

- Type of anode. Anodes with a higher atomic number produce X-ray spectra of greater intensity, higher average and maximum energy and, depending on atomic number, characteristic radiation with higher energies
- Type of rectification. The simplest forms of rectification (the process by which alternating current is converted to direct current) result in pulsating tube voltage (voltage ripple) and the inefficient production of X-rays. Multi-phase (3-, 6- and 12-phase) and high frequency X-ray generators produce a higher tube current as the tube voltage is a near constant maximal, resulting in increased X-ray intensity
- Filtration. Added filtration to the X-ray tube absorbs the low energy X-rays. This increases the quality of the beam and the X-ray spectrum is shifted to the right-hand side as the average energy of the beam is increased. This added filtration is important in reducing the absorbed dose to the patient as it removes the low energy X-ray photons, which will not penetrate the patient or contribute to the useful image.

In a simple X-ray tube (see Figure 1.2), the target is a small rectangle of tungsten approximately 3 mm thick set in a copper block. Copper is a good heat conductor, and so heat is removed from the target by conduction along the copper stem to the cooling fins, which radiate into the surrounding oil bath. The target is set at an angle of about 20 degrees to the vertical (Figure 1.4). This is so that the area of the target struck by the electrons (and therefore the area over which heat is produced) is as large as possible. This area is called the actual focal spot. At the same time, the angulation of the target means that the X-ray beam appears to originate from a much smaller area and this is called the effective focal spot. The importance of having a small effective focal spot (ideally a point source) is discussed below. The design of the target to maximize the actual focal spot size whilst minimizing the effective focal spot size is known as the line focus principle.

Some X-ray machines allow a choice of focal spot size, using two different sized filaments at the cathode.

- The smaller filament produces an electron beam with a smaller cross-sectional area and hence smaller effective and actual focal spots. This is known as fine focus. The emergent X-ray beam arises from a tiny area and produces very fine radiographic definition. However, the heat generated is concentrated over a very small area of target, limiting the exposure factors that can be used.
- The larger filament produces a wider electron beam with larger effective and actual focal spot sizes. This is known as the coarse or broad focus. Higher exposures can be used, but the image definition is slightly less sharp due to the penumbra effect (blurring of the margins related to the geometry of the beam; see Chapter 2). X-ray photons produced at different points on the focal spot travel along slightly different pathways and therefore hit the film or digital recording system in slightly different locations, even though they outline the same anatomical feature. Penumbra is derived from Latin and means 'partial shadow'.

In practice, fine focus is selected for small body parts when fine definition is required (e.g. the limbs) and coarse focus is selected when thicker body parts are to be imaged (e.g. the thorax and abdomen); the latter require higher exposure factors and so the heat generated at the target is higher.

The cathode, anode and part of the copper stem are enclosed in a glass envelope. Within the envelope is a vacuum, which prevents the moving electrons from colliding with air molecules and losing speed and subsequently energy. The glass envelope is bathed in oil, which acts both as a heat sink and as an electrical insulator, and everything is encased in an earthed, lead-lined metal casing. The target produces X-rays in all directions, but only one narrow beam is required, and this emerges through a window in the X-ray tube casing located beneath the angled target. This beam is used to generate the radiographic image and is called the primary beam. X-rays produced in other directions are absorbed by the casing.

Within the X-ray beam are some low energy or 'soft' X-ray photons, which are not sufficiently powerful to pass through the patient, but may be absorbed or scattered by the patient and therefore represent a safety hazard. They are removed from the beam by an aluminium filter placed across the tube window. These filters are a legal requirement as a safety precaution and must not be removed.

With stationary anode tubes, the X-ray output is limited by the amount of heat generated at the target. Overheating the target results in melting and surface irregularity, which reduces the efficiency of the tube; automatic overload devices prevent such high exposures from being used. Stationary anode tubes are found in lower powered, portable X-ray machines. These machines have a limited ability to produce short exposure times for thoracic radiography or high output for larger patients.

More powerful machines require an efficient way of removing heat and this is accomplished using a rotating anode (Figure 1.5). In such tubes, the target area is the bevelled rim of a metal disc (approximately 10 cm in diameter), which is angled at 20

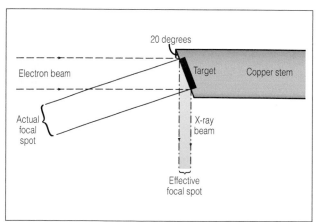

1.4 The line focus principle. Angulation of the target (anode) results in a large actual focal spot and a small effective focal spot. The larger actual focal spot increases the heat capacity of the anode and the smaller projected focal spot increases radiographic definition (image sharpness).

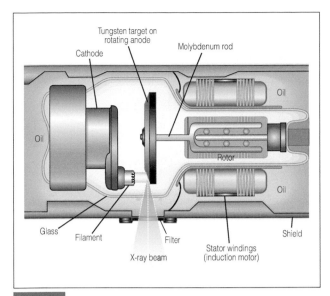

1.5 A rotating anode X-ray tube.

degrees. The target area is made of tungsten or rhenium–tungsten. During the exposure, the disc rotates rapidly, so the target area being struck by the electrons is constantly changing. Therefore, the actual focal spot is the whole circumference of the disc and thus many times greater than that of a stationary anode X-ray tube. The heat generated is spread over a much wider area, allowing larger exposures to be obtained, whilst the effective focal spot remains the same. The disc is mounted on a molybdenum rod and is rotated at speeds of up to 10,000 rpm by an induction motor located at the other end of the rod. Molybdenum is used because it is a poor conductor of heat and therefore prevents the motor from overheating. Heat generated in the anode is lost in this instance by radiation through the vacuum and glass envelope into the oil bath. The size of the emerging X-ray beam must be controlled for safety reasons, otherwise it will spread out over a very large area posing a safety hazard and adversely affecting image quality. This is achieved using a collimation device, usually created by a light beam diaphragm (see Chapter 2 for further details on collimation).

X-ray machine control panel

X-ray machine control panels vary in complexity, but some or all of the following controls are available:

- On/off switch
- Line voltage compensator
- kV control
- mA control
- Timer
- Exposure button
- Activator for a moving grid
- Automatic exposure control (AEC).

On/off switch: As well as a mains socket that can be switched on and off, there is an on/off switch or key on the control panel. Sometimes the line voltage compensator (see below) is incorporated into the on/off switch. When the machine is switched on, a warning light on the control panel indicates that it is ready to produce X-rays or, in the case of panels with digital displays, the numbers are illuminated.

With fixed systems, there may also be a link to a warning sign outside the X-ray room which is illuminated whenever the X-ray machine is switched on. X-ray machines must always be switched off when not in use, so that accidental exposure cannot occur when unprotected people are in the room.

Line voltage compensator: Fluctuations in the normal mains electricity output may occur, resulting in an inconsistent output of X-rays such that the images obtained may appear underexposed or overexposed despite using normal exposure factors. With newer machines, these fluctuations are automatically corrected by an autotransformer wired into the circuit, but in others it is controlled manually. A voltmeter dial on the control panel indicates the incoming voltage, which can be adjusted until it is satisfactory. In such machines the line voltage should be checked before each radiography session.

Kilovoltage control: The kV control selects the kV ('potential difference') that is applied across the tube during the instant of exposure. It determines the speed and energy with which the electrons bombard the target and hence the quality or penetrating power of the X-ray beam produced. Depending on the power and sophistication of the X-ray machine, the kV is controlled in various ways. Ideally, it is controlled in small increments, independent of the mA, but in simple machines there may only be a small choice of kV in 10 kV increments, or it may be linked to the mA. The kV meter is either a dial or digital display.

Milliamperage control: The mA is a measure of the quantity of electrons crossing the tube during the exposure (the 'tube current') and is directly related to the quantity of X-rays produced. Adjusting the mA control alters the degree of heating of the filament and hence the number of electrons released by thermionic emission, the tube current and the intensity of the X-ray beam.

In some portable machines the mA is fixed (e.g. at 20 mA). Alternatively, the kV may be linked to the mA, so that if a higher mA is selected, only a lower kV can be used; there is a single control knob for both kV and mA, and as the kV increases, the mA available decreases. This is not ideal since, for larger patients, a high kV and high mAs may be required at the same time, meaning that long exposure times are needed. In more powerful machines with a higher output, a range of mA can be selected, and in the largest fixed machines this can extend to >1000 mA.

Timer: The quantity of X-rays produced depends not only on the mA but also on the length of time of the exposure (seconds). A given mAs may be obtained using a high mA with a short time or a low mA with a long time. The two variables are multiplied together (e.g. 30 mAs = 300 mA x 0.1 seconds or 30 mA x 1.0 seconds). The effect on the film is the same, except that the longer the exposure, the more likely it is that movement blur will occur. Therefore, the largest mA allowed by the machine for that kV setting should be used in order to minimize the exposure time. This is why a type of machine in which the kV and mA are inversely linked is less than ideal.

The timer is electronic and is usually another dial on the control panel, providing a choice of a wide range of exposure times up to several seconds long. Release of the exposure button terminates the exposure even when long times have been selected. In larger machines, an automatic display of the resulting mAs is also available. Some modern machines with a digital display have a single control for mAs, which automatically selects the shortest exposure time for the selected mAs (see Chapter 2 for more information about choosing exposure factors).

Exposure button: On portable and mobile X-ray machines, the exposure button must be at the end of a cable that can stretch to >2 m to enable radiographers to distance themselves from the primary beam during the exposure. On fixed machines, the button may be on the control panel itself, provided that the panel is at least 2 m from the tube head and/or is separated from it by a lead screen. Most exposure buttons are two-stage devices: depression of the button to a halfway stage ('prepping') heats the filament and rotates the anode (if a rotating anode is present); after a brief pause, further depression of the button causes application of the kV to the tube and an instantaneous exposure to be made. In some machines, only a single-stage exposure button is present. In these cases, there is a slight delay between depression of the button and exposure, during which time the patient may move.

Moving grid: If an under-the-table moving grid (Bucky) is being used, there may be a setting on the X-ray control panel which can be used to turn the Bucky on and off, depending on whether a table top technique or grid is being used.

Automatic exposure control: In modern X-ray machines designed for human radiography, there are often AECs. Small radiolucent detectors are built into the X-ray table and sit between the patient and the X-ray cassette or detector. When an adequate number of X-ray photons have passed through the patient the AEC automatically turns off the X-ray beam. AEC devices are calibrated and positioned specifically for human patients and are not usually suitable for small animal radiography.

Types of X-ray machine
X-ray machines can be divided into three main types: portable, mobile and fixed. X-ray machines require little maintenance, but should be serviced annually by a qualified X-ray engineer who will check both safety issues and calibration of the control buttons.

Portable machines: Portable machines (Figure 1.6) are commonly used in general and peripatetic equine practice. They are relatively easy to move from site to site for large animal radiography and usually come with a special carrying case. The largest weigh approximately 20 kg. The electrical transformers are located in the tube head, which is either supported on a wheeled metal stand or wall-mounted. The tube head must never be held for radiography, as this is very hazardous to the person holding it. The controls may be either on a separate panel or else on the head itself. Portable machines are low powered, producing only about 20–100 mA and often less. In some

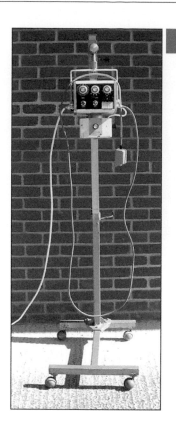

1.6   A portable X-ray machine.

machines, the kV and mA are inversely linked. The relatively low output means that longer exposure times are needed, and thoracic and abdominal radiographs of larger dogs are usually degraded by the effects of movement blur.

Mobile machines: Mobile machines are larger and more powerful than portable machines, but can still be moved from room to room on wheels (Figure 1.7) and some have battery operated motors. The transformers are bulkier and encased in a large box, which is an integral part of the tube stand. Mobile machines usually have an output of up to 300 mA and are likely to produce good radiographs of most small animal patients.

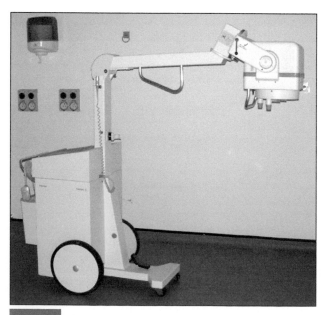

1.7   A mobile X-ray machine.

Fixed machines: The most powerful X-ray machines are built into the X-ray room, being either screwed to the floor or mounted on rails or overhead gantries (Figure 1.8). The tube head is usually quite mobile on its mounting and can be moved in several directions. The transformers are situated in cabinets some distance from the machine itself and connected to it by high-tension cables. The largest fixed machines have an output up to 1250 mA and produce excellent radiographs of all patients, but because of the high cost of purchase, installation and maintenance, they are usually restricted to veterinary institutions and referral practices. However, several companies are now producing smaller, fixed X-ray machines especially for the veterinary market, which are much more affordable. Fixed X-ray machines are often electronically linked to a floating table top and moving grid.

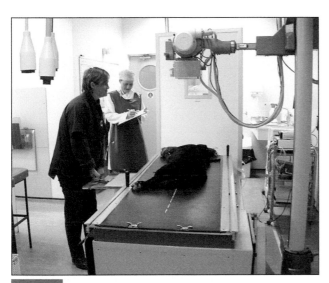

| **1.8** | A fixed X-ray machine. |

High frequency generators: Many older X-ray machines, in particular portable machines, generate X-rays from a pulsating voltage supply. However, modern machines (including portables) use high frequency generators to produce a stable, high voltage supply to the X-ray tube. During this process, the low frequency (50 Hz), low voltage (240 V) mains supply is rectified and smoothed to produce a low voltage direct current (DC). The direct current is then converted into a low voltage, high frequency alternating current using an inverter. This is then converted using a high voltage transformer into a high frequency (kHz), high voltage alternating current. Subsequent rectification and voltage smoothing results in a nearly constant output, similar to that of much bulkier three-phase generators. The advantages of this are that X-ray machines are capable of shorter exposure times, higher exposures and improved efficiency, as well as the fact that the transformer is greatly reduced in weight and size and can be more easily housed within the tube head. Although originally only used for low powered X-ray machines, high frequency generators are now applied to all modern, high voltage systems.

X-ray tube ratings

The maximum kV and mAs produced by an X-ray tube are determined by the amount of heat production it can withstand. If this heat production is exceeded, the tube is said to be 'overloaded' and damage may occur. The majority of X-ray machines have built-in fail-safe mechanisms that prevent these limits from being exceeded and if too high an exposure is selected, a warning light will come on and the machine will fail to make the exposure. However, this may not be the case with older machines and so care should be taken to work within the capabilities of the machine by consulting the manufacturer's details of maximum safe combinations of kV, mA and time. These details are known as rating charts.

Interaction of X-rays with tissues

An X-ray is essentially a 'shadowgraph' or a picture in black, white and shades of grey, created by variations in the amount of attenuation of the X-ray beam by different tissues and hence variations in the amount of radiation reaching the underlying X-ray film or digital detector system (Figure 1.9). The degree of absorption by a given tissue depends on three factors:

- The atomic number (Z) of the tissue or the average of the different atomic numbers present (the 'effective' atomic number)
- The specific gravity of the tissue
- The thickness of the tissue.

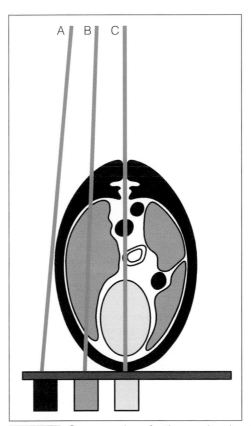

| **1.9** | Cross-section of a thorax showing the formation of an X-ray 'shadowgraph'. X-ray photons passing along path C are largely absorbed, resulting in pale areas on the radiograph, which represent radiopaque structures. X-ray photons passing along path B are only partly absorbed, creating intermediate shades of grey on the radiograph, which represent more radiolucent structures. X-rays passing along path A are outside the patient and so are not absorbed, leading to black areas on the radiograph. |

Bone has a higher effective atomic number than soft tissue and so absorbs more X-ray photons, resulting in paler areas on the radiograph. Soft tissue and fluid have higher effective atomic numbers than fat, allowing differentiation. Specific gravity refers to the density of the tissue or mass per unit volume. Bone has a high specific gravity, soft tissue and fat have medium specific gravity, and gas has a very low specific gravity; hence, gas-filled areas absorb few X-rays and appear nearly black on radiographs. Areas of high absorption are known as radiopaque and areas of low absorption are known as radio-lucent. The combination of effective atomic number and specific gravity results in five characteristic shades seen on radiographs:

- Gas – very dark
- Fat – dark grey
- Soft tissue or fluid – mid-grey
- Bone – nearly white
- Metal – white (as all X-rays are absorbed).

It should be noted that solid soft tissue and fluid have the same radiographic appearance; therefore, fluid within a soft tissue viscus (e.g. urine in the bladder or blood in the heart) cannot be differentiated from the surrounding tissue. Fat is less radiopaque than soft tissue and fluid, so fat in the abdomen is helpful in surrounding and outlining the various organs, enabling serosal detail to be seen.

Overlap in the ranges of grey shades on the radiograph occurs due to the fact that thicker areas of tissue absorb more X-ray photons than thinner areas; hence, a very thick area of soft tissue may actually appear more radiopaque than a thin area of bone. Interpretation of radiographs also relies on assessment of the depth of structures and the effect of superimposition and composite shadows.

Attenuation of the X-ray beam
When the X-ray beam interacts with matter (in this case the tissues of the patient), its intensity is reduced or 'attenuated' by two main processes:

- Absorption – photoelectric effect
- Scattering – Compton effect.

The degree to which these processes occur in different tissues depends on their composition and thickness, and this creates the radiographic image. The relative importance of the two processes is also dependent on the energy of the X-ray beam (i.e. the kV).

Photoelectric effect
If the energy of an incident X-ray photon exceeds the binding energy of an electron in an inner atomic shell (usually the K shell), the electron is ejected from its orbit and the photon gives up all of its energy, thereby being absorbed. The ejected electron or photoelectron travels a short distance within the tissue, creating ion pairs and losing its kinetic energy as heat. The vacancy in the inner orbit creates an unstable situation and so it is quickly filled by an electron from an outer orbit, which falls down into it. The difference between the binding energy of the two orbits is lost as

a photon of X-ray energy, which is characteristic of the two orbits involved and is known as the characteristic radiation of the absorbing material (Figure 1.10). The process is very similar to the production of useful characteristic radiation in the target of the X-ray tube head, although in this instance it does not contribute to the radiographic image as the photon produced has insufficient energy to exit the patient, but it does form part of the patient's radiation dose.

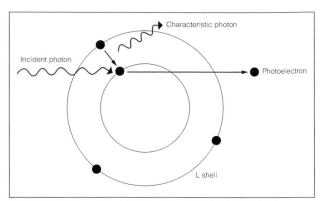

1.10 The photoelectric effect. An incident X-ray photon displaces an electron from an inner orbit and in doing so is absorbed. An electron from an outer shell falls into the vacancy created by the photoelectron and in doing so emits a photon which is characteristic of the absorbing material and the orbit shells involved. The characteristic photon is absorbed within the patient.

The photoelectric effect increases markedly with increasing atomic number or effective (average) atomic number of the absorbing tissue, Z (photoelectric effect varies with kV^3). It therefore creates a high contrast between different tissues as small differences in atomic number result in large differences in attenuation, which is useful for diagnosis. The photoelectric effect is the main cause of beam attenuation at lower kVs (up to approximately 70 kV). This is why a low kV technique results in higher image contrast than a high kV technique. The probability of a photoelectron interaction falls off rapidly with increasing energy of the X-ray beam, which is inversely proportional to the kV^3 (PE α $1/kV^3$). Above 70 kV, photoelectric absorption declines rapidly and the Compton effect predominates.

Compton effect
Although many of the X-ray photons entering the patient during the exposure are either completely absorbed by the photoelectric effect or pass straight through, a certain proportion undergo a process known as scattering (also called the Compton effect). Scattering occurs when incident photons interact with more loosely bound electrons in the tissues of the patient, losing some but not all of their energy and continuing to travel in random directions as photons of lower energy (Figure 1.11). The electron which has been struck is displaced as a Compton or recoil electron and travels a short distance within the tissues releasing heat (in the same manner as the photoelectron). The quantity of scattered photons produced is proportional to the volume of tissue being exposed and the kV. The direction of travel of the scattered photons also varies with kV. As the kV increases, a larger proportion of the scattered photons move in a forward direction

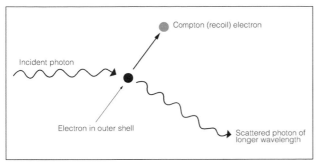

1.11 The Compton effect. An incident X-ray photon collides with a loosely bound electron and ricochets in a different direction at lower energy (longer wavelength).

and therefore scattered photons are more likely to exit the patient and reach the film. At lower kV and when thin areas of tissue are being imaged, the Compton effect is small and most of the scattered radiation produced is low energy and reabsorbed within the patient. Scatter is therefore not a problem when cats, small dogs and the skull and limbs of larger dogs are imaged. However, when a higher kV (>65–70 kV) is used, the amount and energy of the scattered radiation increases and substantial amounts may exit from the body of the patient.

The problems associated with scattered radiation are two-fold:

■ Scatter is a potential hazard to radiographers as it travels in all directions and may also ricochet off the table top, floor or walls. This is not usually a problem in small animal radiography where patients are usually artificially restrained with the examiner standing >2 m from the patient, behind a screen
■ Scattered radiation causes a uniform darkening of the image unrelated to the radiographic image, reducing contrast and definition. The resultant loss of contrast due to film blackening is called fogging (see Chapter 2) and is a major factor in determining the quality of a radiographic image.

Scatter production increases with higher kV, with thicker or denser tissues, and with larger field sizes of the primary beam. The amount of scattered radiation produced, or reaching the film or digital recording system, may be reduced in several ways (see Chapter 2).

Contrast

Contrast is the difference between various radiographic densities (shades of grey) seen on the radiograph. A medium contrast film with a reasonable number of grey shades as well as extremes of white and black on the image is desirable, as this yields most information. A film that shows a very pale image on a black background with few intermediate grey shades to show internal tissue detail has too high a contrast, which is due to the use of too low a kV with insufficient penetrating power. A film without extremes of opacity, showing mainly grey shades, has a very low contrast and is called a 'flat' film. Poor contrast may be due to underdevelopment, over-exposure, overdevelopment and various types of fogging, including scattered radiation. For further information on contrast, see Chapter 2.

Recording and displaying the image

Film–screen (analogue) systems

Once the X-ray beam has passed through the subject and undergone differential absorption by the tissues, it must be recorded in order to create a visible and permanent image. The conventional way of doing this is with X-ray film, which has some properties in common with photographic film, including sensitivity to white (visible) light. It must therefore be enclosed in a light-proof container, either a rigid cassette or a thick paper or plastic envelope, and handled only in conditions of appropriately subdued 'safe lighting' until after processing.

Structure of X-ray film

The part of the film responsible for producing the image is the emulsion, which usually coats the film base on both sides in a thin, uniform layer. The emulsion layers are attached to the transparent polyester film base by a sticky 'subbing' layer and the outer surfaces are protected from damage by a supercoat (Figure 1.12). The emulsion gives unexposed film an apple green, fawn or mauve colour when examined in daylight (obviously an unexposed film examined in this way will then be ruined for X-ray purposes). The emulsion consists of gelatine, in which tiny grains of silver bromide are suspended. The silver bromide molecules are sensitive to X-ray photons and visible light, both of which result in a slight change in their chemical structure.

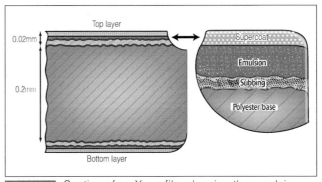

1.12 Section of an X-ray film showing the emulsion coats bound to the base by subbing layers and protected by supercoats.

During a radiographic exposure, X-ray photons passing through the patient cause this invisible chemical change in the underlying film emulsion, but the latent image is not visible to the naked eye and the film will still be spoilt by fogging if exposed to white light. The latent image must be rendered visible to the eye by chemical processing. When film is processed the chemical change in the emulsion continues until those silver bromide grains that were exposed to X-rays lose all of their bromide ions and become grains of pure silver, which appear black when the film is viewed. Some types of film (such as that used for mammography) are coated with emulsion on one side only and are known as single-sided film. Single-sided film provides better image definition because there is a single image, whereas with double-sided (duplitized) film there is superimposition of the images on the two sides. However, single-sided film requires much higher radiographic exposures. Traditionally, single-sided film has been used mainly for orthopaedic and feline radiography. Single-sided film can be recognized as the two sides appear slightly different in reflected light (one being shinier). In the darkroom, when loading the cassette, the active side can be identified by the position of a notch in one corner. Copy film is another example of single-sided emulsion film.

Intensifying screens and cassettes

X-ray film used alone requires a very large exposure to obtain an image and the use of film in this way is unacceptable in most circumstances as it increases the patient's dose of radiation. However, the exposure factors (specifically the mAs) can be greatly reduced for the same degree of blackening if some of the X-ray photons emerging from the patient are converted into visible light photons using intensifying screens (so-called because they intensify the effect of the X-rays on the film). Intensifying screens are flat sheets, coated with crystals of phosphorescent material, held against the X-ray film. Due to the crystalline structure of the phosphorescent material, orbital electrons lie within discrete energy levels. The X-ray photon gives energy to electrons within the crystal, which results in electrons moving from a low energy level to a higher energy level for a short period of time. After a fraction of a second, the electrons fall back to their original low energy state and in doing so emit energy in the form of light.

For many years, the most common phosphor used in the construction of intensifying screens was calcium tungstate, which emits blue light when stimulated by X-rays. In the 1970s a new group of phosphors was first used in intensifying screens; these were the so-called rare-earth phosphors, which produce blue, green or ultraviolet light. It is important that the X-ray film being used is sensitive primarily to the colour of light emitted by the intensifying screen, and for this reason some film–screen combinations are incompatible. One advantage of rare-earth screens is that they are more efficient at converting X-radiation into light than are calcium tungstate screens, allowing exposure factors to be reduced.

The main benefits of intensifying screens are:

- They allow much lower mAs settings to be used and so reduce movement blur, scatter production and patient exposure
- They prolong the life of the X-ray tube since the use of lower exposure factors results in less wear in the tube.

Screens consist of a stiff plastic base covered with a white reflecting surface and then a layer of phosphor. Over the top is a protective supercoat layer. The screens are usually used in pairs and are enclosed in the light-proof metal, plastic or carbon fibre cassette (Figure 1.13) with the film sandwiched between the pair of screens. A single screen only is used with single-sided mammography film. For good detail, the film and screens must be in close contact and so the cassette contains a thick felt or foam pad between the back plate and the back screen.

In areas where there is poor screen–film contact, the image is blurred as the light from the intensifying

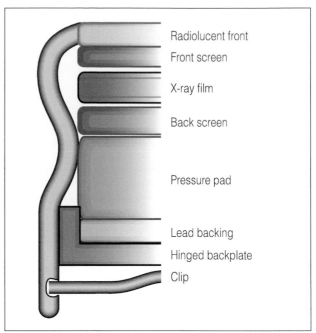

Radiolucent front

Front screen

X-ray film

Back screen

Pressure pad

Lead backing

Hinged backplate

Clip

1.13   Cross-section through an X-ray cassette (note that the lead backing is variably present).

screens spreads out slightly before reaching the film. The top of the cassette must be radiolucent (i.e. allow X-rays through) and the bottom may be lead-lined to absorb the remaining X-rays and prevent scatter being reflected back from the table top (back-scatter) and reaching the film, although this is uncommon with modern cassettes as it makes them very heavy. The cassette must be fully light-proof with secure fastenings and should be robust. Small, flexible, plastic cassettes containing one or two screens may be used for small animal intraoral radiography. Larger non-screen film previously used for intraoral radiography is no longer manufactured, but small, dental non-screen film is available.

Maintenance: Intensifying screens are expensive and delicate and should be treated with care. Scratches and abrasions damage the phosphor layer permanently, resulting in white (unexposed) marks on all subsequent radiographs obtained with that cassette. Screens should not be splashed with chemicals or touched with dirty or greasy fingers. Any dust particles or hairs that fall on to the screen when the cassette is open in the darkroom prevent light from reaching the film and result in fine white specks or lines on the image (even minute particles prevent visible light from the intensifying screens from blackening the film in that area, although they do not interfere with the passage of X-rays). Screens should be periodically cleaned by wiping them gently with soft material in a circular motion using a proprietary anti-static screen cleaning liquid. The cassettes should then be propped open vertically in a dust-free environment to allow the screens to dry naturally. If they are reloaded whilst still damp, the film will stick to the screens and damage them. Cassettes should be handled carefully and never dropped. They should be kept clean, as stains on the front may result in shadow artefacts on the radiograph and fluids seeping in will mark the screens. The catches must not be strained by closing the cassettes when a film is trapped along the edges.

Types of X-ray film

Non-screen film: Non-screen film is film designed for use without intensifying screens (i.e. the image is solely created by X-rays). This type of film requires a very large mAs (usually a long exposure time) but results in extremely fine image definition. The film is wrapped in thick, light-proof paper, rather than being used in a cassette. Non-screen film is now only available as small dental film, which is used for dental radiography and other intraoral views in cats and small dogs. The patient should be anaesthetized for this type of study, so the very high exposure required is not a problem as the radiographer can retire to a safe distance, and movement blur should not occur. The 13 x 18 cm film that was previously popular for intraoral radiography in dogs and for radiography of small exotic species is no longer manufactured; it has been replaced by flexible, plastic cassettes of the same size containing one or two high detail screens. However, the image quality is inferior to that obtained with non-screen film. The flexible nature of these 'cassettes' means that image blurring due to poor screen–film contact occurs if the device is bent in the mouth, but they can be reinforced by taping thick cardboard to them. Care should be taken that the teeth of the patient do not damage the device, so an appropriate level of anaesthesia is required.

Screen film: Screen film is designed for use in cassettes and is used for all other studies. The detail obtained is less than with non-screen film, as the visible light produced by the phosphor crystals spreads out, resulting in blackening of a larger number of silver halide grains than the initial X-ray photon would have done. This effect is called screen unsharpness (Figure 1.14). Monochromatic or blue-sensitive film is for use with calcium tungstate or blue light-emitting rare-earth screens; it is sensitive only to visible light in the blue part of the spectrum. For use with green light-emitting rare-earth screens, the sensitivity of the film emulsion is extended to include green as well as blue light; this is called orthochromatic film. Thus, whilst green-sensitive film can be used with blue light-emitting screens as well (as it is sensitive to both colours), blue-sensitive film can only be used with blue light-emitting screens. One manufacturer produces ultraviolet light-emitting screens, which can only be used with the same brand of film.

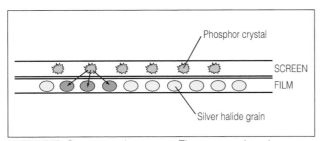

1.14 Screen unsharpness. The arrows show how visible light emitted from each phosphor crystal may affect several silver halide grains, resulting in some loss of definition of the image.

Film and screen speed

The speed of a film, a screen, or a film–screen combination describes the exposure required for a given degree of film blackening. The speed is determined by the size of the silver bromide grains in the film emulsion and the size and shape of the phosphor crystals in the screens, as well as the thickness of the emulsion and phosphor layers. Fast film–screen combinations require less exposure but result in poorer image definition, whereas, slow film–screen combinations require a higher mAs but result in finer detail and are often referred to as 'high definition'. Different manufacturers describe their various films and screens using different terms, making comparison difficult, but most produce films and screens of several speeds (e.g. slow, medium and fast). If a choice of film–screen speeds is available in the practice, then a slow, high definition combination may be used when exposure times are not a problem (e.g. for bone detail in the limbs and skull) but a faster combination should be used where it is important to keep exposure times short in order to reduce movement blur (e.g. for the thorax and abdomen), especially if a grid is used.

Films, screens and cassettes come in a range of sizes (from 13 x 18 cm to 35 x 43 cm). It is wise to have several different sizes available to avoid wasting film by imaging small structures or areas of the patient on large cassettes, although multiple exposures can be obtained using the same film. Hangers of corresponding size must be available if the films are manually processed. Some table top processors do not accept larger sizes of film.

Storage of X-ray film

As unexposed X-ray film is sensitive to light, it must be stored in a light-proof container (either the original film box or a light-proof hopper). Film boxes and loaded cassettes should ideally be kept away from the X-ray area in case they are fogged by scattered radiation; alternatively, they may be kept in a lead-lined cupboard if stored near a source of radiation.

Films are also sensitive to certain chemical fumes and splashes so good darkroom technique is essential with manual processing. Films may be damaged by pressure or folding, so should be stored upright and handled carefully without being bent or scratched. In hot climates, high temperatures or humidity may be a problem, so film may require refrigeration. Film has a finite shelf-life, which varies with the type of film. Therefore, it is sensible to date the film boxes on arrival and use them in sequence, and by the expiry date shown on the box.

Film processing

The latent image on the exposed X-ray film is rendered visible and permanent by a series of chemical reactions known as processing. As with photographic film, this must be conducted under conditions of relative darkness, as X-ray film is sensitive to blackening by white light (fogging) until processing is complete. Although most practices now use automatic processors or digital radiography, an understanding of the principles of manual processing is essential since automatic processors operate in the same manner. In addition, it also aids with the identification of processing faults, which appear similar whether caused by problems with manual or automatic processing.

Manual processing: There are five stages in the procedure of manual film processing: development, intermediate rinsing, fixing, washing and drying.

Development: The main active ingredient in the developing solution is either phenidone-hydroquinone or metol-hydroquinone. These chemicals convert the exposed crystals of silver bromide into minute grains of black metallic silver, whilst the bromide ions are released into the solution. This process is known as reduction and the developer acts as a reducing agent. The length of time the film is immersed in the developer (usually 3–5 minutes) is critical, since longer development times allow some of the unexposed silver bromide crystals to be converted to black metallic silver as well, resulting in uniform darkening of the film (chemical or development fog; see Chapter 2). The developer must be used at a constant and uniform temperature (usually 20°C/68°F). Precise times and temperatures for developing films are provided in the manufacturer's instructions, along with some indication of how the development time may be altered to compensate for unavoidable changes in the temperature of the solution.

Other chemicals present in the developing solution include an accelerator and a buffer, to create and maintain the alkalinity of the solution necessary for efficient development, and a restrainer to reduce the amount of development fog (i.e. the development of unexposed silver bromide crystals by fresh developer). X-ray developing solutions are purchased as concentrated liquids and gloves should be worn when the chemicals are handled. Skin irritation may be observed after handling processing solutions. This may be due either to an allergic reaction or to the alkaline nature of the developer. If the problem is marked, a doctor should be consulted and informed of the chemicals involved.

During the development of each film, a certain quantity of the developer is absorbed into the film emulsion, so the level in the developer tank gradually falls. The solution should not just be topped up with water, as this causes dilution of the chemicals and subsequent underdevelopment of films. The original developer solution is also unsuitable for topping up, as the proportions of the different chemical constituents of the developer change slightly with each film that is developed and topping up with the original solution causes imbalance between the chemical constituents. Instead, special developer replenisher solutions should be used, which take into account, and compensate for, this imbalance. Eventually, the developer will become exhausted as the active ingredients are used up and the solution becomes saturated with bromide ions.

Developer also deteriorates over time due to oxidation, which results in the underdevelopment of films. This process can be slowed by keeping the developer tank covered; with larger replenishment tanks there may also be a floating lid on the surface of the solution. Whether or not the developer is used, it is unlikely to be fit for purpose after 3 months and so the general rule is to change the developer completely either every 3 months or when an equal volume of replenisher has been used, whichever is sooner.

Rinsing: After the appropriate time in the developer, the film and hanger are removed from the solution and quickly transferred to the rinse water tank. Surplus developer should not be allowed to drain back into the developer tank because it will be saturated with bromide ions and contribute to developer exhaustion. The film should be rinsed for approximately 10 seconds to remove excess developer solution and prevent carry-over into the fixer tank. Ideally, the rinse tank should be situated between the developer and fixer to prevent splashes of developer falling into the fixer.

Fixing: Following immersion in the fixer, development is halted and the image is rendered permanent by a process known as fixing. The fixer is acidic and this neutralizes the developer, preventing further development of the emulsion. The fixer also removes the unexposed silver halide crystals, leaving a metallic silver image that can be viewed in normal light. This process is known as clearing. The fixer contains sodium or ammonium thiosulphate, which dissolves the unexposed silver halide, causing the emulsion to take on a milky-white appearance until the process is complete. The time taken for the removal of all the unexposed halide is called the 'clearing time' and depends on the thickness of the film emulsion, the temperature and concentration of the solution, and the degree of exhaustion of the fixer. The fixer becomes exhausted as the amount of dissolved silver halide builds up within it. The exhaustion of fixer occurs more quickly than the exhaustion of developer.

The temperature of the fixer is not critical, but warm fixer clears a film faster than cold fixer. However, staining may occur with temperatures above 21°C/70°F, so the fixer should not be overheated. Fixing can also be speeded up by agitating the film slightly in the fixer. Following immersion in the fixer for 30 seconds, it is safe to switch on the darkroom light and the film may be viewed once the milky appearance has cleared. The total fixing time should be at least twice the clearing time, a total of approximately 10 minutes. Fixing also serves to harden the film emulsion (a process known as tanning), which helps prevent the film from being scratched when handled. In addition to the fixing agent (thiosulphate) and the hardener, the fixer solution also contains a weak acid (to neutralize any remaining developer), a buffer (to maintain the acidity) and a preservative. Fixing solutions are normally made up from concentrated liquids by the addition of water, according to the manufacturer's instructions (as are developing solutions). They should be changed when the clearing time has doubled.

Washing: Following development and fixing, the film must be thoroughly washed to remove any residual chemicals, which would cause fading and yellow-brown staining of the film. Washing is best achieved by immersion of the film and hanger in a tank with a constant circulation of water, using at least three litres per minute so that the film is properly rinsed; static water tanks are much less satisfactory. Washing time should be 15–30 minutes.

Drying: Following adequate washing, the films are removed from their hangers for drying. Films left in channel-type hangers will not dry adequately around the edges. The usual method is to clip the films to a taut line over a sink; care should be taken to ensure that the films do not touch one another. The atmosphere should be dust-free with good air circulation.

Non-screen film: As the emulsion of non-screen film is thicker than that of screen film, it takes longer for the developing and fixing chemicals to penetrate the emulsion. Development time is normally increased by approximately 1 minute and clearing time in the fixer by several minutes. Since the only non-screen film currently available is the very small dental film, it is more practical to process these films in small plastic cups or trays (which can be filled with chemicals taken from the tanks of the manual or automatic processor).

Viewing the radiograph: Although the radiograph may be examined whilst it is still wet (for technical quality or a provisional diagnosis), the image will be somewhat blurred due to swelling of the two layers of wet emulsion. Full interpretation must be delayed until the film has dried, when the emulsion will have shrunk and the image is clearer.

Automatic processing: Automatic film processing has several advantages compared with manual film development, including saving considerable time and effort and producing a dry radiograph that is ready to interpret in a much shorter time. In addition, the films should be processed to a consistently high standard if the processor is operated and maintained correctly. However, with poor use of the automatic processor, film faults may still arise.

Automatic processors are still widely used in general practice, despite increasing use of digital systems. A darkroom is still required to unload and reload the cassettes, but only a dry bench is necessary. The processor may be entirely within the darkroom or the feed tray may pass through the darkroom wall to a processor located outside. Alternatively, a daylight processor (as used in human hospitals) may be used; these automatically unload and process the exposed film and then reload the cassette. Daylight processors do not require a darkroom but do require special cassettes and need regular servicing. Some practices use a daylight processor comprising a small automatic processor with light-proof sleeves into which the forearms are inserted, so that the cassette can be manipulated inside a dark area and the film is fed into the machine by touch.

Construction of an automatic processor: An automatic processor consists of a light-proof container enclosing a series of rollers that pass the film through developer, fixer, wash water and warm air (Figures 1.15 and 1.16). The intermediate rinse is omitted, as excess developer is removed from the film by compression between the rollers. The chemicals are used at a higher temperature (approximately 28°C/82°F) to speed up the process and the solutions are pumped in fresh for each film at a predetermined rate; therefore, there is no risk of poor processing due to the use of exhausted chemicals. A considerable amount of water needs to flow through the unit for the final rinse, so there must be an adequate water supply and

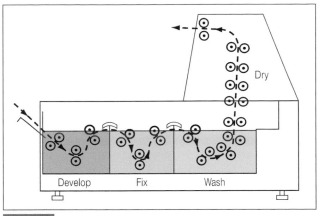

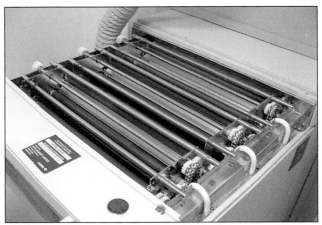

1.15 Essential features of an automatic processor.

1.16 Automatic processor with the lid removed showing the rollers and tanks.

drainage. Finally, the films are dried by a flow of warm air. If the film throughput is high, a silver recovery unit may be attached to the processor to retrieve silver from the waste chemicals.

Maintenance of the automatic processor: Automatic processors usually require a warm-up period of 10–20 minutes prior to use (longer in cold weather). Films processed before the machine has reached its operating temperature will be underdeveloped, although some machines will not accept film until they have reached the correct operating temperature. After the warm-up period, a piece of unexposed film should be passed through to check that the processor is functioning correctly and to remove any dried-on chemicals from the rollers by adherence to the unfixed emulsion. At least ten films per day should be put through the processor to ensure adequate replenishment of the chemicals in the tanks. If necessary these may be old films; although new, unfixed films are better at cleaning the rollers, this is more wasteful and expensive. At the end of the working day, the machine should be switched off and the superficial rollers wiped or rinsed to remove any chemical scum.

Once a week the processor may be cleaned more thoroughly, according to the manufacturer's instructions. This requires a deep sink so that the whole roller assembly for each of the three tanks can be removed and cleaned. An old toothbrush is useful for cleaning around the cogs, especially in hard water areas where limescale can develop. The tanks also need to be cleaned once the chemicals have been drained. An algicide solution (such as 'Milton') can be added to the wash tank to help remove algae from the tank walls and roller assembly, and a limescale treatment may also be required. Care should be taken when handling chemical solutions as they contain substances that are classified as irritant and can also lead to sensitization from cumulative exposure. Cleaning and mixing tasks should always be undertaken using appropriate eye protection and protective clothing. Splashes of developer reaching work surfaces, walls and floors quickly oxidize and become brown; this may cause a permanent stain, so any splashes should be rapidly wiped away.

The chemicals required are produced specifically for automatic processors and are not usually interchangeable with solutions used for manual processing as they are formulated for use at higher temperatures. Since fresh chemicals are pumped in for each film and then discarded, there is no need for developer replenisher solution. The chemicals are made up by mixing concentrated solutions thoroughly with water (in the case of developer there are three concentrates, one acting as a 'starter' solution, and for fixer there are two). The constituents must be mixed in the right order and with the correct amount of water. The developer and fixer solutions are mixed and then stored in tanks, ready to be pumped into the processor. Separate mixing rods must be used for the two solutions.

Alternatively, an automatic mixer unit can be used to mix chemicals for automatic processors. This method provides a safer and more convenient way of mixing and storing chemical solutions. Chemical concentrates for automatic processors are packaged in bottles with plastic seals and screw caps. Mixing is achieved by removing the screw cap and placing the upturned bottle on to the seal opener of the mixing unit. The seal is automatically broken and the contents flow into the tank below, where the correct amount of water is added. The prepared chemicals can be pumped directly from the mixer unit tanks into the processor.

The automatic processor should be serviced regularly by the manufacturer's engineers as breakdowns can be very inconvenient. Most engineers also operate an emergency service, but nevertheless it may be wise to have the facilities to be able to process films by hand, should the occasion arise.

Film quality: Although automatic processing results in films of a consistently good standard, there is always a slight loss of contrast compared with the best images that can be achieved by perfect manual processing. The latter is not often achieved and so an automatic processor is usually of great benefit to a practice with a reasonable throughput of radiographic cases.

Non-screen film: Depending on the nature of the processor, dental non-screen film may be too small to pass through the roller system and may require complete manual development. Putting a large old film through the processor immediately following the dental film can reduce the risk of the dental film becoming stuck in the processor. The film will still need additional fixing after going through an automatic processor and can be placed in a small cup of fixer for several minutes and then manually rinsed and dried. Special small units for the development of dental film are available and may be justified if the practice undertakes a significant amount of dental radiography.

Film faults
Radiographic quality is often degraded by faults arising during exposure or processing of the film. It is important to be able to recognize the cause of film faults in order to correct them (sometimes there may be several possible causes for a given fault). Common film faults, their causes and solutions are discussed in detail in Chapter 2.

Disposal of waste chemicals
Spent chemical solutions should not be poured into the normal drainage system as they can damage the environment. Instead, solutions should be collected and disposed of by a licensed waste disposal company. It is now a legal requirement that the Environment Agency must be notified when hazardous waste (such as used developer and fixer) is produced or removed from any premises. Records of the type and quantity of hazardous waste must be kept for at least 3 years. Certain types of premises, including veterinary practices, are exempt from having to notify the Environment Agency provided that less than a certain amount of hazardous waste is produced per year.

Fixer solution can be collected and reused several times in automatic processors, using a dipstick to test for activity and show when the solution is exhausted. To retrieve the silver content of waste fixer, it can be passed through a silver recovery system; although the cost-effectiveness of this depends upon the world price of silver. Alternatively, the fixer may be taken to a local hospital to pass through their silver recovery unit.

Darkroom design and maintenance
The darkroom is an important part of the radiography set-up within each practice (Figure 1.17). The following factors should be considered in its construction:

- Size
- Light-proofing
- Services
- Ventilation
- Walls, floor and ceiling
- Safe lighting
- Dry and wet areas
- Other darkroom equipment.

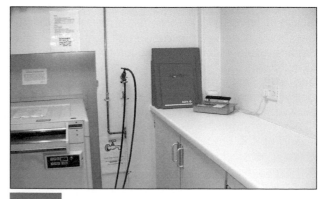

1.17 A darkroom for an automatic processor.

Size: The darkroom should be of a reasonable size to allow for satisfactory working conditions and should not be used for any other purpose.

Light-proofing: The darkroom must be completely light-proof and this must be checked by standing inside the darkroom for about 5 minutes until the eyes become adapted to the dark, as small chinks of light may otherwise go unnoticed. The room must be lockable from the inside to prevent the door being inadvertently opened whilst films are being processed. Light-proof maze entrances or revolving cylindrical doors are used in busy hospital departments so that radiographers have free access to the darkroom.

Services: There usually needs to be a supply of electricity and mains water and a drain, although some table top processors use water in bottles rather than mains water. Access to a sink for cleaning the processor also needs to be considered when designing the room.

Ventilation: Due to the presence of chemical fumes, some form of light-proof ventilation is essential.

Walls, floor and ceiling: The walls and ceiling should be painted in a pale colour (not black) to reflect the subdued lighting and make it easier for those working inside the darkroom to see what they are doing. The walls and floor should be washable and resistant to chemical splashes; it may be wise to tile any wall areas likely to be splashed.

Safe lighting: Since X-ray film is sensitive to white light until the fixing stage, illumination must be achieved using light of low intensity and specific colour (wavelength). This is provided by safe lights which contain low wattage bulbs behind brown or dark red filters. The colour of the light produced must be safe for the type of film being processed (e.g. green-sensitive films require different filters to blue-sensitive films). If the incorrect filter is used, the films become uniformly fogged whilst being handled in the darkroom. Safe light filters must be checked carefully for flaws and damage, as even small pinpricks allow light leakage. The efficiency of the safe lights can be checked by laying a pair of scissors or a bunch of keys on an unexposed film on the work bench for periods of up to 2 minutes and then processing it. If significant fogging is occurring, the metal object is visible on the film. It should be noted that no safe light is completely safe if films are exposed for too long or if the safe light is too close to the handling area. Film manufacturers will advise on the correct filter colour needed for particular types of film. Two types of safe light are available: direct safe lights that shine directly over the working area; and indirect safe lights that shine light upwards, which is then reflected off the ceiling. The number of safe lights required varies with the size of the room, but should be sufficient to allow film handling without fumbling.

Dry and wet areas: If manual processing is used, the darkroom should be divided into two working areas: the dry area and the wet area. If the room is large enough, these areas may be separated by being on opposite sides of the room; however, where this is not possible, they must be separated by a partition to prevent splashes from the wet area reaching the dry bench and damaging the films or contaminating the intensifying screens.

- In the dry area, the films are stored in boxes (preferably in cupboards) or in film hoppers, loaded into and out of cassettes and placed in hangers prior to processing. Films can also be labelled at this stage. Dry hangers should be stored on a rack above the dry bench. There may also be a storage area for cassettes.
- In the wet area, the processing chemicals are kept and used. There should be a viewing box with a drip tray for the initial examination of the films, a wall rack for wet hangers and some arrangement to allow films to dry without dripping over the floor or other working areas.

If few radiographs are processed, the chemicals may be kept in dark, air-tight bottles and poured into shallow dishes for use (as for photographic development). It may also be necessary to employ this technique should the automatic processor break down or for small dental films that cannot be put through an automatic processor. Unused cat litter trays make ideal processing dishes for radiographs and dental film can be processed in small plastic cups. The correct development temperature is achieved either by heating the solution prior to use or by placing the dish on an electric heating pad. The solutions are usually discarded after use as the developer rapidly oxidizes.

Other darkroom equipment: Channel or clip hangers are required for manual processing; each has its advantages and disadvantages. Channel hangers are easier to load but may result in poor development of the edges of the film. Films must be removed for drying and attached to the drying line using clips. The hangers should be washed after the films are removed, as chemicals may otherwise build up in the channels, causing staining of subsequent films. Very large films may not be held securely in channel hangers. Clip hangers avoid these disadvantages but are more fragile and cumbersome to use and may tear the films if not used correctly. A timer with a bell should be available in the darkroom so that the development period can be accurately timed. The timer should ideally be capable of being preset to a given time. A paper towel dispenser and a waste paper bin are also useful additions to the darkroom.

Digital systems

With technological advances, new methods of acquiring and viewing radiographic images have become available. These are based on digital acquisition of the image, whereby the image is created and stored electronically and viewed on a computer monitor rather than a radiographic film. It should be noted that although conventional radiographs can be photographed using a digital camera to produce an image that can be viewed electronically, this is not digital radiography. Digital radiography systems convert the pattern of photons reaching the detector into an electrical signal, which is then digitized. Although the generic term 'digital radiography' is commonly used for all electronically generated images, it consists of two distinct types of technology: computed radiography and digital radiography. The advantages of computed/digital radiography include:

- Tissues with a wide range of attenuation may be seen clearly on the same image (e.g. both bone and soft tissue, and thicker and thinner areas of the patient). This means that fewer exposures are required compared with the use of analogue film
- There is greater tolerance to suboptimal exposure factors. Digital film has a wide latitude (the range of exposures that result in appropriate film blackening/signal) compared with analogue film. This reduces the need for repeat exposures, thereby saving time and money, as well as having safety implications
- The displayed images can be manipulated (post-processing; e.g. zooming the image and altering the greyscale to increase diagnostic sensitivity)
- Radiography is quicker (time savings are greater with direct digital radiography than with computed radiography)
- No requirement for a darkroom, X-ray viewer or film-archiving space. Hard copies can still be made (if desired), using either film that is similar in appearance to X-ray film or high quality paper
- Financial savings on film, processing equipment and chemicals, as well as associated environmental benefits. However, the installation costs of digital radiographic systems can be considerable, depending on the quality of the system
- Images are reliably stored – important radiographs should never go missing!
- Images can be viewed anywhere in the practice where there is an appropriate workstation and can be transmitted off-site for rapid interpretation or referral
- Different types of digital image can be stored on the same network and viewed together (e.g. radiographs, ultrasonograms, computed tomography (CT) images and magnetic resonance (MR) images)
- Digital images can easily be inserted into letters, publications, lecture notes and presentations.

Image acquisition

The digital radiographic image is created from a number of small rectangular picture elements (pixels) arranged in a matrix (Figure 1.18). The spatial resolution of the image is determined mainly by the size of the pixels used to make the image. The smaller the pixel, the higher the spatial resolution; typically, resolution is approximately 5–10 pixels per mm. The spatial resolution of conventional radiographs is often higher than digital radiographs, but due to poorer image contrast, the ability to detect small lesions on conventional radiographs may be no better than lower resolution digital images. For each pixel there is a limited, but large (around 4000), number of potential shades of grey. However, unlike conventional film where the greyscale is limited by the ability of the human eye and brain, the image can be manipulated to use all these potential shades of grey.

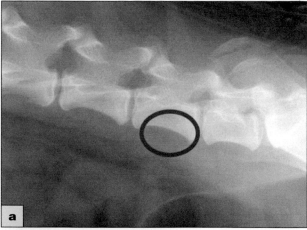

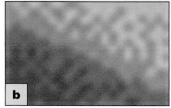

1.18 Digital radiography. **(a)** Lateral radiograph showing the abdomen and spine in a dog. **(b)** Magnification of the circled area in (a) allows the individual pixel elements constituting the matrix, as well as the greyscale, to be recognized.

With conventional radiographs, the relationship between radiographic exposure (number of photons) and optical density (blackness) of the film is known as the characteristic curve and is sigmoidal (S-shaped) (Figure 1.19a). If there are too few (underexposure) or too many (overexposure) photons, the information provided by the pattern of photons is lost. Within the useful (straight) part of the characteristic curve, there is a continuous (but logarithmic) linear relationship between the number of photons and the density of the film. The aim when taking conventional radiographs is to set the exposure to use the useful part of the characteristic curve. Although there are potentially hundreds of shades of grey on the film image, the human eye is limited in its differentiation and can only separate approximately 60 shades.

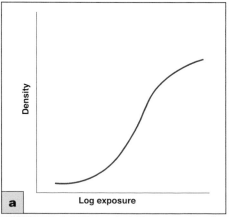

1.19 **(a)** Characteristic curve of radiographic film. The sigmoidal curve reflects the relationship between relative exposure and optical density of the film. Contrast is highest along the linear part of the curve. The toe and shoulder areas of the curve are regions of low contrast. For radiographic film, the linear response extends over a narrow range of exposures. (continues) ▶

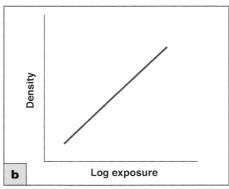

1.19 (continued) **(b)** Digital film has a linear response over a much greater range of radiation exposures. Therefore, structures with a large range of attenuation can all be viewed on the same exposure.

With digital radiographic systems, there is a direct linear relationship between the exposure and signal (Figure 1.19b). This means that there are no 'toe' or 'shoulder' regions where information is lost. In addition, once analogue film is black, extra photons do not result in new information; whereas, in a digital system the extra photons carry useful information. With digital systems, the image can be manipulated after acquisition to alter contrast and brightness. This means it is possible to view areas on the radiograph with marked differences in tissue thickness or to examine the soft tissues and bones without having to take separate images (Figure 1.20).

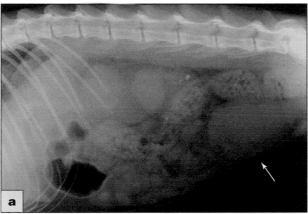

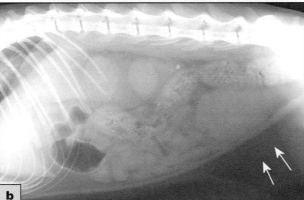

1.20 Lateral abdominal radiographs demonstrating the wide latitude of digital images. **(a)** The bones and thicker soft tissues are visible but the thinner soft tissues and fat along the ventral abdominal wall are overexposed (arrowed). **(b)** Adjustment of the contrast and brightness (window levelling) allows these soft tissues to be seen (arrowed).

Image quality

Image quality with digital systems may not be inherently better than high standard conventional film–screen radiographs, although post-processing manipulation may permit more subtle lesions to be seen. The image quality with some cheaper digital systems is often poorer than that obtained with good conventional radiographs. The method of obtaining the image (generation of the X-ray beam, interaction of the X-ray beam with the patient, and radiographic technique) is the same as for film–screen radiography; it is simply the recording system which differs. The best images are obtained using correct radiographic technique, and failure to do so may result in poor or even non-diagnostic digital images. Image quality also depends on the quality of the acquisition equipment and viewing monitors as well as the software packages used for image manipulation.

Artefacts

Computed/digital radiography systems allow greater flexibility with exposures than do conventional film–screen radiographs, but may create a range of radiographic artefacts (see Chapter 2 for further details).

Labelling

Prior to radiography, the patient details are entered into the workstation computer of the digital system and the type of examination and views are selected (e.g. thorax, abdomen, spine; lateral, dorsoventral, ventrodorsal). This allows the system to apply the correct image reconstruction technique or algorithm for that body part, providing optimum definition and contrast for that area (Figure 1.21). It is important to ensure that the patient details are entered correctly as it may be impossible to alter them after the images have been obtained. Manual entry of patient details has a high error rate and computerized registration of patient details using a modality work list (if available) is preferred as this minimizes mistakes. Failure to retrieve studies, or to retrieve all studies, for a specific patient is the consequence of incorrectly entered patient details. Digital systems can be customized and set up with small animal, equine, exotic or mixed examination algorithms, depending on the needs of the practice. Additional views can be added during the radiographic study where necessary. Once available, the images from a given patient are shown in a list, which identifies each view.

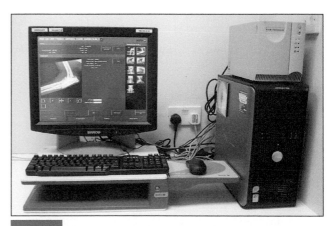

1.21 Computed radiography acquisition workstation.

Computed radiography

Computed radiography replaces the conventional film and intensifying screens with an imaging plate (IP) made from a photostimulable phosphor, most commonly based on europium-activated barium fluoro-halide compounds ($BaFX:Eu^{2+}$). These are similar in appearance to intensifying screens and are contained within cassettes (similar to those used with conventional radiography and available in the same sizes) (Figure 1.22a). They are used with X-ray machines in the same way as film–screen cassettes (i.e. above or below the X-ray table top and with or without a grid). They may be exposed elsewhere (e.g. in an operating theatre or off-site) but should be processed within a few hours of exposure. The thickness, phosphor type and crystalline structure of the phosphor determine the efficiency and resolution of the phosphor. Modern needle crystalline phosphors have greater efficiency than older amorphous crystalline phosphors, almost equivalent to that of digital radiography systems.

During exposure, the photostimulable phosphors (storage phosphors) store energy from the incident X-ray photons in semi-stable 'electron traps', creating a latent image. Following exposure, the cassette is labelled electronically with the patient information and image details before being inserted into an image reader device (digitizer) (Figure 1.22b). The imaging plate is usually automatically removed from the cassette and passed through the reader using rollers. However, in some computed radiography systems the imaging plate is rigid and does not pass through rollers. With some cheaper machines, the phosphor has to be manually unloaded from the cassette and loaded into the reader, but this is not ideal as it increases the risk of artefacts such as dirt on the plate or fading of the latent image due to exposure to light. The phosphor is 'read' by a helium–neon laser, which provides a small amount of energy to the electrons in the 'electron traps', allowing them to move back to their resting state and in doing so release energy in the form of light. The light is released as visible light with a different wavelength to that of the laser used to read the detector. The emitted light is collected by a light guide and converted to an analogue electrical signal before being amplified by a photomultiplier tube and digitized by an analogue-to-digital convertor. The intensity of the light emitted is proportional to the X-ray exposure. The residual image stored on the imaging plate is then automatically erased by exposure to a bright white light, and the imaging plate is replaced in the cassette which is then ejected from the digitizer.

In most computed radiography readers, the phosphor is read using a point scan mechanism whereby the laser repeatedly scans across the phosphor sequentially measuring the signal from each pixel location. Processing the entire image usually takes approximately 1–2 minutes following insertion of the cassette into the digitizer. This is similar to the time taken to process X-ray film using an automatic processor, although time is saved by not having to manually unload and reload the cassette in a darkroom. With more modern computed radiography readers with dual-sided read out and line scan technology, the image can be read in <10 seconds. Automatic computed radiography systems are available that are integrated into a Bucky system and require no manual handling of cassettes. Imaging plates are more sensitive to scattered radiation than are conventional intensifying screens and should be erased prior to use on a daily basis. They should be used in rotation and periodically cleaned with the appropriate computed radiography manufacturer's imaging plate cleaner.

Digital radiography

Digital radiography involves technology that produces an almost instantaneous image on the display screen of the controlling computer without the need for an intermediate 'processing' stage. Some systems convert X-ray energy directly into digitized electrical energy (direct digital radiography) whilst others produce the electrical signal via an intermediate light phase (indirect digital radiography). Digital radiography therefore provides major time savings compared with computed radiography and film–screen radiography. However, the equipment can be much more expensive than that for computed radiography. It is often marketed as an entire package, including the X-ray machine and table, although it may be possible to retro-fit the detectors to an existing system. Digital radiography flat panel detectors contain a thin film transistor array, with the transistors arranged in a matrix, corresponding to the image pixel coupled to a scintillator or amorphous selenium. The image detectors are usually hardwired to the acquisition computer (so the system is less flexible than computed radiography), although portable systems for field use in which the workstation is a laptop computer with a wireless detector are available.

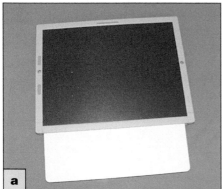

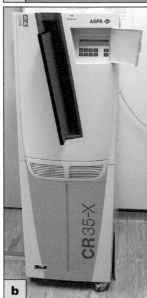

1.22 **(a)** Imaging plate used for computed radiography. The plate is placed within a cassette containing intensifying screens. **(b)** Digitizer for computed radiography with cassette ready to be inserted for reading.

There are three main types of digital radiography system:

- Flat panel detector with direct conversion of the X-ray photon into an electrical charge using a semiconductor (usually amorphous selenium). There is direct conversion of the X-ray photon into an electrical charge
- Flat panel detector with indirect conversion of the X-ray photon into an electrical signal. A scintillator (usually caesium iodide or gadolinium oxysulphide) is built into the flat panel detector, which emits light when struck by the X-ray photon. A photodiode coupled with the thin film transistor array is then used to generate the electrical signal which is used to create the image
- Indirect conversion using a scintillator, which produces light when struck by photons. The light has to be coupled and channelled on to smaller light-sensitive sensors (either charged couple devices or complementary metal oxide semiconductor devices). Compared with flat panel detectors, there is loss of efficiency and with some systems the image quality is poorer.

After the data are acquired, they are processed before being displayed by the computer. If there were no post-processing, the image would be useless with virtually no contrast. The type of post-processing has an effect on the appearance of the final image and specific algorithms are used for different body areas and systems. Post-processing may result in enhancement of edges and reduction in noise of the image.

Digital Imaging and Communications in Medicine

A Digital Imaging and Communications in Medicine (DICOM) image is simply a Tagged Image File Format (TIFF, a lossless image format) image used in medical imaging to which information regarding the patient, radiographic equipment, and protocols for handling, storing, printing and transmitting the image is tagged. The global DICOM system was developed to ensure that different DICOM-compliant digital systems were compatible with respect to image viewing, transmission, storage and printing across all imaging modalities (i.e. radiography, ultrasonography, CT, MRI, nuclear medicine and endoscopy). In 2005, a veterinary DICOM Working Group was established to develop the specifications required in veterinary medicine. These include patient information, owner, species, breed, area imaged and view. DICOM images are embedded with information that is unique to each image and which is near-impossible to alter. Each image has a digital 'header', including a 'unique identifying number', which identifies the source equipment, the patient and the individual view, thus ensuring security and helping to prevent fraud (e.g. with regard to hip dysplasia assessment). The British Veterinary Association (BVA) now accepts digital radiographs for assessment under the Hip and Elbow Dysplasia Schemes, but these must be in DICOM format. Manufacturers now issue a 'DICOM conformance statement' with regard to their equipment, although there is no verification body to oversee this and the purchaser may wish to check DICOM conformance themselves before committing to the purchase. Cheaper digital radiography systems produce images in other formats (e.g. JPEGs and TIFFs) but these are inferior for viewing and should not be used for teleradiology.

Storage and distribution

There is limited storage on computed/digital radiography systems, so it is important that an additional image storage method is used. This can be either offline (on a CD/DVD) or online (typically a central archive). For offline storage, images are copied to a CD/DVD in DICOM/JPEG format; DICOM images normally include a DICOM viewer which allows the CD/DVD to be read on a normal computer. The CD/DVD may be used to store images at the practice, given to a referring veterinary surgeon, or sent away for a second opinion. Images copied in JPEG format are compressed and may not contain the patient detail. In addition, they do not allow full manipulation of the image. JPEG images are useful for insertion into documents or presentations, but may not be of as high a resolution as DICOM images and should not be used for teleradiology or radiological interpretation.

An online archive system is known as a Picture Archiving and Communications System (PACS). It allows images from computed/digital radiography systems (and other digital imaging systems such as CT and MRI) to be saved automatically to a secure location without the manual task of copying to a CD/DVD, as well as retrieval and distribution for viewing. A PACS consists of the imaging modality, an archive server and appropriate routing software, and viewing workstations. It requires a network with reasonable speed, since the images to be transmitted are very large. Veterinary-specific PACSs for different sized establishments have been developed and larger systems can store in excess of 250,000 images. The central archive may connect to a single modality or to several imaging modalities with DICOM output; the initial archive system may be expanded subsequently with procurement of a new imaging modality. A branch practice may install a computed/digital radiography system, but storage at the main practice archive server may be preferred. In these cases, a routing device can be added which encrypts and compresses the images and sends them on to the main practice archive server for storage and distribution across all practice sites. For referred patients, it may be possible to import DICOM or JPEG images or digital photographs acquired elsewhere into the archive from a CD, DVD or memory stick.

Even in a small veterinary practice, it is very useful to be able to access images in consulting rooms, operating theatres and administration offices. An image archive can be supplied with a web browser to enable computers and dedicated viewing workstations within the practice to access the archive server (Figure 1.23). The number of users able to access the web browser simultaneously can be predetermined, depending on the needs of the practice. Staff can search for images using the patient or owner name, animal identification number or date of examination. In human medicine, the PACS is usually integrated with the hospital information system and radiology information system, allowing all patient data to be stored together. This is an ideal situation but is not yet widely available in veterinary medicine,

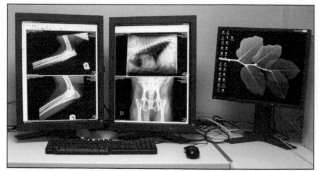

| 1.23 | Digital image viewer simultaneously showing multiple images. |

although the image archive system may be integrated with the practice management system, enabling users to retrieve radiographs using this software.

Teleradiology: This is the ability to transmit digital files (normally in a DICOM format) from one location to another for a veterinary or medical radiologist to interpret, and is a quicker and more efficient system than sending CDs/DVDs. A report is subsequently transmitted back to the practice. This means that expert advice can be obtained quickly from off-site professionals, even working on different continents, therefore providing a 24-hour service. Images are normally sent electronically from the practice PACS to the radiologist using a broadband internet connection or may be downloaded from a secure internet site (e.g. FTP site or commercial file sharing service or file delivery service).

References and further reading

Barrett E (2007) Practice radiography: time to go digital? *In Practice* **29**, 616–619

Bradley K (2006) Digital radiography – considerations for general practice. *UK Vet* **11**, 81–84

Caine A (2009) Practical approach to digital radiography. *In Practice* **31**, 334–339

Mattoon JS (2006) Digital radiography. *Veterinary and Comparative Orthopaedics and Traumatology* **19**, 123–132

Puchalski SM (2008) Digital image processing. *Veterinary Radiology & Ultrasound* **49**, S42–S47

Puchalski SM (2008) Image display. *Veterinary Radiology & Ultrasound* **49**, S9–S13

Robertson I (2007) Image dissemination and archiving. *Clinical Techniques in Small Animal Practice* **22**, 138–144

Wallack S (2008) Digital image storage. *Veterinary Radiology & Ultrasound* **49**, S37–S41

Widmer WR (2008) Acquisition hardware for digital imaging. *Veterinary Radiology & Ultrasound* **49**, S2–S8

Wright MA, Ballance D, Robertson ID and Poteet B (2008) Introduction to DICOM for the practicing veterinarian. *Veterinary Radiology & Ultrasound* **49**, S14–S18

Acknowledgement

The author is grateful to Susan Northwood of Agfa and Visbion for her help.

Principles of radiography

2

Abby Caine and Ruth Dennis

Technique is a critical part of the radiographic study as in many conditions high quality images are required to detect subtle lesions and afford the clinician the confidence that a negative study genuinely means that no pathology is visible. Obtaining high quality radiographs is not difficult but requires an understanding of the fundamental principles of radiography along with patience and attention to detail. The increasing use of digital radiography does not lessen the need for good radiographic technique.

The aim when taking a radiograph is to obtain an image that accurately represents the anatomy of the patient without distortion or unsharpness, which has good contrast and is of high quality and free of artefacts. The clinician must be familiar with which views should be obtained when performing a radiographic study of a specific anatomical region. For many anatomical regions, specific oblique views are required to visualize the anatomy and demonstrate pathology. Before initiating the study, the radiographer should ensure that all equipment required is available and that the animal is appropriately prepared.

The radiographic image represents the pattern of attenuation of the X-ray photons after they have passed through the area of interest. There is superimposition of all structures along the path of the X-ray photon and in order to localize a structure at least two radiographs taken at 90 degrees to one another (orthogonal views) are required.

Patient preparation

Prior to elective studies food should be withheld for 12 hours as in most cases some form of chemical restraint is required and evaluation of the abdomen is easier if the stomach is empty of food. For elective abdominal studies, the patient should have the opportunity to urinate and defecate prior to radiography to reduce the size of the bladder and colon and thus minimize superimposition of these structures on the radiograph. The coat of the animal should be dry and free from dirt, which will otherwise create artefacts on the image. Collars and harnesses should be removed if they will be superimposed on the area being imaged. Additional patient preparation may be required for contrast radiography studies (see Chapter 4).

Patient restraint

Some form of patient restraint is required to facilitate accurate positioning of the animal and prevent motion artefacts, whilst minimizing exposure of veterinary personnel to ionizing radiation. In the UK, manual restraint should not be used, except in exceptional circumstances when there are clinical reasons why an animal cannot be restrained by other means. Restraint can be safely achieved in the majority of cases using a combination of physical and chemical means. A quiet environment and sympathetic handling helps to calm most animals. Many aids are commercially available to facilitate positioning and restraint (e.g. long, loosely filled sandbags).

Very few animals are so medically unstable that it would be unsafe to restrain them with positioning aids or some form of chemical restraint. Some cooperative animals allow thoracic or abdominal radiographs to be taken without sedation or general anaesthesia; restrained only by appropriately positioned sandbags and other positioning aids. It is rare to be able to obtain a diagnostic skeletal radiograph in a conscious animal since muscle rigidity makes it difficult to position the limbs. In addition, even if a thoracic or abdominal radiograph can be obtained in a conscious animal, movement blur (gross movement, panting or shaking) often renders the image non-diagnostic.

Care should be taken to avoid a conscious or lightly sedated animal jumping or falling off the X-ray table and injuring itself. Conscious animals should not have limb ties attached to the X-ray table. Personnel should always be close enough to observe and intervene when a conscious animal is on the table.

Chemical restraint is usually required to obtain good skeletal and most ventrodorsal (VD) radiographs. Some animals are sufficiently relaxed with an opioid alone, particularly if in pain; for others the combination of an opioid with a low dose of phenothiazine or an alpha-2 agonist is necessary (see *BSAVA Manual of Canine and Feline Anaesthesia and Analgesia*). General anaesthesia may be necessary in animals that are uncooperative or for procedures that require complete immobility (e.g. myelography). General anaesthesia is also necessary to obtain inflated radiographs of the thorax, as well as spinal and skull images, and for procedures in which the cassette is placed inside the mouth.

Positioning aids

It is essential to use aids to correctly position the animal. The selection of positioning aids that may be required includes radiolucent wedges, radiolucent troughs and sandbags in a variety of sizes (Figure 2.1). Rope ties are required for some oblique skull views and are used to obtain stressed radiographs of joints. They can also be helpful to retract limbs from the primary beam. The use of rope ties should be reserved for patients that are under general anaesthesia or very heavy sedation as injury may result if the patient struggles whilst restrained in this way.

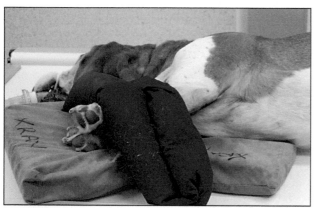

2.1 Radiolucent wedges and a sandbag are used to correctly position this anaesthetized dog for a lateral thoracic radiograph. The wedges are used to elevate the sternum since the thorax is narrower ventrally than dorsally (as is the case in most breeds). The distal limbs are supported by a wedge to avoid rotating the thorax towards the table top when the legs are extended and retracted from the cranial thorax.

Radiolucent wedges are essential to avoid rotation of the animal during positioning (e.g. when obtaining a lateral thoracic radiograph, a wedge is placed under the sternum to prevent rotation due to the ventral thorax being thinner than the dorsal thorax). Wedges are also helpful for padding the mid-cervical and mid-lumbar spine to allow a true lateral view to be obtained when performing spinal radiography. These segments of the spine are prone to 'sag' when the animal is in lateral recumbency. In addition, wedges are required to obtain true lateral and consistent oblique views of the skull.

Radiolucent troughs are very helpful for positioning animals in dorsal recumbency for VD radiographs. However, the edge of the trough will create a radiographic artefact, so it should be positioned with care to avoid superimposition over any area of interest. Sandbags are not radiolucent and must not be included within the area of interest. They are used as an aid to restrain and position the animal. Their weight allows them to 'pull' body parts gently away from the area of interest (e.g. to pull the limbs away from the thorax or abdomen when taking a lateral radiograph). Where possible sandbags should not be included within the collimated beam as they contribute to scatter and reduce image contrast.

Film–screen combinations

Conventional radiography

The choice of film–screen combination and film type has a significant effect on the contrast and spatial resolution of conventional (analogue) radiographs.

- The structure and processing of the film (emulsion thickness, grain size, speed) affects the optical density of the final image. Optical density describes the amount of light transmission through the final processed film (i.e. the degree of blackness). The relationship between the degree of exposure and the optical density is described by the characteristic curve ('H and D curve') of the film. The curve is sigmoid in shape, meaning that the response of the film to X-ray exposure is non-linear (see Chapter 1).
- Film contrast is highest in the linear region of the curve, where small differences in exposure result in large differences in optical density of the film. The steeper the linear region of the curve, the higher is the inherent contrast of the film.
- The speed of radiographic film varies (as with photographic film) with faster films requiring less exposure. Faster film (higher speed film) has larger silver halide grains and results in an image with lower resolution compared with slower speed film.
- Intensifying screens are also available in a range of speeds with faster screens emitting more light for a given exposure than slower screens, but at the expense of having larger crystals and producing images with a lower resolution.
- The film–screen combination used also depends on the output of the available X-ray machine. If only a low output X-ray machine is available, a fast film–screen combination may have to be used to allow for short exposure times and to prevent motion blur. Where high resolution images and fine detail are required (e.g. skeletal radiography, feline thoracic radiography and dental radiography), a slow film–screen combination should be used. For anatomical areas where fine detail is not required, such as the thorax and abdomen of large-breed dogs, a faster film–screen combination can be used to allow for shorter exposure times.

Digital radiography

With digital systems there is not usually a choice of detector, so the spatial resolution of the image cannot be influenced by the operator. The contrast is largely determined by post-processing of the image.

- Direct digital radiography systems have a fixed size detector but with some computed radiography systems a choice of cassette size and resolution may be available. Smaller, higher resolution cassettes (used for mammography in humans) are available, which are suitable for radiography of the extremities.
- The resolution in digital systems is determined by the number of picture elements (pixels) in the image (image matrix). The intrinsic spatial resolution of digital radiography is less than that of conventional radiography, although the effect of this is not apparent in the clinical setting. The

spatial resolution of an image cannot be altered once it has been acquired but the perceived spatial resolution of a digital image can be manipulated by post-processing edge enhancement or smoothing.

- Unlike conventional radiography, the detector response in digital systems is linear, resulting in an increased dynamic range (i.e. the range of exposure times that result in a diagnostic image) (see Chapter 1). This allows a broad scale of contrast such that all anatomical structures have a density value that can be displayed and visualized on the same image. The contrast is determined by the image algorithm selected and by adjusting the brightness and contrast (windowing) of the processed image.

Patient positioning

Good positioning is essential to enable accurate representation of the anatomy of the animal on the radiograph. Recognition of lesions on a radiograph relies on knowledge of normal radiographic anatomy, which is made easier by consistent good positioning. Poor positioning is one of the most frequent radiographic errors. Incorrect positioning necessitates repeated radiographs, increasing costs and radiation exposure levels. Poor positioning can also lead to missed or erroneous diagnoses (Figure 2.2). It is much easier to compare the appearance of a radiograph with that in a textbook or with other examples if the positioning is the same. There are several principles on which correct radiographic positioning is based:

- Minimizing geometric distortion
- Minimizing the penumbra
- Centring
- Magnification.

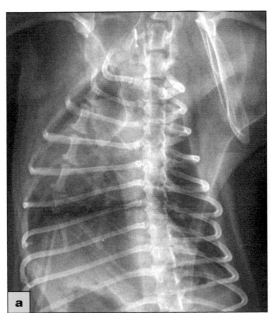

2.2 Incorrect positioning can result in images that display anatomical structures in an unfamiliar way, leading to missed or erroneous diagnoses or difficulty in localizing the abnormalities. **(a)** DV view of the thorax in a dog. Note the marked rotation around the long axis making comparison with examples of normal anatomy in a radiological atlas impossible. (continues) ▶

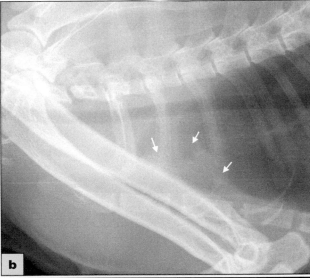

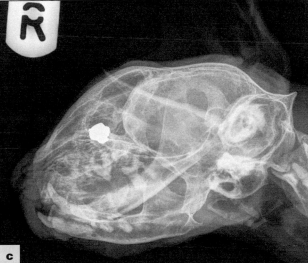

2.2 (continued) Incorrect positioning can result in images that display anatomical structures in an unfamiliar way, leading to missed or erroneous diagnoses or difficulty in localizing the abnormalities. **(b)** Lateral view of the thorax in a cat. Superimposition of the forelimbs on the cranial thorax partially conceals the enlarged sternal lymph node (arrowed). **(c)** Oblique view of the skull of a cat with an airgun pellet injury. This image provides no information about the location of the pellet. Two orthogonal views are required to localize the pellet.

Minimizing geometric distortion

The X-ray beam diverges from the focal spot equally in all directions (Figure 2.3). In addition to the effect on the intensity of the beam (inverse square law), the divergence of the X-ray beam with distance also has an effect on the appearance of the 'shadow' of the object being imaged. Only objects placed parallel with the film, and perpendicular and central to the X-ray beam, are displayed accurately. Objects that are not in the centre of the beam, or not parallel to the film, are distorted due to unequal magnification (as some parts are further away from the film than others). This effect, due to the geometry of the X-ray beam, is known as geometric distortion. Geometric distortion is particularly important in dental radiography as the conformation of the maxilla and mandible, shape of the teeth and multiple roots make it impossible for all teeth to be optimally imaged at the same time.

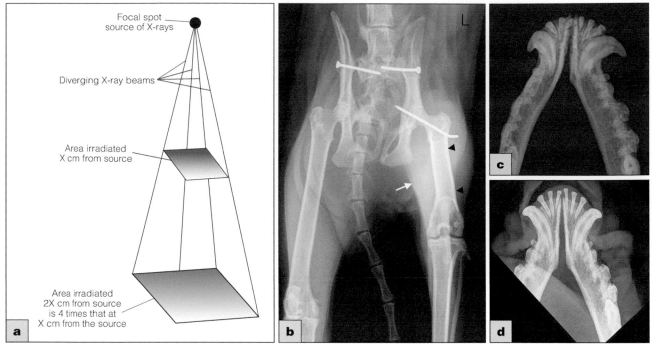

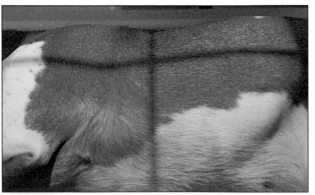
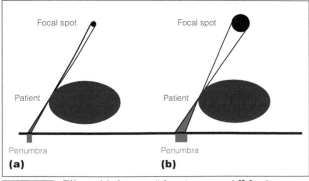

2.3 Geometric distortion. **(a)** The X-ray beam diverges from the focal spot equally in all directions. The further a structure is from the centre of the beam, the greater the geometric distortion. **(b)** VD view of the pelvis of a cat. Foreshortening of the left femur is due to the reduced range of motion in the left coxofemoral joint, preventing the femur from being extended parallel to the X-ray plate. Thus, the left femur appears shorter than the right femur. The foreshortened femur (arrowheads) and surrounding muscles (arrowed) appear more opaque as the depth of tissue penetrated by the X-ray beam is greater. **(c-d)** Dental radiographs of the mandible in a dog. Note the geometric distortion of the teeth when (c) a conventional VD intraoral view is obtained compared with (d) an image taken using the bisecting angle technique.

Minimizing the penumbra

The penumbra is the outer part of the shadow formed around an object, which occurs because the focal spot is not infinitesimally small. If the focal spot were a true point source, the X-ray photons contacting the edge of the object being imaged and reaching the film would result in a sharply marginated shadow with no blurring of the edges. However, since the focal spot is not a point source, the image formed by the X-ray photons is generated from multiple points (Figure 2.4). A photon from one part of the focal spot leads to the shadow of the object being represented at a different location compared with a photon originating from another location within the focal spot. This leads to blurring and loss of sharpness at the margins of the object on the radiograph. The penumbra is greater with a larger focal spot size and with increasing distance between the object and the film. For these reasons, to obtain a sharp image, the body part should be placed as close as possible to the film, and the smallest focal spot available should be selected.

Centring

Each radiograph should be centred to the anatomical area of interest using bony landmarks. This allows for the entire area of interest to be included on the cassette and collimation to be kept as close as possible to the area of interest. Poor collimation is often due to uncertainties about centring points (the tendency is to enlarge the collimated area just to ensure the anatomy is included on the image). The centre of the X-ray beam is shown by a cross in the centre of the light from the light beam diaphragm (Figure 2.5). Penumbra and geometric distortion are smallest at the centre of the X-ray beam and centring

2.4 Effect of **(a)** a small focal spot and **(b)** a large focal spot on image sharpness. The larger the focal spot, the larger the penumbra around an object. The penumbra makes the margin of the object appear less sharp.

2.5 Centring the X-ray beam. The area to be exposed is illuminated by light from the light beam diaphragm. The centre point of the radiograph is indicated by a central cross.

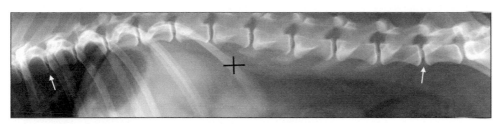

2.6 Lateral thoracolumbar radiograph showing centring for the spine. The disc spaces appear progressively narrower (arrowed) the further away they are from the centre of the beam (+). This is due to divergence.

is of particular importance when imaging the spine and joints. If the spine is correctly positioned, each of the intervertebral disc spaces should be perpendicular to the cassette. However, the X-ray beam diverges from the centre point. This means that the X-ray beam passes parallel to the disc spaces near the centre of the beam, but more obliquely through the disc spaces at the periphery of the radiograph, leading to apparent narrowing of the disc spaces (Figure 2.6). In order to assess disc space width correctly, it is important to obtain multiple views of the spine centred at different levels. When using a grid it is also essential to ensure that the beam is centred correctly and the appropriate focal distance is used to avoid unnecessary grid cut-off (see below).

Magnification

The size of the 'shadow' of an object on a radiograph is determined by the distance between the object and the film (object–film distance) and the distance between the focal spot and the object (film–focal distance) (Figure 2.7). If the object–film difference is small and the film–focal distance is large (approximately 2 m), then the X-ray beam is almost parallel and there is little magnification. The closer an object is to the cassette, the closer it will be to a true size on the image (e.g. for radiography of the extremities, if the limb is placed directly against the cassette, an image with minimal magnification is obtained). There is always some magnification if an under table grid is used, since this increases object–film distance (Figure 2.8). This magnification can be in the region of a 10% increase in apparent size. This can present a problem if accurate measurements are required (e.g. for orthopaedic implants). For this reason, it is useful to have markers of the true size or a ruler (Figure 2.9), which can be placed at the level of interest (e.g. for a total hip replacement implant, placed at the level of the greater trochanter) during radiography so that the degree of magnification can be calculated and corrected for.

Manipulation of digital images after acquisition allows the image to be magnified or reduced in size, but it is important to be able to recognize the original

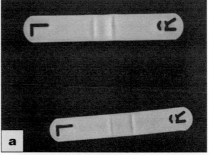

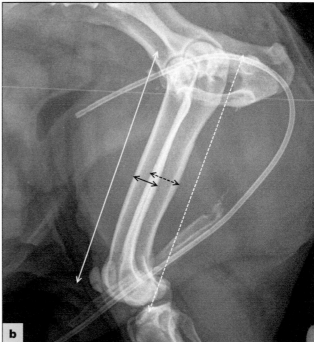

2.8 Magnification. **(a)** The positional marker on the top has been imaged on the table top with the cassette placed under the table. The positional marker on the bottom has been imaged under the table placed directly on top of the cassette. The marker on the top is magnified because of the increased object–film distance created by use of the under table ('Bucky') grid. **(b)** Lateral radiograph of the caudal abdomen of a dog. The effect of magnification is obvious when comparing the length and diameter of the lower (solid arrows) and upper (dashed arrows) limb.

(a)   **(b)**

2.7 Effect of object–film distance on the radiographic image. **(a)** The object is located close to the film, resulting in an accurate representation of the object on the radiograph. **(b)** Increasing the distance between the film and the object results in magnification of the object on the radiograph. If not all parts of the object are parallel to the film (i.e. are not equidistant) there will be uneven magnification of different parts of the same object.

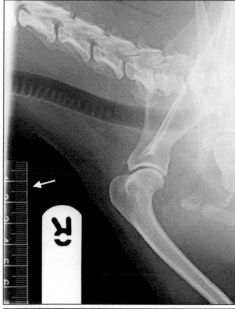

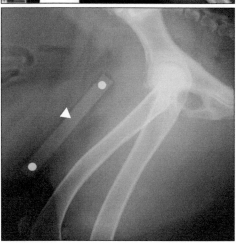

2.9 Radiographic markers. A marker of true size or a ruler (arrowed) with radiopaque measurements should be used where magnification of the image could lead to errors. When taking radiographs for orthopaedic templating, a marker of known length (arrowhead) is positioned at the level of the bone of interest to allow accurate measurements to be obtained.

size of the image. Most Digital Imaging and Communications in Medicine (DICOM) viewers automatically display the image size so that it fits in its entirety on the viewing screen. This means that most images are automatically zoomed or reduced in size. Some DICOM viewers allow images to be displayed at 'True Size' or '100%', but this may require calibration of the viewer settings as the monitor pixel size can affect the True Size display. A True Size or 100% display only shows the image at the size of the imaging plate/phosphor and does not mean that the image genuinely reflects the true size of the anatomical area being imaged since geometric factors still apply with digital images. If measurements are required, a marker of known length should always be used.

Collimation

Collimation is essential for all radiographs, regardless of whether a film–screen or digital imaging system is used. It serves two purposes:

- To improve image quality by reducing scatter
- To aid radiation safety.

To improve image quality, each radiograph taken should be collimated to the area of interest only. For overview radiographs, such as of the thorax and abdomen, collimation to the boundaries of the body cavities (which is not the skin surface in obese animals) is required. Closer collimation is required for skeletal and spinal radiographs, including only the relevant anatomical region within the primary beam. It is also good radiation safety practice to ensure that the collimated beam falls entirely within the film, since the entire area that has been irradiated is then imaged.

Collimation is performed using the variably sized lead shutters within the light beam diaphragm, which can be adjusted by sliders on the front of the tube head. These restrict the area through which the X-ray beam can pass with the collimated primary beam, indicated by a light (projected by mirrors), coinciding with the same area. As part of regular servicing and maintenance, it is good practice to confirm that the area of light from the light beam diaphragm is the same as the irradiated area. This is easily achieved by taking an image of a square with coins placed right in the corners of the collimator light area. The coins should then be seen in the corners of the irradiated area once the film has been processed. If there is a discrepancy, this should be corrected by a service engineer.

Exposure factors

On a correctly exposed radiograph it should be possible to visualize clearly all parts of the anatomy (assuming that it is not obscured by pathology) with bony trabecular detail visible and clear differentiation of fat and soft tissue. The areas of the film outwith the patient and exposed to the primary beam should be black. With conventional radiographs, it may be necessary to use a bright light to assess anatomy in thinner parts of the body (e.g. ventral lung lobes) but the anatomy should still be clearly visible. Underexposure and overexposure appear differently on digital radiographs compared with conventional film and therefore may be missed, but still reduce diagnostic accuracy.

Conventional film–screen combinations have a relatively small range of exposure factors that result in a correctly exposed radiograph and too many or too few X-ray photons reaching the film results in a non-diagnostic or a compromised image. If there are large differences in the depth of the tissue being imaged (e.g. the femur in large dogs where there is a lot more soft tissue proximally compared with distally), it may be impossible to obtain a single radiograph that is properly exposed for all parts of the anatomy. In these cases, separate radiographs need to be taken. Digital radiography systems have much greater latitude than conventional film, which means that a wider range of exposure factors result in a diagnostic image. Although digital systems have a wide latitude, it is still important to use an exposure chart and appropriate exposure technique.

The overall radiographic exposure is created by a combination of milliampere second (mAs) and kilovoltage (kV) factors, which are determined by the settings on the X-ray machine. Factors can be too high (overexposed) or too low (underexposed) or the proportion of the two can be incorrectly balanced leading to incorrect contrast of the radiograph. The degree of contrast can be manipulated by the choice of exposure factors and is to some extent personal preference. An understanding of the contribution made by kV and mAs to image contrast is important in order to prevent the radiographer obtaining images with poor contrast, especially with conventional radiography.

- The mAs value controls the electrical current to the cathode and thereby the temperature of the tube filament. This in turn controls the number of X-rays produced per second. The exposure time is measured in seconds. The mAs determines the total number of X-ray photons produced during the exposure. This is considered the intensity of the emergent beam and is responsible for overall film blackening (which is determined by the number of X-rays reaching the detector). The mAs does not affect radiographic contrast, since this is determined by differential absorption of the X-ray beam (associated with the penetrating power of the beam).
- The kV contributes to both film blackening (overall intensity) and radiographic contrast (penetrating power). Within the diagnostic range for conventional radiography, as the kV increases, the contrast of an image reduces. Conversely, a low kV results in an image with higher contrast as X-ray absorption by the photoelectric effect is maximized (see Chapter 1) and the effect of scatter is reduced. There is a minimum kV that can be used, which depends on the size of the animal as the X-ray photons must have enough energy to pass through the animal and reach the film. If the kV is too low, the film will be underexposed, even if the mAs is increased, as the photons have insufficient energy (Figure 2.10) to penetrate the area being imaged.
- When selecting exposure factors, film blackening must be sufficient so that an adequate image can be seen. This can be achieved by changing both the mAs and kV. Some machines allow only one of these factors to be altered (fixed mA/kV X-ray tubes) but many allow both to be manipulated.

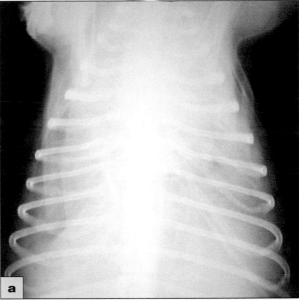

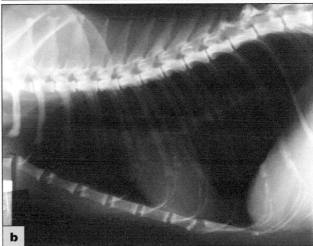

2.10 Exposure factors. **(a)** Underexposed DV thoracic radiograph of a dog taken using conventional (analogue) film. The radiograph needs to be repeated as the amount of meaningful information that can be extracted is limited. For a region such as the thorax with high inherent contrast, the difference between soft tissue structures and air-filled lung is not appreciated. This would suggest that diffuse pulmonary pathology is present and penetration (kV) should be increased by a minimum of 15% (but possibly considerably more). **(b)** Overexposed conventional lateral thoracic radiograph of a cat. The lungs are overexposed and no assessment of the pulmonary parenchyma is possible. Bronchial disease, infiltrate and metastases may all be overlooked. In the cat, pulmonary parenchymal detail is fine, so to assess any changes with confidence, high detail images are required.

The mAs and kV can be altered to maximize radiographic contrast. The abdomen has an inherently low contrast with only small differences in atomic number between the soft tissue or fluid opacity and the abdominal fat separating them. To maximize this difference, a combination of a relatively low kV (45–70) and high mAs (8–20) allows sufficient overall film blackening whilst maximizing contrast. The converse applies to the thorax, where the relatively high inherent contrast between the tissues (ranging from gas to mineral opacity) is compensated for by using a high kV and a low mAs (Figure 2.11), which also reduces the risk of movement blur.

Selecting exposure factors

When selecting exposure factors, the 15% rule is helpful:

- By increasing the kV by 15%, the radiographic density of the film is doubled. In order to maintain the equivalent radiographic density, the mAs is halved (e.g. if you have an exposure of 50 kV and 10 mAs, increasing the kV to 57 and reducing the mAs to 5 results in similar film blackening)
- Conversely, decreasing the kV by 15% can produce similar overall film blackening if the mAs is doubled.

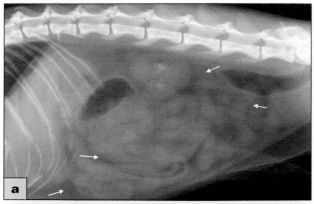

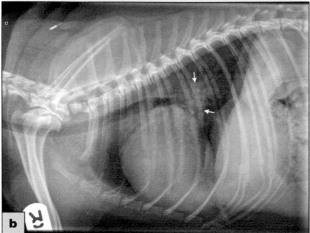

| 2.11 | Inherent contrast. There is inherently less contrast in **(a)** the abdomen than **(b)** the thorax. |

In the abdomen, contrast is due predominately to abdominal fat (arrowed) between the organs. Using a low to intermediate kV and a high mAs maximizes this contrast. In the thorax, there is high contrast between the air-filled lungs and the heart and using a high kV and short exposure time (mAs) limits movement blur. Short exposure times are necessary where conscious radiography is unavoidable, as in this case of a dog with left-sided heart disease (the enlarged left atrium is arrowed) to assess for signs of congestive failure (pulmonary oedema, enlarged lobar veins).

Many X-ray machines do not allow the mA and time to be selected separately, since combined they have the same effect of increasing the quantity of X-ray photons. If the time can be independently controlled, it is worth considering how much the duration of exposure will affect the radiograph. Thoracic radiographs taken in a conscious animal can be particularly affected by long exposure times, resulting in movement blur from breathing. For this reason, the exposure time should be kept to a minimum for thoracic radiography. Exposure time is less of a problem when imaging an area of an animal that will not move (e.g. an extremity radiograph taken under general anaesthesia).

Exposure charts

It is essential to develop a technique chart for use in practice since each radiographic system is unique. Use of an exposure chart reduces the number of radiographs that need to be repeated by standardizing and optimizing the exposure factors used. Reducing the number of repeated radiographs saves time and expense, and also minimizes unnecessary personnel and animal exposure. Since the technique chart needs to be accessible to anyone who is taking radiographs,

it should be simple to understand and the number of variables kept to a minimum. For this reason, the film–focal distance should be standardized (usually 100–115 cm) as altering this variable can alter exposure requirements. Different radiographic techniques are required for different anatomical areas (e.g. table top techniques without a grid for the extremities, skull and small animals compared with use of a 'Bucky' grid in larger animals for the thorax, abdomen, spine and pelvis). The cassettes (with or without screens) should be kept constant for each type of radiograph (in veterinary practice, non-screen radiography is only used in a few circumstances such as dental and intraoral imaging). Separate exposure details should be recorded, depending on whether a grid is used (use of a grid requires an increase in exposure factors).

Digital systems

An exposure chart is still required for digital systems as underexposure is common and results in reduced image quality. Overexposure is less common but also reduces image quality, as well as increasing the dose of radiation to the animal. As the direct relationship between film blackening and exposure factors is lost in digital systems, the degree of exposure is often given by a numerical value (exposure index) on the console. Each equipment manufacturer has their own method of displaying exposure information and usually provides guidelines as to the range of recommended values. The measurement of the number of X-ray quanta on image quality is often expressed as signal to noise ratio (SNR). Images with a low SNR have a grainy, mottled appearance, which may prevent visualization of fine detail. The effect of kV on image quality with digital systems is complex and difficult to measure as the relationship between kV and image contrast is less apparent and affected by multiple factors (e.g. image processing). The sensitivity of the X-ray detector to scattered photons and the effect of X-ray photon energy on detector efficiency varies with detector type and advice should be sought from the equipment suppliers on recommendations on the use of a grid and the choice of exposure factors. Generally, for most digital systems, <100 kV is recommended and the rule varying the kV to optimize image contrast should be followed as for conventional film. Increasing kV may reduce the SNR by increasing noise but not signal. When assessing quality, the images should be reviewed on a diagnostic workstation with an appropriate monitor as subtle changes such as underexposure with poor SNR may not be apparent on the low resolution monitor of the digital radiography console.

Variable kV chart

- The simplest type of exposure chart is a variable kV chart (Figure 2.12). This maintains a constant mAs and only adjusts the kV (increasing with increasing thickness of the tissue). The depth of the tissue being imaged is measured using callipers. The mAs is fixed. If starting from scratch with a new radiography system this can be helpful, although it can be modified later (to maximize the differences for thoracic and abdominal radiography, see below) to improve the quality of the radiographs obtained. Separate charts are required for different body areas as the mAs differs between each region.

Thickness of patient (cm)	kVp	Abdomen/thorax/proximal limbs (mAs)	Spine/pelvis (mAs)	Distal limbs/skull (mAs)	Grid required?
7	58	3.2	5	1.3	No
8	60	3.2	5	1.6	No
9	62	3.2	5	1.6	No
10	64	3.2	6.4	2.5	Yes
11	66	3.2	6.4		Yes
12	68	3.2	6.4		Yes

2.12 An example of a variable kV chart.

- For a variable kV chart, an appropriate mAs is selected (usually the shortest appropriate time so that personnel exposure, animal movement and tube wear are minimized). If using a medium speed system (par 200), a good starting point is an mAs as follows:
  - Abdomen: 7.5–15 mAs
  - Thorax: 5 mAs
  - Spine and pelvis: 10–15 mAs
  - Extremities: 5 mAs.

  When using rapid film (par 400), the mAs can be reduced by half and for detail film (par 100) the mAs can be doubled.
- For radiographs requiring fine detail (extremities or thorax in cats or very small dogs, and skulls) the small focal spot of the X-ray machine is selected, which usually restricts the mA to a maximum of 100–200 mA. For larger animals, 300 mA is usually selected.
- The thickest part of the region being imaged is measured using callipers. If possible, it is ideal to have the thinnest part of the anatomy at the anode end of the tube to make use of the heal effect. The kV is selected using Santé's rule as an initial guide when creating an exposure chart from scratch.
- Once the first exposure has been obtained, the kV is adjusted until the image is optimized:
  - Increase kV by 15% if underexposed
  - Decrease kV by 15% if overexposed.

  This provides the starting point for the exposure chart.
- The chart is then formulated for other animals, increasing the kV with each cm increase in tissue thickness:
  - Increase by 2 kV per cm whilst under 80 kV
  - Increase by 3 kV per cm between 80 and 100 kV.
- With digital systems, because of the greater latitude, it is usually not necessary to alter the kV for every cm but instead for every 5 cm. This simplifies the exposure chart.
- Once the initial exposure chart has been created, it can be fine-tuned to optimize contrast by adjusting the kV and mAs using the 15% rule (see above). In addition to increasing the kV with increasing tissue thickness, the mAs may also need to be increased in large patients and thick body parts.
- It is good practice to update the exposure chart with time. The exposures that result in good images and those that require adjusting should be recorded, and the chart altered accordingly.

- Separate technique charts are compiled for the extremities, thorax and spine/pelvis, as well as the cat, adjusting the mAs and kV as appropriate to optimize contrast.
- If the film–focal distance is altered, the exposure factors need adjusting using the inverse square law.

Santé's rule

kV = ((thickness of the widest part of the patient in cm) x 2) + (film–focal distance in inches)

For example: for a 13 cm thick (at its widest part) dog and a film–focal distance of 40 inches (approximately 1 m, as commonly used), the kV is:

kV = (13 x 2) + 40

kV = 66

Note: if using a grid (as would be the case in this example), then the kV needs to be increased by about 10 (range: 5–15). So in this case, the initial radiograph would be taken using a kV of 76.

Altering the film–focal distance

$$\frac{\text{Initial exposure}}{\text{New exposure}} = \frac{\text{Initial film–focal distance}^2}{\text{New film–focal distance}^2}$$

For example: if the initial film–focal distance is 100 cm with a mAs of 20 and the film–focal distance is changed to 80 cm, the new exposure should be:

$$\text{mAs} = \frac{20 \times (80)^2}{100^2} = \frac{12,800}{10,000}$$

mAs = 12.8

Contrast

Image contrast refers to the difference in brightness or darkness between an area of interest and its surroundings. Image contrast is influenced by radiographic contrast, detector contrast, display contrast and scatter.

Radiographic contrast

The contrast of the final radiograph is largely determined by the number of X-ray photons emerging from the different areas of the animal. Factors which contribute to radiographic contrast include:

- Energy spectrum of the emergent X-ray beam
- Atomic number of the tissues
- Physical density

- Electron density
- Tissue thickness.

It should be noted that whilst kV can be controlled to maximize tissue contrast, the factors within the animal cannot be controlled. When a contrast agent is administered, the composition of the body is altered.

Energy spectrum of the emergent X-ray beam

The energy of the X-ray beam is one of the most important factors controlling image contrast. Photoelectric interactions provide the greatest differentiation between tissue types and maximize tissue contrast. The photoelectric effect predominates at lower X-ray energies whereas Compton interactions predominate at higher proton energies. For soft tissues, which have a low effective atomic number, the photoelectric effect is therefore the main contributor to tissue contrast. The energy spectrum of the X-ray beam is primarily determined by the kV.

Atomic number of the tissues

Soft tissues and fat have low atomic numbers; with that of fat being slightly lower than soft tissue. The small difference in atomic number between fat and soft tissue/water is the main reason why they appear to have different opacities on radiographs (due to the photoelectric effect which varies with the cube of the atomic number). The high effective atomic number of contrast agents is an important factor, resulting in increased X-ray photon attenuation. In addition, although the number of Compton interactions increases with increasing photon energy, the number of photoelectric interactions increases sharply at the K- and L-edges (absorption edges) of materials. Within the range of diagnostic X-ray energies, this corresponds closely to the absorption edges of contrast agents (barium, iodine) used in diagnostic imaging studies. The absorption edges of iodine and barium are in the range of 34–37 kV, which is near the centre of the energy spectrum used for most diagnostic studies. Bone has a higher effective atomic number than soft tissue and fat, and as the photoelectric effect increases with the cube of the atomic number, a combination of greater physical density and effective atomic number means that the photoelectric effect of bone is approximately six times that of the soft tissues and fat (at lower energies). At higher energies, where Compton interactions predominate, the difference is limited.

Physical density

- Air has the lowest physical density, therefore the number of interactions is considerably less than soft tissues, fat and bone.
- Fat is less dense than soft tissue (parenchymatous organs, muscle) and this subtle difference makes a minor contribution to the lower attenuation of fat (but is less important than differences in atomic number). The difference in radiographic contrast between fat and soft tissue is small and can be negated with poor technique.
- Bone has a high physical density which leads to more interactions and higher attenuation.

Electron density

Fat has a higher electron density for a given weight of tissue than either soft tissue or bone as it has a higher hydrogen density. This leads to more Compton interactions per weight of tissue at higher X-ray energies; however, as fat is less physically dense than bone there is no increased attenuation by fat.

Tissue thickness

Differences in tissue thickness allow structures of similar soft tissue attenuation and density to be recognized. A difference in tissue thickness of approximately 3–4 cm is required for a difference in opacity to be recognized.

Detector contrast

This refers to the ability of the detector to convert the X-ray beam exiting the patient into optical density (analogue film) or signal amplitude (digital system) differences.

- For conventional film, the composition and processing (especially developing) of the film affects the contrast of the radiograph. The characteristic curve of the film describes the film contrast and is determined by the range of silver halide grain sizes within the emulsion. A wide range of grain sizes results in a film of lower contrast compared with an emulsion where the grain sizes are uniform. Using intensifying screens results in greater contrast compared with non-screen film. Chemical processing affects image contrast as underdevelopment or overdevelopment reduces contrast.
- The effect of detector contrast is less important with digital systems than conventional film. With digital systems, the very wide dynamic range of the detector means that detector contrast has relatively little effect on the final image contrast, which is largely determined by post-processing of the signal. The construction of the detector and electronics determines the dynamic range and grey shades that can be displayed and are the main determinates of detector contrast on digital systems.

Display contrast

Display contrast refers to window and levelling (displaying pixels according to the values generated by look-up tables). It allows all structures within an object with a wide range of attenuation to be displayed.

Scatter

The production of Compton scatter from the interaction of an X-ray with matter is described in Chapter 1. Compton scatter is disadvantageous for two reasons:

- It can lead to scattered radiation being emitted in any direction, which poses a radiation safety risk for any bystanders
- The scattered photons contain no diagnostic information.

Compton scatter is not representative of attenuation by structures within the animal but does reach the detector, resulting in film blackening (analogue film) or an amplitude recording (digital systems) and reduces contrast. The probability of a Compton interaction is not dependent on the atomic number (Z) in contrast to the photoelectric effect, where the atomic number greatly influences X-ray absorption and image contrast. Compton scattering can occur in any tissue, with the scattered photons reaching the film in an unpredictable manner, leading to a background fog or greyness across the whole film. The two factors that can increase the probability of Compton scattering are the energy of the photon and the density of the tissue.

Reduction of scatter

Since scatter is undesirable, several techniques can be used to reduce it:

- Use of a grid
- Collimation and reducing tissue thickness
- Choice of exposure factors.

Use of a grid: A grid is a device placed between the animal and the cassette, constructed from multiple lead strips separated by radiolucent spacers that are aligned parallel to the primary beam, allowing it to pass through the grid without being attenuated. Any radiation that has passed through the patient and reaches the cassette without interacting with matter will pass through the spacer. The majority of scattered radiation produced within the animal or surrounding objects is no longer moving parallel to the primary X-ray beam and will therefore be absorbed by the lead strips (Figure 2.13).

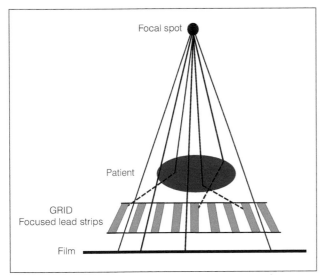

Focal spot

Patient

GRID
Focused lead strips

Film

2.13 A grid comprises multiple lead strips, often angled so that they are parallel to the diverging primary X-ray beam. Scattered or off-focus X-ray photons (dotted lines) cannot pass through the lead strips and are absorbed. Primary beam photons, which are responsible for the useful radiographic image, pass between the lead strips.

- A radiograph taken with a grid has more contrast (typically improved by a factor of 2–3), since the degree of background radiation fog is reduced (Figure 2.14).
- Several types of grid are available: unfocused, focused and crossed. Most grids are focused. These take into account the divergence of the X-ray beam by having the lead strips angled either side of the central line at a radius, the line of convergence of which is the tube head. This requires the grid to be positioned at a specified

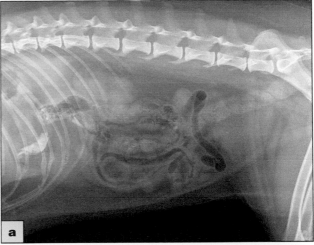

a

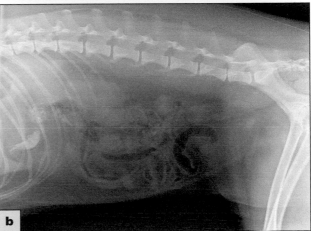

b

2.14 The effect of a grid. Lateral radiographs of the abdomen in a dog taken **(a)** with the use of a grid and **(b)** without a grid. Note the increased contrast of the image taken using a grid.

film–focal distance from the tube head, and the tube head must to be centred to the grid. If focused grids are not positioned correctly, a larger number of X-rays from the primary beam are absorbed. This is most marked at the edges of the image and is known as grid cut-off (Figure 2.15).

- Grids can be positioned underneath, or are built into, the X-ray table. Built-in grids have the advantage of allowing the animal to be positioned and repositioned easily, but care must be taken to ensure that the tube head is aligned to the grid. One disadvantage of a stationary grid is the appearance of very fine lines across the radiograph, coinciding with the position of the lead strips (termed 'grid lines'). The Potter-Bucky moving grid was developed to reduce this artefact. During exposure an electric or spring mechanism oscillates or vibrates the grid from side to side under the table so that the visible grid lines are blurred.
- A further disadvantage of grids is that they absorb some primary radiation as well as scattered radiation. Exposure factors must be increased when a grid is used. This varies with the number of lead strips per mm (grid frequency or grid density) and the ratio of the height of the lead strips to the width of the spacer material (grid ratio). The greater the grid density and grid ratio,

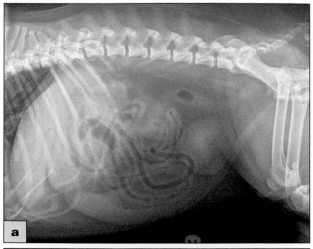

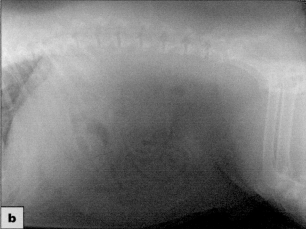

2.15 Incorrect use of a grid. Lateral radiographs of the abdomen in a dog taken **(a)** with a focused grid correctly positioned and **(b)** with a focused grid positioned off-level (i.e. the central X-ray is not perpendicular to the grid). In (b) misalignment of the grid has resulted in an underexposed radiograph and reduced image contrast.

the more efficient is the absorption of scattered and primary radiation. To maintain film density, the mAs must be increased by a factor of 2–3 (manufacturers will advise how much factors must be increased based on the specific design of the individual grid).
- X-rays passing through a thin piece of tissue produce less scatter than those travelling through a thicker piece of tissue. Grids are usually only used when tissue thickness is >10–15 cm.
- Grids are also required for computed/digital radiography and should be used in obese patients and in areas with a tissue depth >10–15 cm. Grid artefacts, in particular interference pattern (Moiré) artefacts, may be present on computed radiography images if a low frequency grid is used. This artefact is more evident when viewing images on a computer monitor because the resolution of the monitor is lower than that of the image. The artefact can be reduced, but not necessarily eliminated, by using a grid with a higher frequency (grid density) or a moving grid. Alternatively, images can be viewed on a high-resolution, clinical-grade monitor. With digital systems the vendor of the system should be consulted to ensure the correct grid type is used.

Collimation and tissue thickness:

- The amount of scatter produced is largely dependent on the volume of tissue irradiated. Therefore, for a given exposure a thinner piece of tissue produces less scatter than a thick piece of tissue. Unfortunately, it is generally impractical to reduce the thickness of a particular part of an animal! Abdominal compression is rarely practical (or safe).
- However, it is possible to control the volume of tissue included in the collimated area. For a given tissue thickness, the ratio of scattered to primary photons increases with increasing area of irradiated tissue. For example: for tissue with a thickness of 20 cm, if an area 400 cm^2 (20 cm x 20 cm) is irradiated, for every one primary photon, three scattered photons reach the cassette (a ratio of 3:1). If the size of the collimated area is reduced to 25 cm^2 (5 cm x 5 cm), the ratio of primary photons to scattered photons is reduced to 2:1.
- It is particularly important to reduce the size of the collimated area when radiographing anatomical areas with thick soft tissues such as the shoulder joint or spine. Close collimation reduces the amount of scatter produced and results in improved radiographic contrast. Failure to collimate appropriately is often due to lack of knowledge of centring points or difficulty in palpating centring points. If the centring point cannot be felt, there is a tendency to increase the size of the collimated area just to ensure the area of interest is included on the radiograph.

Choice of exposure factors: The effect of exposure factors on scatter is complex, but overall increasing the kV increases the amount of scatter reaching the film and reduces image contrast. With increasing kV the mean energy of the scattered photons increases. The scattered photons are more likely to exit the patient and reach the film. The direction of scatter also changes with kV. As the kV increases, more scattered radiation is moving in a forward direction (away from the X-ray tube head) and is more likely to reach the film. The actual number of scattered photons reduces with increasing kV, but the scatter which is produced is more likely to reach the film; therefore, the overall effect of increasing kV increases the effect of scatter on the film. Reducing the kV increases contrast by reducing the effect of scatter.

Labelling

- Adequate labelling of the radiograph is required to identify the patient and provide directional markers and information about beam orientation. Radiographs are considered part of the medical records, and as such are required to be identified accurately and stored safely in case they are required for future review.
- Labelling should be applied at the time of the radiographic examination since this reduces the likelihood of mislabelling. Several methods are available:
  - A radiopaque marker can be placed in the primary beam during exposure (either lead

letters or disposable write-on tape)

- Alternatively, with conventional films, a light marker can be used prior to processing. The film has a small area protected from exposure during radiography that is exposed to a light (to which the film is sensitive) in the darkroom. The radiograph is then processed as usual.
- For digital images, it is good practice to label all radiographs before processing.

■ All radiographic labelling should identify the practice, the animal and owner name, and date of the radiographic examination.

■ In addition to identifying the patient, labels should be used to indicate the position of the animal:

- A left/right marker is placed within the primary beam on the appropriate side of the patient for dorsoventral (DV) and VD radiographs of the thorax, abdomen and axial skeleton, so that pathology can be localized accurately.
- The side of the patient that is dependent on a lateral radiograph (i.e. the part closest to the film) is indicated by a left/right marker.
- For oblique radiographs of the trunk and spine used to separate paired structures such as the ureters or highlight the left and right side of the spinal cord, respectively, the film must be correctly labelled. Therefore, for a right ventral–left dorsal oblique view of the abdomen, the right marker should be placed dorsal to the spine and the right ureter displayed dorsal to the left ureter.
- All limb radiographs should be labelled according to whether they are of the left or right leg.

■ There are specific requirements for labelling the BVA/Kennel Club Hip and Elbow Dysplasia Scheme radiographs (see www.bva.co.uk/chs to ensure these are fulfilled).

- Digital images may be submitted as DICOM files.
- Only one dog may be included per disc submitted.
- The Kennel Club registration number, microchip or tattoo number, and date of the radiographic examination must be included, using either radiopaque tape at the time of exposure or by annotating the image using the desktop software that operates the digital system.
- Images may be printed as laser printed images or as high quality photographs.
- Image size must not vary from the original by more than 10% for printed film.
- A known millimetre scale must be included on the image at the time of radiography.

Digital imaging processing algorithms

Appropriate image processing is required with both computed and digital radiography systems to produce diagnostic images. Without any image processing, the digital radiograph would lack contrast and be non-diagnostic. With both computed and digital radiography systems, the aim of image processing is to maximize contrast in the area of interest and discard information outside the collimated area. During image processing, the boundary of the collimated area is automatically detected. The pixel values for the area within the collimation are analysed (usually by histogram analysis) and then undergo data processing to optimize contrast and sharpness, which varies with anatomical area. The post-processed pixel values are then used for the image display. A variety of computer algorithms and techniques are used for post-processing and vary between manufacturers. The type of image processing has a huge impact on the appearance of digital images and it is important that appropriate algorithms are selected for each body area. Poorly set-up algorithms (e.g. too much edge enhancement) can lead to misdiagnosis (e.g. lysis around surgical implants or the false impression of a trabecular pattern where none exists on skeletal radiographs).

Radiographic artefacts and film faults

An artefact is a manmade object (i.e. something not found in nature). In radiographic terms, this means anything that appears on the radiograph that is not purely formed by the passage of X-rays through the body of the animal. Technically, any manmade object seen on the radiograph can be considered an artefact. These are usually quite easy to spot. Some can be avoided (e.g. taking care not to allow drip lines or electrocardiography leads to drape across or under the part of the animal being imaged); however, others are unavoidable (e.g. endotracheal tubes or microchips) and must simply be recognized.

Other radiographic artefacts are created by inappropriate technique, including:

■ Inadequate or incorrect choice of exposure factors
■ Inappropriate centring, collimation or use of a grid
■ Incorrect/faulty processing.

Digital radiography has unique radiographic artefacts, which may be related to hardware or software. Artefacts due to poor patient preparation and other patient factors, and poor positioning, collimation and centring have the same appearance and remedy for both conventional and digital radiography. Figure 2.16 summarizes some of the common technique-based artefacts and suggests how these can be corrected.

Exposure artefacts

Conventional systems
The overall combination of mAs and kV must be selected to result in appropriate blackening of the film.

Underexposure: A radiograph that is underexposed will be too light overall (see Figure 2.10a). An underexposed radiograph occurs due to either too few photons reaching the film (mAs too low), insufficient energy of the photons (kV too low) or a combination of both. In most cases, underexposure is due to insufficient penetration (kV too low), resulting in an inability to visualize anatomical detail, although the collimated area around the animal will be black since there is little attenuation by the air surrounding the patient. If there is adequate penetration (kV) but insufficient beam intensity (mAs

Fault	Cause	Correction
Exposure and development		
Area of interest too light on image; any area outside the animal but within the primary beam is dark	Underexposed	Increase kVp or mAs
Whole film too light (including any area outside the animal but within the primary beam)	Underdeveloped	Increase time in developer, replenish developer and check temperature is high enough
Film too dark, except under lead markers	Overexposed	Decrease kVp or mAs
Whole film too dark (including under lead markers)	Overdeveloped or fogged	Reduce time in developer, check developer temperature not too high, check for causes of fogging
Patchy opacity across film	Patchy development	Stir developer, if manual processing ensure film agitated in developer
Film turns brown with time	Inadequate washing or fixing procedure	Correct washing/fixing
Contrast		
'Flat' film without any contrast (usually with evidence of exposure beyond the limits of the collimation)	Too much scatter	Reduce kV, use grid, collimate, ensure film not fogged or underdeveloped
Film darkening unrelated to exposure to the primary beam (areas under lead markers may show image blackening). Results in reduced contrast and, if severe, film too dark	Fogging	Store film carefully to avoid light, chemical and radiation fogging, keep darkroom light tight, use film whilst in date, check safelight, check no light leakage in cassette. Light leakage within the cassette due to a faulty catch, or exposure of an edge of the film whilst within the box, results in blackening of one edge of the film
Whole film too light or too dark leading to a lack of contrast	Overdevelopment or underdevelopment	Correct inadequate development
Black and white film ('soot and whitewash' appearance) with inadequate X-ray penetration of the patient	Underexposed with kV too low	Increase kVp
Unsharpness		
Movement blur	Movement of patient, cassette or tube head	Keep equipment static, restrain patient, reduce respiratory blur, reduce exposure time
Poor image resolution with loss of definition of fine detail and slightly indistinct margins to all structures (no marked blurring in contrast to movement blur)	Large focal spot, fast film–screen combination, long object–film distance	Depends on cause: replace X-ray machine, use detail film–screen combinations, alter radiographic technique to reduce magnification and penumbra
Conventional imaging processing errors		
Splashes	Dark splashes	Developer splashes
	White splashes	Fixer splashes
	Grey splashes	Water splashes
Crescentic black lines	Crimp marks	Handle film gently, avoid bending or placing pressure on the film
Light lines with a palpable defect on the emulsion	Scratches	Clean rollers within the automatic processor, handle film gently
Parallel lines across film	Roller marks	Clean rollers as part of routine maintenance
Digital imaging processing errors		
Poor image contrast	Look-up table/incorrect algorithm	Select correct anatomical area prior to processing/ speak to supplier of system if consistently incorrect
Alternating bands of dark and light across entire image when viewed on computer monitor. The bands move and change direction and width as the image is zoomed	Moiré	Do not use grid, check grid ratio is appropriate for system, use moving grid
Lucent halo around an orthopaedic device	Uberschwinger	Check processing algorithm (reduce edge enhancement), correct level of unsharp masking, contact vendor
Linear white line across entire computed radiography image	Dirt on light guide of computed radiography digitizer	Clean light guide as per manufacturer instructions
Image has a grainy appearance (including any area outside the animal but within the primary beam)	Underexposure	Increase kVp and/or mAs
Thinner areas of animal are black with no detail visible	Overexposure or clipping	Reduce exposure factors, repeat process using a different algorithm

2.16 Common film faults and how to correct them. (continues) ▶

Fault	Cause	Correction
Linear bands on digital radiography image and image too dark	Planking on digital radiography image due to overexposure	Reduce exposure factors
Repeat or periodic lines on digital radiography image	Radiofrequency interference	Check no source of radiofrequency next to the detector and cables to the detector. If persists, contact vendor
Faults common to both conventional and digital imaging		
White specks or lines on image	Dirt or animal hair in cassette	Have regular cleaning regime of cassettes

2.16 (continued) Common film faults and how to correct them.

too low), peripheral blackening is generally adequate and some anatomical detail is present. Gross underexposure can be corrected by applying Santé's rule or increasing the kV by at least 15% (which doubles film blackening). For less severe underexposure, where some anatomical detail is present, doubling the mAs or increasing the kV by at least 5% can be used as a starting point to improve the image.

Overexposure: An overexposed radiograph will be too dark (see Figure 2.10b). However, the areas protected by the lead markers will remain white. If the film is too black, but bones are clearly visible and unexposed parts of film are white, then the mAs should be halved and processing should be checked for overdevelopment. If the film is too black and bones are indistinct, the kV should be reduced by 10–15% and the mAs halved. With both underexposure and overexposure, the film–focal distance should be checked to ensure that it has not been altered inadvertently, as this will influence the intensity of the beam and affect the exposure factors required.

Digital systems

Digital radiography copes much better with a wide range of exposures than conventional radiography. Underexposure and overexposure do occur with digital systems, but have quite a different appearance to similar problems that occur with conventional radiography (Figure 2.17).

- Underexposure results in a grainy or 'noisy' appearance, called quantum mottle. This is due to an insufficient signal (photons) reaching the detectors, so the system is unable to differentiate the inherent electronic noise from the low level signals created by the X-ray photons. This leads to non-uniformity of opacity, even in quite uniform organs. Any attempt to manipulate the image to improve the greyscale quality amplifies the quantum mottle and the graininess persists. Underexposed grainy radiographs have reduced radiographic contrast.
- Digital radiography tolerates overexposure relatively well. Overexposed images have low quantum mottle and remain of diagnostic quality due to the ability of the digital systems to rescale the high signals within the visible greyscale range. With extreme overexposure there will still be some detail visible, but the areas with the lowest radiographic density may be displayed as completely black without any discernible anatomy. This is because during pre-processing the look-up table assigns certain pixel values to monitor brightness. Pixel values beyond the range chosen

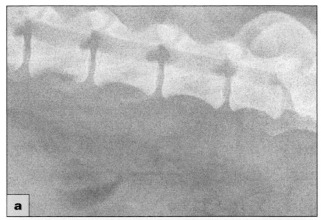

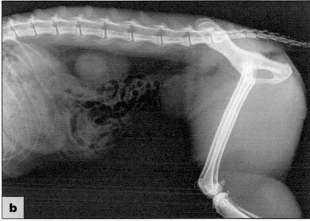

2.17 Effect of exposure on digital images. **(a)** Underexposure and **(b)** overexposure. The wide dynamic range of digital radiography allows the structures within the abdomen to still be visible on both images. (a) This image has a grainy or 'salt and pepper' appearance due to quantum mottle. Insufficient information (number of X-ray photons) has reached the detection system. (b) In this image the thinner parts of the patient are displayed as completely black. All pixels in these areas have been assigned the maximum value. Altering image brightness or contrast will not generate any useful information about these regions.

for display are all shown as black. This results in 'clipping' of the image with poorly attenuating areas (e.g. thin soft tissues at the margin of bone, the lungs or the ventral abdominal wall) all displayed as black. No amount of post-processing will recover these areas.

> Underexposure and overexposure may be indicated by the exposure index being outside the recommended range. Increasing or decreasing the kV by 10–15% is a good starting point to correct underexposure and overexposure, respectively.

Unsharpness

The most common cause of image unsharpness is motion blur, the appearance of which is the same for conventional and digital radiography. This is most commonly due to patient motion (Figure 2.18); however, it can also be due to tube head motion if the tube head is not properly fixed. Motion blur can be minimized by taking radiographs during the respiratory pause (or by taking manually inflated radiographs under general anaesthesia). Other causes of unsharpness are related to equipment and physical factors.

- Focal spot size – a larger focal spot generates a greater penumbra (see above) and leads to greater image unsharpness.
- Object–film distance – a greater object–film distance also results in a greater penumbra, so a sharper image is obtained by having the area of interest as close to the film as possible.
- Film speed – a 'faster' film speed (using the par system: the higher the par, the faster the film) means each crystal in the film is larger. This allows the image to be generated from a lower number of X-ray photons reaching the film; however, the resultant image is inherently less sharp. A 'rapid' film is faster than a 'detail' film. The concept of film speed does not apply to digital radiography where resolution is not determined by film crystal structure but by pixel size.
- Screen speed – in the same way, the large crystals in the faster screens emit light over a larger area than the smaller crystals in a slower screen. Larger crystals produce an image that is less sharp than that produced by smaller crystals.

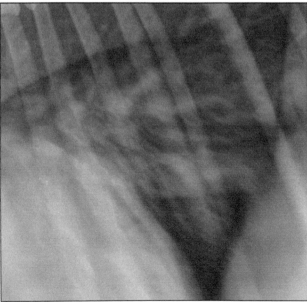

2.18 Lateral radiograph of the thorax in a dog. The motion blur (most evident in the mid-section of the ribs, the larger caudal lobar vessels and the diaphragm) is due to rapid panting.

Artefacts affecting conventional film processing

Manual processing tends to generate more film faults than automatic processing. Despite this, even with automatic processors, poor maintenance or machine error leads to film faults.

Development

Underdevelopment and overdevelopment are common faults, which occur when the film is retained for the incorrect period of time, or at the incorrect temperature, in the developer solution. Exhausted developer also results in underdeveloped films.

- Underdevelopment leads to a film with an image and background that are too light. When illuminated by the X-ray viewer, fingers placed between the film and the X-ray viewer can be seen through the exposed area outside the patient (Figure 2.19). In comparison, on underexposed films the area outside the animal is usually adequately blackened.
- Overdevelopment leads to a film that is too dark, even in areas that should have been protected from radiation (e.g. under a lead shield/marker). A radiograph may become overdeveloped if it becomes stuck in the developer whilst passing through the automatic processor (Figure 2.20).
- Fixing and washing errors can both lead to the radiograph developing a brown or yellow appearance over time (Figure 2.21).
- An incompletely fixed film may have a grey background. This background is not transparent.
- Splashing of developer (Figure 2.22) and fixer/water on to unprocessed film is more common with manual processing and leads to dark or pale splash marks on the film, respectively.

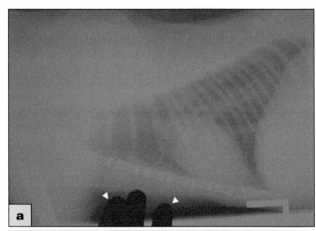

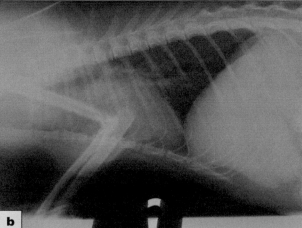

2.19 **(a)** The underdeveloped film is too light across both the image and the background. When held to a light box, fingers can be seen through the background (arrowheads), which is not the case in **(b)** an adequately developed radiograph.

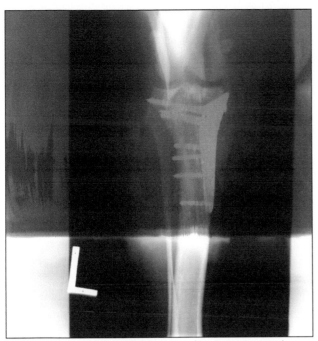

2.20 Overdeveloped film. The film became stuck during automatic processing and the top part of the radiograph is overdeveloped. It is too dark, even in the parts which have not been exposed (e.g. underneath the orthopaedic implant).

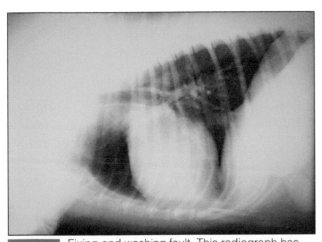

2.21 Fixing and washing fault. This radiograph has become yellow/brown due to inadequate fixing or washing of the film at the time of processing. The fault can be corrected by reprocessing the film.

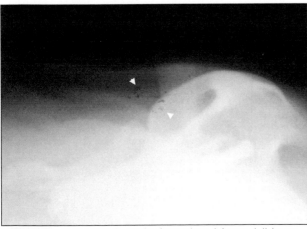

2.22 Dark splash marks (arrowheads) are visible on this radiograph. This is due to developer splashing on to the radiograph prior to processing.

Damage to the film

- Careless handling or kinking of the film before processing leads to fingernail-shaped dark crimp marks where the film is bent and the emulsion damaged, allowing the developer solution to penetrate more easily (Figure 2.23).
- Dirt on the rollers in the automatic processor results in parallel marks on the film (Figure 2.24).
- Incorrectly aligned rollers or rough handling of the film leads to scratch marks (Figure 2.25).
- Dirt, particularly animal hairs, in the cassette leads to white specks or lines on the film (Figure 2.26).

Fogging

Film fogging is recognized as a general grey–black haze (increase in film density) across the radiograph, which degrades the image quality and reduces contrast.

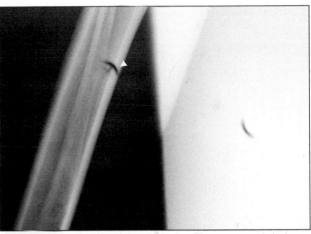

2.23 Crimp or pressure marks. These curved dark lines (arrowhead) are caused by bending or kinking of the film due to careless handling prior to processing. This results in areas of the film being overdeveloped because the film emulsion is damaged, allowing developer to penetrate into the emulsion.

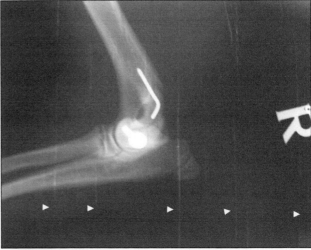

2.24 Roller marks. The regularly spaced parallel lines (arrowheads) across the radiograph are due to dirt on the rollers. The areas of film under the dirt are undeveloped.

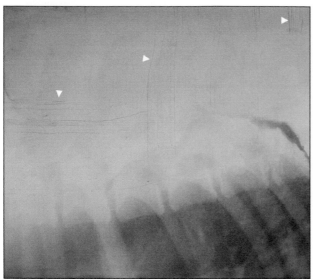

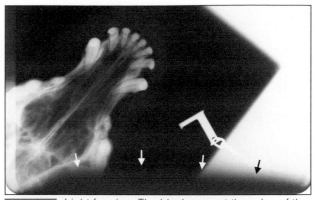

2.27 Light fogging. The black zone at the edge of the radiograph (arrowed) is due to light fogging. The protective plastic envelope that encloses the flexible cassette was damaged along the seam and white light has caused fogging of the film. Important diagnostic information has been lost. A similar appearance occurs along the top edge of film within an incompletely sealed storage packet. Any visible white light (e.g. from mobile phones being used in the darkroom or damaged indicator lights on the automatic processor) can lead to fogging of the film.

2.25 The surface emulsion of the film has been scratched (arrowheads) during handling or processing. This leads to sensitized areas of the film and overdevelopment.

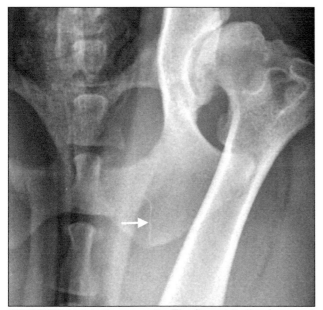

2.26 Hair in the cassette. The fine white line (arrowed) is caused by a hair within the cassette located between the film and the intensifying screen. Any debris between the screen and the film results in a white mark on the image as it attenuates light produced by the intensifying screen. The artefact is sharply marginated due to the proximity of the dirt to the film surface. Note: hair attenuates light and not the X-ray beam directly.

- Film fog results from exposure to radiation, white light (Figure 2.27) or chemicals.
- Unexposed film should be stored away from radiation sources, preferably in a separate darkroom or storage room. Cassettes loaded with conventional film and unexposed computed radiography plates should be kept at a distance from the X-ray tube until required to avoid scattered radiation creating film fogging.
- Film fog produced as a result of scatter from the patient can be minimized by collimating to the region of interest and using a grid where appropriate.

- Exposure to white light before processing is avoided by careful storage of films in a lead-lined, light-safe hopper and by following correct darkroom procedure. White light from mobile phones, digital watches and incompletely light-proofed darkrooms can lead to film fog. Film should be used before the expiry date to avoid 'storage fog'.

Artefacts affecting digital image acquisition

Due to the differences in image creation, the artefacts associated with image detection and formation are different for computed and digital radiography systems.

Computed radiography

Dirt on the phosphor or within the reader: This is a common artefact with computed radiography systems and results in white marks on the image (Figure 2.28), which are visible on multiple exposures. The dirt prevents light emitted from the phosphor from reaching the photodetector in the computed radiography reader.

- Dirt on the phosphor results in small focal white marks. Most dirt on the phosphor within the cassette can be identified by inspecting the surface.
- Dirt on the rollers or light guide results in linear white marks. Dirt within the computed radiography reader requires initiation of the cleaning process, as recommended by the manufacturer. If this is not sufficient, the dirt will need to be removed by an engineer.

Delayed scanning of cassettes: A long delay (>24 hours) between acquisition and processing results in fading of the image. Fading of the image may also occur due to exposure of the phosphor to light in computed radiography systems where the phosphor is manually removed from the cassette for processing.

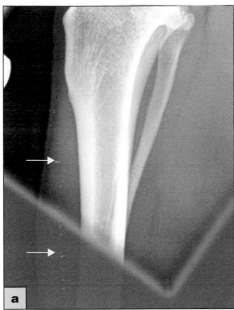

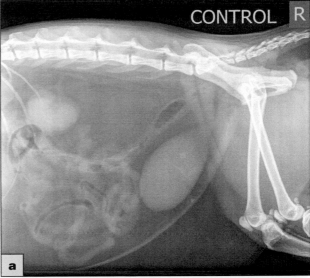

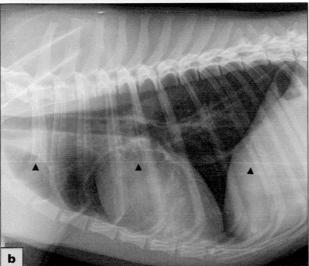

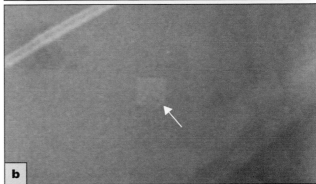

2.28 Dirt on **(a)** the imaging phosphor and **(b)** the light guide. (a) The white spots (arrowed) across the image are due to dirt on the imaging phosphor, which prevents light from reaching the detector during processing. (b) The white line (arrowheads) across the radiograph is caused by dirt on the light guide of the computed radiography digitizer.

Reader artefacts, digitization errors and data transfer errors: These result in artefacts with abrupt geometric shapes or lines (Figure 2.29). These artefacts may be intermittent, but if they persist an engineer is required to evaluate the electronics and calibrate the system.

Look-up table errors

- Common artefacts seen on digital images are associated with look-up table errors. During the image processing phase, the look-up table is necessary to allow the raw data on the imaging phosphor to be converted into an image that can be viewed. The look-up table contains data detailing how bright the pixel should be on the monitor, for that amount of phosphor excitation. Many systems have packaged the appropriate look-up table with other automatic image

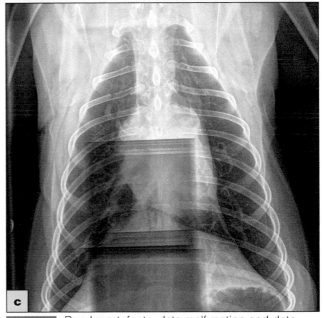

2.29 Reader artefacts, data malfunction and data transfer artefacts may appear as geometric shapes or lines, which can mimic pathology. **(a)** Reader artefact mimicking a bladder calculus. **(b)** Magnified view of (a); the artefact is denoted by the arrow. **(c)** Data transfer artefact. The central areas of the image have been incompletely digitized or corrupted during data transfer.

processing tools (such as edge enhancement), so that the technique for 'thorax' can be selected and should be optimized for thoracic radiographs. Care must be taken to select the appropriate body part to be used as the processing algorithm.

■ Inadequate or no collimation of the region of interest can result in an artefact where parts of the image are not displayed or are 'blacked' out (Figure 2.30). This occurs because the software attempts to apply automatic collimation to the straight lines identified on the image and, occasionally, inadvertently collimates to straight lines in the patient (e.g. the spine). Reapplying the collimation during processing allows the software to 'find' the margins and the correct image to be displayed.

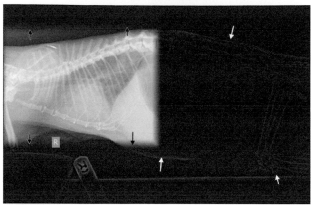

2.30 Inadequate or no collimation. If no collimation is applied, the software defines the margins of the 'patient' (black arrows) based on pixel intensity and excludes or rejects useful information (white arrows). Manually reapplying the collimation allows the useful information in the image to be retrieved.

Uberschwinger and Moiré artefacts

■ Uberschwinger (rebound) artefacts result from an image processing error (usually an overly edge enhancing algorithm), which allows portions of the radiograph with large differences in radiopacity between adjacent pixels to be excessively enhanced. This is most commonly seen with orthopaedic implants, where the edge enhancement causes a lucent halo around the implant (Figure 2.31). This halo may be mistaken for loosening of the implant or low grade infection.

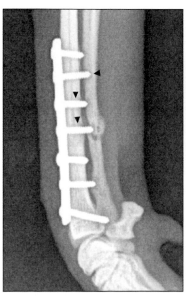

2.31

Uberschwinger artefact. The radiolucent halo around the screws in the radius (arrowheads) is an artefact created by incorrect processing of the data due to large density differences between the metal and surrounding bone. The inappropriate filtering can be avoided by selecting algorithms that do not produce edge enhancement. Note: there is marked quantum mottle from underexposure.

■ Moiré artefacts (alternating dark and light bands across the image) are seen on the computer monitor if a static grid has been used for computed or digital radiography, or if the grid is aligned with the readout of the computed radiography cassette (Figure 2.32). Moiré artefacts occur due to interference by the grid lines and the monitor display, and are more common with low resolution monitors and coarse grids. This can be corrected by using a Potter-Bucky moving grid or choosing a grid with >180 lines per inch (manufacturers can advise the correct grid ratio for each system).

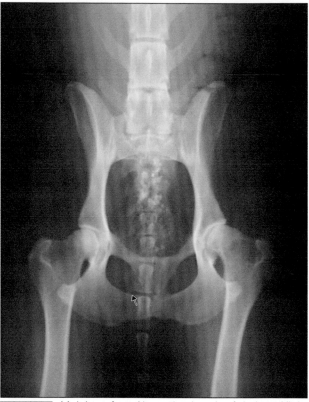

2.32 Moiré artefact. Alternating bands of dark and light are present across the radiograph where a static low frequency grid was used. During processing, alignment of the computed radiography laser with the grid lines results in this interference pattern. Moiré artefacts are more obvious when images are viewed on a low resolution monitor and can be avoided by using a high frequency or moving grid and viewing images on a high resolution clinical grade monitor.

Legislation and safety procedures

In 1985, the law governing the use of radiation and radioactive materials was revised and updated with the publication of T he Ionizing Radiations Regulations (IRR) 1985, which has subsequently been updated as The Ionizing Radiations Regulations (revised) 1999. This legal document covers all uses of radiation and radioactive materials, including veterinary radiography. As it is written in legal terms and is somewhat lengthy, a second booklet was published at the same time which attempted to explain the Regulations and is called the Approved Code of Practice for the Protection of Persons against Ionizing Radiation arising from any Work Activity. The Code of Practice does contain some specific references to veterinary radiography, but is also rather long and complex, and so guidance notes explaining the law as it applies to veterinary radiography were published by the British Veterinary Association in 2002 (Veterinary Guidance Notes for the Ionizing Radiations Regulations 1999). These cover premises, equipment, personnel and procedures, and aim to minimize the radiation dose received by veterinary staff.

Principles of radiation protection

Protection follows three basic principles:

1. Radiography should only be undertaken if there is definite clinical justification for use of the procedure.
2. Any exposure of personnel should be kept to a minimum. The three words to remember are time, distance and shielding (i.e. reduce the need for repeat exposures and therefore the time exposed to radiation, keep as far away as possible during the exposure, and wear protective clothing or stand behind a lead screen).
3. No dose limit should be exceeded.

Radiation Protection Supervisor

A Radiation Protection Supervisor (RPS) must be appointed within the practice and is usually the principal or another senior member of the veterinary or nursing staff. The RPS is responsible for ensuring that radiography is carried out safely and in accordance with the Regulations, as well as the Local Rules, but the person need not be present at every radiographic examination.

Radiation Protection Adviser

Most practices also need to appoint an external Radiation Protection Adviser (RPA). RPAs must hold a certificate of competence issued by an appropriate body stating that they have the knowledge, experience and competence required to act as a veterinary RPA. They are usually medical physicists, although holders of the RCVS Diploma in Veterinary Radiology who have undertaken appropriate further training may also be eligible. The RPA provides information on all aspects of radiation protection, the demarcation of the controlled area, and advises on drawing up the Local Rules and instructions for safe working.

Local Rules and written arrangements

The Local Rules are a set of instructions drawn up by the practice's RPA which detail the equipment, procedures and restriction of access to the controlled area for that practice. The written arrangements form part of the Local Rules and include the sequence of actions to be followed for each exposure, including the method of restraint of animals for radiography and the precautions to be taken should manual restraint be necessary. A copy of the Local Rules should be given to anyone involved in radiography and should also be displayed in the X-ray room.

Controlled area

A specific room should be identified for small animal radiography and should have sufficiently thick walls that no part of the controlled area extends outside it (single brick is usually adequate; thin walls may be reinforced with lead ply or barium plaster). The room should ideally be large enough to allow people remaining in the room to stand at least 2 m from the primary beam. If this is not possible, a protective lead screen should be provided, unless the radiographer can routinely step outside the room and stand behind a brick wall during the exposure. Unshielded doors and windows may be acceptable if the workload is low and the room is large enough. Special recommendations are made for flooring in cases where there may be an occupied area below the radiography room. If horizontal beam radiography is going to be performed then the RPA needs to be consulted to ensure that the walls of the controlled area are sufficient to stop the primary beam.

Technically, the controlled area is the area around the primary beam within which the average dose rate of exposure exceeds a given limit of 7.5 μSv per hour. The controlled area for a typical practice is within a 2 m radius from the beam, but usually needs to be defined by the RPA. Since the controlled area must be physically demarcated and clearly labelled, it is usually simpler to designate the whole X-ray room as a controlled area and to place warning notices on the doors to exclude people not involved in radiography. When the radiographic examination is complete, the X-ray machine must be disconnected from the power supply; the room then ceases to be a controlled area and may be entered freely.

A warning sign should be placed at the entrance to the X-ray room, consisting of the radiation warning symbol and a simple legend. For permanently in-stalled equipment there should also be an automatic signal at the room entrance indicating when the X-ray machine is in a state of readiness to produce X-rays. This signal usually takes the form of a red light or an illuminated sign. Whilst not a legal requirement for portable and mobile X-ray machines (which comprise the majority of practice X-ray machines), many practices install red lights outside the radiography room to warn when a radiographic examination is in progress and prevent accidental entry, and this is to be recommended.

In addition, all X-ray machines should have lights visible from the control panel indicating (a) when they are switched on at the mains and (b) when exposure is taking place. Sometimes instead of a light, a noise such as a beep or buzz is used to indicate when exposure is occurring. Illuminated signs outside the X-ray room may also have two different legends; for example, one showing in yellow light when the X-ray machine is switched on and the other in red light when an exposure is taking place (Figure 2.33).

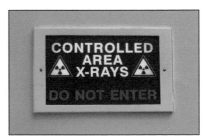

2.33 Illuminated warning sign outside an X-ray room containing a fixed X-ray machine. The yellow lettering is illuminated whenever the machine is switched on and the red lettering is illuminated during the preparation and exposure stages.

X-ray equipment

Suppliers of X-ray machines have a responsibility to ensure that they are safe and functioning correctly, and they should provide a report to this effect when installing the equipment. Leakage of radiation from the tube housing must not exceed a certain level and the beam filtration must be equivalent to not less than 2.5 mm aluminium. All machines must be fitted with a collimation device, which is typically a light beam diaphragm. The position of the exposure button must allow the radiographer to stand at least 2 m from the primary beam or behind a protective lead screen (Figure 2.34). Servicing of X-ray machines is a legal requirement and should be carried out at least once a year by a qualified engineer. The radiation safety features of the X-ray machine should be checked during the service.

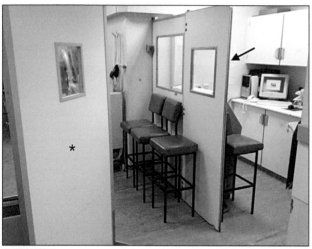

2.34 X-ray room with a mobile lead screen (*) and a permanent lead screen (arrowed) behind which the operating console of the X-ray machine is mounted. The radiographer remains in the room behind the permanent screen when the exposure is taken and can observe the animal through the lead glass window. The exposure button is mounted on the operating console. The mobile lead screen is used to shield any person required to stay within the room close to the patient (e.g. for the purpose of manual inflation of the lungs for thoracic radiography).

The X-ray table must be lead-lined, or else a sheet of lead 1 mm thick and larger than the maximum size of the beam should be placed on, or below, the table to absorb the residual primary beam and reduce scatter. Many practices now use purpose-built X-ray tables that are not only lead-lined but also fitted with hooks to aid in patient positioning; some also contain a built-in grid and cassette holder.

Film and film processing

The Regulations recommend the use of fast film–screen combinations in order to reduce exposure time. They also stress the importance of correct processing techniques in order to minimize the number of non-diagnostic films and avoid the need for repeat exposures. Digital radiography has important safety benefits as the number of repeat exposures required is reduced, since exposure factors chosen are less critical, and both bone and soft tissue can be seen adequately on the same exposure of a given area.

Recording exposures

It is necessary to record each radiographic exposure taken. This is achieved using a daybook for radiography and should include the following details for each exposure:

- Date
- Animal identification
- Exposure factors used
- Quality of image
- Means of restraint.

If the animal has had to be held during radiography, the name(s) of the person(s) doing so must be recorded. If horizontal beam radiography is performed this must also be recorded.

Protective clothing

Protective clothing consists of aprons, gloves, sleeves and neck (thyroid) protectors and comprises rubber impregnated with lead. The thickness and efficiency of the garment is described in millimetres of lead equivalent (LE) (i.e. the thickness of pure lead that would afford the same protection). It is important to remember that protective clothing is only effective against scatter and does not protect against the primary beam.

Lead aprons should be worn by any person who needs to be present in the X-ray room during the exposure, unless they are behind a protective lead screen. They cover the trunk (especially the gonads) and should reach at least to mid-thigh level. They should be at least 0.25 mm LE thick; some are 0.35 mm LE or even 0.5 mm LE, although the latter are rather heavy to wear. Single-sided aprons covering the front of the body with only straps at the back are cheaper, but provide less protection than double-sided aprons that cover both the front and back, and are also less comfortable to wear for long periods of time. Aprons are expensive items and should be handled carefully. When not in use they should be stored on coat hangers or on rails (Figure 2.35); they must never be folded as this can lead to undetected cracking of the material.

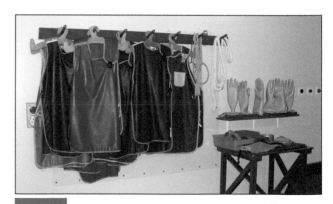

2.35 Correct storage of lead aprons and gloves.

Lead gloves, open-palm mitts and hand shields must be available for use in those cases where manual restraint is unavoidable. Lead sleeves are tubes of lead rubber into which the hands and forearms may be inserted as an alternative to gloves. Single sheets of lead rubber draped over the hands are not adequate as they do not protect against back scatter. Gloves, hand shields and sleeves should be at least

0.35 mm LE and must never appear in the primary beam, as they offer inadequate protection against the high energy primary X-rays. It is important to remember that, although a lead glove may appear completely opaque on a radiograph, the film is protected by two layers of lead rubber but the hand by only one (Figure 2.36). Lead rubber neck guards for protection of the thyroid gland may also be used and are held in place using Velcro.

All items of protective clothing should be checked frequently for signs of cracking. A small defect may not allow many X-ray photons through, but will always be over a similar area of the body. If in doubt, the garment may be imaged or examined with fluoroscopy to check for cracks (Figure 2.37).

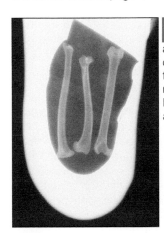

2.36 Radiograph of bones covered by a single layer of lead rubber: compare with the edge where there are two layers of lead rubber and all the primary beam appears to have been absorbed.

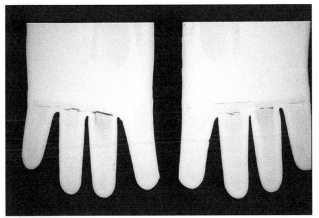

2.37 Radiograph of gloves showing cracking of the lead rubber at the base of the fingers (typical site). These gloves should be discarded.

Dosimetry

All personnel involved in radiography should wear small monitoring devices or dosemeters to record any radiation to which they are exposed. Dosemeters can be obtained from dosimetry services such as the National Radiological Protection Board (NRPB) or the local hospital and should be sent off for reading every 1–3 months, depending on the radiographic caseload. The main dosemeter should be worn on the trunk beneath the lead apron, but an extra dosemeter may be worn on the collar or sleeve to monitor the level of radiation received by unprotected parts of the body. Extremity ring or finger stall dosemeters are available for wearing on the hands beneath lead gloves and are used for large animal radiography, for work with radioactive materials (e.g. during scintigraphy) and for handling cats undergoing radioiodine treatment. Each dosemeter should be worn only by the person to whom it is issued and must not be left in the X-ray room whilst not being worn or exposed to heat or sunlight. Dosemeters should only be worn on the veterinary premises (or when performing off-site large animal radiography), as it is important that they reflect accurately any radiation dose received at work and not false readings due to other factors. There are two types of dosemeter available:

- Film badges which contain small pieces of X-ray film and are usually blue. They comprise small metal filters that allow assessment of the type of radiation to which the badge has been exposed
- Thermoluminescent dosemeters which contain radiation-sensitive lithium fluoride crystals. On exposure to radiation the electrons in the crystals are rearranged, thus storing energy. During the reading process the crystals are heated and give off light in proportion to the amount of energy that they have stored. This provides a quantitative reading.

Dosemeters may also be used to monitor radiation levels in the X-ray room or in adjacent rooms by mounting them on the wall. They can also be used to check the adequacy of protection offered by internal walls and doors. The exact arrangements for dosimetry in the practice should be made in consultation with the RPA, and the records must be filed for easy retrieval or available for new employers if a staff member leaves. Anyone whose badge reveals a reading should be informed, so that the cause can be identified if possible and working practices adjusted accordingly. Dose records must be retained as they may be required by future employers if staff members leave.

Dose limits

Dose limits are amounts of radiation that are thought not to constitute a greater risk to health than those encountered in everyday life. Legal limits have been laid down for various categories of person and for different parts of the body. Maximum permitted doses (MPDs) are laid down for the whole body, for individual organs, for the lens of the eye and for pregnancy. 'Classified' persons are those working with radiation who are likely to receive >30% of any relevant MPD. However, in veterinary practice these levels should not be reached and so veterinary workers rarely need to be designated as classified persons, provided that they are working under formal written arrangements drawn up by the practice's RPA.

Personnel

The Local Rules must include a list of designated persons authorized to carry out radiographic exposures. It should be remembered that nurses and other lay staff aged 16 or 17 have a lower MPD than do adults aged 18 or over and therefore their involvement in radiography should be limited. Young people under 16 years of age should not be present during radiography under any circumstances. Owners should not routinely be present as they are members of the general public and are neither trained in radiography nor wearing dosemeters, although their presence may be necessary in emergency situations or during equine radiography. The Local Rules should ensure that doses to pregnant women are well within the legal limit, but nevertheless it is wise to avoid the involvement of pregnant women in radiography whenever possible.

The general rule is that the minimum number of people should be present during radiography. When the animal is artificially restrained (as is usual), only the person taking the exposure need be present, and this should be the case in the majority of radiographic studies. Usually the radiographer is able to stand behind a protective screen or outside the room during the exposure.

Radiographic procedures and restraint

Whenever possible, the beam should be directed vertically downwards on to an X-ray table. The minimum number of people should remain in the room and should either stand behind lead screens or wear protective clothing. All those present must obey the instructions given by the person operating the X-ray machine. The beam must be collimated to the smallest size practicable and must be entirely within the borders of the film. Grids should only be used when the body part being imaged is >10 cm thick, as their use necessitates an increase in the exposure.

The method of restraint is of paramount importance. The Approved Code of Practice states that 'only in exceptional circumstances should a patient or animal undergoing a diagnostic examination be supported or manipulated by hand'. These exceptional circumstances may include severely ill or injured animals for whom a diagnosis requires radiography but for whom sedation, anaesthesia or restraint with sandbags is dangerous (e.g. very young puppies and kittens, or animals with congestive heart failure, ruptured diaphragm or other severe traumatic injuries). In these cases, the animal may be held, provided that those restraining it are fully protected and that no part of their hands (even in gloves) enters the primary beam. A light beam diaphragm is essential for manual restraint. The majority of patients may be positioned and restrained artificially using positioning aids under varying degrees of sedation or general anaesthesia, and sometimes with no chemical restraint at all.

Establishing a practice radiographic facility

Setting up a radiography facility in a new or refurbished practice presents an ideal opportunity to ensure that all safety features are incorporated, whilst at the same time ensuring the ease and efficiency of workflow is optimized. The practice's RPA should be consulted for advice at an early stage of planning. A number of factors must be considered, including the room to be used and its demarcation, the equipment to be purchased and the records which need to be kept.

Radiography room

Ideally, the room should be used only for radiography, so that it may be performed without impacting on other work activities. Its position relative to other parts of the practice (such as the operating theatre or ward)

should be considered, as patients often need to be moved between areas whilst anaesthetized. The room must be large enough to allow free movement around the X-ray table and for manoeuvring other items of equipment such as anaesthetic machines and trolleys. It should be possible to place the animal in both left and right lateral recumbency for radiography and to have the head at either end of the table.

The thickness and construction of the walls, doors and windows must be adequate to prevent detection of significant amounts of radiation outside the room, and in this respect the advice of the practice's RPA must be sought. Stud walls are inadequate and brick or breeze block is necessary; increasing the radiation protection of walls with lead ply or barium plaster is possible but extremely expensive. Special consideration must be given to the protection of adjacent rooms and, in the unusual instance of the radiography room not being on the ground floor, of rooms beneath. The occasional necessity for use of a horizontal X-ray beam should also be considered.

It is a legal requirement that the radiographer stands at least 2 m from the primary beam or behind a protective lead screen. Indeed, even when the room is large enough to permit the 2 m distance, a portable or fixed lead screen is highly recommended. One option is to stand outside the room during the exposure, especially if the patient can still be observed through a window in the door. However, this is not recommended for animals that are artificially restrained but not anaesthetized.

As an animal undergoing a diagnostic examination may only be manually restrained in exceptional circumstances, and no part of any person involved in the radiographic procedure is to be included within the primary beam, the importance of scattered radiation must be considered. Scattered radiation created within the animal or the structures surrounding the animal is an important source of potential absorbed dose for personnel involved with radiography (Figure 2.38). Scattered radiation is primarily 'soft' or of low intensity

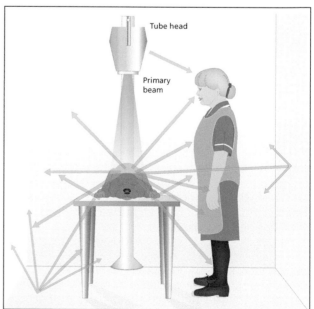

Tube head

Primary beam

2.38 Sources of radiation hazard, including both leakage of primary radiation from a damaged tube head and scattered radiation from the patient, table top and floor.

and is predominately absorbed by those parts of the body not protected by shielding. Exposure to scattered radiation can be minimized by distancing and shielding personnel from the patient during exposure, avoiding manual restraint and using efficient film–screen or screen–detector combinations.

Warning signs and lights

The requirements for warning signs ± lights are detailed above. There is a legal requirement for the controlled area (usually the whole X-ray room) to be identified as such whenever the X-ray machine is switched on. The RPA should be consulted during the planning stage for a new facility, but this is an ideal opportunity to install a foolproof system with an illuminated warning sign wired to the X-ray machine (see Figure 2.33).

Equipment

X-ray machine

The types of X-ray machine available are described in Chapter 1. The highest output machine consistent with other constraints (including cost) should be purchased, as better and therefore more diagnostic radiographs will be produced. Buying a low powered machine on the basis of cost alone is a false economy. Other factors to consider include:

- The nature of the radiography to be performed
- Whether the machine must be portable
- The efficiency of any post-purchase backup from the supplying company.

It is wise to view and compare X-ray machines at large veterinary conferences and, if possible, obtain advice from colleagues in other practices.

Analogue versus digital: If the practice opts for a film–screen system, other equipment is required including cassettes, viewers and processing facilities. A darkroom will also probably be needed. However, the last few years have seen a large move towards digital radiography and it is likely that most veterinary practices installing new radiography facilities will opt for this technology. Tailor-made veterinary practice packages are offered by many vendors, with a wide range of purchase costs. Digital systems have many advantages over conventional radiography, but it is a common fallacy that digital images are always better than conventional images. Poor quality digital systems may produce images significantly worse than a good conventional radiograph.

When considering a new digital system, it is important to trial the system prior to purchase and to look critically at images obtained from a range of patient sizes and body regions. Again, viewing the systems at conferences and talking to colleagues is recommended. The vendor should be asked to supply contact details for practices that have already installed their equipment, and the purchaser is well advised to take up such references about its value and user-friendliness. Pre-purchase consideration should be given not only to the digital acquisition system, but also the viewing monitor, Picture Archiving and Communication System (PACS) and after-sales support. All digital systems should be DICOM compliant

and the vendor should be able to produce a DICOM compliancy statement for the equipment. If images are going to be sent electronically for review, then the ease of exporting or saving the DICOM files should be checked. If the radiographic facility is being upgraded to digital from analogue, the redundant darkroom may make an ideal digital viewing and reporting office.

X-ray table

The X-ray table must be large and strong enough to support giant-breed dogs, and not too high as some animals will need to be lifted up from the floor. Purpose-made X-ray tables should be appropriately lead-lined and some have an in-built cassette holder (a Bucky), which can be linked to a moving grid built into the table. Strategically placed hooks for positioning ties are helpful.

Record keeping

Meticulous records must be kept of various aspects of radiography, since it is a potentially hazardous procedure and the Health and Safety Executive have the power to make unannounced inspections. The RPA will confirm the nature of the records that must be kept, including details of X-ray machine servicing, exposures made and dosimetry.

Summary

Good radiographic technique is vital to maximize the diagnostic utility of radiographs. An understanding of the basic principles of radiography, patience and attention to detail are required to take good images. Prior to radiological interpretation, the radiograph should be assessed for quality and if there are technical problems with the image then these should be addressed and the radiographs repeated if necessary. When considering whether a radiograph is of adequate quality to allow a diagnosis to be made, the mnemonic *P*ink *C*amels *C*ollect *E*xtra *L*arge *A*pples can be used as a checklist of all the factors that need to be assessed:

- P = patient preparation and positioning
- C = centring
- C = collimation
- E = exposure
- L = labelling
- A = artefacts.

References and further reading

Armbrust LJ (2009) Comparing types of digital capture. *Veterinary Clinics of North America: Small Animal Practice* **39(4)**, 677–688

Armbrust LJ (2009) PACS and image storage. *Veterinary Clinics of North America: Small Animal Practice* **39(4)**, 711–718

Ballance D (2008) The network and its role in digital imaging and communications in medicine imaging. *Veterinary Radiology & Ultrasound* **49(Suppl. 1)**, S29–S32

Balter S (1993) Fundamental properties of digital images. *Radiographics* **13(1)**, 129–141

Bushberg JT, Seibert JA, Leidholdt EM and Boone JM (2002) *The Essential Physics of Medical Imaging, 2nd edn.* Lippincott, Williams and Wilkins, Philadelphia

Cesar LJ, Schueler BA, Zink FE *et al.* (2001) Artefacts found in computed radiography. *The British Journal of Radiology* **74**, 195–202

Curry TS, Dowdey JE and Murry RC (1990) *Christensen's Physics of Diagnostic Radiology.* Lea and Febiger, London

Daniel GB (2009) Digital imaging. *Veterinary Clinics of North America: Small Animal Practice* **39(4)**, 667–676

Dendy PP and Heaton B (1999) *Physics for Diagnostic Radiology, 3rd edn.* Taylor and Francis Group, New York

Dennis R, Kirberger R, Barr F and Wrigley R (2010) *The Handbook of Small Animal Radiology and Ultrasound*. Elsevier, Oxford

Drost WT, Reese DJ and Hornof WJ (2008) Digital radiography artifacts. *Veterinary Radiology & Ultrasound* **49(Suppl. 1)**, S48–S56

Hammerstrom K, Aldrich J, Alves L and Ho A (2006) Recognition and prevention of computed radiography image artifacts. *Journal of Digital Imaging* **19(3)**, 226–239

Jiménez DA and Armbrust LJ (2009) Digital radiographic artifacts. *Veterinary Clinics of North America: Small Animal Practice* **39(4)**, 689–709

Jiménez DA, Armbrust LJ, O'Brien RT and Biller DS (2008) Artifacts in digital radiography. *Veterinary Radiology & Ultrasound* **49(4)**, 321–332

Körner M, Weber CH, Wirth S *et al.* (2007) Advances in digital radiography: physical principles and system overview. *Radiographics* **27(3)**, 675–686

Krupinski EA, Williams MB, Andriole K *et al.* (2007) Digital radiography image quality: image processing and display. *Journal of the American College of Radiology* **4(6)**, 389–400

Lo WY and Puchalski SM (2008) Digital image processing. *Veterinary Radiology & Ultrasound* **49(Suppl. 1)**, S42–S47

Puchalski SM (2008) Image display. *Veterinary Radiology & Ultrasound* **49(Suppl. 1)**, S9–S13

Robertson ID and Saveraid T (2008) Hospital, radiology, and picture archiving and communication systems. *Veterinary Radiology & Ultrasound* **49(Suppl. 1)**, S19–S28

Robertson ID and Thrall D (2012) Digital radiographic imaging. In: *A Textbook of Veterinary Diagnostic Radiology, 6th edn*, ed. D. Thrall, pp. 22–37. Saunders Elsevier, St. Louis

Schaefer-Prokop CM, De Boo DW, Uffmann M and Prokop M (2009) DR and CR: recent advances in technology. *European Journal of Radiology* **72(2)**, 194–201

Schueler BA (1998) Clinical applications of basic X-ray physics principles. *Radiographics* **18**, 731–744

Seymour C and Duke-Novakovski T (2007) *BSAVA Manual of Canine and Feline Anaesthesia and Analgesia, 2nd edn*. BSAVA Publications, Gloucester

Shetty CM, Barthur A, Kambadakone A, Narayanan N and Kv R (2011) Computed radiography image artifacts revisited. *American Journal of Roentgenology* **196(1)**, W37–W47

Thrall D (2012) Introduction to radiographic interpretation. In: *A Textbook of Veterinary Diagnostic Radiology, 6th edn*, ed. D Thrall, pp. 74–86. Saunders Elsevier, St. Louis

Thrall D and Widmer WR (2012) Radiation protection and physics of diagnostic radiology. In: *A Textbook of Veterinary Diagnostic Radiology, 6th edn.*, ed. D Thrall, pp. 2–21. Saunders Elsevier, St. Louis

Wallack S (2008) Digital image storage. *Veterinary Radiology & Ultrasound* **49(Suppl. 1)**, S37–S41

Walz-Flannigan A, Magnuson D, Erickson D and Schueler B (2012) Artifacts in digital radiography. *American Journal of Roentgenology* **198(1)**, 156–161

Widmer WR (2008) Acquisition hardware for digital imaging. *Veterinary Radiology & Ultrasound* **49(Suppl. 1)**, S2–S8

Williams MB, Krupinski EA, Strauss KJ *et al.* (2007) Digital radiography image quality: image acquisition. *Journal of the American College of Radiology* **4(6)**, 371–388

Principles of radiological interpretation

Elizabeth Baines and Andrew Holloway

Radiological interpretation is the process by which a radiographic study is critically evaluated and the imaging findings correlated with the clinical presentation, with the aim of advancing the management of the patient. Radiological interpretation is not easy and, although the basic principles can be taught, development of expertise requires examination of a large number of radiographs. Critical comparison of the radiological diagnosis with surgical findings, or the interpretation of the same images by an experienced radiologist, helps develop the skills required for sound radiological interpretation.

Viewing the radiograph

The radiograph should be viewed in a standardized fashion. Viewing conditions must be such that the observer can concentrate on the whole radiograph (Figure 3.1). Errors are more likely to occur when the interpretation is rushed or the observer is tired or distracted.

- Radiological viewing stations, whether light boxes or monitors, must be in a quiet, darkened room and radiographs should be viewed with a dark-adapted eye (i.e. the observer should allow their eyes time to adapt to the darkened conditions before starting to view the images).
- Radiographs should be positioned on the viewer or screen in a consistent manner. The convention is usually for lateral views to be oriented with the head of the animal towards the left, and for ventrodorsal (VD) and dorsoventral (DV) views to be oriented with the animal's left to the observer's right and the cranial aspect (head/neck) at the top (Figure 3.2). Radiographs of the extremities are viewed with the proximal part of the limb at the top and the cranial or dorsal aspect to the left.
- The images should be arranged in exactly the same way each time, whether on a viewer or a monitor. For example, for a three-view thoracic study, when facing the viewing boxes, the left lateral view should be displayed on the left-hand side, the DV/VD view in the middle and the right lateral view on the right-hand side. For the

Conventional radiographs	Digital radiographs
Always use a quiet, darkened room	Always use a quiet, darkened room
Have at least two uniformly illuminated light boxes available	Have at least two diagnostic monitors available
Use a bright light to study relatively overexposed areas	Use appropriate adjustment of brightness and contrast (windowing) to study areas relatively poorly exposed. However, do not use this as a substitute for poor radiographic technique
Mask the edges of the light box not covered by the radiograph	Images should be masked appropriately before viewing
View the radiograph from both 15 cm and 2 m away	View the radiograph from both 15 cm and 2 m away
Use a magnifying glass to examine small areas	Use the magnifying function to examine small areas

3.1 Viewing conditions required for conventional and digital radiographs.

extremities, it is often useful to display radiographs of the contralateral joints side-by-side to allow direct comparison. It should be noted that comparison of size on analogue films is straightforward, whereas when viewing digital radiographs the magnification factor must be identical to avoid overlooking any variation between the extremities or between studies obtained on different days.

- Conventional film–screen (analogue) radiographs should be viewed on a light box.
  - The brightness of the light box is a very important factor in radiographic interpretation (with analogue film the contrast between adjacent structures is determined by the difference in transmission of light from the viewer through the film).
  - Good quality viewers with a sufficient number of panels (at least two but preferably four) should be used. Faulty light box tubes must be replaced.
  - A bright light should be used for spot-checking overexposed areas to identify small mineral opacities or gas in the soft tissues. However,

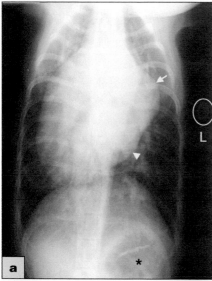

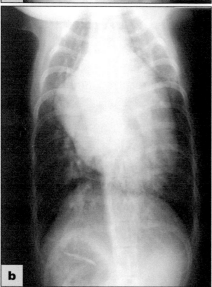

3.2 Orientation of a DV radiograph of the thorax of a dog using positional markers. **(a)** The indistinct positional marker (L) is correct (circle). This can be confirmed by the position of gas within the stomach in the left cranial abdomen (*). If the radiograph is oriented correctly, with the left of the animal to the observer's right, then the findings of enlarged pulmonary artery (arrowed), left auricular appendage (arrowhead) and left ventricle are clearly visible. **(b)** However, if the film is flipped horizontally, the radiograph appears more 'normal' with the cardiac apex superimposed on the 'left' hemithorax, but the enlarged pulmonary artery and atrium might then be missed. Diagnosis: patent ductus arteriosus.

when using a bright light, it is important not to turn it on unless a dark part of the film is covering it, as this can lead to overstimulation of the retina and, ultimately, solar retinopathy. In addition, any part of the light box not covered by an exposed part of film should be masked off to avoid flooding the retina with light, making it much harder to detect low contrast lesions on the film. Masking the uncovered parts of the viewer is of particular value when the film has any degree of overexposure.

- A magnifying glass may be used to look at fine detail on a film, particularly when assessing feline pulmonary patterns and the trabecular patterns of bone.

- Monitors used for viewing digital films should be of diagnostic quality.
  - The computed radiography/digital radiography acquisition workstation LCD monitor available on many digital systems to evaluate radiographic quality of the image at the time of acquisition is often also the one and only monitor used for interpretation. The image quality and resolution of these and conventional personal computer monitors are not sufficient to be used as a reporting station. High specification monitors are an expensive but worthwhile investment. Such monitors vary in size and resolution, and their quality is reflected in their price. A diagnostic viewing workstation consisting of at least two monitors (dual, side-by-side) allows multiple images and studies to be reviewed at the same time. Subtle abnormalities may become apparent during comparison. There is the temptation when evaluating digital radiographs to view one radiograph at a time, negating the benefit of side-by-side comparison. Multiple viewing monitors allow images to be viewed at full size.
  - The images should be masked to remove any white borders, and it may be necessary to use the windowing tool to alter brightness and contrast. However, care must be taken to avoid overuse of this tool as it may hide poor radiographic technique.
  - The zoom or magnifying function is very useful on digital systems as it allows assessment of small areas and fine details.
- When interpreting a contrast study, the films should be ordered according to the timing of the study, beginning with the survey films, before moving on to the contrast images. With a gastrointestinal contrast series, the two views taken at each time point must be assessed first, then all the serial lateral views should be compared, and then all the serial VD views should be compared.

Routine radiographic assessment

Before beginning to interpret the radiographic series, the films must be assessed and appraised for technical quality and completeness (Figure 3.3).

- An initial check should be made to ensure that the radiograph (or all radiographs if more than one) is from the patient being examined, and the date of the study should also be checked.

- Ensure radiographic study matches patient
- Check date(s)
- Ensure study is complete (minimum: two (usually orthogonal) views of each area studied)
- Identify views provided and ensure all are labelled correctly
- Assess technical quality of film, including degree of inspiration on thoracic views
- Ensure previous films are available for comparison

3.3 A radiographic appraisal should be performed to check the technical quality and completeness of the radiograph.

- There should be a minimum of two orthogonal views for each area in the study. If the study is not complete, non-diagnostic views should be repeated, where possible. If it is not possible to obtain a complete study, this should be noted and the reason recorded (e.g. the patient is dyspnoeic and so cannot be placed in lateral recumbency; hence only a DV view of the thorax was taken).
- The views should be identified and any positional markers checked. It is very important that the right and left sides or limbs of the animal are labelled correctly to avoid errors in interpretation and lesion localization.
  - When using *X-Rite* tape (X-Rite Ltd, UK), the writing on the tape will be normally oriented on the mediolateral view of any right limb when the display convention (i.e. proximal part of the limb at the top, and cranial or dorsal aspect to the left) is used, but the writing will be reversed on the mediolateral view of the left limb using the same convention. This aids in identifying the correct limb.
  - For a VD view of the thorax or abdomen, the writing on the X-Rite tape should be readable when the radiograph is viewed according to the conventions above and reversed for the DV view.
  - In addition, when viewing VD/DV views of the thorax, the position of the cardiac apex (normally located to the left of the midline) and the stomach should be noted.
  - On a DV view, gas should be visible in the gastric fundus (located in the left cranial quadrant of the abdomen). On a VD view, gas should be present in the body of the stomach (which runs perpendicular to and traverses the spine in the cranial abdomen).
  - When viewing VD radiographs of the abdomen, the position of the stomach and descending colon (to the left of the midline), as well as the relative position of the kidneys (right cranial to left), should be noted.
  - Although pathological changes, such as organomegaly, displacement, torsion and situs inversus (where the position of the visceral organs is reversed, e.g. the stomach and spleen are located on the right side of abdomen), can affect these structures, it is worth acquiring the habit of looking for normality on radiographs as the majority of images that are interpreted will be normal.
- Radiographic technique, other technical factors and patient positioning should be assessed (see Chapter 2). A radiographic study of diagnostic quality is one that includes the entire area of interest, is correctly exposed and is developed to assess the tissues of interest. For example, on overexposed abdominal radiographs, the details of the ventral abdomen are easily lost and this can lead to errors of interpretation when assessing for small intestinal or bladder disease. If, when looking at a radiograph, one's overwhelming instinct is to close one's eyes against the glare originating from the parts of the light box not covered by exposed film, then it is likely that the radiograph is overexposed. However, it is important to identify whether the lack of correct exposure is secondary to a disease process. For example, a thoracic radiograph may appear underexposed if pleural effusion is present. Once the presence of the pleural fluid has been recognized, it should be removed by thoracocentesis before any adjustments to the radiographic technique are made.
- For the majority of thoracic studies, radiographs taken at full inspiration are preferred and an assessment of the degree of inspiration should be made at the point of exposure. The radiographic features of expiratory views are frequently misinterpreted as pulmonary disease. Cranial displacement of the diaphragm by large volumes of abdominal fluid, fat accumulation, flatus (gas), faeces and large abdominal mass lesions restricts inflation of the lungs. It is essential that the radiographic study is properly performed to prevent the clinician being distracted by artefacts that mimic disease. It is then possible to advance the investigation of the patient by identifying genuine abnormalities or, if the films are normal, to allow some of the differential diagnoses to be eliminated.
- If the animal has been imaged before, the previous films should be available for comparison and review.
- For contrast studies, an assessment of the technique should be made, including adequacy of patient preparation and the completeness of the study.

Basic approach to radiological interpretation

Once the study has been assessed as being of diagnostic quality and complete, interpretation can commence. There is some merit in performing an unbiased assessment of a radiograph; however, in a busy general practice, the clinician is almost inevitably aware of the clinical presentation and other findings. Therefore, the radiological interpretation in these cases can be termed 'hypothesis driven', and is used to confirm or disprove a range of anticipated findings. However, it must be emphasized that this does not represent a weakness as, in any animal at any stage, an informed review of the radiographs, taking into account the history, progression of the disease and more recent images, may be necessary. It is important that the radiographic interpretation is performed in a systematic and thorough fashion with minimal assumptions regarding diagnosis by the clinician.

Generally, a detailed radiological assessment involves a series of steps:

- A recognition phase ('search')
- A descriptive phase ('report')
- An interpretive or analysis phase ('diagnosis or differential diagnoses').

The method used to evaluate radiographs is a matter of preference. A systematic or rigid search pattern is favoured by some, whereas an approach emphasizing the importance of what represents normal radiographic anatomy is advocated by others.

The best approach is to be consistent, which inevitably equates to using a combination of both methods, benefiting from the discipline imposed by a systematic search pattern and becoming sensitized to detecting changes that vary from normal anatomy.

Training is important for the recognition and descriptive phases and experience will improve decision-making. The clinician should never be afraid to ask for a second opinion or be embarrassed to admit when unsure. One of the advantages of radiographic studies is that the image is a permanent record and can be reviewed (by the original examiner, by colleagues or by a specialist) when required. Continued practice at radiological reporting, in association with critical reflection and discussion with experienced radiologists, will allow interpretive skills to improve.

Recognition phase

Systematic search pattern

Each radiograph is evaluated or 'read' systematically using either an 'organ approach', studying each body system in turn, or an 'area or concentric circles approach', starting at the periphery and working inwards (Figure 3.4). Each observer tends to develop their own system, but the important principle is that the entire radiograph must be interpreted, with no region or structure overlooked. This directed search approach may need to be adapted depending on the region being assessed. For example, in the thorax, using a systems approach the observer may begin with the cardiovascular system, move on to the respiratory system (lungs and airways), then the cranial abdomen and finally the skeleton. Alternatively, using a concentric circles approach, the areas beyond the primary beam, underexposed areas and overexposed areas (Figure 3.5) may be assessed first, followed by the skeletal structures, then the cranial abdomen and finally all the intrathoracic structures (cardiovascular and respiratory structures) together.

The benefit of a directed search pattern is that the observer avoids being distracted by an obvious or conspicuous lesion and so the assessment of the radiograph is not prematurely suspended. This is important in traumatized patients where multiple injuries may be present (Figure 3.6), or in older animals in which more than one disease can be present.

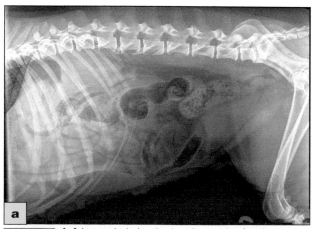

3.4 **(a)** Lateral abdominal radiograph of a dog presented with reluctance to move. The intra-abdominal structures are unremarkable. (continues) ▶

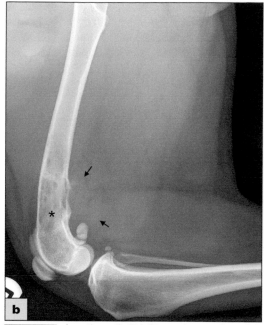

3.4 (continued). **(b)** Closer inspection of the periphery of the film reveals a large soft tissue mass (arrowed) and associated destructive changes in the distal right femur (*).

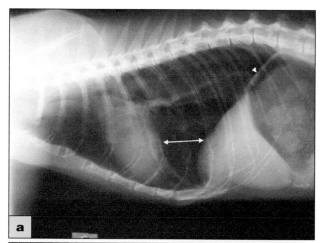

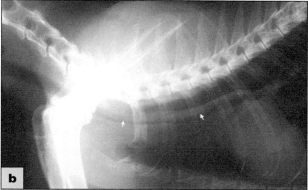

3.5 Lateral thoracic radiographs of a dyspnoeic cat. **(a)** The lungs are hyperinflated: the diaphragm is flattened (arrowhead), the distance between the cardiac silhouette and diaphragm is increased (double arrow) and the lungs have rounded margins and extend past the last rib. A cause for the air-trapping is not evident at first, but closer inspection of the relatively underexposed cranial thorax and inlet reveals that the air column in the trachea is not of even diameter throughout. **(b)** With the forelegs pulled forwards and the exposure increased, a plaque-like soft tissue mass within the dorsal trachea (arrowed) is visible. Diagnosis: tracheal neoplasia (carcinoma).

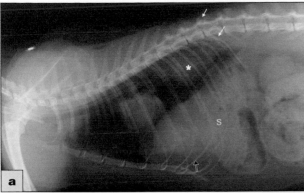

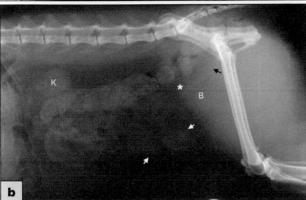

Axial and appendicular skeleton

- Alignment
- Bones
- Cartilage and joints
- Devices (implants)
- Soft tissues (gas, foreign bodies)

Abdomen

- Air (free gas, abnormal bowel gas patterns)
- Bones and bladder (intact?)
- Contrast (fat and fluid – serosal detail: fluid, haemorrhage, peritonitis, urine)
- Displacement (location of disease)
- Size (effect of disease)

Thorax

- Airways (upper, lower, larynx, trachea, lungs)
- Bones (chest wall, spine, limbs)
- Cardiac (size, vasculature, evidence of failure)
- Diaphragm (and cranial abdomen)
- Fluid (pleural space)
- Mediastinum
- Soft tissues (mass lesions invading thorax, gas)

Skull and neck

- Airspaces (nasal chambers, paranasal sinuses, nasopharynx, bullae)
- Bones (symmetry)
- C1–C2 alignment
- Dentition
- Soft tissues (swelling, foreign bodies)

3.6 Lateral radiographs of **(a)** the thorax and **(b)** the abdomen of a cat following trauma. (a) There is pulmonary consolidation (*), presumed to be haemorrhage, diaphragmatic hernia (outlined black arrow) with cranial displacement of the stomach (S), rib fractures and a small volume pneumothorax (white arrows). (b) Overexposure of the ventral abdomen at the periphery of the film obscures the herniation of intestinal loops through an abdominal wall defect (white arrows), avulsion of the prepubic tendon (black arrow) and the 'empty' caudal abdomen (*) with herniation of the urinary bladder (B) into the inguinal region. The left kidney (K) is small. These images emphasize the importance, especially in trauma cases, of not suspending the search until all films have been assessed and the periphery and overexposed areas of the radiograph have been evaluated. (Courtesy of Frean and Smyth Veterinary Surgeons)

3.7 Interpretive checklist using the ABCDS system. (Modified from Chan and Touquet (2007) with permission from the publisher)

easily. The concept of positioning the animal such that the diseased portion is further away from the cassette is contrary to the fundamental radiographic principle that the area of interest should be as close as possible to the cassette (Figure 3.8).

It may be tempting on occasion, for reasons of speed, economy or forgetting the importance of orthogonal views, to take a single radiograph of the

Peripheral or unexpected lesions have less chance of being overlooked using this approach. An interpretive checklist (Figure 3.7) can be produced and posted adjacent to the viewer or monitor to assist the observer. This may be helpful when assessing complex areas of anatomy.

Lesion localization
It should be remembered that a radiograph is a two-dimensional (2D) representation of a three-dimensional (3D) object, so there will always be superimposition by the overlying structures, which can make lesion localization a challenge. Hence the need for orthogonal views to be obtained in all cases.

Thorax: Orthogonal views of the thorax usually comprise a DV view and either a right or left lateral view. Routinely, a right lateral recumbent view is obtained, but the DV view should be assessed first and, if disease of the right hemithorax is suspected based on this view, a left lateral view should be acquired initially, as the lung in the uppermost hemithorax will be better inflated and hence show pathological changes more

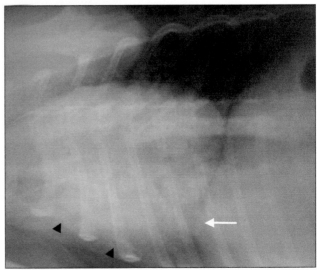

3.8 Decubitus VD thoracic radiograph showing the effect of collapse of dependent lung lobes. The cardiac silhouette has descended toward the dependent thoracic wall as a result of the reduction in lung volume (arrowheads). The dependent hemidiaphragm has moved cranially (arrowed). It should be noted that the pathology, whether diffuse or metastatic nodules, within the dependent lung is difficult to distinguish from the collapsed lung tissue.

thorax. This should be avoided if at all possible, but if only a single view is feasible, then a DV view should be taken as this allows limited assessment of both hemithoraces, whereas a single lateral recumbent view does not allow evaluation of the dependent hemithorax (Figures 3.9 and 3.10). The limitation of a single view can be appreciated when assessing a thoracic radiograph on which a conspicuous soft tissue opacity is visible, superimposed on the caudal thorax (Figure 3.11). There is no difficulty in recognizing the pathological change. However, the lesion may be located at any point along the pathway of the primary beam. The orthogonal view is required to demonstrate that the structure actually lies on the midline, which is a crucial observation as it narrows the list of differential diagnoses to an abnormality arising from the caudal mediastinum and indicates appropriate further tests to be performed.

The same principle may apply to differentiating a suspected radiopaque foreign body from the contents of the colon, and determining the significance of foreign bodies or missiles embedded within the patient

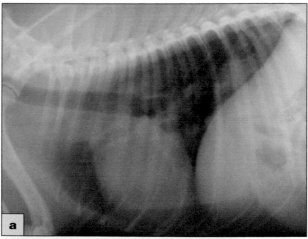

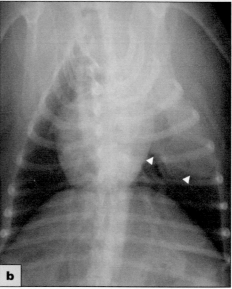

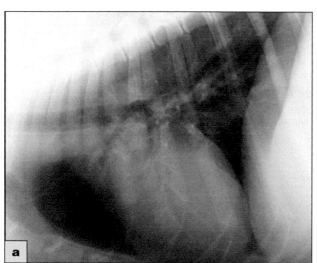

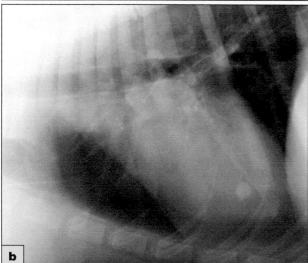

3.9   **(a)** Right and **(b)** left lateral thoracic radiographs of a dog with mammary adenocarcinoma. No abnormalities are visible on the right lateral view but there is a clear soft tissue nodular opacity superimposed on the cardiac silhouette on the left lateral view. The nodule is consistent with pulmonary metastasis within the right lung. Significant pathology within the poorly inflated dependent lung lobe will be overlooked on lateral recumbent views unless two, preferably three, views are obtained.

3.10   **(a)** Lateral and **(b)** DV thoracic radiographs of a dog presenting with a cough. No abnormalities are evident on the left lateral view, but complete consolidation of the left cranial lung lobe (arrowheads) is apparent on the DV view. Extensive consolidation or large mass lesions in the lung may not be distinguished without a sufficient number of radiographic views.

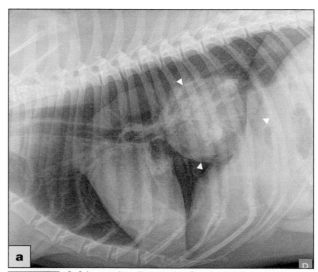

3.11   **(a)** Lateral radiograph of a dog with a thoracic mass. On this view, the large mass (arrowheads) could be located at any point in the direction of the X-ray beam and involve the chest wall, pulmonary parenchyma or the mediastinum. (continues) ▶

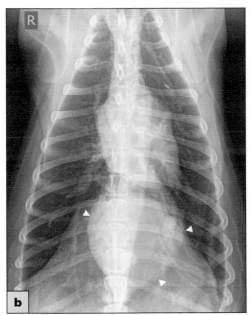

3.11 (continued) **(b)** DV thoracic radiograph of a dog with a thoracic mass. This view localizes the mass (arrowheads) to the midline. The list of differential diagnoses is narrowed to a caudodorsal mediastinal mass lesion (e.g. oesophageal mass, mediastinal abscess or primary mediastinal neoplasia).

adjacent to vital structures such as the eyes, spine, heart and abdominal organs (Figure 3.12). A thoracic study for the investigation of pulmonary metastases comprises both right and left lateral views, in addition to a DV or VD view.

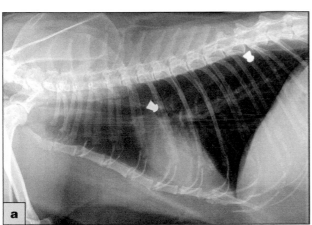

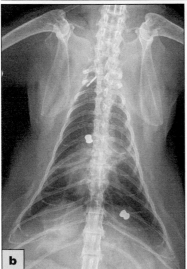

3.12 **(a)** Lateral and **(b)** DV thoracic radiographs of a cat. Relying on a single view, it is not possible to determine whether both air-gun pellets lie within the thorax. Assessment of orthogonal views, together with the location of the entry wounds, can indicate which important structures may have been damaged along the path of the pellet.

Abdomen: Orthogonal views of the abdomen comprise a VD view and either a right or left lateral view. The appearance of the stomach can be very different between the two lateral views. On the right lateral view, any gas in the stomach will be in the fundus and the pylorus appears as a rounded soft tissue opacity, whereas on the left lateral view any gas will be in the pylorus. There is often value in obtaining both right and left lateral views where there are concerns about the pyloric region or descending duodenum (Figures 3.13 and 3.14).

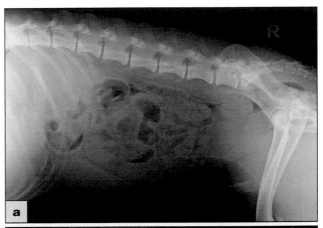

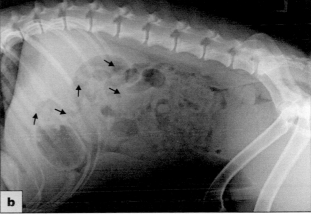

3.13 **(a)** Right and **(b)** left lateral radiographs of a dog presenting with vomiting. On the right lateral view, the abnormal mixed gas and soft tissue opacity caudal to the stomach may be the transverse colon. However, on the left lateral view, the lumen of the duodenum is highlighted with gas (black arrows). It has a tortuous or zigzag path across the abdomen. Other dilated small intestinal loops are of soft tissue opacity. Diagnosis: small intestinal linear foreign body.

Identification: Identifying views and checking positional markers can be useful to highlight the part of the body that might be affected.

- Thoracic radiographs – if the disease is seen on the right lateral view, it is more likely to be present in the left hemithorax.
- Abdominal radiographs – if a right lateral view is known to have been obtained but gas is present in the pylorus, the possibility of gastric torsion should be considered (Figure 3.15).

Descriptive phase
The purpose of radiological description is to identify and describe all the changes seen on a radiograph.

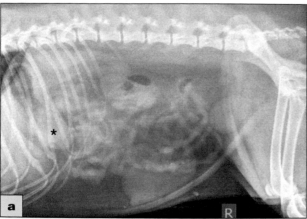

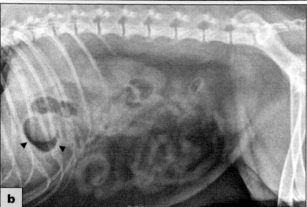

3.14 **(a)** Right and **(b)** left lateral abdominal radiographs of a dog presenting with vomiting. On the right lateral view, the pylorus is of soft tissue opacity (*) and distinguishing between 'normal' fluid within the dependent pylorus and disease (mass or intraluminal foreign body of a soft tissue opacity) is not possible. On the left lateral view, a sharply demarcated soft tissue structure in the pylorus is surrounded and highlighted by gas (arrowheads). This appearance is consistent with an intraluminal gastric foreign body. Two bouquet garni muslin bags were removed at surgery. (Courtesy of Palmerston Veterinary Group)

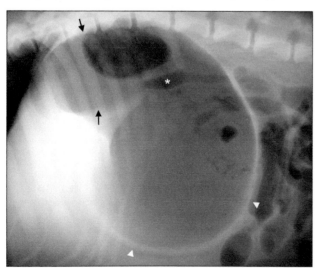

3.15 Right lateral radiograph of the abdomen of a large-breed dog. There is a large bilobed gas-filled viscus in the region normally occupied by the stomach. Both the body of the stomach and the pylorus are filled with gas (and quite a large amount of fluid). The fundus (arrowheads) is located ventrally and the gas-filled pylorus (arrowed) is located dorsally, indicating malpositioning of the stomach. The descending duodenum (*) is not usually visible on the right lateral view, but can be seen here due to rotation of the stomach to the left. Diagnosis: gastric dilatation–volvulus.

Abnormalities should be classified according to defined radiological changes. These are known as Röntgen signs. These changes should then be evaluated to produce an interpretation relevant to the current problem.

It is important to remember that radiological findings may be due to changes that have occurred in the past and which may be unimportant, or related to the current problem. As discussed above, it may be difficult for the clinician to be unaware of the clinical problem or findings, but the initial description should identify all abnormalities present, regardless of the clinical problem. It is at the interpretive stage that the history, clinical findings and results of any additional investigations should be considered with the radiological findings to reach a diagnosis or differential diagnosis list with suggestions for appropriate further investigations.

The ability to discern different tissues and structures depends on adequate contrast on the radiograph. The appearance of each tissue is referred to as its radiopacity. Without differential absorption of the primary X-ray beam by different tissues and the resulting different radiopacities, plain radiography would be of little value as a diagnostic tool.

Röntgen signs

The Röntgen signs used to describe changes seen on a radiograph are size, shape, contour or margination, number, position and opacity (Figure 3.16). Some idea of function may also be deduced, but a radiograph is an anatomical study rather than a functional study. Each structure should be assessed in terms of each Röntgen sign and evaluated to determine whether it is:

- A feature of normal anatomy
- A composite shadow caused by superimposition of structures
- An artefact created by inaccurate positioning or poor technique
- A pathological lesion.

Röntgen sign	Change	Possible cause
Size	Increased	Hypertrophy Hyperplasia Inflammation Neoplasia Oedema Congestion Torsion Cystic change
	Decreased	Atrophy Hypoplasia Congenital anomaly
Contour/shape	Localized or diffuse	Trauma Hypertrophy Hyperplasia Neoplasia Necrosis Ulceration
Number	Increased	Accessory ossification centres Congenital anomaly
	Decreased	Congenital anomaly Ectopia (relative)

3.16 Röntgen signs and the causes of associated changes. (continues)

Röntgen sign	Change	Possible cause
Position	Displacement	Pulsion (mass effect) Traction Torsion Ectopia Hernia/rupture
Opacity	Increased	Fluid or soft tissue within a normally air-filled structure Calculi Mineralization within soft tissues (dystrophic, metastatic)
	Decreased	Abnormal gas Osteopenia
Internal architecture	Alteration	Inflammation Neoplasia Rupture
(Function)	Alteration in pattern	Inspiratory *versus* expiratory films
(Contrast studies)	Alteration in time	Gastrointestinal tract transit

3.16 (continued) Röntgen signs and the causes of associated changes.

The need for comprehensive knowledge of the normal radiographic appearance of the dog and cat cannot be emphasized enough, as the identification of abnormalities on a radiograph relies on the ability of the interpreter to appreciate normality. It may be difficult to determine whether an abnormality exists, as there is a wide range of normal variants, and it is impossible to remember (or even to see) all the normal variations, so reference should be made to textbooks, atlases of normal radiographic anatomy, normal radiographs, tissue specimens and the contralateral limb. Suitable adjectives should be used to provide further descriptive information about the lesion. There is the temptation, particularly when beginning to produce radiological reports, to describe findings just based on opacity, but the other Röntgen signs should not be ignored.

Size: Alteration in the size of an organ or tissue affects the appearance of its silhouette on the radiograph (Figures 3.17 and 3.18). It can be very difficult to judge changes in size, particularly if only one view is available, as an alteration in organ size or structure in one dimension may not be visible on the particular view being assessed. Changes in position may also give the appearance of a change in size. Any measurements are best made relative to another structure on the same radiograph, in order to avoid magnification being a factor in the measurements.

Gross organomegaly can usually be appreciated, but small changes can be subjective and the experienced observer will tend to have a 'rule of thumb' about the size of structures, rather than any hard and fast rules.

- Cardiac size is influenced by breed conformation, phase of respiration, concurrent therapy (diuretics) and type of cardiac disease. Cardiac size in small-breed dogs with a shallow chest conformation is exaggerated, and over-interpretation is likely if the lateral view is relied on alone. Considering the variability in the factors

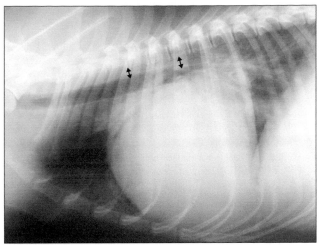

3.17 Röntgen sign: size. Lateral thoracic radiograph of a dog showing marked cardiomegaly. Moderate to marked cardiomegaly can usually be distinguished from a normal cardiac silhouette; however, differentiating mild cardiac enlargement is difficult given the variability of chest conformation in the dog. Not all 'classic' signs of left-side enlargement, such as elevation of the trachea (arrowed), are recognized in all dogs (e.g. in deep-chested breeds, such as the Dobermann, the trachea may remain divergent from the spine even in advanced disease).

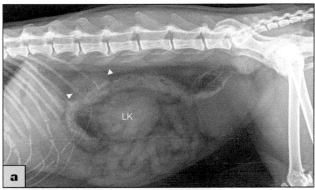

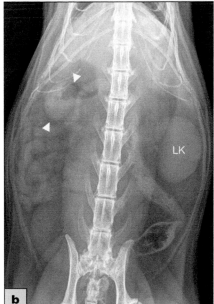

3.18 Röntgen sign: size. **(a)** Lateral and **(b)** VD abdominal radiographs of a cat with unequally sized kidneys. The right kidney (arrowheads) is small and irregular, representing hypoplasia or end-stage disease. In comparison, the left kidney (LK) is moderately enlarged due to secondary renal hypertrophy.

noted above, distinguishing mild enlargement from normal size is therefore impossible. Confidence increases with moderate to severe enlargement, but some significant cardiac diseases (e.g. ventricular septal defect and pulmonary hypertension) demonstrate only subtle changes and therefore the insensitivity of radiography for these diseases should be noted.

- Neoplasia is a common cause of increased size; however, cystic transformation, inflammation and hypertrophy should also be considered.
- Changes in size can be physiological (e.g. urinary or faecal retention if the patient has not had the opportunity to void, gastric distension (aerophagia) due to dyspnoea, and splenomegaly due to phenothiazines or general anaesthesia). Interpretation may be hampered by physiological changes and radiography should be repeated following an enema, catheterization of the bladder or the opportunity to void.
- A change in size in the appendicular skeleton, usually bone length but occasionally diameter, is best made by comparison with the contralateral limb (Figure 3.19).

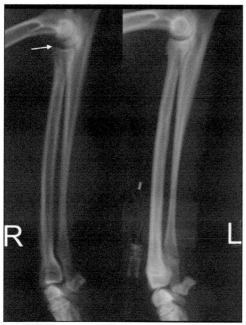

3.19 Röntgen sign: size. Mediolateral radiograph of the right antebrachium of a dog with shortening of the radius (arrowed). Comparison with the normal left limb is helpful to confirm the reduced length and compare the degree of subluxation of the radial head.

Shape and contour/margination: The shape and contour of an organ should be assessed (Figure 3.20). Changes in shape may be seen if there are pathological changes within the organ (such as a renal tumour causing deformity of the normal kidney contour). An alteration in shape does not always imply disease or abnormal function. Malformation may be an incidental finding. This is common in the vertebral column (e.g. block vertebrae, hemivertebrae and fused spinous processes).

Indistinct margination may be a sign of disease (e.g. indistinct caudal aspect of the liver silhouette due to the presence of peritoneal fluid, irregular bladder

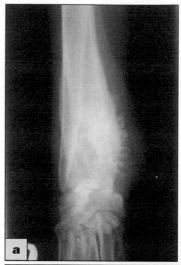

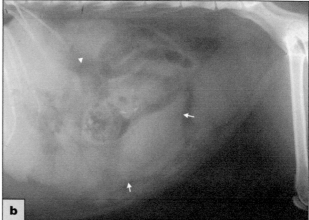

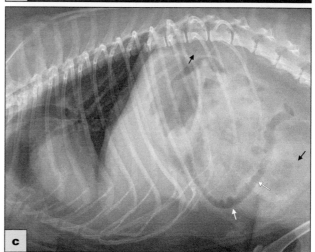

3.20 Röntgen sign: contour and shape.
(a) Dorsopalmar radiograph of the carpus of a dog with irregular spiculating new bone on all aspects of the distal radius. The appearance of the periosteal reaction is used to categorize the changes as that of aggressive disease. Diagnosis: primary malignant bone tumour.
(b) Lateral radiograph of a cat with a lemon-shaped soft tissue opacity (arrowed) in the mid-ventral abdomen, representing expansile change from a structure such as the intestine or, in this case, the tail of the spleen. Diagnosis: splenic mass. **(c)** Lateral radiograph of the caudal thorax and cranial abdomen of a dog with an intestinal perforation. The intestinal loop crossing the abdomen has a corrugated margin (white arrows). This change, which is consistent with bowel irritation and spasm, is indicative of severe inflammation. Taking into consideration the free abdominal fluid, reduced serosal detail, and free gas (black arrows), the most likely cause is septic peritonitis.

margin following loss of integrity due to bladder rupture, and indistinct renal margins due to retroperitoneal fluid). Corrugation (tightly undulating margin) of the serosal surface of the intestines is suggestive of irritation or spasm of the intestinal wall. When associated with loss of peritoneal detail of the serosal surfaces or free abdominal fluid, it is suggestive of peritonitis due to either aseptic (pancreatitis, uroabdomen) or septic causes.

Number: The number of each organ or structure should be assessed (Figures 3.21 and 3.22). This may be considered a straightforward sign, but unfortunately intrinsic patient factors and poor radiographic technique can conspire to obscure structures that should normally be visible. For example, it can be difficult to recognize the kidneys, particularly the right kidney, on a VD view of the abdomen due to the superimposition of the gastrointestinal tract, especially

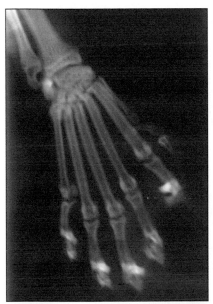

3.21 Röntgen sign: number. Dorsopalmar radiograph of the manus of a cat with six digits. The change is of no clinical significance and consistent with congenital polydactyly.

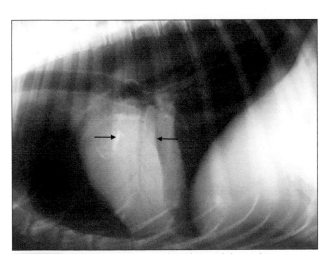

3.22 Röntgen sign: number. Lateral thoracic radiograph of a dog showing complete consolidation of the right middle lung lobe (arrowed). The loss of normal air-filled lung is easily overlooked as it is completely superimposed on the cardiac silhouette.

if it is filled with ingesta. If the orthogonal view is also inconclusive, then alternative imaging techniques, such as an intravenous contrast study, repeat radiography or ultrasonography, may be needed to verify that both kidneys are present. It is often more difficult to recognize that something is absent than that it is present. All structures expected to be visible on a radiograph should be actively searched for and, if not seen, should be considered of potential significance and accounted for in the differential diagnosis list.

Position: Familiarity with normal radiographic anatomy is required to appreciate displacement of structures from a normal position or orientation (Figure 3.23). Changes in position may occur due to a primary disease within that organ (e.g. pyloric displacement in gastric torsion) or secondary to disease elsewhere (e.g. displacement of the bladder ventrally through an abdominal wall rupture or dorsal displacement of the trachea by left atrial enlargement).

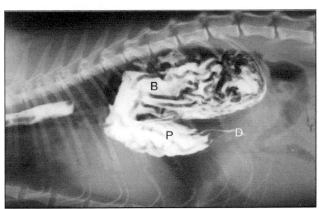

3.23 Röntgen sign: position. Lateral thoracic radiograph of a cat following oral administration of barium suspension. The gastric body is displaced cranially into the thorax. Diagnosis: diaphragmatic rupture. B = fundus; D = duodenum; P = pylorus.

Opacity: There are five relative radiographic opacities (Figure 3.24): gas, fat, soft tissue/fluid, mineral and metal.

Material	Effective atomic number (Z)	Density (g/cm³)	Radiographic appearance
Gas	7.8	0.001	Black
Fat	6.5	0.92	Dark grey
Water	7.5	1.00	Mid-grey
Soft tissue	7.6	1.04	Mid-grey
Mineral	12.3	1.65	Light grey/white
Lead	82	8.7	Bright white

3.24 Appearance of different materials that may be visible on radiographs.

Gas: This is the most radiolucent material visible on a radiograph. On survey radiographs, gas provides inherent contrast, especially within the lungs on thoracic images, in the nasal chambers and paranasal sinuses on skull images and within the gastrointestinal tract on abdominal images. Gas in abnormal locations, such as extra-pulmonary gas in cases of pneumomediastinum or pneumothorax and free peritoneal gas, should not be overlooked. Free peritoneal gas may be very difficult to detect where intra-luminal gas shadows overlap with free gas. Even large volumes of gas can be overlooked (Figure 3.25). The serosal surfaces of the oesophagus, abdominal organs and viscera, and the peritoneal surface of the diaphragm, are not normally visible. Gas within the soft tissues is easily overlooked on overexposed radio-graphs. Analogue films, especially areas with soft tissue swelling, should be bright-lit to rule out small amounts of gas. The wide latitude of digital film usu-ally allows adequate assessment of the soft tissues.

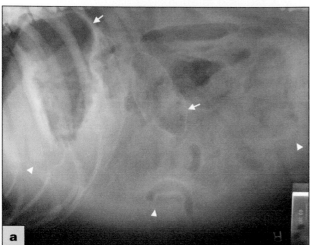

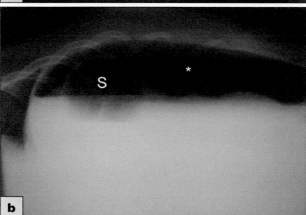

3.25 Röntgen sign: gas opacity. **(a)** Lateral and **(b)** right decubitus VD horizontal beam abdominal radiographs of a dog with sudden collapse. (a) The abdomen is distended and serosal detail is poor, indicating a large abdominal effusion. The large gas bubble superimposed on the abdominal contents is easily overlooked as the margin is indistinct (arrowheads). The serosal surfaces of the stomach and colon are highlighted by gas (arrowed). These are additional signs that there is free gas in the abdomen. (b) The volume of free gas (*) collects under the costal arch and surrounds the fundus of the stomach (S). A fluid–gas interface is present due to the large volume of free abdominal fluid.

Fat: This is more radiolucent than bone or soft tissue, but more radiopaque than gas. This relative radio-lucency provides contrast, allowing soft tissue struc-tures surrounded by fat to be visualized. Without peritoneal fat, plain abdominal radiography would be very unrewarding, as fat in the falciform, umbilical, mesenteric and retroperitoneal areas enables visual-ization of the serosal surfaces of all the abdominal viscera. In musculoskeletal radiography, fat allows the fascial planes to be visualized, enabling assessment of muscle size and, in places, the location of tendons and ligaments. Displacement of the fascial planes is used to assess for the presence of joint effusion and synovial enlargement. In addition, fat in the pericar-dium may allow limited assessment of cardiac size and position in the presence of pleural fluid.

Soft tissue and fluid: Soft tissue and fluid have the same radiographic opacity; thus, a hollow viscus filled with fluid (such as the bladder) and a solid paren-chymatous organ (such as the liver) have the same radiographic opacity. Differences in the thickness of the soft tissues leads to variation in the opacities on a radiograph: soft tissue structures of greater thickness appear more opaque than thinner structures (Figure 3.26). For example, on a VD view of the abdomen of a cat, the body of the spleen may be clearly seen as a triangular structure, as it curves round, with the thinner, flatter head and tail running cranially and cau-dally, respectively, less well visualized (Figure 3.27).

Mineral or bone: Mineral is the most opaque or 'whitest' physiological opacity seen on a radiograph: tooth enamel has the greatest opacity, but all normal bony structures are markedly more opaque than the soft tissues. There are normal variations in the radio-pacity within a bone and between different bones, because of the difference in density between com-pact and spongy bone, trabecular bone and inter-trabecular spaces, and cortical bone and the medullary cavity. Diseased bone may be more opaque (sclerotic) or less opaque (penic) than normal bone (Figure 3.28). Approximately 30–50% of mineral content must be lost before any alteration is seen in the radiographic opacity of the bone.

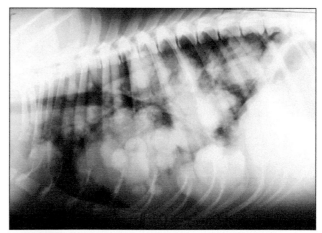

3.26 Röntgen sign: soft tissue opacity. Lateral thoracic radiograph of a dog with multiple soft tissue opacities throughout the lung fields. Summation of multiple nodules results in a marked increase in opacity. Some of the summated nodules are equal to or greater in opacity than the thin bones such as the ribs. As neither the physical density nor the effective atomic number of the soft tissue nodules change, the increase in opacity is entirely due to the increase in the thickness of the tissues through which the X-rays must pass. The combined effect of greater physical density of bone and larger effective atomic number means that an equal thickness of bone attenuates X-rays six times more than soft tissue. Therefore, the increase in thickness of the soft tissue needs to be considerable for the opacity to be similar to that of bone. Diagnosis: pulmonary metastases.

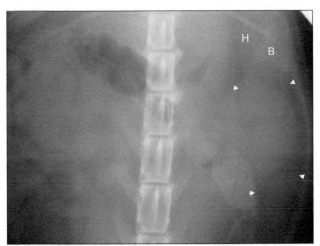

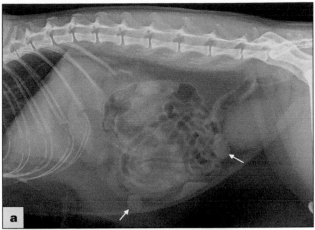

3.27 Röntgen sign: soft tissue opacity. VD abdominal radiograph of a cat. The body (B) of the spleen is a relatively radiopaque soft tissue triangle, visible craniolateral to the left kidney. The head (H) and tail (arrowheads) of the spleen are less well defined and less opaque oblong radiopacities extending medially from the body of the spleen. The increase in thickness of the body of the spleen as it curves round results in the increased opacity.

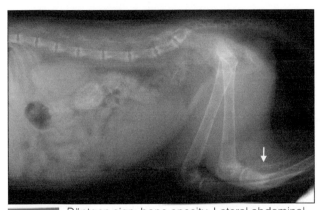

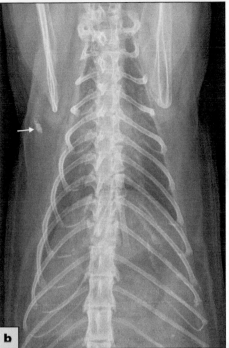

3.28 Röntgen sign: bone opacity. Lateral abdominal radiograph of a dog with generalized osteopenia and a folding fracture (arrowed) of one tibia. The flat bones of the pelvis are almost unrecognizable, and the soft tissue structures are more conspicuous and opaque compared with the bones. Diagnosis: nutritional secondary hyperparathyroidism.

Dystrophic mineralization (Figure 3.29) is mineralization of degenerated or necrotic tissue. Metastatic mineralization occurs when there is a systemic mineral imbalance (usually hypercalcaemia) that leads to mineralization of the soft tissues. Dystrophic mineralization has an irregular appearance, whereas metastatic mineralization often has a geometric appearance depending on the affected structure (e.g. linear in blood vessel walls or undulating when involving the gastric mucosa). Unusual forms of mineralization may occur with certain diseases, such as ossifying myositis, or as peripheral 'egg-shell' mineralization of the wall of paraprostatic cysts or nodular fat necrosis in the cat. The latter is an incidental finding most commonly seen in older cats. Lesions with this appearance are most likely to be incidental findings and should not be confused with neoplastic abdominal masses. Mineralization of the coronary arteries and aortic valves in dogs and the adrenal glands of older cats are usually incidental findings.

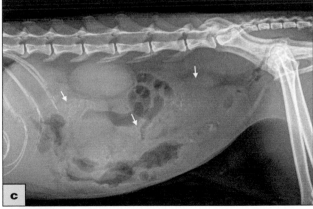

3.29 Röntgen sign: dystrophic mineralization.
(a) Lateral abdominal radiograph of a cat. The discrete rounded structures (arrowed) with fine mineralization of the periphery are due to fat necrosis (a form of dystrophic mineralization). They are usually single and may be attached to the mesentery or free floating within the abdomen. **(b)** DV thoracic radiograph of a cat with dystrophic mineralization of the soft tissue lateral to the spine. The dystrophic mineralization has a fine granular appearance (arrowed). The cause is unknown but tissue damage from a bite wound or trauma is suspected.
(c) Lateral abdominal radiograph of a cat with extensive mineralization of markedly enlarged visceral lymph nodes. Diagnosis: metastatic carcinoma. (continues) ▶

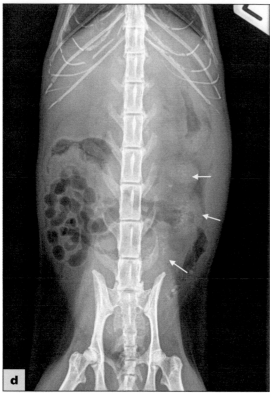

3.29 (continued) Röntgen sign: dystrophic mineralization. **(d)** VD abdominal radiograph of a cat with extensive mineralization of markedly enlarged visceral lymph nodes (arrowed). Diagnosis: metastatic carcinoma.

Metal: This is the most opaque opacity seen on a radiograph. Common examples include orthopaedic implants, microchips, metallic foreign bodies and artefacts such as metal on collars or electrocardiogram needles.

High atomic number elements: Non-metallic substances containing high atomic number elements, such as barium ($Z = 56$) and iodine ($Z = 53$), used as positive contrast medium agents are markedly opaque. However, the opacity is affected by concentration. Water-soluble, iodine-containing contrast agents are concentrated within the renal tubules, accounting for the gradual increase in opacity within the renal pelves and bladder.

Function/integrity/internal architecture: Assessment of function requires dynamic studies, usually using contrast agents. Fluoroscopy, stressed radiographs of joints, inspiratory and expiratory radiographs and angiography are dynamic studies that provide variable information relating to function and integrity (Figure 3.30). Within a soft tissue structure of homogeneous opacity (such as parenchymatous organs or muscles), little change in the internal architecture can be appreciated unless there is also a change in opacity, whereas the internal architecture of bony structures can be seen and change appreciated. Hollow soft tissue structures (such as the stomach or intestines) may show changes in internal contents due to abnormal ingesta or gas patterns, which are of clinical significance (Figure 3.31).

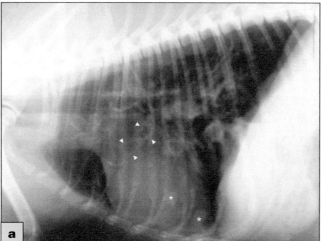

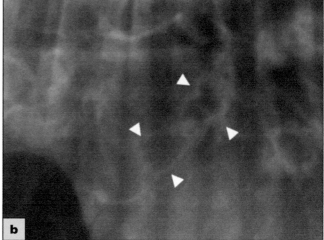

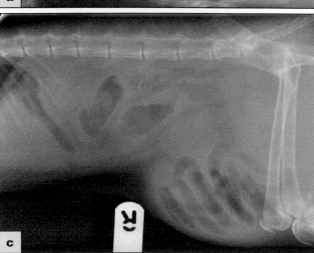

3.30 Röntgen sign: architecture/integrity. **(a–b)** Lateral thoracic radiographs of a dog. The normal tapering air-filled bronchi are lost and have been replaced by a sacculated dilated bronchial pattern (arrowheads). Although the function of the bronchi cannot be directly assessed, the bronchial pattern represents an irreversible change in architecture (bronchiectasis) and this indirectly suggests abnormal clearance by the bronchi. Some of the bronchi are filled with exudate and mucus and appear as soft tissue nodules (*), which should not be mistaken for metastases. **(c)** Lateral abdominal radiograph of a cat showing loss of the normal contour of the caudoventral body wall and loops of gas-filled small intestine located cranial to the stifles. Diagnosis: body wall rupture.

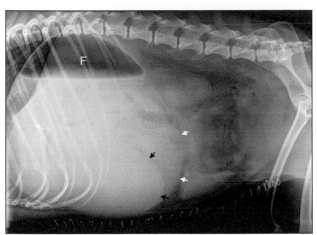

3.31 Lateral abdominal radiograph of a dog presenting with vomiting following surgery for bile duct obstruction (cholelith). Ultrasonography demonstrated that the stomach was distended with fluid and ruled out post-surgical pancreatitis. Radiography provided a better assessment of the degree of gastric distension. The pylorus (black arrows) and body (white arrows) are markedly dilated, extending almost to the umbilicus, and have displaced the contents of the small intestines caudally. The small intestinal loops are not dilated. This pattern is consistent with a gastric outflow obstruction in this dog (due to adhesions) and is similar in appearance to that seen with congenital or acquired pyloric stenosis. There is no need for a barium study in this dog. Restraint of the dog in lateral recumbency was not possible, hence the radiograph was obtained using a horizontal beam. F = fundic gas cap.

Factors influencing contrast

Border effacement: In order to be able to distinguish the borders of two objects of similar radiopacity on radiographs, they must be separated by a substance of different opacity. Border effacement (also known as positive silhouetting) is the term used when two structures of similar radiopacity are in contact with one another, and thus their margins at the point of contact cannot be identified. The liver and diaphragm both have soft tissue opacity, and where they come into contact their individual outlines are not normally visible. In the normal animal, small pulmonary vessels can be seen superimposed on the cardiac silhouette as they are separated from the cardiac tissue by air in the lungs (Figure 3.32). Similar sized coronary vessels cannot be distinguished as they are in contact with the cardiac tissue. Cranial mediastinal vessels cannot be distinguished from adjacent soft tissue structures with which they are in contact, unless a contrasting substance (usually air due to pneumomediastinum) is present. The presence of unexpected border effacement can be a useful indicator of pathology. For example, pleural fluid causes border effacement of the ventral border of the cardiac silhouette on a DV thoracic radiograph (Figure 3.33) whereas, if a VD view is obtained, the cardiac margins are more visible as the fluid pools dependently around the spine.

Surrounding contrasting substances: Some normal structures (e.g. the prepuce or nipples) appear strikingly radiopaque relative to other soft tissue opacities on the radiograph. This is partly because they are highlighted by air, so they are more visible

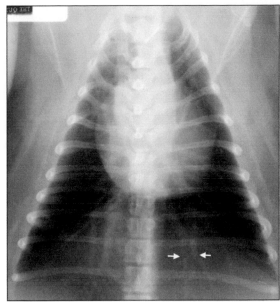

3.32 DV thoracic radiograph of a dog. The pulmonary vessels (arrowed) can be clearly seen, even over the cardiac silhouette, as they are separated from the heart by air-filled lung. The coronary vessels cannot be seen as they are in contact with the heart.

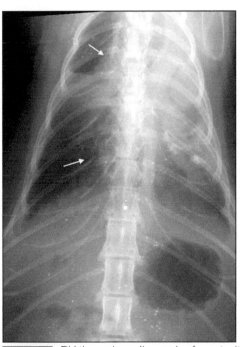

3.33 DV thoracic radiograph of a cat with border effacement of the cardiac margins due to pleural fluid. The cardiac margins cannot be clearly seen as the opacity of the fluid and the heart is the same (arrowed).

than the adjacent soft tissue structures, but also their margins are parallel to the primary beam and so are well defined (Figure 3.34). In addition, the perceived appearance of structures alters as their surroundings alter (e.g. if surrounded by contrast medium) (Figure 3.35).

Tissue thickness: Increasing tissue thickness leads to greater attenuation of the X-ray beam. This applies to all tissues but is most relevant for soft tissue. An increase in soft tissue thickness may be due to an

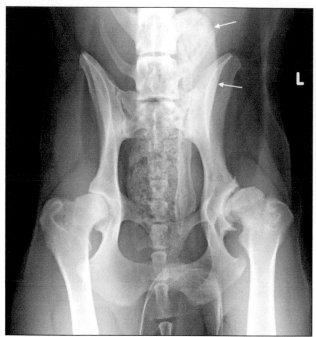

3.34   VD radiograph of the pelvis of a male dog with marked unilateral hip dysplasia and secondary osteoarthritis. The prepuce (arrowed) can be clearly seen to the left of the caudal lumbar spine, due to the sharp interface between air and the soft tissue and because the margins are parallel to the beam.

increase in the size of the tissue or organ under investigation, the result of superimposition of several structures (see below) or the accumulation of fluid within the thorax or abdomen.

Composite shadows: Composite shadows are formed when parts of the patient in different planes are superimposed. Often these composite shadows are created by the superimposition of normal structures

(e.g. on lateral abdominal radiographs, the cranial pole of the left kidney and the caudal pole of the right kidney are often superimposed), resulting in a relatively more radiopaque area, which may be mistaken for a mass (Figure 3.36). Pulmonary blood vessels can be mistaken for pulmonary nodules either when viewed end-on, when they appear as obvious circular soft tissue opacities, or when they cross the ribs. Inexperienced observers may see the oblong region of increased opacity at the rib/vessel intersection, but miss the linear soft tissue (vessel) and bony (rib) opacities extending out from the 'nodule' (Figure 3.37). Distinguishing composite shadows of normal structures from those due to pathology is dependent upon:

- Comparison with additional (usually orthogonal) views
- Adequate inflation of the thorax and/or adequate serosal detail in the abdomen
- Contrast studies or cross-sectional imaging (computed tomography (CT), ultrasonography).

Superimposition: The effect of superimposition has been discussed above (see Lesion localization).

Artefacts and optical illusions: Perception errors can influence the contrast of structures within a radiograph. However thoroughly the radiograph is assessed, the observer can be misled if their eyes and brain do not accurately perceive the appearance of structures. The most frequent perception error is the Mach Phenomenon. Mach lines are optical illusions that appear as radiolucent or radiopaque lines at sharp boundaries between structures with large differences in opacity. Mach lines are present throughout the radiographic image, but are important when evaluating skeletal disease as they can mimic pathology, particularly fractures (Figure 3.38). If the line can be made to

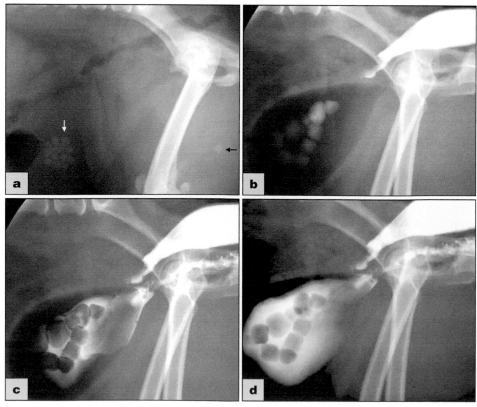

3.35   Lateral abdominal radiographs, illustrating change in relative opacity. **(a)** Survey radiograph of a male dog with radiopaque cystic (white arrow) and urethral (black arrow) calculi. **(b–d)** Retrograde vaginourethrogram series showing the change in appearance of cystic calculi as the nature and opacity of the surrounding substance alters. The calculi are markedly opaque compared with gas, lucent when surrounded by a small volume of iodine, but become more opaque as the surrounding volume of iodine increases, partially obscuring them. This emphasizes the importance when performing a double-contrast cystogram (see Chapter 4) that neither the concentration nor the volume of the contrast medium should be so great as to obscure small lesions.

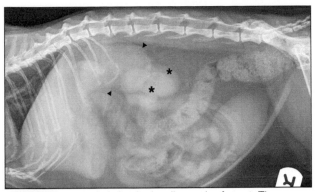

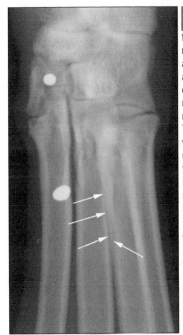

3.36 Lateral abdominal radiograph of a cat. The composite shadow in the craniodorsal abdomen ventral to L2–L3 is caused by the overlapping of both kidneys (∗). Note that one kidney is smaller than the other and a large right adrenal gland mass (arrowheads) is present.

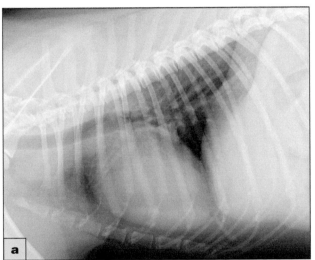

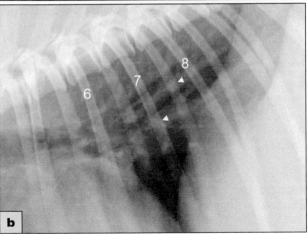

3.37 Lateral thoracic radiographs of a dog. **(a)** Superimposition of the ribs and pulmonary vessels creates the impression of nodules. **(b)** These 'nodules' (arrowheads) are particularly visible in the caudodorsal thorax at the sixth, seventh and eighth ribs.

3.38 Dorsoplantar radiograph of the tarsus of a dog. Fine radiolucent lines (arrowed) are apparent where the abaxial and axial cortices of the third and fourth metatarsal bones respectively, overlap. These are Mach lines, which may be misinterpreted as fissure fractures. They are optical illusions that appear at the sharp boundaries between structures with large differences in opacity. A similar effect is produced when using computed or digital radiography systems (see Chapter 2) only the appearance is the result of image processing.

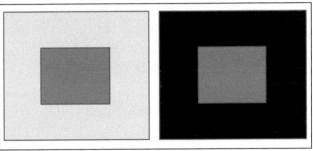

3.39 Effect of background on perceived opacity. The squares in the centre are of the same opacity, but the one on the right appears less opaque due to the darker background.

disappear by masking the area adjacent to a perceived fracture, then it is a Mach line. Masking removes the boundary between adjacent bright–dark structures and the veracity of the visible line is established. Mach lines are also responsible for the perception of pneumothorax where soft tissue folds are superimposed on the thorax. Other optical illusions include the effect of background opacity on the perceived opacity of a structure (Figure 3.39). Structures superimposed on a lighter background appear more opaque than those structures superimposed on a dark background.

Digital radiography: Digital images have the advantage of an inherently wide dynamic range, so the contrast and brightness of an image can be adjusted at the workstation to suit the tissue or organ being assessed. For conventional film, the linear region of the characteristic curve is smaller; therefore, the range of exposures which produce the same contrast in a diagnostic radiograph is limited, whereas the response of digital detectors is linear across a wider range of exposures. The linear region of the characteristic curve is in the order of 1–2 orders of magnitude for conventional film, whereas for digital film it is in the order of 5–10 orders of magnitude. This has the advantage of enabling suboptimal exposure choice to produce an image of diagnostic quality, although this should not be used as a substitute for selection of proper exposure factors (for further information, see Chapter 1).

Measurements

Many studies have reported definitive measurements for assessing organ dimensions on radiographs, including cardiac size, intestinal wall thickness, small intestinal loop diameter (serosa to serosa), prostate size, trachea to thoracic inlet ratio, and kidney size. However, the drawback is breed variation, particularly in dogs. Measurements should be used with care and in conjunction with the patient's clinicopathological data, rather than as definitive judgements. For example, the normal length of the cardiac silhouette is often described as less than two-thirds the height of the thorax with divergence of the trachea from the thoracic spine. This may be valid for breeds with an 'average' chest conformation, such as the Labrador Retriever, but for many normal small-breed dogs this ratio is often exceeded and the trachea never diverges. Deep-chested breeds, such as the Dobermann, may have marked cardiomegaly and not exceed this ratio or have tracheal elevation. The most common use of measurements is for comparison within the same patient, where several radiographic studies obtained at different times are available. One of the most practical examples of this application is monitoring cardiac size in a dog receiving treatment for heart disease. Specific methods of measurement are covered in the relevant chapters.

Anatomical comparison

The difficulty encountered with an approach in which the radiograph is compared with normal anatomy is the enormous difference in size, shape and configuration of almost all areas (skull, skeleton, thorax and abdomen) between dog breeds. This potentially creates an almost infinite set of possibilities for normal anatomy and is only partially overcome using consistent positioning and radiographic technique. Whilst there is generally less variation between breeds of cat, extremes do remain. These factors emphasize the necessity for a systematic search pattern and developing a sound familiarity with radiographic anatomy. Atlases of radiographic anatomy are available and some have examples of different breed types and shapes. The thorax, and therefore cardiac silhouette, of a deep-chested breed such as the Dobermann has a very different shape to that of a breed such as the Labrador Retriever, which has a more compact 'barrel-chested' thorax. The forelimbs of a Dachshund appear grossly abnormal if compared with those of a Border Collie. It is difficult and somewhat pointless to try and compare a radiograph of the skull of a Bulldog with an image of a normal skull of a Springer Spaniel in an anatomy atlas, so efforts must be made to build up a practice library of images of various different types of breed to enable easier comparison in the future.

Interpretive phase

Having decided upon the radiological abnormalities present, the radiologist/clinician should generate a list of possible differential diagnoses for each abnormality. These radiological differential diagnoses should be evaluated in conjunction with the signalment, history, clinical findings and results of other investigations to determine the clinical significance. A differential diagnosis list, ordered from most to least likely, should then be created. For example, if microhepatica is identified on abdominal radiographs from a dog, but there are no clinical signs of liver disease and liver enzyme concentrations and post-prandial bile acids are normal, then it is likely that the radiological findings are insignificant. A dog with hypercalcaemia and

a cranial mediastinal mass on radiography should have the differential diagnoses lymphoma and thymoma more highly ranked than mediastinal cyst.

If a number of radiological abnormalities have been identified, differential diagnoses that are common to all abnormalities should be placed higher up the differential diagnosis list. In many cases this 'consensus diagnosis' that ties all abnormalities together is the correct diagnosis. For example, an elderly dog with hepatomegaly and sublumbar lymphadenopathy (Röntgen sign: increase in size of the liver and sublumbar lymph nodes) may have hyperadrenocorticism and anal sac metastases to the sublumbar lymph nodes as the respective differential diagnoses, but infiltrative neoplasia (lymphoma) should be ranked higher as it is common to both differential diagnosis lists. Secondary ranked differential diagnoses may be important, particularly in older animals that more often have multiple diseases, to help identify the further imaging studies and clinical investigations required to narrow the list of differential diagnoses.

When creating a differential diagnosis list for the radiological abnormality identified, such as an abdominal soft tissue mass, the approach should be two-fold: the organ or tissue of origin and the nature of the mass (e.g. tumour, cyst, abscess, granuloma, haematoma) should be considered. It is rare for a definitive diagnosis to be made based on radiological appearance alone (e.g. a splenic mass may be a tumour or a haematoma, but the correct diagnosis can only be made with histopathology). Exceptions occur when the recognized Röntgen sign is pathognomonic, including:

- Ruptures or hernias (Röntgen sign: change in position of the herniated organs or change in contour of ruptured structure)
- Fractures (Röntgen sign: change in shape or contour) – but care should be taken to determine whether the fracture is traumatic or pathological.

Radiological interpretation should not be simplified into generating endless differential diagnosis lists, but an approach synthesizing and integrating the radiological findings with the clinicopathological data should be used. Differential diagnosis lists are most useful for ensuring possible diagnoses have not been overlooked once a radiological diagnosis has been reached. For example, if thoracic radiographs have been obtained to evaluate for pulmonary metastases in an elderly cat with oral squamous cell carcinoma, and a soft tissue mass is identified in the mediastinum cranial to the cardiac silhouette, then the differential diagnoses for the cranial mediastinal mass should include benign as well as neoplastic conditions. As mediastinal metastasis would be unusual with this presentation, the differential diagnosis list should reflect this analysis. Incidental cranial mediastinal cysts are uncommon, but not rare, in the older cat and should rank higher on the list, together with ectopic thyroid tissue and other neoplastic masses (thymoma and lymphoma). Other diagnostic tests, including ultrasonography and tissue sampling, are required to reach a definitive diagnosis in these cases (see Chapter 4). The clinician/radiologist should not be afraid to reconsider the differential diagnoses in the face of conflicting results from further tests or new information.

Radiological abnormalities should fit with the clinical findings, but it should be remembered that, based on probability, it is more likely that an unfamiliar radiological finding is an unusual manifestation of a common disease rather than representative of a rare disease. For example, Kartagener's Syndrome is a rare but well known inherited condition associated with bronchial ciliary dyskinesia and situs inversus; however, before reaching this diagnosis, correct placement of the positional markers should be verified as well as the position of the stomach and spleen, as it is more likely that the film has been incorrectly labelled.

The analytical phase of radiographic interpretation takes the longest to develop. Guidelines published in textbooks often imply a degree of certainty in diagnosis that is impossible to achieve from radiography alone. It should always be remembered that there is a large overlap between normal and abnormal. Many 'abnormalities' are not associated with clinical signs and, equally, in many diseases there are no radiological abnormalities. The magnitude of diagnostic error rates in veterinary radiology is not known, but factors that influence it include the diagnostic quality of radiographs, the quality of teaching or experience, and the subtlety of the lesions.

Radiological report

Creating a written report should be an integral part of every radiological interpretation. The radiological report is an important part of the clinical notes and for each patient the date of the study, the region imaged and the views obtained should be recorded. Radiographs can be lost, even with a digital Picture Archiving and Communications System (PACS), and a written report within the clinical notes ensures that some record of the radiological findings is retained. Medical audio transcription software is available but time needs to be invested to achieve consistent coherent results.

Purpose and content of the report

The radiological description should include sufficient detail to enable someone to view the radiograph and see what the original observer was describing, without the original observer being present to point it out. The report should focus on the most important findings (Figure 3.40). Use of the Röntgen sign terminology enables an accurate description of the radiological changes to be given. Structures considered to be normal should be mentioned to confirm that

they have been evaluated. All abnormalities should be listed and prioritized in terms of likely significance. The report should also suggest appropriate differential diagnoses and suitable further investigations (e.g. further diagnostic imaging studies, endoscopy and biopsy).

Terminology

Anatomical and radiographic terminology must be consistent. Standard directional terms should be used: cranial and caudal for the trunk, neck and limbs proximal to the carpus and tarsus, and dorsal and palmar or plantar used for the distal limbs.

Radiographic views

Views should be named according to the direction of the primary beam, taking into account the direction of entry and exit through the body region.

- For a mediolateral view, the medial aspect of the limb faces the X-ray tube with the lateral aspect of the limb resting on the cassette.
- For a VD view of the thorax, the animal is placed in dorsal recumbency with the sternum facing toward the X-ray tube.
- Oblique views, where the X-ray beam enters the body at an angle to one of the usual directions (mediolateral, craniocaudal, DV), should include (where possible) the angle of obliquity (e.g. dorso 45 degrees lateral–palmaromedial oblique, D45°L–PaMO). Small animals are often rotated using positioning aids, such as foam wedges, to enable oblique views to be taken. These views are most useful for the skull (e.g. when imaging the tympanic bullae or temporomandibular joints) and limbs (particularly when imaging the metacarpal or metatarsal bones), to try and overcome the superimposition encountered on a true lateral view.

When describing lateral views of the thorax and abdomen, the convention in the UK is to describe the position of the animal, rather than the direction of the primary beam (i.e. 'right lateral' or, more descriptively, 'right lateral recumbent' view). Although differences in radiographic anatomy usually allow views to be recognized retrospectively, it is important to identify which lateral views have been taken as occasionally this may be of diagnostic significance (e.g. when localizing the lesion to a specific lung lobe) or may be valuable when comparing radiographs from serial studies. More than two views may be required of some areas, such as the limbs or skull, to remove superimposition of overlying structures (oblique views) and identify dynamic instability (stressed views of joints).

Colloquial terms

Many colloquial terms have found their way into the radiological vocabulary, either as descriptive terms for reporting findings or for defining interpretive strategies and errors. Care should be taken when using these terms in a report. The term 'gravel sign', for example, is used to describe a collection of particulate mineralized material within the gastrointestinal tract, proximal (or orad) to a lesion causing chronic partial intestinal obstruction. It is acceptable to use the term in this setting, but use of the term to describe any collection of mineralized material is inappropriate.

- Identify subject (if not part of a known clinical record, note the species, breed/type, age and gender) and record date of study, region imaged and views obtained. Record whether any contrast studies were performed
- Appraise radiographic quality (centring, collimation to area of interest/film, exposure, processing, labelling and artefacts)
- Assess radiological findings (Röntgen signs)
- Develop list of differential diagnoses for each sign
- Integrate knowledge from the signalment, history, clinical findings and other tests to refine diagnoses
- Suggest further investigations if diagnosis not definitive

3.40 Contents of a radiological report.

Limitations of radiography

Radiography has inherently poor specificity and sensitivity for many diseases. The absence of abnormalities on a radiograph does not equate with normal; if none of the Röntgen signs are altered by pathology, then abnormalities will not be detected. In addition, there is an enormous amount of individual variation and great overlap between a normal organ and a mildly (structurally) affected abnormal organ. In addition, abnormalities that are detected on a radiograph may be due to previous disease or may not be clinically significant. Disease states are rarely static and for changes identified on an image, of which the significance is unknown, repeat or serial radiography performed after a period of time will provide additional information, based on the assumption that significant findings will usually have altered.

Even when present, radiographic change indicates structural or anatomical change in an organ, tissue or structure, but plain radiography rarely provides information on function. Exceptions include complete bone fractures or gastric dilatation–volvulus, when it is obvious that the affected structure will no longer function normally. The identification of cardiomegaly on a radiograph provides no information about cardiac function and, equally, a normal sized heart can be in failure; however, evidence of pulmonary venous congestion or a perihilar alveolar pattern indicating pulmonary oedema allows a diagnosis of congestive heart failure to be made. Serial radiographs are very useful to monitor the degree of failure and the response to treatment.

Since a radiograph is a 2D representation of a 3D object, it provides a composite image of a region with superimposition of all structures and tissues included in the field of view. Cross-sectional imaging modalities (such as CT and ultrasonography) allow more detailed assessment of individual organs without superimposition. In addition, CT and magnetic resonance imaging (MRI) can demonstrate exquisite contrast in regions not well served by radiography, such as the brain and spinal cord. However, the resolution of film–screen radiography is superior to that of CT and MRI and is excellent at providing an overview of large regions of the body, such as the thorax and abdomen, as well as structural information with particular regard to the skeletal system.

Further investigations

Repeat radiography

Serial radiographic studies can be very useful. Previous films from a patient, where available, should always be reviewed alongside current studies. Interpretation is aided by comparing similar views, preferably side-by-side on the light box or monitor. Some radiological findings may be more (or less) significant, depending on how they have altered over time. Equally, if the findings are equivocal, it may be worth repeating films after a period of time. Disease states are dynamic and the appearance of a disease will alter over time (disease in transition). For example, a dog developing congestive heart failure will initially show just pulmonary venous congestion, which, if left untreated, will progress to interstitial oedema (visible on the radiograph as an increased interstitial pattern in the lungs) before progressing to true pulmonary oedema (visible as an alveolar pattern).

The time interval between serial studies varies according to the area of interest; when assessing gastrointestinal distension it may be appropriate to repeat radiographs after only a few hours, whereas when assessing more slowly progressive lesions, such as long bone changes, there is little point in repeating radiographs within 2–3 weeks of the initial examination.

Serial radiography can also be used to monitor the response to treatment, particularly in cases with suspected heart failure, bronchopneumonia, lung contusion and pleural effusion. In most dogs with pulmonary oedema due to congestive heart failure, if an alveolar or interstitial pattern is detected on the initial radiographs, reduction in the severity of the pattern should occur within a few hours of administration of appropriate diuretic treatment. Failure of the alveolar pattern to decrease in severity should alert the clinician to revisit their diagnosis and treatment (perhaps alter the diuretic or consider other differential diagnoses for the alveolar pattern such as pneumonia, haemorrhage or neoplasia).

If findings are equivocal, additional radiographs may be taken to try and clarify the situation. This is particularly useful in the musculoskeletal system, when radiography of the contralateral limb often provides information as to whether the finding is an artefact or a normal anatomical variation (such as a nutrient canal or a separate centre of ossification). However, it should be remembered that some diseases can be bilaterally symmetrical, such as carpal hyperextension or elbow dysplasia. In these cases, clinical examination should differentiate bilateral pathology from an anatomical variant.

Other diagnostic tests

It is uncommon for any imaging modality to provide a definitive diagnosis. Generally, a list of differential diagnoses can be generated which, when considered with other clinical data, can assist in suggesting the most likely diagnosis. Frequently, further investigations are required in order to achieve a definitive diagnosis. If the abnormality is a gross structural change (e.g. an ectopic ureter, portosystemic shunt or mitral valve dysplasia) then further imaging studies such as radiographic contrast studies or ultrasonography will provide the diagnosis. For other presentations, such as the radiological diagnosis of generalized hepatomegaly, the list of differential diagnoses cannot be refined further, even following ultrasonography, and the clinician must recognize the limitations of imaging studies and that a definitive diagnosis can only be determined by obtaining a representative tissue sample.

The radiological report should include suggestions for further diagnostic tests, such as ultrasonography, cerebrospinal fluid (CSF) analysis, dynamic endocrine tests or biopsy. The considerable improvement in equipment and the skills of the clinician has led to ultrasonography superseding or completely replacing abdominal radiography. Ultrasonography and radiography both have advantages and disadvantages (Figure 3.41) but are complementary techniques. Misdiagnosis and missed diagnoses may occur with both techniques and, reassuringly, both may provide the same answer where there is doubt (Figure 3.42).

Parameter	Radiography	Ultrasonography
Cardiac disease	Demonstrates pulmonary venous congestion or oedema in left-sided congestive heart failure	Demonstrates venous congestion in right-sided congestive heart failure. Excellent for defining structural changes in cardiac disease. Allows rapid assessment for pericardial fluid and mass lesions
Respiratory disease	Defines the distribution and pattern	Limited value for general assessment of pulmonary disease unless consolidation or infiltrate is extensive. Used for focused evaluation of masses or infiltrate identified on radiographs
Gastrointestinal disease	Identifies gastric torsion and radiopaque foreign bodies	Identifies wall thickening and mass lesions more reliably than radiography
Free gas in the abdomen or thorax	More reliable than ultrasonography; positional radiography invaluable	Experience required to recognize free gas
Free fluid	Small volumes easily overlooked	Rapidly identified
Lesion localization	Provides a general overview and targets for the ultrasound examination	Significant lesions easily identified. Localizes changes to specific organs or viscera. Internal structure of organs and viscera can be assessed. Integrity of the body wall, diaphragm and bladder easily overlooked or significance under-interpreted
Multiple lesions	Valuable for general overview and identifying skeletal involvement	Valuable for identifying lesions for which no radiological changes or abnormal Röntgen signs are evident
Other	Contrast studies demonstrate the location and integrity of viscera, ureteral ectopia and duct obstruction (e.g. lacrimal duct)	Ultrasound-guided aspiration of lesions or therapeutic drainage of effusions

3.41   Comparison of the uses of radiography and ultrasonography.

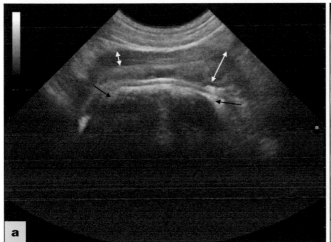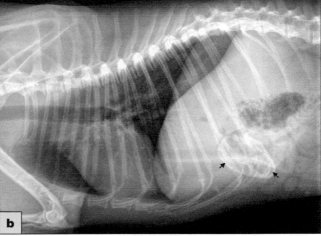

3.42   **(a)** Ultrasonogram and **(b)** right lateral radiograph of the abdomen of a dog with marked weight loss and chronic vomiting. (a) Foreign material (black arrows), creating distal shadowing, was identified within the stomach on the ultrasonographic study, but the amorphous shape and strong shadowing limit a confident assessment of the extent and significance of the material. The white arrows denote the stomach wall. (b) The radiographic study confirms the ultrasonographic findings and that the foreign material (arrowed) is radiopaque and of such size to be clinically significant. A large mass of plastic material was removed at gastrotomy and the clinical signs resolved. (Courtesy of Mandeville Veterinary Hospital)

Errors in interpretation

Errors in radiology are common and often multifactorial, and may involve problems with radiographic technique, evaluation of the radiograph and interpretation of any findings. Clinical audit and following up the outcome of cases, along with correlating radiological findings with other information such as surgical findings, are important in recognizing radiological errors.

Search errors
Search errors occur when the observer fails to spot a lesion as a consequence of not evaluating the whole film.

- Missing the lesion during the visual search of the radiograph. This is usually due to lack of experience (failure to assess all areas of the radiograph; peripheral lesions in particular are easily overlooked) and unfamiliarity with normal radiographic anatomy (Figure 3.43). It cannot be emphasized enough that abnormalities can only be identified when the normal radiographic appearance is known and can be recognized.
- Failing to complete the search when the 'answer' is found. The observer is satisfied based on finding an abnormality and review of the film is stopped. For example, in the case shown in Figure 3.44, pleural fluid is recognized as the cause of the

dyspnoea, but the cause of the pleural fluid (a destructive rib lesion) can also be identified if the search is completed and not terminated early.
■ Becoming distracted by obvious but less significant findings, such as pulmonary heterotopic bone in a coughing dog, when the mineral opacities are obvious due to their radiopacity but of no clinical significance.

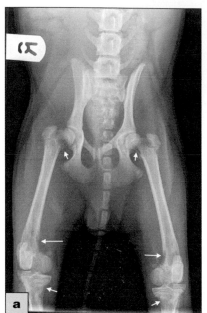
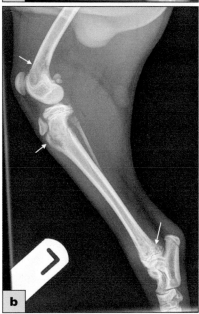

3.43 **(a)** VD radiograph of the pelvis and **(b)** mediolateral radiograph of the right stifle of a 16-week-old puppy with pyrexia, lethargy and reluctance to move. Neurological disease was suspected and radiographs of the spine (including the pelvis) were obtained. Close scrutiny of the pelvis revealed irregular areas of lysis within the proximal and distal metaphyses of both the left and right femur. A full survey of the appendicular skeleton revealed similar changes in other metaphyses (arrowed), including the proximal and distal tibia. The changes are consistent with metaphyseal osteomyelitis (an aggressive haematogenous osteomyelitis). Two important radiographic principles are demonstrated in this case: firstly, all areas of the radiograph were assessed, allowing the peripheral lesions to be recognized, and secondly, the metaphyseal lesions must be differentiated from the normal appearance of the physes in a dog of this age.

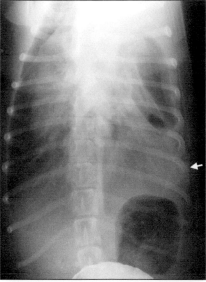
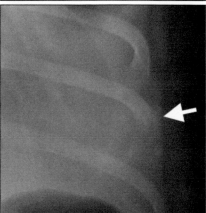

3.44 DV thoracic radiograph of a dog with dyspnoea. A cursory examination of the film reveals pleural fluid; however, a thorough search reveals a left thoracic wall lesion (destruction of the tenth rib; arrowed), which is the likely cause of the pleural effusion.

■ Overlooking the absence of a normal structure (e.g. retroflexed or ruptured bladder, reduced liver size due to herniation).
■ Missing lesions in overexposed areas as a result of not using a bright light, masking any uncovered areas of the light box or suboptimal viewing conditions (see Figure 3.1).
■ Failing to evaluate fully regions of complex anatomy or with marked superimposition.
  • Lesions in the mediastinum obscured by superimposition of the sternum and spine on DV/VD views of the thorax are easily overlooked.
  • Intestinal content (gas and mineral opacities) superimposed on VD views of the lumbar spine and sacrum can mimic or obscure lesions involving the vertebrae.
  • The numerous bones, air-filled cavities, dentition and soft tissue structures (such as ear folds) of the skull represent an area of complex anatomy and superimposition. Lesions, both small and large, are easily overlooked.
■ Overreliance on pattern recognition (or 'radiology snap'). It can be tempting to use pattern recognition to make a diagnosis based on a radiograph having a similar appearance to one

previously examined. However, different diseases frequently have a similar radiological appearance, such as pneumonia, *Angiostrongylus* infection and pulmonary oedema. In addition, it is impossible to remember the appearance of every disease, and a disease not previously encountered will not be recognized. It is far better to use a systematic approach with Röntgen signs and to develop differential diagnosis lists for each abnormality detected.

Search errors can be avoided by adopting a methodical approach to every film and using a bright light to evaluate any overexposed areas of film. Multiple structures such as the ribs or vertebrae are often overlooked, particularly when viewing the thorax or abdomen. The ribs and vertebrae should be routinely counted to ensure that these areas are closely examined. Some clinicians find that changing the orientation of the radiograph (e.g. rotating a lateral view of the thorax and viewing it with the cranial end at the top of the light box) aids in remembering to assess the whole film. On computer monitors, the digital image greyscale can be inverted to create an image similar to that seen with fluoroscopy or Polaroid X-ray film, projecting bones as black and air as white, which may help to ensure that no structure is overlooked.

Judgement or analysis errors

Judgement errors represent flawed reasoning or failure to correctly integrate data. An experienced clinician should also have an excellent knowledge of physiology and pathophysiology to avoid judgement errors. Experience should lead to fewer errors in judgement, but it can be difficult to eradicate them all. Continued critical reflection and comparison of definitive diagnoses (based on histopathological findings) with radiological diagnoses, and discussion with specialists, should help reduce judgement errors. Judgement errors can be broadly divided into three groups:

- Under-reading
- Over-reading
- Faulty reasoning.

Under-reading

Under-reading is when a significant lesion is either not seen (i.e. search errors) or erroneously classified as being of no significance.

- Failure to recognize a lesion due to poor radiographic quality or technique. Limitations of the radiographic technique (Figure 3.45) should be recognized. Contributing factors that lead to lesions being overlooked include rushing the assessment, failing to evaluate all films, overexposed films and poor viewing conditions. Even large lesions may be missed if image quality is poor.
- Lack of knowledge. Under-reading may occur due to deficits in knowledge or lack of experience with certain conditions. For example, an emphysematous pattern within a consolidated lung lobe accompanied by pleural fluid is highly

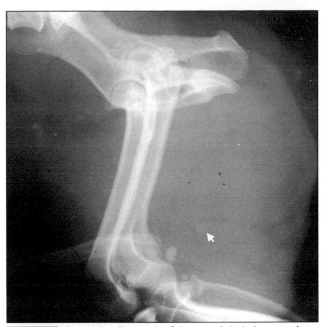

3.45 Lateral radiograph of the caudal abdomen of a male dog. There is an ill defined mineral opacity (arrowed) superimposed on the soft tissues caudal to the os penis. This may be considered a displaced fabella or an artefact, but was confirmed as an urethral calculus. Calculi and other lesions within the penile urethra may be overlooked if the pelvis is not included when imaging male dogs presenting with signs of lower tract disease. An additional view with the hindlimbs pulled forward should be obtained for a complete assessment of the urethra.

suggestive of lung lobe torsion, but those clinicians less familiar with these radiographic features may not realize their significance. These errors are associated with uncommon or rare conditions. These errors become less common with time as, with increased experience, the clinician is more likely to be familiar with the changes.

- Committing to a diagnosis before performing the radiographic study. It is essential to avoid preconceived ideas regarding the diagnosis to prevent the temptation to try and match radiographic changes to a likely diagnosis (Figure 3.46). For example, in anticipation of a diagnosis of bronchopneumonia in a coughing dog with pyrexia, lung changes may be interpreted as an inflammatory infiltrate, overlooking features which point to the presence of a nodular lung pattern. This is one of the reasons why some radiologists prefer to examine radiographs without the relevant history to begin with, to avoid being persuaded along a certain path. The radiographic study should always advance the diagnostic investigation. The differential diagnosis list generated before the radiographic study should be revisited once the findings have been identified and compared with clinical expectations.
- Interpreting a certain combination of radiological findings as indicating a specific diagnosis (e.g. always diagnosing effusion in the stifle as cruciate ligament rupture, although other differential diagnoses could include haemarthrosis, polyarthritis or septic arthritis). This is an

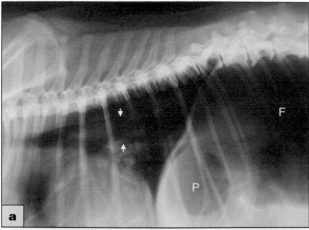

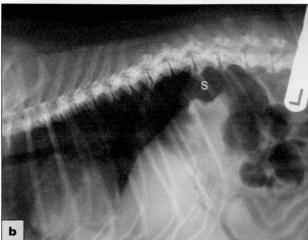

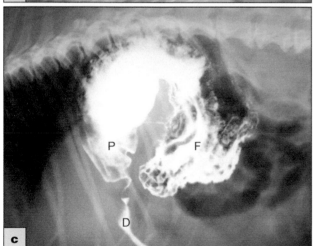

3.46 **(a)** Right and **(b)** left lateral thoracic radiographs and **(c)** left lateral barium gastrogram of a Cavalier King Charles Spaniel receiving treatment for congestive heart failure. Recent unproductive coughing and retching unresponsive to further diuresis was reported. (a–b) Radiography was performed but not considered to demonstrate pulmonary congestion. On review of the radiographs, dilatation of the caudal oesophagus (arrowed) was noted. The body of the stomach (F) is dilated with air, as is the pylorus (P); the latter is an abnormal finding on the right lateral view. On the left lateral view, the stomach has an abnormal C-shape with caudal rotation of the body and fundus (S). (c) Barium administration confirmed a chronic gastric torsion. This case emphasizes the importance of evaluating all parts of the film, correlating the radiograph with clinical expectations and the value of reviewing the films. D = duodenum. (Courtesy of Frean and Smyth Veterinary Surgeons)

approach with which many radiologists are familiar and is termed the 'Aunt Minnie' approach to radiological diagnosis. The analogy compares recognition of incontrovertible radiological features associated with a particular condition to one's absolute familiarity with family members, in this case a favourite aunt, the eponymous 'Aunt Minnie'. However, there are few classic radiological signs which are regarded as so specific and typical of a condition that when they are recognized no other differential diagnosis need be considered. The approach can lead to the observer focusing on more obvious findings, under-reading the film by suspending the search early, and committing to a single diagnosis whilst excluding plausible alternatives.

- Failing to revisit the differential diagnosis list in the face of new evidence. The differential diagnoses should be reassessed if additional information becomes available. For example, survey thoracic radiography may reveal generalized cardiomegaly, leading to a differential diagnosis list including cardiac disease and pericardial effusion. However, if abdominal radiographs subsequently demonstrate a small liver, the possibility of a diaphragmatic defect with herniation of the liver into the pericardial sac should be considered, resulting in the addition of peritoneo-pericardial diaphragmatic hernia to the list of differential diagnoses.

Over-reading

Over-reading is the diagnosis of an abnormality when none exists. Attributing greater significance to a lesion or faulty reasoning are common errors. The inexperienced clinician is prone to this error of judgement, perhaps due to the false expectation that most radiographs will demonstrate a significant finding.

Misinterpretation of normal anatomy: Misinterpretation of normal anatomy for pathology (Figure 3.47) is probably the most common judgement error.

- Failing to identify breed variations as normal. Some findings considered normal in certain dog breeds may be considered to represent

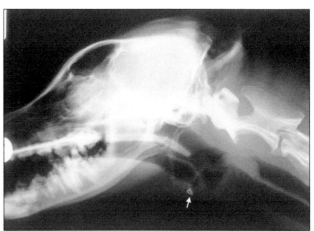

3.47 Lateral view of the skull of a dog. The basihyoid bone (arrowed) can be seen as a relatively radiopaque structure ventral to the tip of the epiglottis. It can be confused with a foreign body.

pathological changes in other breeds (see above). Hence, familiarity with the variation in radiographic appearance between breeds is an essential component of meaningful interpretation. Examples of breed variations include:
- Rounded heart shape in barrel-chested dogs may be mistaken for cardiomegaly
- An upright, narrow heart shape in deep-chested dogs may be mistaken for hypovolaemia
- Short, curved legs in chondrodystrophoid breeds may be mistaken for growth abnormalities
- A relatively narrow trachea in brachycephalic breeds may be mistaken for tracheal collapse
- A widened mediastinum in Bulldogs may be mistaken for a mediastinal mass.
- Mistaking end-on pulmonary blood vessels for pulmonary nodules.
- Misinterpreting retraction of the lung lobes in obese animals (usually dogs) for retraction of the lung lobes from the periphery of the thorax due to pleural effusion.
- Misinterpreting poor serosal detail associated with young or emaciated animals for peritoneal fluid.
- Over-interpreting intestinal wall thickness on plain radiographs (Figure 3.48).
- Over-interpreting pulmonary patterns seen on digital films. The logarithms used for digital images result in sharper definition of the bronchial walls, thoracic vascular structures and pulmonary markings compared with analogue films. This should not be misinterpreted as disease.
- Misinterpreting pericardial fat for right-sided heart enlargement on DV views.
- Misinterpreting intra-abdominal fat with the small intestines gathered in the centre of the abdomen in the cat for a linear foreign body (despite the expectation that an abnormal gas pattern and plicated intestine would be present).

- Over-interpreting a poor contrast study (Figure 3.49). Improper patient preparation and retention of faeces can result in indentation of the bladder wall, which may be mistaken for a filling defect due to a bladder wall mass.
- Mistaking a nutrient canal for a long bone fracture.
- Mistaking ossification centres for avulsion fracture fragments (C1–C2).

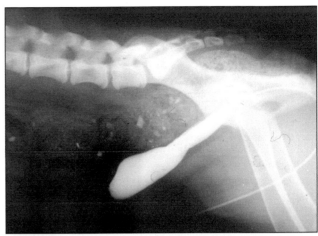

3.49 Lateral abdominal radiograph of a male dog following positive-contrast cystography. The bladder is poorly filled with contrast medium. There has been inadequate patient preparation as the colon is still filled with a large volume of faeces. The quality of this study is poor and the resulting artefacts might be misinterpreted as a structural abnormality of the bladder.

Classification of an incidental finding as a significant abnormality:

- Mistaking incidental pulmonary heterotopic bone for metastatic pulmonary nodules (Figure 3.50).
- Mistaking incidental omental/mesenteric fat necrosis for a clinically significant mineralized abdominal mass.

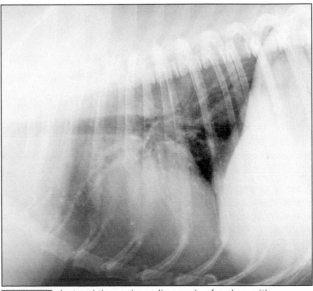

3.50 Lateral thoracic radiograph of a dog with multiple small mineral opacity nodules throughout the lung fields. These are consistent with pulmonary heterotopic bone and should not be mistaken for metastatic disease.

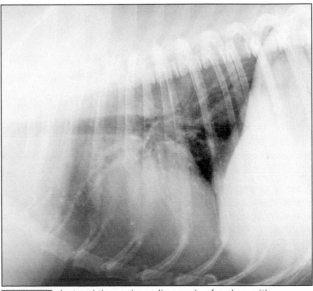

3.48 Lateral abdominal radiograph of a dog showing apparently thickened small intestinal walls (arrowed) highlighted by gas within the lumen. This artefact is commonly misinterpreted as pathology. The appearance is caused by the fluid contents of the small intestine silhouetting with the walls, with a gas cap on top, creating apparent wall thickening. Intestinal wall thickness should only be measured after contrast medium administration or with ultrasonography.

Mistaking artefacts for pathology:

■ The effect of radiographic technique (underexposure), poor inflation of the lungs (Figure 3.51) and obesity may result in increased lung opacity. This can resemble disease where none is actually present, or appear more dramatic than, and obscure, the changes produced by the underlying pathology.

■ Deviation of the intrathoracic trachea due to flexion of the head and neck or rotation of the thorax on DV views could result in the mistaken diagnosis of a cranial mediastinal or heart base mass. Retraction and flexion of the forelimbs with superimposition of the triceps muscles on the cranial thorax can contribute to this appearance.

■ Mach lines may be misinterpreted.

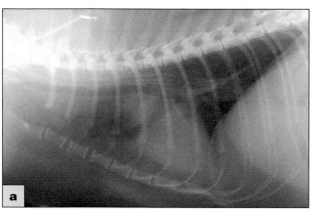

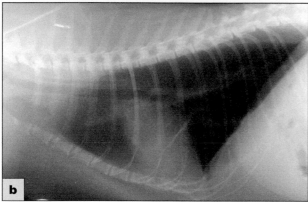

3.51 Lateral thoracic radiographs of a cat: **(a)** expiratory and **(b)** inspiratory views. (a) On the expiratory view, pleural fluid and possibly even a cranial mediastinal mass might be suspected. In addition, any pathological changes in the lungs would not be detected. (b) The inspiratory view shows a normal thorax. Poor inflation is usually considered to be a technical error in larger patients, but these images demonstrate that this artefact may also occur in the cat.

Faulty reasoning

Faulty reasoning leads to incorrect conclusions and differential diagnoses, and often involves aspects of one or more interpretive errors. The lesion may be correctly identified but incorrectly localized, leading to faulty reasoning and inappropriate differential diagnoses. For example, a large mass lesion arising from a rib within the cranial thorax may be mistaken for a mediastinal mass if the clinician fails to recognize the involvement of the rib. The differential diagnosis list created as a result of incorrect conclusions may lead to inappropriate management of the patient.

Common mistakes

Lateral thoracic radiograph of a dog with lobar pneumonia that has been used in undergraduate teaching to demonstrate common mistakes made in interpretation. The same mistakes are consistently made. The absence of air-filled lung over the cardiac silhouette is overlooked (unfamiliarity with normal radiographic appearance). The prominent mineral opacities superimposed over the cardiac silhouette (most likely to be incidental aortic or coronary mineralization) are noted and the search is terminated. The air-filled bronchus seen coursing dorsoventrally across the cardiac silhouette is identified, but described as being a coronary artery (erroneous interpretation of opacities).

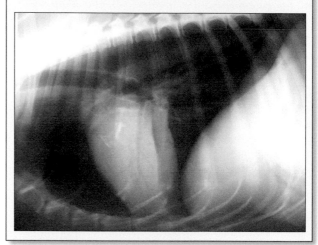

Summary

To summarize, good radiological interpretation only comes with practice and relies upon:

■ Recognizing the importance of a high quality, complete radiographic study
■ Understanding the significance of the different radiographic opacities
■ Acquiring excellent knowledge of radiographic anatomy
■ Performing a thorough review of the radiograph
■ Being able to identify deviations from the normal
■ Integrating the findings with clinical knowledge to advance the investigation of the patient.

In human trauma radiography, these principles are usually summarized as the 'rules of two' (Figure 3.52), which apply equally to veterinary patients.

■ Two views – one view is one view too few. Obtain the opposite lateral or an orthogonal view
■ Two joints – include joints above and below a long bone
■ Two sides – compare with the other side (for paired and symmetrical structures)
■ Two abnormalities – look for a second abnormality. More than one disease may be present or an underlying cause evident elsewhere
■ Two animals – compare anatomy with normal control of similar breed and age

3.52 'Rules of two'. (Modified from Chan and Touquet (2007) with permission from the publisher (continues) ▶

- Two occasions   compare current radiographs with previous films (for pulmonary and cardiac disease, and bone healing)
- Two films – repeat the study after a procedure (postoperative film) or therapy (thoracic films)
- Two opinions – ask a colleague or specialist for a second opinion
- Two records – record clinical and radiographic findings
- Two modalities – radiography complements other imaging modalities

3.52 (continued) 'Rules of two'. (Modified from Chan and Touquet (2007) with permission from the publisher

References and further reading

Alexander K (2010) Reducing error in radiographic interpretation. *Canadian Veterinary Journal* **51(5)**, 533–536

Berry CR and Thrall DE (2007) Introduction to radiographic interpretation. In: *Textbook of Diagnostic Radiology, 5th edn*, ed. DE Thrall, pp. 78–92. Elsevier, St. Louis

Brook OR, O'Connell AM, Thornton E *et al.* (2010) Anatomy and pathophysiology of errors occurring in clinical radiology practice. *Radiographics* **30**, 1401–1410

Chan O and Touquet R (2007) General principles: how to interpret radiographs. In: *ABC of Emergency Radiology, 2nd edn*, ed. O Chan, pp. 5–12. Wiley Blackwell, Oxford

Chasen PH (2001) Practical application of Mach band theory in thoracic analysis. *Radiology* **210**, 596–610

Coulson A and Lewis ND (2008) *An Atlas of Interpretative Radiographic Anatomy of the Dog and Cat, 2nd edn*. Wiley Blackwell, Oxford

Cruz R (2008) Digital radiography, image archiving and image display: practical tips. *Canadian Veterinary Journal* **49**, 1122–1123

Doubilet P and Herman PG (1981) Interpretation of radiographs: effect of clinical history. *Radiology* **17(1)**, 1055–1058

Drost WT (2011) Transitioning to digital radiography. *Journal of Veterinary Emergency and Critical Care* **21(2)**, 137–143

Drost WT, Reese DJ and Hornof WJ (2008) Digital radiography artifacts. *Veterinary Radiology & Ultrasound* **49**, S48–S56

Griscom NT (2002) A suggestion: look at the images first, before you read the history. *Radiology* **223**, 9–10

Jimenez DA, Armbrust LJ, O'Brien RT and Biller DS (2008) Artifacts in digital radiography. *Veterinary Radiology & Ultrasound* **49**, 321–332

Lamb CR, Parry AT, Baines EA and Chang Y (2010) Does changing the orientation of a thoracic radiograph aid diagnosis of rib fractures? *Veterinary Radiology & Ultrasound* **52(1)**, 75–78

Lamb CR, Pfeiffer DU and Mantis P (2007) Errors in radiographic interpretation made by veterinary students. *Journal of Veterinary Medical Education* **34(2)**, 157–159

Puchalski SM (2008) Image display. *Veterinary Radiology & Ultrasound* **49**, S9–S13

Robinson PJA (1997) Radiology's Achilles' heel: error and variation in the interpretation of the Röntgen image. *The British Journal of Radiology* **70**, 1085–1098

Contrast radiography

Andrew Holloway

The limitation of plain radiographic studies is that many structures or organs have similar soft tissue opacity. Contrast media are used to address this lack of inherent contrast by selectively absorbing more X-ray photons than the soft tissues and appearing white, or transmitting more X-ray photons than the soft tissues and appearing black. Contrast media with a radiographic density different to that of the soft tissues can be introduced into blood vessels, viscera, cavities, joints or the thecal sac. The information gained from contrast studies relates to anatomy (size, shape, position, margination, internal detail), integrity and to some extent, directly and indirectly, function. Despite the widespread availability of diagnostic ultrasonography and cross-sectional imaging techniques, contrast radiographic procedures remain relevant. To obtain the maximum amount of information from contrast procedures, the objective, technique and interpretation of each study should be understood.

Types of contrast media

Contrast media should ideally:

- Attenuate the X-ray beam differently to soft tissues
- Be non-irritant and non-toxic
- Define the organ or viscus being investigated
- Persist for a time sufficiently long enough to be demonstrated on radiographs
- Be eliminated from the body.

Negative contrast agents

Negative contrast agents are gases. They are useful because they have a very low physical density and therefore appear radiolucent. Room air is the most commonly used negative contrast agent; however, fatal air embolism may occur. Carbon dioxide and nitrous oxide are occasionally used, as they are more soluble in the blood and thus safer than room air or oxygen. Negative contrast agents provide poor mucosal detail and are often used to define the location of a viscus rather than obtain detailed anatomical information.

Positive contrast agents

Positive contrast agents are media that have a high atomic number and attenuate the X-ray beam more within the viscus, organ or cavity into which they have been introduced than do adjacent structures. Positive contrast media appear more opaque than the surrounding tissue. The most commonly used agents are barium (atomic number = 56) and iodine (atomic number = 53).

Barium

Barium sulphate is used only in gastrointestinal studies.

- It is a chemically inert heavy metal and therefore is insoluble (i.e. is not absorbed or digested). It does not dissociate but remains particulate. Most dogs tolerate the administration of barium by stomach tube or with food (most barium preparations are palatable). Cats tolerate the administration of barium less well. Barium sulphate may have a therapeutic effect in animals with diarrhoea by coating and protecting the inflamed mucosa. Constipation is a possible side-effect.
- Following oral administration, aspiration of barium into the bronchi and lungs may occur (Figure 4.1), particularly in animals with swallowing disorders, laryngeal paralysis or in the struggling patient. When barium is to be administered by stomach tube, a small volume of water should be passed through the tube first. If a cough is elicited, the tube is incorrectly placed in the trachea and must be removed and replaced. Aspiration of a small amount of barium is not usually a concern as it is inert and with time (months to years) the lungs and bronchi will clear. Coughing usually clears most of the barium. Aspirated barium is phagocytosed by macrophages and can be seen in the local tracheobronchial lymph nodes many months to years after the event. The significance of aspirated barium usually relates to the volume and whether gastric contents are present in the aspirated material. The latter may lead to bacterial infection and aspiration pneumonia. Acute aspiration of a large volume of barium should be managed by positioning the animal head down and attempting to clear the aspirated material from the alveoli

(e.g. via coupage or inducing coughing). Aspiration of hyperosmolar iodinated contrast agents (see below) is more of a clinical concern as they can lead to pulmonary oedema.

- Leakage of barium into the mediastinum or peritoneum leads to granulomatous mediastinitis and peritonitis, respectively, with adhesions and fibrosis. Where possible, the body cavity should be decontaminated and flushed to remove as much of the leaked material as possible.
- A barium study should not be performed <24 hours before endoscopy.

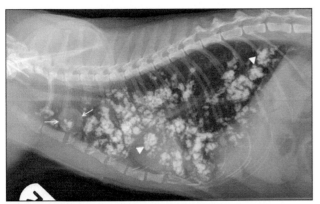

4.1 Lateral radiograph of the thorax of a cat. Aspirated barium (arrowheads) within the alveoli of the lungs results in multiple coalescing, markedly opaque patches in all lung lobes. This radiograph was obtained many years after aspiration. The discrete, round, soft tissue opacity in the cranial mediastinum (a mediastinal cyst, arrowed) is an incidental finding.

Preparations: Barium sulphate is available in the following preparations (Figure 4.2):

- Colloidal suspension – administered by stomach tube, syringe or mixed with food. Used for swallowing and oesophageal studies, gastric and small intestinal tract studies and occasionally as an enema to evaluate the colon. Colloidal suspensions should be shaken before use. Prepared effervescent solutions (e.g. Baritop 100) are widely used but should be mixed well to avoid artefacts created by gas bubbles
- Paste for pharyngeal and oesophageal (ulceration) studies
- Powders are available, but clumping of the barium may occur, which can reduce the quality of the study unless it is well mixed
- Barium impregnated spheres (BIPS) – these are capsules containing small (1.5 mm diameter) and large (5 mm diameter) spheres impregnated with barium (Figure 4.3):
  - They can be administered without food
  - They can potentially be used to evaluate for obstruction or to assess gastrointestinal motility and intestinal transit times
  - The information gained about transit times and bowel patency is not specific. Interpretation of findings where the spheres are spread throughout the bowel or with partial obstructions can be difficult. Furthermore, as the bowel is not distended with contrast media, no information about wall thickness or the mucosa is available

Formulation	Trade name	Comments
100% w/v suspension	Baritop 100	300 ml can
100% w/v liquid barium suspension 105% w/v liquid barium suspension	Polibar	1900 ml
60% w/v liquid barium suspension	Liquid EZ-Paque	1900 ml
Barium impregnated polyethylene spheres	BIPS	Large (5 mm diameter) and small (1.5 mm diameter) combined in capsules
Barium sulphate powder	Barium sulphate BP	500 g

4.2 Commonly used barium contrast media. Trade names given are examples.

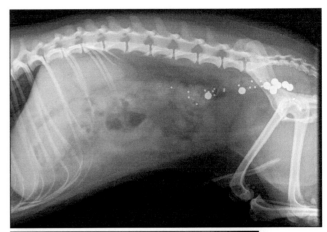

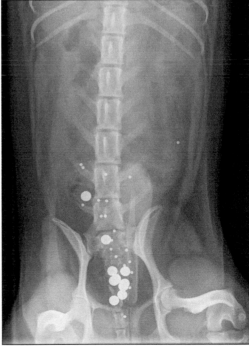

4.3 BIPS. The small and large spheres have collected within the colon 24 hours after administration, ruling out complete obstruction. This, together with the normal diameter of the small intestinal loops, indicates that complete obstruction cannot be present and partial obstruction is unlikely. The BIPS do not provide any information about intestinal wall thickness or mucosal integrity.

- One practical use is in animals suspected by the owner to have ingested a foreign body when neither the clinical examination nor survey radiographs support a diagnosis of obstruction. If BIPS are administered and all are gathered within the colon on a radiograph taken 12–24 hours later, this indicates that a complete obstruction cannot be present and that a partial obstruction is unlikely. Thus, further conservative management may be a reasonable clinical judgement.

Iodine

Iodinated contrast agents are used for:

- Intravascular studies (e.g. upper urinary tract and angiography of the cardiovascular and portal systems)
- Lower urinary tract
- Joints (arthrography)
- Salivary glands (sialography)
- Lacrimal sac and duct
- Investigation of peripheral sinuses and fistulae
- Myelography
- Lymphangiography.

All iodine-containing contrast media are derived from organic tri-iodinated benzoic acids. They are water-soluble and are excreted by the kidneys. When they are used to evaluate the gastrointestinal tract, they can be difficult to administer as they are unpalatable, provide poor contrast and become diluted as they transit the bowel.

Preparations: Water-soluble iodinated contrast media are available in ionic and non-ionic forms (Figure 4.4).

Ionic (hyperosmolar) contrast media:

- These agents are monomers derived from the sodium or meglumine salts of iothalamic, diatrizoic or metrizoic acid. As salts they are ionic and dissociate in solution; therefore, they are hyperosmolar (1000–2000 mOsm/kg). This can lead to hypertonicity, ionicity and allergic reactions. The sodium salts of these acids are more toxic, whereas the meglumine salts are less toxic but more viscous; some media (e.g. sodium meglumine diatrizoate) are a combination of both.
- These agents are viscous and should be warmed to body temperature prior to use.
- They are contraindicated in hypotensive or dehydrated patients and those with severe renal failure. Ionic agents should not be used for myelography.
- In veterinary practice, ionic agents are mainly used for cardiovascular and urinary tract studies.

Non-ionic (low osmolar) contrast media:

- Non-ionic agents do not dissociate in solution and are considered iso-osmolar to blood plasma (even though their osmolality ranges from 1 to 3 times that of blood plasma).
- As they do not dissociate they do not have a charge and therefore direct chemotoxicity is reduced. Furthermore, as they carry no charge they can be used for myelography.
- Non-ionic agents are considered to be associated with fewer allergic reactions (the iodine molecules are shielded) but they are more expensive than ionic agents.
- The most commonly used agents in veterinary practice are the monomers iohexol and iopamidol but dimers with an even lower osmolality but higher iodine content are available (iotrolan).
- In veterinary practice, non-ionic agents are mainly used for myelography and arthrography. They are also used in cardiovascular and urinary tract studies, where the status of the patient dictates their use and ionic media are contraindicated.

Side effects: Contrast reactions can be divided into non-idiosyncratic reactions, which are dose-dependent and idiosyncratic reactions, which are independent of the dose administered. Non-idiosyncratic reactions are associated with the hyperosmolality and ionicity of these iodine-containing contrast agents and therefore are more common and severe with ionic agents than non-ionic agents. Whilst blood has an osmolality of approximately 290 mOsm/kg, the osmolality of ionic agents is 1000–2100 mOsm/kg. Non-ionic agents are approximately iso-osmolar.

Constituent	Properties	Trade name examples	Uses			Formulations (mg iodine/ml)
			Spinal	Vascular; urinary	Gastrointestinal	
Iothalamic acid	Monomer; ionic; high osmolar	Conray	–	+	–	141; 202; 280; 400
Sodium meglumine diatrizoate	Monomer; ionic; high osmolar	Urografin	–	+	–	146; 325; 370
	Monomer; ionic; high osmolar	Gastrografin	–	-	+	370
Ioxaglate	Dimer; ionic; low osmolar	Hexabrix	–	+	–	320
Iohexol	Monomer; non-ionic; low osmolar	Omnipaque	+	+	+	140; 180; 240; 300; 350
Iopamidol	Monomer; non-ionic; low osmolar	Niopam	+	+	–	150; 200; 300; 340; 370
Iopromide	Monomer; non-ionic; low osmolar	Ultravist	–	+	–	150; 240; 300; 370
Iomeprol	Monomer; non-ionic; low osmolar	Iomerol	–	+	–	250; 300; 350; 400

4.4　Commonly used iodinated contrast media.

Non-idiosyncratic reactions: These reactions may be acute (occur within 5–10 minutes following administration) or delayed. The most severe reactions are cardiovascular or respiratory in nature.

- Contrast-induced nephrotoxicity:
  - This is associated with renal vasoconstriction, renal hypoxia and a direct toxic effect on the renal tubular epithelial cells. Iodine-containing contrast agents are freely filtered by the kidneys and are not resorbed from the renal tubule. Renal tubular epithelial cells are highly metabolically active and as contrast media is concentrated in the tubule, it may exert a direct toxic effect on these cells. The necrotic cells accumulate in the tubules, resulting in tubular obstruction
  - Nephrotoxicity can be recognized in some cases by a persistent nephrogram which does not progress to a normal pyelogram. Contrast-induced nephrotoxicity is usually an acute reaction and the nephrogram should be monitored carefully during the early period of the study to ensure that contrast medium is being excreted into the lower urinary tract
  - Predisposing factors include dehydration, hypotension and pre-existing renal disease. All dehydrated and hypotensive patients should be stabilized *before* an intravenous study using either ionic or non-ionic water-soluble iodine-containing contrast agents is performed. Where possible, non-ionic agents should be used in these patients. Renal failure *per se* is not a contraindication for the use of these media but is a risk factor. Severe renal failure is a contraindication. In the dog, a threshold volume of 90 ml has been associated with an increased risk of contrast-induced nephrotoxicity
  - Contrast-induced nephrotoxicity can occur with any intravenous technique using iodinated contrast media (e.g. mesenteric portovenography and angiography). The kidneys in these patients should be assessed to ensure excretion of the contrast medium proceeds normally.
- As ionic media are hyperosmolar, they should not be administered orally to volume-depleted animals as this can lead to hypovolaemic shock when water is drawn into the intestinal tract. Similarly, leakage of hyperosmolar agents into a body cavity can lead to volume depletion due to a shift in extracellular fluid volume. Within the lungs, aspiration of hyperosmolar media can cause pulmonary oedema.
- Cardiovascular effects include bradycardia, hypertension and hypotension.
  - Bradycardia is presumed to be a vasovagal effect, as well as an initial hypertensive response to the injection of a hypertonic agent.
  - Hypotension is due to the direct (physiochemical) effect on the peripheral vasculature, which results in vasodilation. This may be severe. Hypotension may also occur due to hyperosmotic diuresis. Hence, patients undergoing intravascular studies usually receive fluid support during the procedure.

- The use of ionic media should be avoided in patients with congestive failure as hyperosmolality can lead to fluid retention and aggravation of the pre-existing disease.
- Nausea and vomiting may occur and are due to a direct effect on the brain or a vasovagal reaction. These effects may be minimized by performing the procedure under general anaesthesia (where possible) or at least under sedation.
- The neurotoxicity of ionic contrast agents is due to their osmotic effect, viscosity and ionicity. Ionic media should never be used for myelography. Ionic agents may also lead to an increase in permeability of the blood–brain barrier, which can result in seizures. Ionic agents should not be used intravenously if disruption of the blood–brain barrier is suspected.
- Extravasation of ionic contrast media into the subcutis can cause irritation. They should always be administered through an intravenous catheter. Where rupture of the urethra or bladder is suspected, and a positive contrast study with an iodine-containing contrast medium is being used to confirm the diagnosis, non-ionic media should be used. Extravasation of ionic contrast media into the abdomen or periurethral soft tissues may lead to fluid being drawn into the abdomen, which can potentially cause hypovolaemic shock or soft tissue damage.
- Miscellaneous side effects of ionic contrast media include potentiation of prothrombotic states, due to endothelial damage in the peripheral circulation, as well as anticoagulant effects. Bronchospasm and skin reactions may occur in patients with known allergic disease.

Idiosyncratic reactions: These represent anaphylactic or allergic-type reactions as antibodies to contrast agents have not been demonstrated. These reactions are evident immediately following intravenous administration and present as severe respiratory signs associated with laryngeal oedema, bronchospasm and pulmonary oedema, or as cardiovascular collapse (hypotension, decreased cardiac output). Urticaria may also be recognized. Idiosyncratic reactions occur with a test dose of contrast medium, whereas non-idiosyncratic reactions do not (as they are dose-dependent). In humans, a mortality rate of 1:40,000 has been reported with the use of intravenous contrast agents. Intravenous procedures using iodine-containing contrast agents should be performed under general anaesthesia and crash trolley equipment should be at hand.

Management of adverse reactions: Details regarding the specific management of contrast media reactions should be sought in texts on emergency care. However, the following summarizes the management strategies for the most important side effects:

- Bradycardia – administer anticholinergics (e.g. atropine sulphate/glycopyrrolate)
- Hypotension – administer crystalloid fluids
- Apnoea – mechanical ventilation
- Seizures (usually on recovery from myelography) – administer diazepam

- Contrast-induced renal failure – administer bolus fluids, furosemide, mannitol and dopamine
- Pulmonary oedema – administer oxygen, furosemide and corticosteroids.

Gastrointestinal studies: Iodinated contrast media can be used to evaluate the gastrointestinal tract where perforation and leakage are potentially present and hence the use of barium is contraindicated. In practice, alternative methods (e.g. positional radiography, ultrasonography or computed tomography (CT)) to demonstrate leakage should be considered first.

- Ionic contrast media for gastrointestinal use (e.g. Gastrografin) are available, but as the solutions are hypertonic and unpalatable, difficulties may arise. Aspiration of the media can result in pulmonary oedema. In dehydrated patients, absorption of water from the circulation into the bowel lumen or, where perforation is present, into the peritoneum can result in circulatory collapse. The contrast media provide poor mucosal detail and, as they are hypertonic and draw water into the bowel, become diluted. Thus, contrast (especially distally within the gastrointestinal tract) is poor. Ionic contrast media are irritant to the intestinal mucosa and cause hyperperistalsis and rapid transit of the gastrointestinal tract contents.
- Non-ionic contrast media can be used for evaluation of the gastrointestinal tract where perforation is suspected. Their limitation is that the volume of contrast medium required to perform a satisfactory study is exorbitantly expensive. Furthermore, mucosal detail is poor and dilution still occurs to some extent. One of the circumstances where non-ionic contrast media may be used is to evaluate the integrity of the stomach following placement of a percutaneous endoscopic gastrostomy (PEG) tube.
- One of the limitations of using iodine-containing contrast agents in the gastrointestinal tract is that leakage of a small volume of contrast medium may be overlooked.
- Iodinated contrast media are also used if endoscopy is going to be performed soon after the contrast study, as they do not prevent visualization of the mucosal surfaces.

Techniques

General

- Contrast studies should only be performed if the clinical status and temperament of the patient allows a diagnostic study to be obtained without compromising the welfare of the animal. For example, withholding food overnight may not be appropriate in very young animals.
- Informed consent should be obtained from the owners. Contrast studies are not without risk and the goals of the study and the potential complications should be discussed with the owners. Contrast studies are expensive, as, with the exception of upper gastrointestinal studies, they

are typically performed under general anaesthesia and frequently require intravenous fluid support and (in many cases) numerous radiographic exposures. Owners should be counselled that they may not lead to a definitive diagnosis and that the findings may be inconclusive.
- Survey radiographs must be obtained in orthogonal planes. Contrast studies are used to confirm findings recognized or suspected on survey radiographs. Therefore, the radiographic technique (patient positioning, exposure factors) must be satisfactory *before* proceeding with the study. The information sought on the plain films includes:
  - Is a diagnosis evident on the survey films? Will management of the condition be improved if a contrast procedure is performed? For example, if there is firm evidence of bowel obstruction and a foreign body is visible, then a barium contrast study is not indicated
  - Is a contrast study contraindicated? As many studies are performed under general anaesthesia, are there any findings on the survey films (e.g. aspiration pneumonia) that suggest that general anaesthesia would represent an unacceptable risk to the patient?
  - Is patient preparation (particularly for urinary tract studies) adequate? Poor technical quality is one of the main reasons for frustrating, non- or poorly diagnostic contrast studies
  - Is the contrast agent and technique being used appropriate to address the clinical presentation?
  - The survey films *must* be compared with those of the contrast study.
- Where body fluids are withdrawn as part of the study (e.g. cerebrospinal fluid (CSF) for myelography, joint fluid for arthrography or urine for studies of the urinary tract), these samples should always be submitted for analysis, regardless of the expected diagnosis.
- The clinician should establish whether any medications are being administered that may interfere with the study.

Double-contrast procedures

Double-contrast procedures combine both positive and negative contrast agents and are used to assess mucosal surfaces so that small filling defects, calculi or wall thickening are not overlooked. Double-contrast procedures of the colon and stomach can be performed, but have been superseded by endoscopy and ultrasonography. Thus, for practical purposes, the bladder is the viscus most commonly studied using double-contrast procedures.

Limitations

- Contrast studies may be normal despite the presence of disease.
- Findings are rarely specific (except for foreign body obstruction) and biopsy may still be necessary.
- The reasons for a non-diagnostic study are usually improper patient positioning, insufficient administration of contrast medium and an insufficient number of films obtained (Figure 4.5).

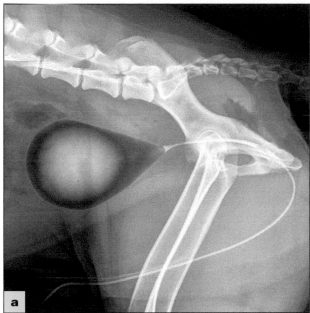

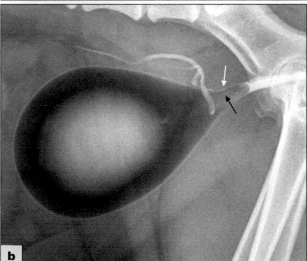

4.5 Retrograde urethrography in a 3-year-old neutered male dog with urinary incontinence. **(a)** The initial study was unremarkable. **(b)** The study was repeated with a slightly larger volume of contrast medium. There is better distension of the proximal urethra, which has resulted in retrograde filling of both ectopic ureters (black and white arrows). At the level of the trigone of the bladder, the terminal ureters are relatively normal in appearance but continue caudally within the bladder wall (intramural) to terminate in the proximal urethra. This study emphasizes the importance of repeating contrast studies, particularly swallowing and oesophageal studies, and those evaluating the lacrimal ducts, salivary glands, lower urinary tract, sinuses and fistulas.

Urinary tract studies

The three most common procedures used to evaluate the urogenital system are:

- Intravenous urography (also known as excretory urography) for the evaluation of the kidneys and ureters
- Cystography
- Retrograde vaginourethrography (female) or urethrography (male).

General principles and patient preparation

- Urine samples for routine urinalysis, culture and sensitivity should be obtained prior to the contrast study. Contrast media alter the urine specific gravity, and the concentration of iodine used for intravenous urography may inhibit the growth of some bacteria.
- Intravenous urography should be performed under general anaesthesia. Although the procedure could be performed under sedation, the benefits of general anaesthesia include better consideration of patient welfare and more consistent radiographic technique. General anaesthesia limits patient anxiety and the signs of nausea, drooling, retching and tactile sensations which may occur, in particular with rapid injection of the contrast medium. Patient positioning can be performed more accurately, consistently and efficiently, limiting the duration of the study. Inappropriate restraint should not be used as an excuse for an improper study.
- Subject to the clinical status of the patient, food should be withheld for 24 hours. The bowel (especially the colon) should be clear of ingesta or faeces to avoid artefacts that mimic pathology or obscure the termination of the ureters. An oral bowel cleansing solution containing an osmotic laxative can be given by stomach tube the day before the examination to assist in evacuating the bowel. However, animals may find the solution distasteful and the stomach tube distressing. Alternatively (and usually preferably), a warm water enema should be administered the day before, as well as 1–2 hours prior to, the contrast procedure using a Higginson (enema) pump.
- The patient should be offered the opportunity to void on the morning of the procedure. This is especially relevant in hospitalized patients.
- Contrast medium should be administered via a peripheral intravenous catheter. Extravasation of ionic contrast media can cause irritation and swelling of the soft tissues surrounding the catheter as well as rendering the study non-diagnostic.
- Contrast media reactions, although uncommon, do occur and preparations should be made to manage these (see above).

These procedures are time-consuming and hence intravenous urography should be recognized as an elective procedure. It may be helpful to draw up a standard operating procedure (SOP), which can be kept in the radiography exposure book, to ensure that all steps are followed.

Intravenous urography

This technique provides an anatomical assessment of the kidneys and ureters, although evaluation of the renal parenchymal changes may be limited. This type of study also provides a limited, indirect assessment of renal function; however, it must be recognized that abdominal perfusion and excretion of the contrast medium by the kidneys may be affected by one or more pre-renal (hypotension, dehydration, obstruction of the renal artery), renal (primary or contrast-induced pathology) or post-renal factors.

Indications:

- Suspected kidney disease associated with a change in:
  - Number
  - Size
  - Shape
  - Margination
  - Renal pelves
  - Integrity
  - Presence and significance of mineralization within the kidney.
- Suspected disease of the ureters associated with a change in:
  - Size (obstruction, ectopia or infection)
  - Integrity
  - Number
  - Location of the ureteral termination
  - Presence and significance of mineralization in the region of the ureters.
- Suspected trauma to the urinary tract.
- Haematuria and pyuria suspected to arise from an upper urinary tract infection.
- Incontinence.
- Assessment of the potential involvement of the kidneys and ureters with abdominal masses.

Contraindications: Renal failure *per se* is not an absolute contraindication for intravenous urography, but is a risk factor associated with contrast-induced side effects or complications. The dose of contrast medium may need to be increased by at least 10–15% to obtain a diagnostic study. However, hypotension and dehydration are contraindications, as is severe renal failure. Unstable patients should be stabilized and rehydrated prior to the procedure.

Complications: Idiosyncratic and non-idiosyncratic reactions (see above).

Technique: Two techniques can be used for intravenous urography:

- A bolus technique (small volume, high concentration) is used to evaluate the renal parenchyma structures and ureters
- An infusion technique (high volume, low concentration) is usually performed together with a pneumocystogram to evaluate the ureters, as distension and cranial displacement of the bladder neck allows the termination of the ureters to be identified.

Bolus technique:

- The study is performed under general anaesthesia.
- Lateral and ventrodorsal (VD) survey radiographs are obtained. A cassette large enough to include the cranial abdomen, kidneys and pelvis should ideally be used.
- A pneumocystogram (see below) is performed (the lateral view is obtained with the patient in left lateral recumbency) so that the termination of the ureters can be assessed.
- The bulb of the urinary catheter is advanced to the centre of the bladder. If it is pulled caudally into

the neck, the ureteric orifices may be distorted or obscured.

- For an intravenous urography study, the patient is placed in dorsal recumbency (usually in a radiolucent cradle) with the legs in a neutral (frog-legged) position. The initial 2–3 exposures are obtained with the patient in dorsal recumbency (without being moved) so that the kidneys can be evaluated without being superimposed on each another. Lateral views are usually only obtained once the clinician has evaluated and is satisfied with the initial VD films.
- The dose of iodine required is 600–800 mg iodine per kg. This approximates to 2 ml/kg of a solution containing 300–400 mg iodine per ml. Both ionic and non-ionic iodine-containing contrast media suitable for intravenous administration can be used. For high risk patients or those with pre-existing disease, non-ionic agents (although more expensive) should be used. Contrast media should be warmed to body temperature before administration.
- An immediate film (0 minutes) is taken at the end of the contrast medium injection. Radiation protection requirements should be observed. An extension set that has been prefilled with contrast medium can be used. The volume of contrast medium required to fill the extension tubing must be calculated and added to the volume to be injected into the patient. This is particularly important in smaller patients. It is helpful to start a timer when the contrast medium is administered so that the timing of the exposures is accurately recorded. For analogue film, the time at which the exposure was made should be marked on the film immediately with a permanent marker pen. Digital films should be similarly annotated using the workstation software.
- Subsequent exposures are obtained with the patient in dorsal recumbency at 1 and 5 minutes. After 5 minutes, the patient can be turned into lateral recumbency, with further VD and lateral exposures obtained at 10, 15 and 20 minutes. Where poor renal function is present, glomerular filtration may be delayed and exposures obtained after 20 minutes may be necessary.
- Intravenous fluid is usually administered following completion of the bolus injection.
- VD views are used to assess the kidneys and lateral views are helpful to assess the ureters as they opacify.

Infusion technique:

- The study is performed under general anaesthesia.
- Lateral and VD survey radiographs are obtained. A cassette large enough to include the cranial abdomen, kidneys and pelvis should ideally be used.
- A pneumocystogram (see below) is performed (the lateral view is obtained with the patient in left lateral recumbency) so that the termination of the ureters can be assessed.
- A 150 mg/ml solution of iodine is used. This is available as a ready-to-use infusion (Urografin 150, Bayer Schering) or can be made by diluting a more concentrated solution to the required

concentration with 0.9% saline. The total dose of iodine required is 1200 mg iodine per kg, which equates to 8 ml/kg, and the solution is infused over 10–15 minutes. Contrast media should be warmed to body temperature.

- The first exposure is usually obtained approximately 5–10 minutes after the start of the infusion or when the calculated volume of contrast medium has been completely infused, whichever occurs first. Subsequent exposures are obtained at 10, 15 and 20 minutes. As for the bolus technique, the initial exposures at 5 and 10 minutes are obtained with the patient in dorsal recumbency. A lateral view is useful as, depending on the location of the bladder neck, superimposition of the pelvis may make identification and assessment of the termination of the ureters difficult.
- Oblique views (45 degree lateral oblique view) of the abdomen can also be obtained to overcome the difficulties posed by superimposition of the

pelvis on the terminal ureters. Both left and right oblique views are obtained. The patient is placed in lateral recumbency with the upper hindlimb elevated and tied back out of the primary beam, and the abdomen axially rotated to approximately midway (45 degrees) between the vertical and table top. The ureter on the dependent side will lie ventral to the upper ureter and a positional marker is placed ventral to the body wall to show the dependent side (see Figure 6.78).

- Although centred on the kidneys, the initial exposures are collimated to include the caudal abdomen (including the pelvis, where possible) as early accumulation of contrast medium within the urethra, vagina or on the perineum is a useful indicator that an ectopic ureter is present.
- Where the purpose of the study is to investigate urinary incontinence, intravenous urography should be followed by a retrograde study (e.g. vaginourethrogram or urethrogram).

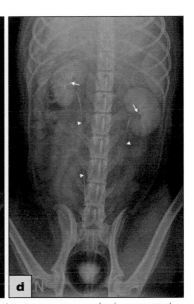

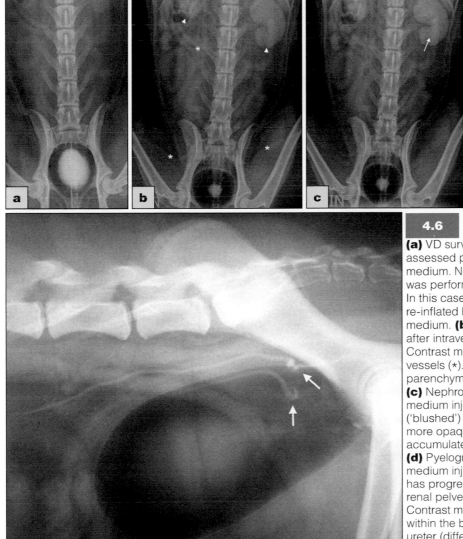

4.6 Intravenous urography in a normal bitch using the bolus technique.
(a) VD survey radiograph. Patient positioning is assessed prior to the injection of contrast medium. Note that double-contrast cystography was performed prior to intravenous urography. In this case, the bladder was drained and re-inflated before the administration of contrast medium. **(b)** Angiogram phase – immediately after intravenous contrast medium injection. Contrast medium is present within the large vessels (*). Early enhancement of the renal parenchyma is present (arrowheads).
(c) Nephrogram phase – 1 minute after contrast medium injection. The kidneys have enhanced ('blushed') homogeneously. The medulla is more opaque as contrast medium starts to accumulate within the renal tubules (arrowed).
(d) Pyelogram – 3 minutes after contrast medium injection. The nephrogram (still present) has progressed and contrast medium fills the renal pelves (arrowed) and ureters (arrowheads). Contrast medium has started to accumulate within the bladder. **(e)** The terminations of the ureter (different case to the bitch in a–d) at the trigone have a 'hook' or 'crook' shape (an ectopic ureter is not present).

Interpretation:

Normal: The following phases can be recognized during intravenous urography (Figure 4.6):

- Arterial phase:
  - Opacification of the aorta and other abdominal arteries (coeliac, cranial mesenteric and its branches, and renal) may be identified on immediate exposures. Early renal opacification (of the cortex) may also be present. A mild, generalized, overall increase in opacity of the abdomen may also be recognized due to contrast medium within the highly vascularized gastric and small intestinal mucosa.
- Nephrogram phase:
  - Characterized by gradual opacification of the renal cortex and medulla. This opacification should increase gradually over 3–5 minutes and be followed by contrast medium appearing in the collecting system of the kidneys (pyelogram phase). The nephrogram then gradually decreases.
- Pyelogram phase:
  - Characterized by the concentration of contrast medium within the collecting system. The appearance of the renal pelvis is quite variable and the pelvic recesses may not be visible in all patients. They may be better visualized using the infusion technique (Figure 4.7). The renal pelves should be mirror-images of each other. The renal pelvis and proximal ureter should taper and the ureters should be even in diameter along their length, although focal

narrowing or the absence of contrast medium may occur due to peristalsis. This can be confirmed by repeating the exposure to assess whether the segment being evaluated fills with contrast medium on the subsequent exposure.

Abnormal:

- Arterial phase:
  - Failure of one or both kidneys to opacify may be due to ischaemia, hypotension or renal artery thrombosis (Figure 4.8).
- Nephrogram phase:
  - Failure of the kidney to opacify may be due to renal ischaemia, severe hypotension or severe chronic renal obstruction
  - Failure of the nephrogram to progress to a pyelogram or ureterogram phase may occur due to pre-existing or contrast-induced hypotension or contrast-induced renal failure (Figure 4.9). The appearance is of a nephrogram in which renal opacification gradually increases and persists, but contrast medium is not recognized in the ureters or in the bladder. It is important that this condition is recognized and dealt with

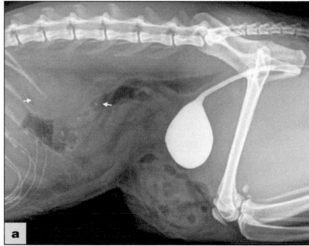

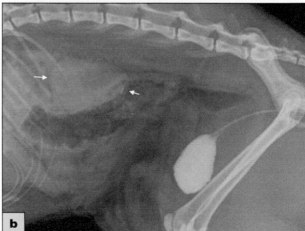

4.8 Intravenous urography in a cat following trauma. **(a)** Lateral survey radiograph. Retrograde urography has been performed and reveals that although the bladder has herniated through a ventral body wall defect, it remains intact. The kidneys are arrowed. **(b)** Lateral radiograph taken immediately after intravenous contrast medium injection. There is no arterial phase or early enhancement of the kidneys (arrowed). (continues) ▶

R 15 MINUTES PI

4.7 Intravenous urography using the infusion technique. The renal diverticula (white arrow) are filled with contrast medium and the termination of the ureters are well defined and distinct (black arrow).

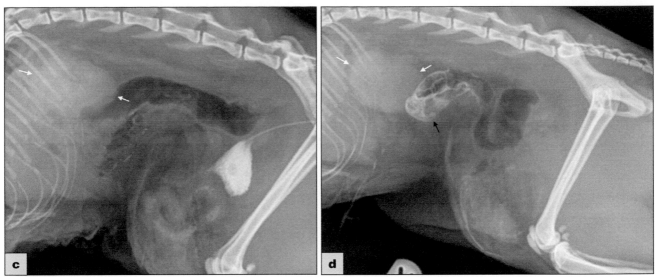

4.8 (continued) Intravenous urography in a cat following trauma. **(c)** Lateral radiograph taken 25 minutes after contrast medium injection. The kidneys remain unopacified (arrowed). **(d)** Lateral radiograph taken 24 hours after contrast medium injection. The iodinated contrast medium is located within the colon (black arrow) as it has undergone hepatobiliary excretion following the failure of renal excretion. The failure of the kidneys (white arrows) to opacify may be due to hypotension, renal ischaemia or renal infarction.

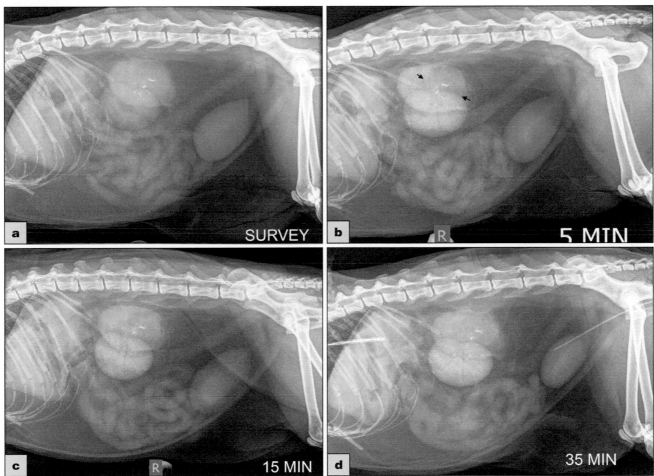

4.9 Contrast-induced renal failure in a cat. **(a)** Survey abdominal radiograph. The left kidney is slightly larger with an irregular margin and multiple irregular foci of mineralization are superimposed on the region of the renal pelvis. Soft tissue streaks radiating from the capsular margin suggest perirenal/retroperitoneal fluid. **(b)** Lateral radiograph taken 5 minutes after contrast medium injection. Both nephrograms have a quite markedly opaque appearance but there has been no progression to a normal pyelogram phase. The cranial pole of the left kidney is opacified, but an ill defined area of poor opacification (arrowed) occupies most of the caudal pole. A very small amount of contrast medium has entered the bladder. **(c)** Lateral radiograph taken 15 minutes after contrast medium injection. The kidneys remain markedly opaque, despite aggressive fluid and supportive therapy. The pyelogram phase has still not been reached and the size of the bladder is unchanged, indicating little if any urine production. **(d)** Lateral radiograph taken 35 minutes after contrast medium injection. Note that the intensity of nephrogram opacification increases from (b) to (d). A urinary catheter has been placed to monitor urine production. Renal function and urine function were eventually re-established. Final diagnosis: infiltrative renal carcinoma.

immediately (see above). These changes are usually bilateral, whereas if this pattern is recognized with acute renal obstruction, the changes are usually unilateral
- A poor nephrogram (poor opacification), but one in which contrast medium can be recognized accumulating in the ureters and bladder, and in which the nephrogram phase fades rapidly is usually associated with polyuric renal failure or an insufficient dose of contrast medium
- A nephrogram in which the renal parenchyma is mottled with areas of persistence of the contrast medium usually indicates severe generalized (interstitial) disease and/or ischaemia
- Filling defects may be due to renal masses, cysts or hydronephrosis (Figure 4.10).

- Pyelogram phase:
  - Failure to progress to the pyelogram phase (see above)
  - Dilated pelvis with an irregular, distorted or rounded shape due to inflammation (Figure 4.11), infection or ureteral ectopia. Blood clots or purulent material may result in filling defects within the renal pelvis
  - Dilated renal pelvis due to an obstruction within the ureters or lower urinary tract. Ureteric obstruction may be the consequence of 'calculi' masses or adhesions arising within the retroperitoneal space.

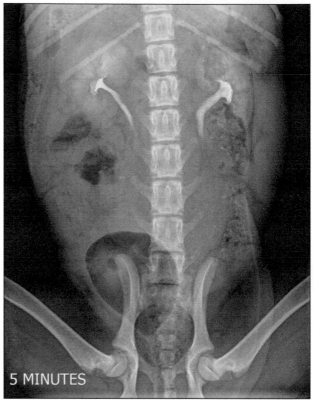

4.11 Intravenous urography in a puppy with chronic pyelonephritis. The pyelogram is abnormal. The renal pelves are dilated with irregular margins. Poor filling of the peripheral right renal pelvis is due to the accumulation of exudate. Note the irregular renal margins and patchy nephrogram, which is consistent with interstitial nephritis. The proximal ureters are dilated.

Cystography

Indications:

- Haematuria.
- Dysuria.
- Urinary retention.
- Incontinence.
- Assessment of bladder location and integrity (trauma).
- Assessment of the bladder wall and mucosa.
- Examination for the presence of calculi.

Technique:

- General preparation is as for intravenous urography (see above).

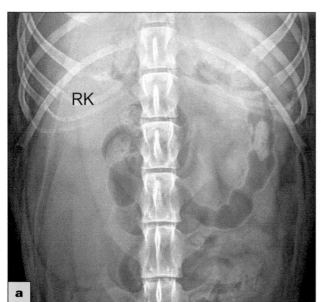

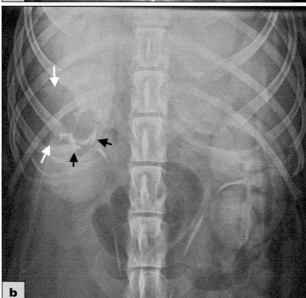

4.10 Intravenous urography in a dog with a renal tumour. **(a)** VD survey abdominal radiograph. The shape and size of the kidneys are unremarkable. **(b)** VD radiograph taken 1 minute after contrast medium injection. The cranial and caudal poles have opacified normally, but an irregular lobulated filling defect (white arrows) occupies the central region of the right kidney (RK). The pelvis is distorted and displaced (black arrows) with irregular filling, indicating extension of the mass into the renal pelvis. Diagnosis: renal haemangiosarcoma.

- The study is performed under general anaesthesia.
- Orthogonal survey radiographs centred on the pelvis are obtained.
- Bladder size is assessed by palpation and correlated with the volume of urine drained. This provides an estimate of the volume of contrast medium that can be administered safely to the patient.
- The catheter should be placed in as aseptic a manner as possible. For bitches, catheter placement can be challenging, even in an anaesthetized patient (see *BSAVA Guide to Procedures in Small Animal Practice* for information on correct placement technique). The procedure is considerably easier if a speculum with a suitable light source is used. In bitches, a suitably sized Foley catheter with a guide wire is used. The bulb is slowly inflated with water and a radiograph obtained to confirm correct placement of the catheter tip. Inflation of the bulb within the urethra can lead to urethral rupture, especially if urethral disease is present. Blood pressure and heart rate can be monitored whilst the bulb is inflated. If either hypertension or tachycardia is noted, the bulb should be deflated and the catheter repositioned. The bulb can be pulled gently into the neck of the bladder to avoid leakage of the contrast medium around the catheter and through the comparatively wide urethra in the bitch.
- The length of the catheter required can be estimated before being placed, which helps avoid trauma to the bladder wall or knotting of the catheter (rare, but prevents the catheter from being withdrawn).
- Oblique views are rarely obtained.

Pneumocystography

Indications: Pneumocystography is used primarily to identify the location of the bladder and, together with intravenous urography or retrograde vaginoure-throgivraphy/urethrography, to assess the distal ureters. Assessment of mucosal detail is poor compared with a double-contrast study and small lesions and calculi may be overlooked. Large soft tissue masses can be recognized but small areas of mucosal irregularity may be overlooked.

Contraindications: Pneumocystography should not be used when the bladder is ruptured or if there is gross evidence of mucosal trauma or fresh haemorrhage, including that induced by catheterization. Mucosal trauma allows direct access to the venous circulation with the attendant risk of air embolism, especially if bladder pressure is increased by the procedure and the bladder is poorly distensible.

Complications:

- Bladder rupture.
- Air embolism.
- Trauma to the bladder wall by the urinary catheter.

Air embolism

- Air embolism occurs when air gains access to the systemic circulation via the venous drainage of the bladder.
- The condition and integrity of the bladder mucosa are important predisposing factors.
- Pneumocystography should be avoided if there is evidence of recent gross haemorrhage, ulcerative cystitis or trauma.
- The patient should be placed in left lateral recumbency for radiography. Any air embolus produced may become trapped in the right atrium (uppermost aspect of the right heart in left lateral recumbency) and gradually absorbed into the circulation.
- Air embolism is recognized by a sudden decrease in cardiac output and oxygenation. Without turning the animal, radiographs of the thorax and abdomen should be obtained to identify air within the caudal vena cava and the heart.
- The animal should remain in left lateral recumbency for 60 minutes to allow the embolus to be absorbed.

Technique:

- The patient is placed in left lateral recumbency to minimize the effect of air embolism should it occur.
- Room air is administered through a catheter using a three-way tap. Carbon dioxide (CO_2) or nitrous oxide (N_2O) can be used instead of room air, and these gases are considered safer as they are more soluble in blood. A volume of CO_2/N_2O can be collected from a cylinder in a sterile glove or balloon and used to fill a syringe.
- Usually 5–10 ml/kg (25 ml in the cat) of gas is sufficient. The bladder is gently palpated as the gas is injected. When the bladder feels moderately distended (but not turgid) an exposure is taken. An additional volume of gas should be injected if the degree of distension of the bladder on the radiograph is not considered adequate. An estimate of whether sufficient gas has been injected can be made by direct palpation, sensing back pressure on the syringe plunger or the reflux of air around the catheter. Extensive distension, especially in a diseased bladder, can lead to pain, discomfort and even air embolism. Subtle lesions of the bladder wall may be less conspicuous if the bladder is over-distended.
- Lateral views usually suffice as the neck and parts of the bladder may be obscured by the spine and pelvis on VD views.
- The catheter should be withdrawn so that the tip does not distort the wall and lies in the bladder neck or proximal urethra if pathology within the neck of the bladder is suspected.

Interpretation:

Normal:

- Can be combined with intravenous urography to assess the location of the terminal ureters.

- Position of the bladder and bladder neck:
  - The whole of the bladder, including the vesicourethral junction, should lie within the abdomen cranial to the pubis.
- Shape:
  - In the bitch, the bladder is pear-shaped and the neck tapers gradually towards the urethra. In the cat, the transition to the urethra is more abrupt (Figure 4.12).
- Opacity:
  - The gas opacity is homogeneous.
- Bladder wall:
  - The bladder wall should be of even thickness (2–3 mm). However, pneumocystography is less informative than double-contrast cystography and the mucosal detail is less well visualized.

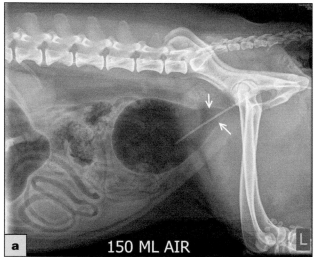

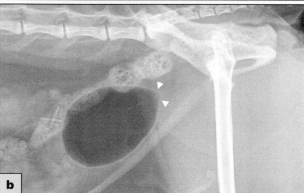

4.12   Pneumocystography. **(a)** A normal bitch. The bladder is moderately well distended. The bladder neck (arrowed) lies within the caudal abdomen and tapers gradually towards the pelvis. **(b)** A normal tom cat. The bladder neck tapers abruptly (arrowheads) and the urethra is long. Patient preparation in this case is inadequate: an enema should have been administered.

Abnormal:

- Size:
  - The chronically inflamed bladder may be poorly distensible
  - Chronic distension of the bladder (e.g. secondary to reflex dyssynergia) may result in a bladder which requires a greater volume of gas to achieve adequate distension (Figure 4.13).
- Position of the bladder and bladder neck:
  - Intrapelvic bladder and short urethra (Figure 4.14)

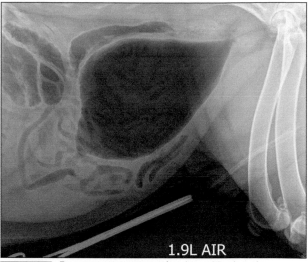

4.13   Pneumocystogram of a dog with chronic distension of the bladder due to reflex dyssynergia. The bladder still has a flaccid appearance despite the large volume of air administered.

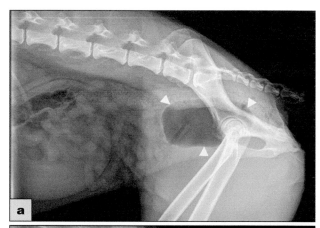

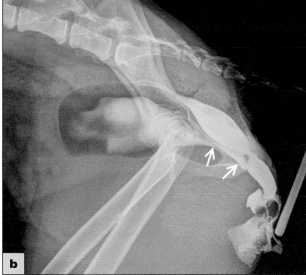

4.14   Pneumocystography in an incontinent bitch with an intrapelvic bladder neck. **(a)** The bladder is reasonably well distended with gas (arrowheads). The neck has a rounded (or 'gourd-like') appearance and lies within the pelvis. **(b)** Retrograde vaginourethrography demonstrates that the urethra (arrowed) is shortened. The vagina and vestibule fill normally. The position of the bladder neck together with the short urethra, contribute to urethral sphincter mechanism incompetence. Note that the bitch has not been adequately prepared as the colon is filled with semi-formed faeces.

- Retroflexion into a perineal hernia or herniation through a body wall defect
- Ureteral involvement relative to mass lesions.
- Shape:
  - Intraluminal and mural filling defects and diverticula
  - Distorted shape due to urachal remnants, adhesions or displacement by extravesicular masses.
- Opacity:
  - Filling defects, submucosal gas (mucosal slough) and leakage from the bladder.
- Bladder wall:
  - Inflammation, neoplasia or ureterocele may affect the thickness of the bladder wall.

Positive-contrast cystography

Indications:

- Primarily used to demonstrate changes involving the bladder wall, including defects and integrity due to congenital or acquired abnormalities (e.g. urachal remnants, acquired diverticula) or trauma.
- Demonstrate communication between the bladder and other abdominal structures.
- To identify the location of the bladder neck relative to the pelvis.

Compared with pneumocystography, this technique provides a better assessment of the mucosa; however, small mural lesions or luminal pathology can be obscured by the contrast medium and easily overlooked.

Complications:

- Bladder rupture due to incorrect technique (overdistension of the bladder) and poor ability of the bladder to distend secondary to underlying disease.
- Iatrogenic trauma to the bladder wall by the catheter.

Technique:

- A solution containing 150 mg iodine/ml is usually sufficient and can be produced by diluting a more concentrated solution with 0.9% saline.
- A dose of approximately 5–10 ml/kg of the solution is used in the dog. If the bladder is chronically inflamed, a considerably lower volume may be required. In the cat, 25 ml reflects the approximate volume required, but this should be assessed by palpation.
- Reflux of contrast medium into the distal ureters is a normal finding in some dogs, especially in younger patients and when bladder distension is significant.

Interpretation:

Normal:

- Size, position and shape of the bladder are as seen on a pneumocystogram.
- Opacity:
  - The bladder appears as a homogeneous, highly attenuating 'white' opacity.
- Bladder wall:
  - Mucosal detail is superior to that seen with pneumocystography (Figure 4.15).

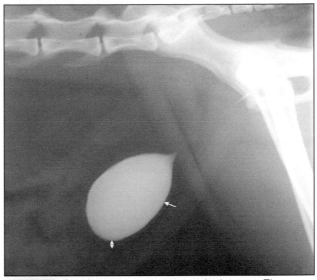

4.15 Positive-contrast cystography in a cat. The mucosal surface of the bladder is smooth (arrowed). The wall of the bladder at the vertex is slightly thicker (double-headed arrow) than it is dorsally and ventrally, suggesting moderate distension. Filling of the proximal urethra usually indicates adequate distension (compare with the cats in Figures 4.16 and 4.18).

Abnormal:

- Position of the bladder and bladder neck:
  - As seen on a pneumocystogram. Positive-contrast cystography provides better detail to assess involvement of the trigone region and proximal urethra when a bladder mass is identified.
- Shape:
  - Intraluminal and mural filling defects and diverticula (Figure 4.16)

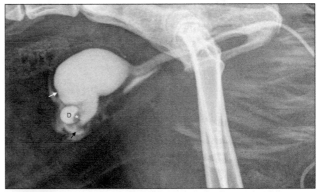

4.16 Positive-contrast cystography in a cat with a cyst-like diverticulum. A discrete ex-vagination (D) cranioventral to the vertex of the bladder is filled with contrast medium. It is smooth with an oval filling defect (*) caudally (due to a large calculus, which was evident on the survey film). The bladder wall is thickened and flattened cranioventrally (white arrow) due to chronic cystitis. The bladder is small and appears poorly distensible and turgid. The curvilinear streaks of contrast medium (black arrow) surrounding the vertex and diverticulum and ventral to the urethra are due to submucosal extension of contrast medium secondary to the poor distensibility of the bladder. They do not represent rupture and the bladder remains intact. Positive-contrast cystography is useful to demonstrate the communication between the cyst-like diverticulum and the bladder.

- Distorted shape due to congenital urachal remnants, adhesions or displacement by extravesicular masses.
- Opacity:
  - Intraluminal filling defects. Leakage of contrast medium through defects (Figure 4.17) or filling of diverticula.
- Bladder wall:
  - Thickening is usually due to inflammation, neoplasia or a ureterocele (intramural, cyst-like dilatation of the terminal (usually ectopic) ureter. If positive-contrast cystography is combined with intravenous urography, it allows for a good assessment of the trigone region.

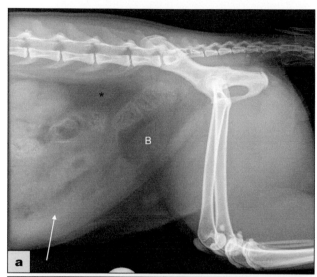

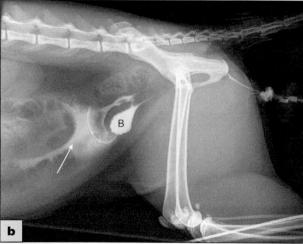

4.17 Positive-contrast cystography in a cat with rupture of the bladder. **(a)** Lateral survey radiograph of the abdomen. Free abdominal fluid results in poor serosal detail in the mid-ventral abdomen (arrowed). The bladder (B) is small. Retroperitoneal detail is normal (*). **(b)** Contrast medium has leaked widely into the caudal abdomen (arrowed). The bladder (B) is small and the margin is irregular and distorted due to inflammation and spasm. Positive-contrast cystography is the technique of choice to demonstrate leakage of urine from the bladder.

Double-contrast cystography

Indications: Double-contrast cystography provides good assessment of mucosal detail, allowing fine lesions not recognized using gas or contrast medium alone to be identified. Although ultrasonography has superseded cystography for the identification of many bladder diseases, contrast procedures can still be useful (e.g. for assessing the margins of a mass lesion relative to the ureters).

Technique:

- The bladder is drained of urine. A dose of 5–20 ml of 150 mg iodine/ml contrast medium solution is injected into the bladder, followed by gas (as for pneumocystography). The gas is injected slowly to avoid creating air bubbles.
- If double-contrast cystography is to be performed after pneumocystography, then the patient is gently rolled to ensure that the bladder wall is coated with the contrast medium.
- If double-contrast cystography is to be performed after intravenous urography, then the bladder is emptied of contrast medium and gas, and gently re-inflated. Additional contrast medium should not be necessary as the kidneys will continue to excrete contrast medium into the bladder.
- The central pool of contrast medium in the dependent aspect of the bladder should not be so large as to obscure pathology.

Interpretation:

Normal:

- Position and shape of the bladder:
  - The whole of the bladder, including the vesicourethral junction, should lie within the abdomen cranial to the pubis.
- Opacity:
  - Large peripheral gas opacity
  - Small central, moderately opaque, pool of contrast medium (Figure 4.18).

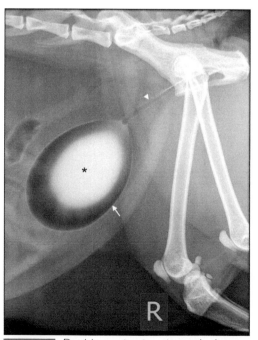

4.18 Double-contrast cystography in a normal cat. The bladder is adequately distended. This is suggested by the rounded shape and distension of the proximal urethra (arrowhead). The bladder wall (arrowed) is of even thickness throughout. The pool of contrast medium (*) should not be so large as to obscure small lesions. Patient preparation is adequate and although some faecal material remains it does not obscure the area of interest.

- Bladder wall:
  - Double-contrast cystography provides excellent mucosal detail.

Abnormal:

- Position of the bladder and bladder neck:
  - Intrapelvic bladder and short urethra
  - Retroflexion of the bladder into a perineal hernia or herniation through a body wall defect
  - Ureteral involvement relative to mass lesions can be evaluated when double-contrast cystography is combined with intravenous urography.
- Shape:
  - Intraluminal and mural filling defects and diverticula.
- Opacity:
  - Intraluminal and mural filling defects (Figure 4.19).
- Bladder wall:
  - Double-contrast cystography can be used to assess subtle mucosal irregularities associated with inflammation or neoplasia.

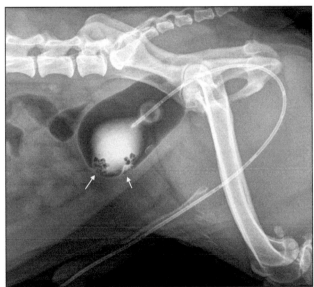

4.19 Double-contrast cystography in a dog with polypoid cystitis. The bladder is well distended with gas and a small pool of contrast medium fills the bladder cranioventrally. Several cauliflower-like defects are present at the edge of the contrast medium pool arising from the cranioventral bladder wall (arrowed). The adjacent bladder wall is moderately thickened.

Retrograde urethrography

Indications:

- Persistent haematuria.
- Dysuria.
- Urinary incontinence.
- Lower urinary tract obstruction.
- Prostatic disease.
- Disease of the os penis (trauma, neoplasia or callus).
- Urethritis or neoplasia.
- Urethral discharge.
- Urethral tear (traumatic, iatrogenic).

Complications:

- Rupture of the urethra. The nature of the pre-existing disease (neoplasia/trauma) is a predisposing factor. The volume of contrast medium injected should be strictly observed.
- Introduction of infection.
- Iatrogenic trauma.

Technique:

- The patient is prepared using warm water enemas to ensure that the colon is free from faecal material.
- The study is performed under general anaesthesia.
- The catheter is placed using routine aseptic technique.
- The bladder is emptied of urine or, if intravenous urography has been performed, urine and contrast medium are removed. A pneumocystogram is performed. Occasionally, a full bladder is preferred to allow better distension of the urethra or vagina by resistance from the increased bladder volume. This is not advised if a urethral tear is suspected.
- A small diameter, soft polypropylene catheter with an inflatable balloon is used. Care should be taken to ensure that the cuff is inflated only sufficiently to prevent the retrograde flow of contrast medium, and to avoid trauma to the urethra. If a bulb tip catheter is not available, a lubricated rigid plastic dog catheter can be used, but care must be taken to ensure that the urethral mucosa is not damaged. The preputial fold can be clamped gently across the tip of the penis using atraumatic bowel clamps, clips or a peg to prevent the retrograde leakage of contrast medium.
- The catheter is prefilled with contrast medium. A volume of 5–10 ml of a 150–200 mg iodine/ml water-soluble contrast medium is injected. Ionic contrast media may be irritant, hence in most animals non-ionic contrast media are used. Radiographs should be taken at the end of the first and midway through the second contrast medium injection. This allows variations in the contrast medium column due to factors such as bladder filling or spasm to be assessed. The injection of contrast medium against a distended bladder is an alternative method to provide better distension of the urethra, but, due to the high pressure, subtle stenosis may be overlooked. Alternatively, equal volumes of contrast medium and sterile KY jelly can be mixed well and used (this should be mixed the day before the examination to allow the air bubbles to dissipate). Some radiologists consider this mixture allows the contrast medium column to persist within the urethra for a longer period of time.
- The tip of the catheter is placed just distal to the segment of the urethra within which the pathology is suspected to be located. Where this is not known, the tip of the catheter is placed initially within the distal penile urethra. Based on the findings of the initial radiograph, the tip of the catheter can be advanced for subsequent exposures.

- Radiographs are obtained with the legs pulled cranially to assess the segment of the urethra between the ischial arch and the caudal aspect of the os penis, and caudally to assess the pelvic and prostatic urethra.
- Fluoroscopic assessment may be useful in cases with stenosis.

Interpretation:

Normal:

- The mucosa should be smooth without irregularities (Figure 4.20).
- The contrast medium column is usually slightly thinner over the ischial arch.
- The diameter of the pelvic urethra can be quite variable, and in some cases even dilated.
- In some normal dogs, the pelvic urethra has an undulating or sigmoid appearance.
- The holes of the catheter may contain gas bubbles, which also resemble calculi.
- The presence of contrast medium in the prostate gland is not necessarily abnormal. The pattern is usually that of radiating linear accumulations of contrast medium.
- Extravasation of contrast medium into the peri-preputial vessels may occur with a high volume or excessive pressure.

Abnormal:

- Persistent irregularity of the mucosa, masses, filling defects, stenosis and the leakage of contrast medium (Figures 4.21 and 4.22).
- Filling defects due to pathology usually persist, whereas artefacts are transient.
- Gas bubbles may mimic calculi. However, gas bubbles do not displace the urethral wall, whereas calculi may.
- Irregular, extensive contrast medium extravasation within the prostate gland is more likely to represent pathology.

Retrograde vaginourethrography

Indications:

- Suspected ectopic ureters.
- To assess for vaginal or urethral tears.
- Vaginal stenosis.
- Vaginal discharge.
- To assess mass lesions within the pelvis or vagina.

Complications:

- Rupture of the vagina. The nature of the pre-existing disease (neoplasia/trauma) is a predisposing factor. The volume of contrast medium injected should be strictly observed.
- Introduction of infection.
- Iatrogenic trauma.

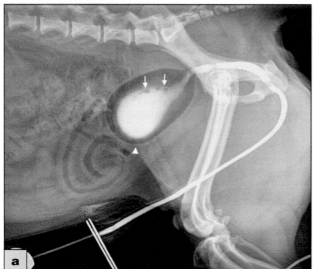

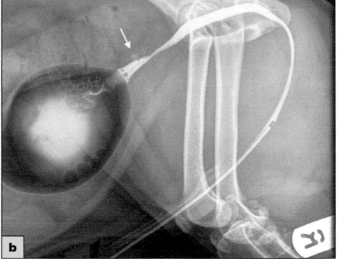

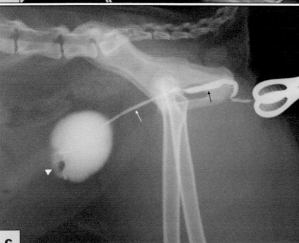

4.20 **(a)** Normal retrograde urethrography in a neutered male dog. Pneumocystography has also been performed. The urethra is evenly and well distended along its length and the contrast medium margins are smooth. Irregular filling defects are present in the dorsal contrast medium pool (arrowed) and the cranioventral bladder wall is mildly thickened (arrowhead). The differential diagnoses for the former include focal wall thickening (polypoid cystitis), blood clots or early neoplasia. **(b)** A small volume of contrast medium extravasation into the prostate gland can be normal (arrowed) as in this dog with prostatic hyperplasia. **(c)** Normal retrograde urethrography in a cat. The increased diameter of the pelvic urethra (black arrow) is a normal finding. The proximal urethra is long and narrow (white arrow). The filling defect at the apex (arrowhead) is due to a partial tear of the bladder wall.

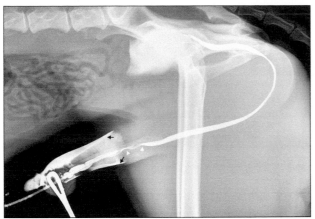

4.21 Retrograde urethrography in an entire male dog with a penile haemangiosarcoma. A soft tissue mass arising around the base of the os penis has resulted in urethral stenosis. Narrowing of the urethra is due to two adjacent focal extramural compressive areas (arrowheads). The luminal margin of the urethra remains smooth. Contrast medium has also refluxed into the preputial sac, resulting in a large filling defect in the caudal region of the prepuce (arrowed) as a result of the penile mass.

Technique:

- Patient preparation includes the administration of one or more warm water enemas to ensure that the distal gastrointestinal tract is empty.
- The study is performed under general anaesthesia.
- Survey orthogonal views of the caudal abdomen and pelvis are obtained.
- The tip of a bulbed (Foley) catheter is cut off. The bulb is placed in the vestibule so that the contrast medium is injected at the level of the urethra. The catheter may need to be pulled downwards to facilitate filling of the urethra. The vulva lips can be gently clamped around the catheter using atraumatic bowel clamps.
- The catheter is prefilled with a water-soluble, iodine-containing contrast medium. The solution should contain 150–200 mg iodine/ml. The volume of contrast medium injected is usually not more than 1 ml/kg, as rupture may occur if this volume is exceeded or forceful pressure is used. The contrast medium is injected over 5–10 seconds and an exposure taken at the end of the injection.

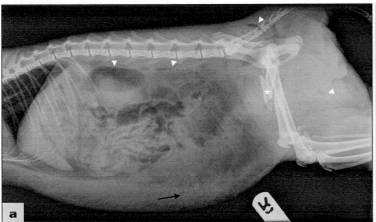

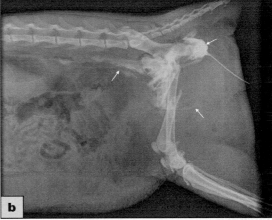

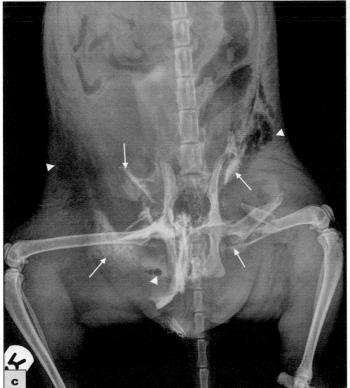

4.22 **(a)** Lateral survey and **(b)** lateral and **(c)** VD abdominal radiographs following retrograde urethrography in a cat with a urethral rupture. (a) There is marked swelling of the subcutis of the ventral abdominal wall and inguinal regions (arrowed). The subcutis has a streaky appearance (chemical cellulitis). Free gas (arrowheads) is present within the subcutis overlying the swollen area, caudal to the tail base, and superimposed over the dorsal abdomen (within the retroperitoneal space). A comminuted mid-shaft femoral fracture (*) is also present. (b–c) Following urethrography, contrast medium has leaked (arrowed) extensively around the perineal urethra, tracked into the caudal retroperitoneal space and distally into the mid-femoral area. Subcutaneous emphysema (arrowheads) is also present. Some of the contrast medium within the fascial planes may be within the lymphatic system draining the area. No contrast medium enters the bladder.

- The lateral view is the most important. The VD view is of limited use unless a large vaginal or pelvic mass lesion is present, or an ectopic ureter is identified, in which case the orthogonal view is required to lateralize the lesion.
- Fluoroscopy may be useful to evaluate filling of the urethra as it can be difficult to demonstrate this on an individual film.
- Retrograde vaginourethrography is rarely performed in the cat as the vagina is small and the images are difficult to assess and interpret.

Interpretation:

Normal:

- The vagina, vestibule, cervix and urethra are all demonstrated (Figure 4.23).
- The entire length of the urethra can be assessed without artefacts due to the urinary catheter.
- The caudal urethra is usually wider than the cranial urethra.
- Focal narrowing between the vestibule and vagina is a normal finding. The ratio of the height of the vestibulovaginal junction to the maximum height of the vagina can be calculated on lateral views. A ratio >0.35 is considered anatomically normal; a ratio of 0.26–0.35 is considered indicative of mild stenosis; a ratio of 0.20–0.25 is considered indicative of moderate stenosis; and a ratio <0.20 is considered indicative of severe stenosis. However, care should be taken when applying these ratios as muscular contractions can mimic vaginal stenosis.
- The vagina is larger in intact bitches and those receiving oestrogen therapy for incontinence. This may lead to poor filling of the urethra. This enlargement or 'ballooning' of the vagina may lead to a false diagnosis of vestibulovaginal stenosis.
- The normal cervix has a 'spoon' or 'corkscrew' appearance.
- The uterine horns may fill with contrast medium in intact bitches.

Abnormal:

- Ectopic ureters may be demonstrated.
- Rupture of the vagina or urethra (secondary to disease, excess pressure or volume of contrast medium).
- Irregularity or strictures of the mucosal folds of the vagina and vestibule (vaginal stenosis, vaginitis, neoplastic masses).
- Luminal filling defects arising from the vaginal wall (neoplasia, granulomatous inflammation) (Figures 4.24 and 4.25).
- Communication between the vagina, urethra or cervix/uterus and the colon.

Antegrade nephropyelography

In severe obstructive renal disease, as can occur secondary to ureteral obstruction or accidental ligation of the ureter at ovariohysterectomy, contrast medium may not accumulate sufficiently for a diagnostic pyelogram to be produced. Therefore, demonstration of the cause of the ureteric obstruction is not possible. To overcome these difficulties, contrast medium can be injected directly into the renal pelvis of the affected kidney. This technique is termed antegrade nephropyelography (Figure 4.26). The procedure is rarely performed and case selection is crucial. The technique requires experience. Irreversible damage to the

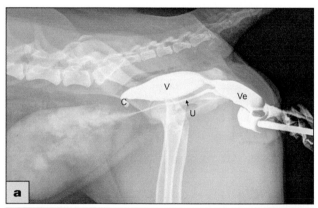

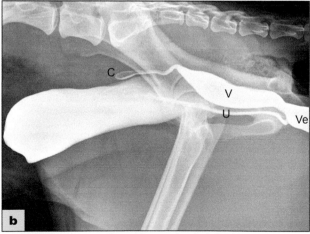

4.23 Retrograde vaginourethrography in two normal bitches. **(a)** The vestibule (Ve) and vagina (V) are well filled with smooth margins. The slight narrowing between the vagina and the vestibule is normal. The urethra (U; arrowed) is of even diameter and well filled with contrast medium along its length. In this bitch, the bladder has not been emptied, which can help distend the urethra. The tip of the bulb of the Foley catheter has been cut off and lies below the distal urethral orifice. **(b)** The 'spoon'-shape of the cervix (C) is normal.

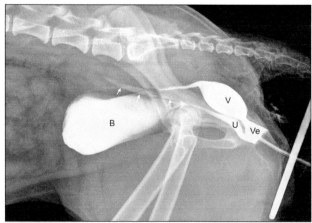

4.24 Retrograde vaginourethrography in an entire bitch with urinary incontinence. A large diameter tubular ectopic ureter (arrowed) entering the proximal urethra has filled with contrast medium following vaginourethrography. B = bladder; U = urethra; V = vagina; Ve = vestibule.

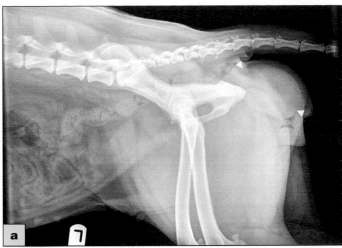

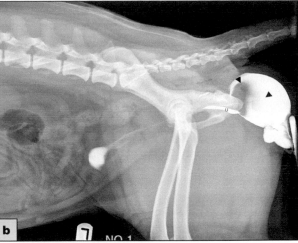

4.25 Retrograde vaginourethrography in an entire bitch with a vaginal mass (leiomyoma). **(a)** Lateral survey view of the pelvis. The large oval soft tissue mass is easily recognized (arrowheads). **(b)** The retrograde study is performed to determine the extent of the mass. Note that although the mass is large and causes a large filling defect (arrowheads), the vagina is still able to fill significantly with contrast medium. There is no involvement of the urethra (U).

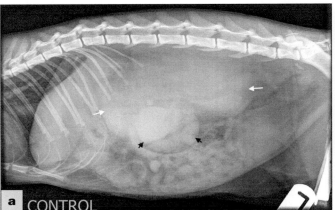

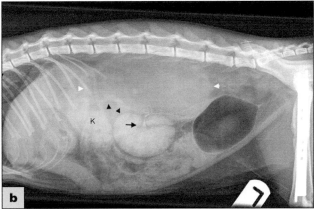

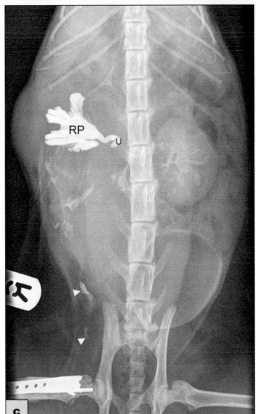

4.26 Antegrade nephropyelography in a cat with severe hydronephrosis of the right kidney due to a urinoma. **(a)** Lateral survey abdominal radiograph. A large, smoothly marginated homogeneous soft tissue mass (white arrows) occupies the dorsal abdomen. One of the kidneys (black arrows) is displaced ventrally by the mass. **(b)** Lateral radiograph taken following intravenous urography. The ventrally displaced kidney and ureter opacify normally (black arrow). There is poor enhancement of the other kidney (K) and ureter (black arrowheads). The large dorsal mass (white arrowheads) does not enhance. **(c)** VD radiograph taken following antegrade nephropyelography. A volume of 3 ml of contrast medium was injected directly into the dilated pelvis (RP) of the right kidney. The proximal ureter (U) is dilated and terminates abruptly. The remainder of the ureter is not filled apart from the terminal saccular dilatations (arrowheads). The wispy contrast medium caudal to the kidney is due to leakage from the injection site. The study confirms that the right kidney and ureter do not communicate with the dorsal mass. The right ureter is not just displaced but almost completely, and irreversibly, obstructed. A urinoma is a large cystic pararenal mass in the retroperitoneal space due to leakage of urine from the kidney or ureter, usually as a result of trauma, and leads to ureteric obstruction.

already compromised renal parenchyma and laceration of the renal vasculature are possible complications. Leakage of contrast medium along the needle tract and around the kidneys complicates interpretation.

Gastrointestinal tract studies

Ultrasonography and endoscopy have superseded contrast radiographic studies as the techniques of choice for evaluation of the gastrointestinal tract. However, radiographic and fluoroscopic (dynamic) studies using barium as a positive-contrast agent remain important diagnostic tools for examination of the oropharynx, oesophagus and stomach. Fluoroscopy is the modality of choice for assessing swallowing disorders and is used when a functional disorder is suspected.

As barium studies of the stomach and intestine (also known as 'barium follow-through studies') are rarely performed these days (they are time-consuming, expensive, generate a low diagnostic yield and have been superseded by other techniques), it is important for the clinician to be familiar with the features of a normal diagnostic study so that pathology can be recognized.

Studies of the gastrointestinal tract (excluding the colon) are usually performed with the patient conscious. Sedation may occasionally be necessary in some patients, but the potential effect on gastric emptying and the risk of regurgitation or aspiration should be considered. Barium should never be administered orally to an anaesthetized animal. The study will be non-diagnostic and there is an increased risk of aspiration of barium.

Health and safety considerations

The radiation safety implications of fluoroscopy need to be considered. Occupational exposure (i.e. to those staff involved in performing the examination) is greater than that for conventional radiographic examinations in small animal practice. Occupational exposure is closely related to the length of time that screening occurs. In addition, with fluoroscopic studies of the gastrointestinal tract, a horizontal beam is almost always used and staff are usually in close proximity to the tube in order to restrain the animal. Therefore, fluoroscopic studies should be reserved for animals in which there is a high index of suspicion for a disease that can be confirmed using fluoroscopy, and for cooperative patients in which screening can be kept to a minimum. Interpretation can be challenging and therefore studies should only be performed if the image can be recorded for review.

Oesophagus

Indications:

- Regurgitation.
- Retching.
- Haematemesis.
- Hypersalivation and pain associated with suspected ulceration/oesophagitis.
- Aspiration/recurrent bronchopneumonia.
- Dysphagia.

A suspected oesophageal foreign body (i.e. one not evident on survey films and where there is no evidence of oesophageal perforation) can be considered an indication for a contrast study of the oesophagus. However, endoscopy should be considered the preferred diagnostic technique where available.

Contraindications: Barium should not be administered to animals where there is the possibility of oesophageal perforation as leakage of barium into the mediastinum or pleural space results in potentially catastrophic fibrogranulomatous mediastinitis or pleuritis. There is no justification for the use of barium in the investigation of suspected pharyngeal stick injuries. Trauma to the pharynx and larynx can lead to temporary dysfunction of the coordinated swallowing movements and aspiration of barium. If perforation of the pharynx or oesophagus has occurred barium may leak into the fascial planes of the neck.

Complications:

- Aspiration of barium into the airways and lungs.
- Leakage of barium into the mediastinum or pleural space.

Technique:

- Orthogonal survey radiographs are obtained. These films are inspected for evidence of aspiration pneumonia. The presence and severity of the aspiration pneumonia should dictate whether the contrast study is delayed and the patient managed medically (fed from a height, antibiosis) until stabilized. The risk of further aspiration in debilitated patients usually outweighs the necessity for an immediate oesophageal contrast study.
- Barium can be administered as a suspension, paste or with food. It is usually difficult to administer a sufficiently large volume of barium liquid by syringe into the buccal fold and to position the patient before the barium is rapidly propelled into the stomach. Thick barium paste placed on the tongue or hard palate usually persists long enough for radiographs to be obtained. However, paste is not appropriate for demonstrating the presence or extent of oesophageal dilatation. It is usually more convenient to mix a soft or semi-liquid food with 30 ml of barium liquid and allow the patient to eat most of the mixture before positioning and obtaining the required views. Most patients with oesophageal disease associated with regurgitation are hungry, especially after food has been withheld for 12 hours, and will eat readily. This technique consistently demonstrates oesophageal dilatation and the location of any oesophageal narrowing.
- Lateral views centred on the cervical and thoracic oesophagus usually suffice. The cervical view should include the oropharynx, and the thoracic view should include the thoracic inlet and stomach (to assess for hiatal hernia). It is usually impossible to obtain VD views.
- Where patient cooperation permits, the oesophageal study is repeated 2–3 times as the study is dynamic and changes may only be evident on one film.

■ With some diseases, mild focal stenosis may be overlooked when liquid barium or barium mixed with soft or semi-liquid food is used. A barium meal consisting of larger food chunks or biscuit may be required.

Interpretation:

Normal:

■ A bolus of barium or a barium–food mixture is pushed from the base of the tongue into the pharynx. Once accumulated, and depending on the texture of the contrast medium, this action may take several seconds. The pharynx is moderately distended by the developing bolus, but there should be no reflux into the nasopharynx or aspiration into the cranial cervical trachea. The pharynx is pushed forward, the cricopharyngeal sphincter opens and the bolus is pushed into the cranial oesophagus by the pharyngeal muscles. Opening of the cricopharyngeal sphincter is transient and almost never recognized. Consistent visualization of the contrast bolus within the sphincter is abnormal.

■ The oesophageal bolus is usually shaped like a short, fat sausage and is rapidly propelled to the stomach. It may be delayed transiently above the diaphragm before the lower oesophageal sphincter opens. A small amount of streaky barium may persist in places along the oesophagus (Figure 4.27), but secondary peristaltic waves usually move this towards the stomach so that no contrast medium remains after approximately 30 seconds.

■ There should be no reflux of material into the oesophagus from the stomach. If only a single exposure is taken, the chance of identifying reflux is limited.

■ Contrast medium should not adhere to the wall of the oesophagus, particularly after all primary and secondary peristaltic waves have been completed.

■ All of these features are better recognized on fluoroscopy than radiography.

Abnormal:

■ Reflux into the nasopharynx, aspiration into the trachea or gastro-oesophageal reflux.

■ Adherence or persistence of barium may suggest the presence of ulceration or neoplasia.

■ Pooling of barium indicates abnormal oesophageal motility, which can vary from hypomotility to generalized megaoesophagus (Figures 4.28 and 4.29).

■ Leakage of contrast medium into the mediastinum or airways (but study choice would be inappropriate in this case).

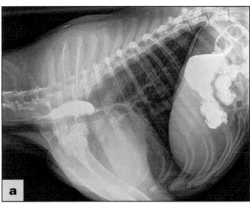
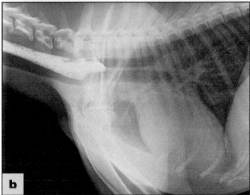
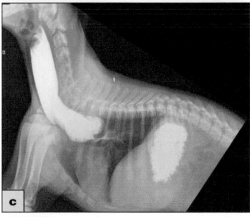

4.28 Oesophageal contrast studies in three dogs with **(a)** normal oesophageal function, **(b)** mild hypomotility and **(c)** a severe segmental dilatation of the oesophagus, respectively. (a) The bolus is discrete and sausage-shaped. (b) There is moderate dilatation of the caudal cervical and cranial thoracic oesophagus and the bolus is elongated. Oesophageal hypomotility in this dog improved with age. (c) The entire cervical and cranial thoracic segments of the oesophagus are dilated. The sacculation narrows abruptly dorsal to the base of the cardiac silhouette due to a persistent right aortic arch. There is dilatation caudal to the narrowing, but the barium meal passes into the stomach. Compare the location of the narrowing in this case with that in Figure 4.29.

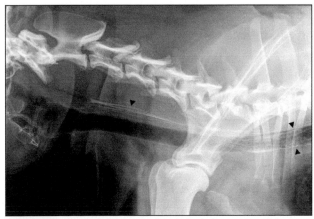

4.27 Oesophageal contrast study in a normal dog. The barium has collected temporarily in the linear smooth muscle folds (arrowheads). In the normal dog, further secondary peristaltic waves of contraction strip any retained barium caudally and into the stomach.

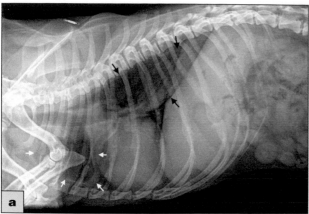 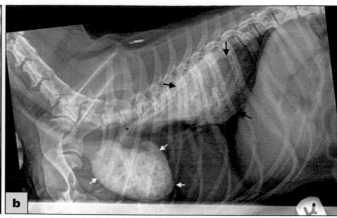

4.29 **(a)** Lateral survey thoracic radiograph and **(b)** barium contrast study in a French Bulldog with recurrent regurgitation due to a large oesophageal diverticulum. (a) A triangular structure of gas opacity is superimposed over the ventral thorax cranial to the heart (white arrows). Particulate mineral material suggestive of a 'gravel sign' overlies the ventral third to fourth intercostal spaces. Note that the cranial thoracic trachea does not deviate ventrally. The caudal oesophagus is also dilated (black arrows). (b) Following contrast medium administration, a large diverticulum in the cranial thorax fills with barium (white arrows). The dilated caudal oesophagus also partially fills with barium (black arrows). Note that the location of the 'normal' oesophagus at the caudal extent of the diverticulum is at the level of the second rib (*). For most vascular ring anomalies, the oesophagus is narrowed at the cranial heart base (which lies at the fourth to sixth intercostal space) and is an important distinguishing feature in this dog.

Stomach and small intestine

Indications:

- To assess the location of the stomach in relation to the liver, diaphragm or cranial abdominal masses.
- Persistent vomiting, especially where accompanied by weight loss.
- Haematemesis or melaena.
- Abdominal discomfort or swelling.
- To assess a palpable abdominal mass associated with the gastrointestinal tract.

Contraindications:

- Swallowing disorders predisposing to the aspiration of barium.
- Suspected gastrointestinal tract perforation.
- Suspected oesophageal foreign body.
- Obvious foreign body (lucent or opaque) or convincing signs of obstruction on survey films.
- Suspected linear foreign body.

Complications:

- Aspiration of barium into the lungs.
- Peritonitis if there is leakage of barium into the abdomen.

The investigation of recurrent or episodic vomiting or diarrhoea not associated with weight loss by means of barium contrast studies is often unrewarding. The signs in these patients are usually best evaluated with ultrasonography.

Types of study:

- Pneumogastrogram – primarily used to assess the location of the stomach and large mass lesions.
- Positive-contrast gastrogram – primarily used to assess the location of the stomach, and to evaluate gastric emptying and large mass lesions involving the stomach (small mass lesions may be obscured).

- 'Barium follow-through study' (small intestine) – primarily used to assess for partial or complete obstruction suspected on survey radiographs, evaluate for mass lesions or ulcers resulting in melaena, and to determine the location of the small intestinal loops (herniation, incarceration).

Technique:

- Food is withheld for 24 hours where possible.
- Survey films (including the thorax to rule out the presence of an oesophageal foreign body) are obtained. These should include both left and right lateral recumbent, VD and dorsoventral (DV) views centred on the cranial abdomen. If necessary, an enema should be administered.
- Ideally, the study is performed with the patient conscious, but where necessary neuroleptanalgesia (acepromazine and/or butorphanol/buprenorphine) may be used to facilitate patient cooperation. The effect on intestinal motility is usually minimal and may be less than the delay caused by anxiety in a nervous patient. A satisfactory study usually requires 8–10 exposures (orthogonal views). Thus, such studies are unsuitable for all but the most relaxed and cooperative of cats.
- For examination of the stomach, a volume of 5–10 ml/kg of a 30–50% w/v barium sulphate liquid suspension is used. The barium used for gastric and small intestinal studies can be mixed with warm water and semi-liquid food to improve palatability, but the consistency should be liquid. The use of barium–food mixtures (chunks or biscuit) is usually limited to oesophageal studies.
- The liquid barium mixture is usually administered into the buccal pouch via syringe or a plastic bottle fitted with a nozzle. In cooperative patients, the use of a gag and stomach tube is usually efficient and well tolerated. However, it should be noted that as this procedure is performed less frequently, clinicians may be less practiced at

placing a stomach tube in the conscious patient.

- Following the administration of contrast medium, four radiographic views (as used for the survey films) are immediately obtained.
- These views should be repeated at 10–15 minute intervals, depending on the rate at which gastric emptying is observed. In most patients, gastric emptying starts immediately and is advanced by 30 minutes. In patients with delayed emptying due to structural disease, functional disease (pylorospasm) or in nervous animals, this can take up to 2–3 hours, and the need for further exposures should be adapted accordingly.
- A barium study of the small intestine ('barium follow-through study') follows the positive-contrast gastrogram, either as the principal purpose of the study or as a continuation of the study if no lesion is indentified in the stomach. For the small intestine, lateral and VD views suffice. Films are obtained every 15 minutes until the barium has reached the colon. A radiograph must be taken 24 hours after the administration of barium (Figure 4.30) to demonstrate that all the contrast medium has reached the colon and that no barium has been retained in the stomach or small intestine, which could represent a foreign body or retention in damaged mucosa.

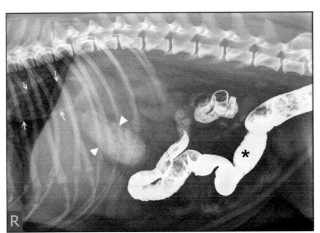

4.30 Lateral abdominal radiograph of a dog with chronic vomiting. Barium has been administered previously, almost all of which has reached the colon (*) within 24 hours. Indistinct barium retained in the stomach is incorporated within foreign material (arrowheads). The caudal oesophagus is dilated with gas (arrowed). A sock foreign body was removed at surgery. Films should be obtained 24 hours after contrast medium administration to rule out foreign material obscured by barium during the examination. Residual barium retained by, or adhered to, foreign material can be recognized on delayed films.

Interpretation:

Normal:

- If survey films demonstrate marked retention of ingesta in the stomach, then the goal of the study should be reconsidered. A positive-contrast study may still be appropriate for assessing gastric emptying, but filling defects should not be mistaken for masses or foreign bodies.
- A positive-contrast gastrogram does not usually result in complete filling of the stomach with

barium. A volume of air almost inevitably remains, resulting in radiographic features of a double-contrast gastrogram.
- The appearance and location of the pool of barium within the stomach varies with the position of the animal and volume of contrast medium administered (Figure 4.31):
  - With the patient in right lateral recumbency, the fundus and body are uppermost and the pylorus is dependent and will fill with barium. The pylorus appears as a roughly rounded pool of barium in the cranioventral abdomen. Smooth U-shaped filling defects, 2–4 mm wide and 4–6 mm deep, represent rugal folds viewed end-on. There is variable filling of the fundus and body of the stomach, depending on the volume of barium administered
  - In left lateral recumbency, barium pools in the fundus and body, and the pylorus is filled with gas. The mucosa is well defined due to barium coating the mucosa and gas in the lumen (double-contrast effect). The location of the duodenal sphincter may be recognized. The proximal duodenum is usually angled craniodorsally before turning sharply caudodorsally beneath the right kidney
  - On the DV view, the barium pools in the body of the stomach which lies perpendicular to the thoracic spine. The amount of filling of the fundus and pylorus varies depending on the volume of contrast medium administered, the rate of emptying of the stomach and the conformation of the animal. The pylorus is more likely to fill with contrast medium in shallow-chested dogs
  - On the VD view, the barium pools in the fundus (dependent portion of the stomach) and variably in the pylorus. The descending duodenum may also fill contrast medium.
- As opening and closing of the sphincter is transient, the pyloric sphincter itself is rarely identified. In animals with ileus, the sphincter may be visualized as a constant, focal smooth narrowing or 'pinching' between the pylorus and the duodenum.
- Liquid barium is emptied from the stomach more rapidly than food.
- Peristaltic waves are seen as transient (i.e. not recognized on subsequent films), smoothly marginated, focal areas of gastric narrowing.
- Mucosal folds (rugae) should be smoothly marginated, deep rather than wide, and occur more frequently in the body than in the fundus.
- The following guidelines regarding gastrointestinal motility apply:
  - In many patients, the stomach starts to empty immediately or at least within 15 minutes. The more distended the stomach, the more rapid the onset of gastric emptying. The stomach is normally empty by the time the contrast medium reaches the colon. In nervous animals, or those in pain, gastric emptying may be delayed by up to several hours
  - Barium should reach the colon within 4 hours of administration
  - All barium should have reached the colon within 24 hours of administration.

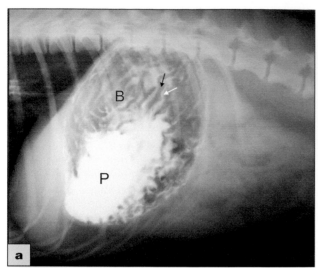

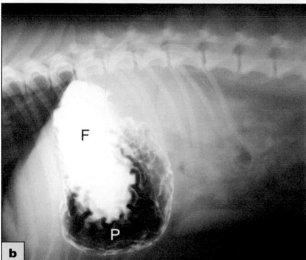

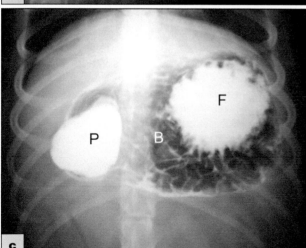

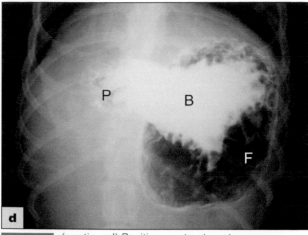

4.31 (continued) Positive-contrast gastrogram. **(d)** DV view. The body (B) is dependent and filled with barium. The appearance of the pylorus (P) depends on the volume of barium administered and the orientation of the stomach in relation to the conformation of the animal (the stomach is more upright in deep-chested dogs). It should be remembered that the body is the largest part of the stomach, thus the air-filled area (F) includes part of the body. (Courtesy of Cambridge Veterinary School)

- A small intestinal contrast study in a normal animal should demonstrate:
  - A smooth continuous column of contrast medium with intestinal loops of even diameter. The intestinal loops should be sinuous or tightly looped (Figure 4.32). The contrast medium column should not be interrupted. The location of the small intestine should be visible from the pylorus, along the right body wall ventral to the kidney, caudal to the root of the mesentery at L1–L2 (caudal duodenal flexure), to the mass of small intestines within the mid-abdomen. The ileocolic junction is recognized in almost all dogs to the right of the midline at the level of L2–L3. The caecum has a bilobed or corkscrew appearance

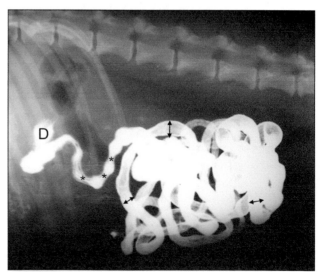

4.32 'Barium follow-through study' of the small intestine. The barium column is continuous, and the intestinal loops are all of a similar diameter (double-headed arrows) and form tight bends. The mucosal surfaces are smooth. The proximal duodenum (D) continues distally into the descending duodenum and several peristaltic waves (*) are visible.

4.31 Positive-contrast gastrogram. **(a)** Right lateral recumbent view. Barium fills the dependent portion of the stomach (pylorus, P) with air in the body and fundus (B). The degree of filling of the body and fundus depends on the volume of contrast medium administered. The rugal folds (black arrow) in the body are parallel, sinuous and thick. The interrugal areas (white arrow) are filled with barium. **(b)** Left lateral recumbent view. The pylorus (P), and a large proportion of the body (as the volume of barium administered is small), are filled with gas. The rugal folds in the pylorus and distal body are less numerous. The fundus (F) is filled with barium. **(c)** VD view. The pylorus (P) and fundus (F) are dependent and filled with barium. The body (B) is filled with gas. (Courtesy of Cambridge Veterinary School) (continues) ▶

- Normal findings in the dog include shallow flattened indentations along the anti-mesenteric border of the duodenum due to Peyer's patches, and in the cat the descending duodenum may have a segmented appearance ('string of pearls') due to peristalsis. In some dogs, a fine fimbriated appearance along the mucosal margin may be appreciated as a normal finding where barium has extended between the villi.

Abnormal:

- Areas of the stomach that do not distend evenly or adequately may reflect areas of wall thickening due to mass lesions, infiltration or spasm. Wall thickness should be assessed in these regions.
- Failure of the stomach to empty can indicate complete obstruction of the pylorus or proximal duodenum, but retention of barium within the stomach can be prolonged and dramatic in very nervous animals or those in pain. Mass lesions (Figure 4.33) and most foreign bodies can usually be seen, but obstruction as a result of linear foreign bodies or stenosis due to adhesions can be challenging to identify.

- Irregular or patchy areas of contrast medium accumulation ('flocculation') may occur where there is pathology or pooling of gastric secretions, which mix poorly with barium. Retention of barium consistently in the same area of the stomach on more than one exposure, and preferably on more than one view, when most of the barium has emptied from the stomach can indicate ulceration (primary, inflammatory or associated with neoplasia).
- In the stomach, filling defects represent areas in which contrast medium is expected to pool but does not, and therefore they appear radiolucent. Filling defects can be due to intraluminal material (foreign bodies) or mural lesions.
- Any pathology or filling defect should be recognized on more than one exposure and, preferably, on more than one view to be considered reliable.
- The location of gastrointestinal structures within the abdomen, especially the highly mobile small intestine, can provide an indication of the presence of other pathology within the abdomen or body wall. Conditions localized outside the gastrointestinal tract (e.g. retained surgical swab, abscess or cyst within the mesenteric root, hernia

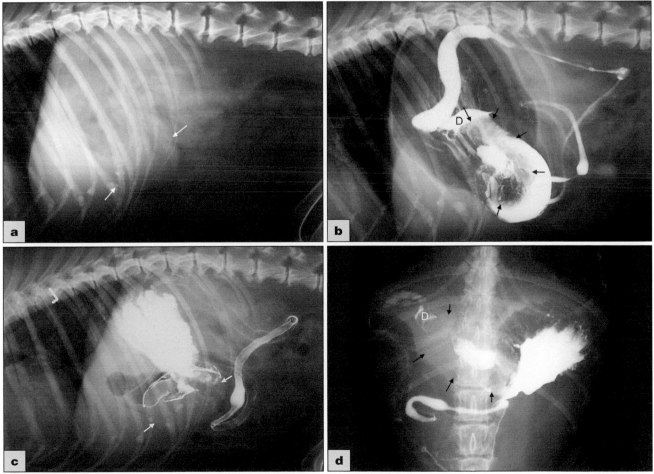

4.33 **(a)** Right lateral survey radiograph of a dog with a gastric mass. The mass is indistinguishable from the fluid-filled pylorus (arrowed). **(b–d)** Double-contrast gastrogram. (b) Right lateral view. The mass appears as a doughnut-shaped filling defect (arrowed) within the craniodorsal aspect of the pylorus. The mass probably extends into the proximal duodenum (D). (c) Left lateral view. The pylorus should be filled with gas but instead is filled with a soft tissue mass. The caudoventral aspect of the body is irregular (arrowed). (d) DV view. The pyloric mass is large (arrowed) and extends into the body to the left of the midline and into the proximal duodenum (D). The mass prevents the pylorus and body filling with barium, except for a small amount superimposed on the midline. (Courtesy of Cambridge Veterinary School)

(diaphragmatic, umbilical, paracostal or inguinal) or adhesions) may be responsible for the clinical signs (chronic or acute) which lead to the barium study being performed. Under these circumstances, the displacement of the gastrointestinal tract structures is better visualized and appreciated, and may help to narrow the list of differential diagnoses.

- Pathology of the small intestine which can be recognized on barium studies includes:
  - Leakage of contrast medium into the abdomen
  - Dilatation of small intestinal loops
  - Filling defects (intraluminal or mural, eccentric or concentric)
  - Abnormal patterns (e.g. two 'populations' of small intestine, intestinal plication, intussusception)
  - Wall thickening.

Large intestine

Endoscopy is generally considered the technique of choice for evaluating the colon. Ultrasonography can provide valuable information, but artefacts and technical ability can be limiting factors. However, contrast radiography may still be appropriate in certain circumstances. It is useful for identifying cecocolic intussusception, suspected masses (including polyps) and fistulas (see Figure 6.39). A pneumocolon procedure is useful where the extent and location of the colon needs to be confirmed. Findings from colonic contrast studies may complement colonoscopy findings (e.g. a barium enema can be useful for evaluating narrowing of the lumen and strictures as it allows better assessment of the degree to which a segment of colon can be distended than endoscopy). A positive-contrast or double-contrast enema can provide fine detail for the detection of mucosal changes, but it is technically difficult and rarely performed.

Indications:

- Tenesmus.
- Haematochezia or melaena.
- Chronic diarrhoea (intussusception).
- Large caudal abdominal or pelvic mass where the location of the colon is not clear or is uncertain.
- To rule out stricture of the colon.

Contraindications:

- Perianal fistulae.
- Risk of colon rupture (localized peritonitis may be suspected on survey films).

Complications:

- Rupture of the colon.
- Haematochezia due to iatrogenic trauma to the mucosa.

Technique:

Pneumocolon:

- Food is withheld for 24 hours. The animal should be offered the opportunity to void and empty its bladder.

- A rectal examination must be performed to ensure that it is safe to perform the procedure.
- A warm water enema is administered several hours before the procedure. If survey radiographs indicate that patient preparation is inadequate, then a further 2–3 warm water enemas should be administered.
- The procedure is, ideally, performed under general anaesthesia.
- A bulb-tipped catheter (Foley catheter with a 'Christmas tree' adaptor for a Luer tip syringe) is used. The bulb must be gently inflated. If there is an air leak, a purse-string suture can be used to make an air-tight seal.
- The colon is slowly insufflated using 5–10 ml/kg of air. The colon should be palpated and more air added, if necessary, based on the exposures.
- Lateral and VD radiographs are obtained. Oblique views can be quite useful to asses intrapelvic structures obscured by the pelvic bones.

Barium enema: This technique is also known as a positive-contrast study.

- Patient preparation is as for a pneumocolon procedure.
- The colon is slowly insufflated with 5–15 ml/kg of a 15–20% w/v barium solution. This solution can be made by diluting a 100% suspension with water.
- Colloidal suspensions rather than barium powder should be used as clumping occurs more readily with powder and could be misinterpreted as pathology.
- The barium suspension is warmed to body temperature to avoid artefacts caused by spasm of the colon.
- A positive-contrast study should not be carried out if rupture of the colon is a possibility or risk.

Interpretation:

Normal:

- Pneumocolon:
  - The diameter of the colon should be even along its length
  - With adequate distension, gas fills all segments of the colon
  - Peristalsis results in transient smooth concentric narrowing of the colon
  - It is possible to distinguish the colon from the small intestine.
- Barium enema:
  - The mucosal lining should be smooth. There are no villi in the colon, so once distended the mucosal surface is very smooth
  - With adequate distension, wall thickness can be evaluated.

Abnormal:

- Pneumocolon:
  - The cranial (orad) aspect of a mass may be demonstrated (this may not be possible endoscopically if the endoscope cannot be advanced alongside and past the mass)

- Stenosis, strictures and poorly distensible segments may be identified (Figure 4.34)
- It may be possible to evaluate whether a mass is intraluminal or extraluminal.
- Barium enema:
  - Significant findings, in particular focal narrowing to concentric disease (e.g. carcinoma) should be consistent
  - Wall thickening, mucosal irregularity, ulceration or masses
  - Stenosis, strictures or poorly distensible segments may be indentified
  - Subtle changes may be missed or inadequate preparation misinterpreted.

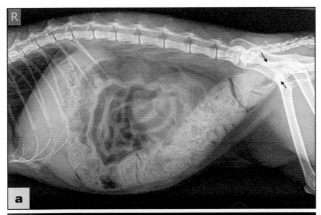
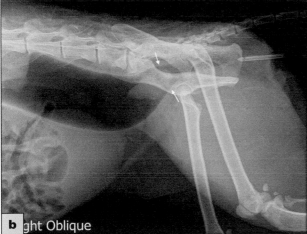

4.34 **(a)** Lateral survey abdominal radiograph of a cat with severe obstipation. Almost the full length of the colon is distended with dense faecal material. The obstipation appears to terminate at the pelvic inlet (arrowed) without substantial accumulation of faeces within the rectum. **(b)** The pneumocolon study (lateral oblique) demonstrates that there is no underlying soft tissue or bony stenosis (arrowed) causing the obstipation.

Miscellaneous procedures

The following contrast procedures are either uncommonly performed, technically challenging or require very specific indications. Only the important indications, specific technical principles or limitations, and advantages and disadvantages are covered here.

Arthrography

The shoulder is the joint most commonly assessed using arthrography. Magnetic resonance imaging (MRI) and CT are also widely used, but arthrography remains a rapid and technically simple procedure, which can be followed by arthroscopy if indicated.

Indications:

- Investigation of shoulder disease.
- Occasionally used to demonstrate disruption of the joint capsule or communication with external wounds.

Technique:

- Arthrography is performed under general anaesthesia.
- Orthogonal survey radiographs are obtained. For the shoulder, this includes a skyline (cranioproximal–craniodistal) view of the bicipital groove.
- The site of the injection is aseptically prepared. Synovial fluid is withdrawn and submitted for analysis.
- Without removing the needle, a volume of 1–5 ml of a diluted (100–150 mg iodine/ml) non-ionic, water-soluble contrast medium is injected. Undiluted contrast medium may mask subtle lesions. Ionic media should not be used as they are irritant.
- The joint is flexed gently to distribute the contrast medium throughout the joint space.
- A poorly performed study may be non-diagnostic due to:
  - The use of undiluted contrast medium
  - Too great a volume of contrast medium being injected, resulting in over-distension of the joint
  - Leakage of contrast medium from the joint
  - The introduction of air bubbles
  - A delay between contrast medium administration and obtaining radiographs, as the contrast medium is rapidly reabsorbed.

Interpretation:

Normal:

- Defines the articular cartilage surfaces, synovial borders and pouches.
- The biceps tendon has a smooth margin and tapers towards its origin from supraglenoid tubercle and sheath (Figure 4.35).

Abnormal:

- Subchondral bone defects, attached cartilage flaps and detached joint mice.
- Bicipital tendon disease:
  - Effusion in the tendon sheath and poor filling with chronic disease
  - Swelling of the tendon
  - Filling defects of the tendon sheath due to swelling of the tendon, joint mice, adhesions or osteophytes in the bicipital groove
  - Total or partial rupture of the tendon or tendon sheath and the orientation of the tear.

Mesenteric portovenography

Indications:

- To confirm the morphology and location of suspected portosystemic anomalous communications.
- To identify intra- and extraportal obstructions (thrombus, mass).

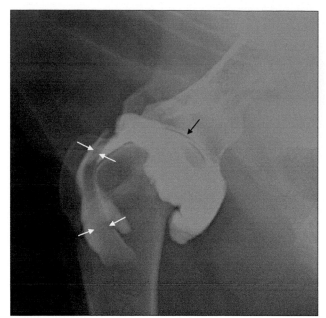

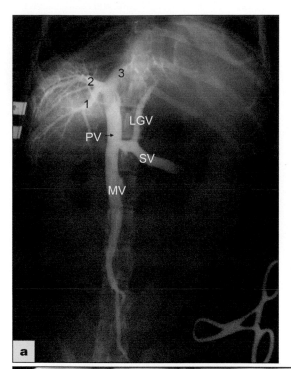

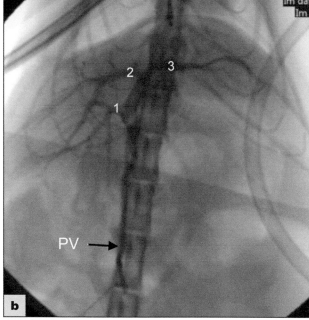

4.35 Normal arthrogram of the shoulder of a dog. There is good filling of the joint and bicipital tendon sheath with contrast medium. There are no filling defects or leakage of contrast medium. The cartilage surfaces are smooth and of even thickness, and appear lucent compared with the contrast medium and subchondral bone (black arrow). The bicipital tendon sheath is evenly filled and the margins of the tendon and tendon sheath are smooth (white arrows). Overfilling of the joint obscures cartilage surfaces in the caudal aspect of the joint. (Courtesy of the University of Bristol)

Technique:

- Mesenteric portovenography is performed intraoperatively under general anaesthesia.
- A mesenteric vein is catheterized.
- VD and lateral survey radiographs are obtained.
- The technique can be performed 2–3 times, usually pre- and post-ligation studies are performed. Either ionic or non-ionic, water-soluble, iodinated contrast media (240–300 mg iodine/ml) can be used. Non-ionic contrast media are safer, but the cost in large-breed dogs may be exorbitant. A maximum dose of 6 ml/kg should not be exceeded.
- A liver biopsy is usually performed. This is particularly important if an anomalous communication cannot be identified on the portovenogram or on gross inspection.

Interpretation:

Normal: In the normal patient, the cranial and caudal mesenteric veins join and from the confluence with the splenic vein, the extrahepatic portal vein is formed. The gastroduodenal vein enters the portal vein just before the porta hepatis. At the porta hepatis, the portal vein divides into a right branch, which branches into the caudate and right lateral liver lobes. The continuation of the portal vein curves to the left, with branches to the right medial, quadrate and, finally, left medial and left lateral liver lobes (Figure 4.36). The diameter of the portal vein increases gradually as it approaches the porta hepatis.

4.36 **(a)** Radiographic and **(b)** fluoroscopic views of a normal portovenogram. (a) The water-soluble, iodinated contrast medium appears white. (b) Contrast medium within the splanchnic vessels appears black (opposite to a conventional radiographic image). The portal vein (PV) divides into a right branch, which branches to the caudate and right lateral (1) liver lobes. The continuation of the portal vein curves to the left with branches to the right medial (2), quadrate, left medial and left lateral (3) liver lobes. Multiple smaller intrahepatic branch ramifications are visible. LGV = left gastric vein; MV = mesenteric vein; SV = splenic vein. (b, Courtesy of Bristol University)

Abnormal:

- In patients with portosystemic shunts (Figures 4.37 and 4.38), portovenography demonstrates an anomalous vessel connecting the portal vein, or one of its tributaries, to the caudal vena cava or right side of the heart (portoazygous shunt).

- The identification of shunting vessels may be challenging, especially with intrahepatic shunts. Differentiation of intrahepatic shunts from extrahepatic shunts can also be difficult in some instances.
- Poor filling of large shunts (particularly intrahepatic shunts) due to the size of the shunt, insufficient volume of contrast medium injected, early or delayed radiographic exposures, or injection of contrast medium over too long a period can all lead to the shunt not being demonstrated by the study.
- Hypoplastic portal vein.
- Acquired shunts, tortuous vessels in the dorsal abdomen entering the caudal vena cava directly or via the left renal or gonadal vein.
- Rarely, thrombi or mass lesions invading the portal vein can be identified.

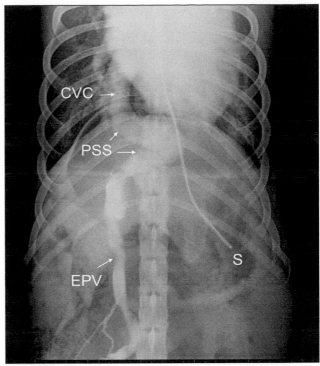

4.38 VD portovenogram of a dog with an intrahepatic portosystemic shunt (PSS). The shunt forms a large sigmoid curve to the left (left divisional shunt or patent ductus venosus) and drains into the caudal vena cava (CVC) at the level of the diaphragm. Note that because of the large diameter of the vessel, the contrast medium has a diluted appearance. EPV = extrahepatic portal vein; S = stomach.

Peripheral lymphangiography

Indications:

- Evaluate swelling of the distal limb due to suspected lymphoedema.
- Not commonly performed.

Technique:

- Direct catheterization of a distal lymphatic vessel is technically challenging. The alternative of injecting 1–2 ml of a 240–300 mg iodine/ml, non-ionic, iodinated contrast medium solution into the subcutis distal to the swelling usually allows diagnostic radiographs to be obtained. In the limbs, contrast medium is injected into the subcutis between the pads.
- The contrast medium is rapidly absorbed and serial radiographs are obtained immediately after injection.
- If there is doubt as to the significance of a lesion, contrast medium can be injected into both limbs. If the disease is unilateral, the normal limb serves as a control.

Interpretation:

Normal:

- The lymphatic vessels appear as undulating linear structures resembling vasculature (Figure 4.39). They drain into the local lymph nodes, which also opacify.
- Contrast medium injected into the hindlimbs can occasionally be followed via the cisterna chyli into the thorax and right atrium.

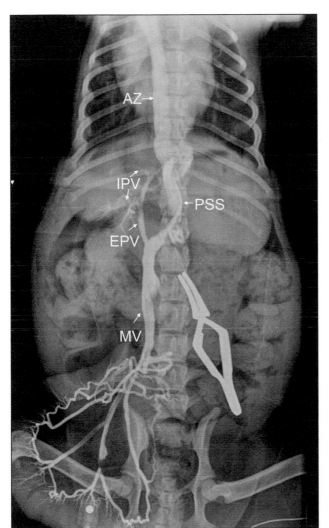

4.37 VD portovenogram of a dog with an extrahepatic shunt (portoazygous). The large diameter shunting vessel (PSS) is superimposed on the spine from T11–L1 and continues within the thorax via the enlarged right azygous vein (AZ). The distal extrahepatic portal vein (EPV) is reduced in diameter compared with the shunting vessel. There is poor opacification of the intrahepatic portal veins (IPV) with only the caudate, right medial and right lateral primary branches visible. The material to be used to restrict the diameter of the shunt, in this case a cellophane band which is not visible on the radiograph, has been preplaced around the shunt and secured with metal forceps. MV = mesenteric vein.

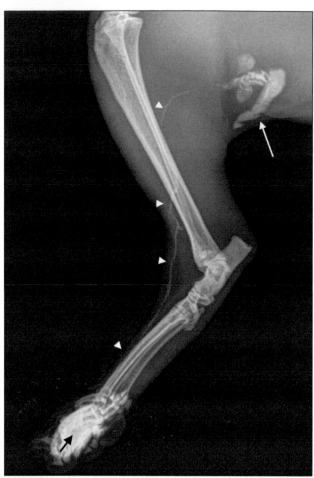

Abnormal:

- Abnormal lymphatic vessels, which can be dilated and distorted (Figure 4.40).
- Interruption of proximal drainage.

Mesenteric lymphangiography

Indications:

- To visualize the thoracic duct in cases of chylothorax.
- This procedure is technically challenging and not commonly performed.

Technique:

- A mesenteric lymphatic vessel is catheterized and a non-ionic, iodinated contrast medium administered.
- Contrast medium is rapidly absorbed into the lymphatic vessels/cisterna chyli and radiographs are obtained immediately following injection.

Interpretation:

Normal:

- It can be difficult, or impossible, to recognize contrast medium within the thoracic ducts if a large volume of pleural fluid remains.
- The cisterna chyli extends from the mid-lumbar vertebra through the diaphragm.

Abnormal:

- Multiple abnormal lymphatic vessels within the thorax.

4.39 Lymphangiography. Contrast medium has been injected into the subcutis of the paw (black arrow). The lymphatic vessels (arrowheads) are rapidly filled and drain into the local lymphocentre (in this case, the popliteal lymphocentre; white arrow). The lymph nodes have a flattened, elongated appearance.

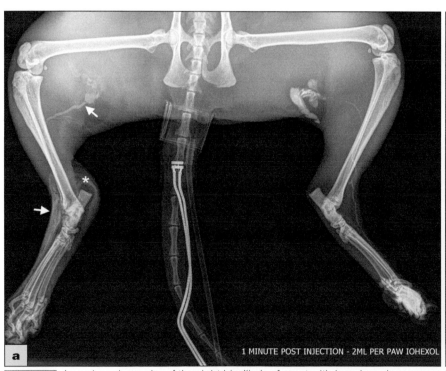
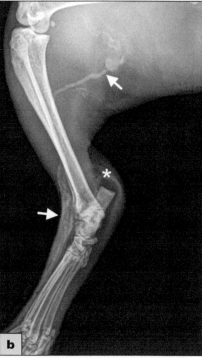

1 MINUTE POST INJECTION - 2ML PER PAW IOHEXOL

4.40 Lymphangiography of the right hindlimb of a cat with lymphangiosarcoma. This is the same cat as in Figure 4.39. **(a)** There is marked swelling of the distal right limb (*). The lymphatic vessels are dilated and tortuous with focal sacculations in places (arrowed). Multiple vessels are present. The nodes of the lymphocentre are rounded and poorly circumscribed compared with those of the left limb. **(b)** Magnified view.

Sinography and fistulography

These techniques have generally been superseded by cross-sectional imaging.

Indications and interpretation:

- These techniques can be used to investigate draining tracts in the pharyngeal/cervical or flank regions. As multiple tracts can be superimposed on one another, not all tracts are demonstrated, and the identification of a foreign body is often impossible.
- In a limited number of cases, these techniques are still useful (e.g. to demonstrate a communication between two cavities, viscera or anatomical areas) (Figure 4.41).
- If a communication between two viscera is suspected (e.g. rectovaginal fistula), then a non-ionic, water-soluble contrast agent is injected into the sterile/less contaminated viscus (i.e. the vagina not the rectum) to avoid introducing infection.

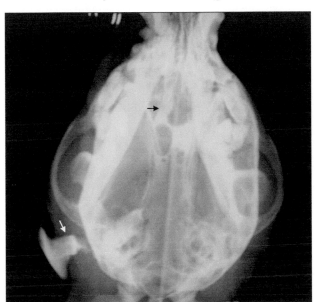

4.41 Sinography in a dog with a draining tract beneath the right ear and concurrent reverse sneezing following bulla osteotomy. Water-soluble contrast medium has been injected into the sinus (white arrow) beneath the right ear and has collected in the nasopharynx (black arrow). Note the large air bubbles in the contrast medium pool. Sinography and fistulography can be useful to demonstrate a functional connection between viscera or cavities. (Courtesy of Cambridge Veterinary School)

Technique:

- Bulb tip catheters are used to avoid leakage of contrast medium.
- The opening of the sinus tract is marked with a metal probe or marker.

Dacryocystography

This technique is also known as dacryocysto-rhinography.

Indications:

- Investigation of chronic conjunctivitis and epiphora, and to confirm the patency of the lacrimal duct.

- Investigation of facial swellings associated with epiphora and conjunctivitis.

Complications:

- Rupture or the introduction of infection.

Technique:

- Dacryocystography is performed under general anaesthesia.
- The diseased side of the head is placed closest to the cassette for survey radiographs, but for contrast studies is placed closer to the X-ray tube to facilitate the administration of contrast medium.
- The nose can be tilted downwards to promote drainage via the lacrimal duct and to avoid retrograde flow into the nasal chambers and posterior nares.
- The superior (usually) or inferior punctum can be catheterized using a nasolacrimal catheter. The remaining punctum can be closed using digital pressure. A well placed catheter is usually quite stable or can be taped to the adjacent skin. The catheter is advanced as far as possible to prevent retrograde movement during the contrast medium injection.
- A volume of 0.5–2 ml of undiluted iodine-containing, water-soluble, non-ionic contrast medium is administered.
- A lateral view, centred on the maxilla and including the nares, is obtained immediately following injection of the contrast medium. Repeating the radiographs after removing any contrast medium that has leaked is very important to demonstrate consistent findings, particularly if an intraluminal structure is suspected or filling is not adequate. Additional views which may be useful include an intraoral DV view of the nose, a ventro 20 degrees rostral–caudodorsal oblique (V20°R-DCdO) view and a lateral 30 degrees ventrodorsal oblique (L30°VDO) view (see Chapter 8).
- Poor filling is often due to inadequate technique.

Interpretation:

Normal: On lateral or lateral oblique views, the lacrimal duct extends ventrally from the lacrimal sac, caudal to the maxilla, and then turns sharply rostrally at the level of the maxillary recess. The duct extends rostrally, at the level of the mid-nasal chamber, is superimposed on the proximal root of the mandibular canines and empties into the nasal vestibule. The duct is of even diameter. Occasionally, both the upper and lower lacrimal canaliculi and the lacrimal sac are filled with contrast medium (Figure 4.42), if a sufficiently large volume has been used. On DV or VD oblique views, the duct extends the length of the nasal cavity medial to the maxillary recess and maxillary premolars and canines to enter the nasal vestibule.

Abnormal:

- Occlusion may be partial or complete and due to discharge, foreign material, stenosis as a result of scarring or mass lesions (Figure 4.43).

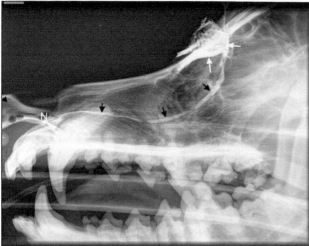

4.42 Dacryocystography in a normal dog. The upper and lower canaliculi (white arrows), lacrimal sac and lacrimal duct are well filled with contrast medium. The lacrimal duct (black arrows) curves sharply ventrally and then extends rostrally to open within the nasal vestibule (N), just rostral to the maxillary canine. Contrast medium also fills the nares and has refluxed into the ventral nasal meatus and surrounds the rostral turbinates. Reflux can be limited by positioning the nares lower than the rest of the nose and suspending the contrast medium injection as soon as there is leakage from the nares.

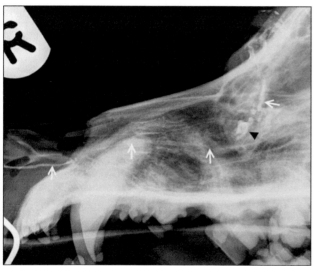

4.43 Dacryocystography in a dog with epiphora due to obstruction of the lacrimal duct. Although contrast medium has accumulated within the nasal vestibule demonstrating patency of the duct, the duct itself is poorly filled along its length (arrowed). Pockets of contrast medium (flocculation) are present in the segment of the duct dorsal to the maxillary recess (arrowhead). This suggests poor filling of the duct and the accumulation of discharge, or a foreign body. A grass seed foreign body was removed.

- Dilatation of the duct proximal to a complete obstruction or stenosis. Intraluminal obstruction results in a filling defect, but the cause of the obstruction is challenging to identify.
- Extraluminal causes can be recognized by demonstrating the presence of the primary mass and broad-based obstruction of the duct.
- Stenosis appears as a consistently non-distended segment of the duct.
- Lacrimal cysts are large cystic cavities which communicate with the lacrimal system and fill with

contrast medium. These can cause localized lucent or lytic areas due to pressure necrosis of the overlying bone.

Sialography

Studies are rarely performed as they usually do not contribute to the management of suspected salivary mucoceles, tumours or abscesses. The presence of sialoliths is not an indication for sialography, unless they are accompanied by swelling or clinical signs.

Indications:

- Demonstrate whether soft tissue masses in the pharyngeal region communicate with one of the salivary glands.
- Demonstrate obstruction of the salivary ducts.

Technique:

- Survey radiographs are obtained.
- The punctum of the salivary gland being investigated is catheterized (see Chapter 8 for a description of the location of the punctae). This can be technically difficult, but is facilitated by initial catheterization of the duct with a thin piece of rigid nylon suture material over which the catheter can be advanced.
- A volume of 0.5–3 ml of diluted (approximately 150 mg iodine/ml), non-ionic, iodinated contrast medium is administered. The volume of contrast medium should be adjusted based on the requirements of the study (evaluation of the duct requires a smaller volume of contrast medium compared with examination of the glands for which a larger volume of contrast medium is required). Injection of an excessive volume of contrast medium can be associated with discomfort.
- Lateral and VD views are obtained.

Interpretation:

Normal:

- The salivary ducts appear as thin tubular structures of even diameter.
- The glands fill with contrast medium and appear rounded to trapezoidal or U-shaped, depending on the gland. The contrast medium within the gland creates a coalescing cobblestone pattern.

Abnormal:

- Pathology is difficult to interpret, but there may be:
  - Duct obstruction, leakage from a ruptured duct, filling defects in the duct or displacement of the duct by external masses (Figure 4.44)
  - Other filling defects due to mass lesions, abscessation or displacement and distortion of the appearance of the gland due to an external mass effect
  - Extravasation into a homogeneous cavity due to a mucocele
  - Rupture of the gland, which can be recognized by extravasation of contrast medium.

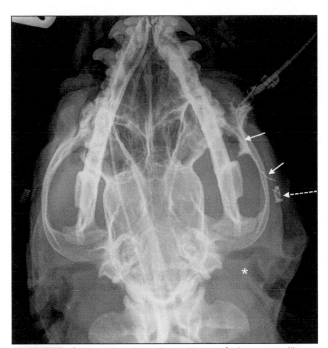

4.44 Sialography in a dog with a soft tissue swelling of the left side of the face at the angle of the jaw. The opening of the parotid duct has been catheterized and the terminal duct has filled normally (block arrows). The duct is focally dilated with an irregular filling defect (dashed arrow) and neither the proximal duct nor the parotid salivary gland is filled with contrast medium. The duct is obstructed. On MRI, the proximal segment of the duct was markedly dilated and filled with material due to granulomatous inflammation as a result of obstruction by a grass seed.

Myelography

Myelography has been widely superseded by cross-sectional imaging (CT/MRI), which is considered more sensitive and specific for demonstrating pathology associated with spinal cord disease. However, poor quality CT/MR images may provide less information than a good quality myelogram in breeds in which clinical signs are predictably associated with degeneration and extrusion (e.g. Dachshunds). Myelography is often still the technique of choice in large dogs, particularly where lesion localization is equivocal and access to MRI is limited to low field systems. Myelography allows the entire subarachnoid space to be evaluated and is useful for demonstrating some nerve root lesions. Myelography is of limited value for assessment of the lumbosacral junction and provides little information about the status of the spinal cord.

Indications:

- Ataxia, paresis or paralysis due to spinal cord pathology.
- Spinal pain.

Technique:

- Survey radiographs are obtained in orthogonal planes and include the entire segment of the spine, as determined by neurolocalization.
- Non-ionic contrast media should be used.
- Contrast medium can be administered by cisternal or lumbar puncture. The injection site is determined by the clinical presentation. In animals

with malformation of the caudal fossa, occipital condyles or C1 vertebra, cisternal puncture should be avoided. In some patients, both cisternal and lumbar puncture may be required.
- CSF should always be collected for analysis.

Interpretation:

- The purpose of myelography (Figure 4.45) is to demonstrate whether pathology is present and whether it can be localized to the extradural space, the intradural–extramedullary space or the medulla (see Chapter 9).
- Localization of the changes to areas overlying the intervertebral disc space or within the length of one or more vertebral bodies is an important principle of interpretation. The former is typically associated with intervertebral disc disease or nerve root

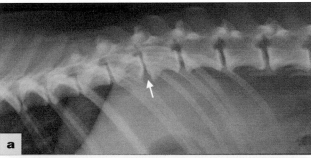

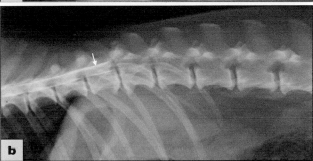

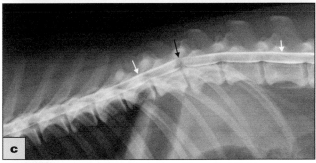

4.45 Myelography in a dog with ambulatory paraparesis. **(a)** Survey radiograph of the vertebral segment of interest (based on neurolocalization). The T12–T13 intervertebral disc space is narrowed (arrowed). Survey radiographs must be obtained prior to myelography. **(b)** The contrast medium, which was injected via a cisternal puncture, terminates abruptly dorsal to the T12–T13 intervertebral disc space (arrowed). The flow of contrast medium is interrupted, but whether the obstruction is due to an extradural or intradural lesion cannot be established on a single view. In addition, the caudal aspect of the lesion is not demonstrated. **(c)** Contrast medium has been administered via a lumbar puncture at L5, allowing the contrast medium to flow forwards. The dorsal (white arrows) and ventral subarachnoid spaces are filled with contrast medium, but the dorsal column is thinned dorsal to the T12–T13 intervertebral disc space (black arrow). (continues) ▶

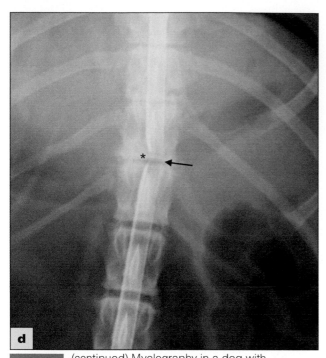

4.45 (continued) Myelography in a dog with ambulatory paraparesis. **(d)** The VD view demonstrates that the spinal cord is displaced to the left by a large volume of extradural material (*). This compressive lesion, presumed to be extruded disc material lying lateral to the spinal cord on the right, thins both the right and left contrast medium columns (arrowed). (Courtesy of the Stowe Veterinary Group)

lesions, whereas changes within the length of the vertebral body in an extradural location can be due to extension of vertebral masses, inflammatory disease or intradural lesions.

Angiocardiography

Angiocardiographic studies were widely used in the past to investigate congenital cardiac disease, but have now been largely superseded in this area by echocardiography. Angiocardiography involves an intravascular or intracardiac injection of water-soluble, iodinated contrast medium to opacify the chambers of the heart and great vessels. Studies are ideally performed using fluoroscopy, to allow real-time imaging, with spot films obtained as required. The use of angiocardiography may increase again in the future as interventional procedures become more widely used in the veterinary field.

For a non-selective angiogram, contrast medium is injected into a peripheral vein, which subsequently (in a normal animal) passes through the right side of the heart, the pulmonary vasculature, the left side of the heart and the aorta. This technique was used to diagnose conditions such as septal defects and patent ductus arteriosus, as the aorta (± the left side of the heart) would opacify at the same time as the pulmonary artery. Selective angiography involves the injection of contrast medium into a specific cardiac chamber or vessel to minimize dilution of the contrast agent as it passes through the circulatory system. The need for cardiac catheterization means that this is a more invasive technique, but has the advantage of being targeted, so it can provide more information about a specific anatomical area.

References and further reading

Baines E (2005) Practical contrast radiography 3: urogenital studies. *In Practice* **27**, 466–473

Bradley K (2005) Practical contrast radiography 2: gastrointestinal studies. *In Practice* **27**, 412–417

Dennis R and Herrtage ME (1989) Low osmolar contrast media: a review. *Veterinary Radiology* **30(1)**, 2–12

Gleeson TG and Bulugahapitiya S (2004) Contrast-induced nephropathy. *American Journal of Roentgenology* **183**, 1673–1689

Holt PE (2008) *Urological Disorders of the Dog and Cat: Investigation, Diagnosis and Treatment*. Manson Publishing, London

Kieves NR, Novo RE and Martin RB (2011) Vaginal resection and anastomosis for treatment of vestibulovaginal stenosis in 4 dogs with recurrent urinary tract infections. *Journal of the American Veterinary Medical Association* **239(7)**, 972–980

Latham C (2005) Practical contrast radiography. *In Practice* **27**, 348–352

Wallack ST (2003) *Handbook of Veterinary Contrast Radiography*. San Diego Veterinary Imaging, California

Radiology of the thorax

5

Kate Bradley

There are many indications for thoracic radiography, both for the diagnosis of intrathoracic disease and as a means of screening to determine the extent of systemic diseases. This makes it an essential technique in the clinical investigation of many animals. However, despite the frequency with which thoracic radiographs are taken, the thorax remains one of the most challenging areas of veterinary radiography, in terms of the technical aspects of obtaining a diagnostic image and the subsequent radiological interpretation. A combination of an optimal radiographic technique and a logical approach to interpretation will maximize the clinical information that can be gained from thoracic radiographs.

Indications

Tracheal, airway and lung disease

- Coughing.
- Dyspnoea.
- Collapse.
- Abnormal respiratory noise.
- Cervical or thoracic trauma.
- Assessment of any secondary consequences of cardiac disease.
- Pyrexia of unknown origin.
- Staging of suspected or known neoplastic disease.

Cardiac disease

- Investigation of cardiac murmurs.
  - In young animals where the clinical significance of the heart murmur is unknown.
  - In older animals with clinical signs that could be caused by a cardiac condition.
- Exercise intolerance or collapse.
- Differentiating cardiac from non-cardiac causes of coughing.
- Staging heart failure.
- Assessing the progression of known cardiac disease.
- Unexplained alterations in cardiac rate and/or rhythm.
- Screening (e.g. hyperthyroid cats prior to isolation for ^{131}I treatment).

Mediastinal disease

- Dyspnoea.
- Suspected trauma (including to the pharyngeal and cranial oesophageal regions).
- Reduced chest wall compliance on clinical examination.

Thoracic wall and pleural space disease

- Assessment of traumatic injuries.
- Investigation of palpable masses.
- Investigation of discharging sinuses.
- Characterization of thoracic wall deformities.
- Muffled heart and lung sounds.
- Tachypnoea/dyspnoea.

Oesophageal disease

- Chronic or persistent dysphagia.
- Regurgitation.
- Excessive salivation.
- Retching or gagging.
- Aspiration pneumonia or recurrent respiratory infection.
- Suspected foreign body ingestion.

Restraint and patient preparation

Sedation is highly recommended for thoracic radiography because in addition to reducing the 'stress' of the procedure and helping restraint, the respiratory rate is usually lower in a sedated animal and this helps to minimize movement blur. General anaesthesia is also commonly used, eliminating any resistance on the part of the animal to optimal positioning. However, general anaesthesia can lead to increased atelectasis of the dependent lung, which causes decreased volume and increased radiographic pulmonary opacity, a significant hindrance when interpreting lung changes. Although a potential disadvantage of general anaesthesia, atelectasis can usually be minimized by inducing anaesthesia whilst maintaining the animal in sternal recumbency and obtaining the dorsoventral (DV) view prior to the lateral view(s). General anaesthesia-related atelectasis can also be reduced by manual inflation of the lungs prior to the radiographic exposure. For radiography of the cervical trachea, the patient should be extubated and any collar removed.

In animals presenting with severe dyspnoea, it is usually possible to improvise some means of restraint that is adequate to obtain a 'screening' radiograph without the need for general anaesthesia or sedation. For example, a small dog or cat may be placed in a cardboard pet carrier or other radiolucent box. There may be some clinical circumstances where it is better to delay radiography and stabilize the patient first. Ultrasonography can be used to rule in or out pathology, such as pleural effusion or a large thoracic mass, quickly and non-invasively.

Standard radiographic views

A thoracic radiographic investigation should comprise at least two views: usually a lateral recumbent view and either a DV or ventrodorsal (VD) view. This combination of views is necessary to localize any observed changes accurately (Figure 5.1). The combination of views required depends on the suspected pathology and the clinical condition of the animal.

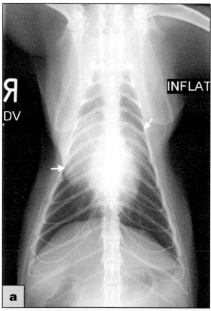

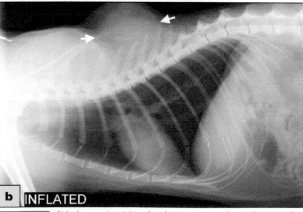

5.1 It is important to obtain two, usually orthogonal, views for lesion localization in thoracic radiography. **(a)** DV view of the thorax of a cat with increased soft tissue opacity over the cranial cardiac silhouette and adjacent lung (arrowed). **(b)** The lateral view demonstrates that this change is actually extrathoracic and is due to a dorsally located subcutaneous mass (arrowed).

- A dyspnoeic animal should not be placed on its back and may not even tolerate lateral recumbency, so a DV view may be the only option in these cases (unless a horizontal beam approach is used).
- The caudal lobar vessels are best visualized on the DV view.
- The VD view is preferred for assessment of the accessory lobe and the ventral aspects of the lung parenchyma.

However, in some clinical situations two lateral views (right and left), in addition to a DV/VD view, are recommended. In an animal positioned in lateral recumbency, the dependent lung will collapse to some extent but the uppermost lung remains well aerated, allowing potentially good contrast between any pathology and the aerated lung. By relying on a single lateral view of the thorax, significant pathology within the partially collapsed dependent lung may not be visible due to border effacement between the lesion and the atelectatic lung (see Figure 3.10). Examples where two lateral views are advisable include screening for metastatic lesions, as aerated lung provides good contrast for any small nodular lesions present, and assessing lungs for evidence of aspiration pneumonia, as small areas of alveolar filling are not seen in dependent, collapsed lobes.

Laterolateral views

If a single lateral view is to be taken, it is best to be consistent in order to become familiar with the expected 'normal' appearance of structures, particularly the cardiac silhouette, caudal vena cava and diaphragm. A right lateral view is preferable in many instances – the cardiac silhouette lies in a more consistent position due to the 'cardiac notch' of the right lung (the division between the cranial and right middle lobes) and the diaphragm obscures less of the caudodorsal lung field. A left lateral view is useful when the pathology is primarily right-sided, as the right lung will be better aerated in this position and hence radiological changes will be easier to detect. The cranial lobar pulmonary vessels may also be easier to recognize and assess on a left lateral view. When evaluating a lateral thoracic radiograph for diagnostic quality, the degree of patient rotation can be assessed by looking at the ribs. If the thorax is axially rotated, such that the spine and sternum are not equidistant from the table top, the costochondral junctions will not be at the same level, and the rib heads will not be superimposed. Several pairs of ribs at the level at which the X-ray beam is centred should be superimposed on one another. However, the divergence of the X-ray beam may mean that not all the rib pairs will be superimposed on one another, even if the thorax is perfectly straight.

- The animal is positioned in lateral recumbency (on its right side for a right lateral view and on its left side for a left lateral view).
- The forelimbs are pulled cranially and secured with sandbags (or ties in an animal under general anaesthesia) to minimize superimposition of the triceps muscle over the cranial thorax.
- The forelimbs are supported with a foam pad or sandbags to avoid axial rotation.

- The head and neck are gently extended.
- The spine and sternum should lie at the same height above the tabletop (Figure 5.2a).
  - A foam wedge under the sternum may be needed to achieve this in some animals, especially deep-chested breeds.
  - In a few barrel-chested breeds, the sternum may be higher than the spine and a foam wedge may be needed under the spine to prevent rotation.
- The hindlimbs should remain in a neutral position.
- The X-ray beam is centred at the level of the caudal border of the scapula (usually around the level of the fifth rib) and midway between the sternum and the vertebral bodies of the thoracic spine (usually one-third of the way up the chest from the sternum) (Figure 5.2b).
- The X-ray beam is collimated to include the thoracic inlet, the thoracic vertebral bodies (*not* the entire height of the spinous processes and the skin), the entire diaphragm and the sternum.

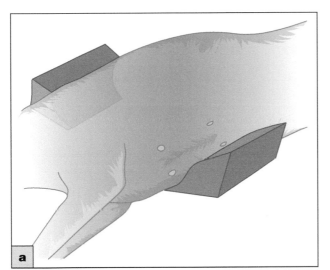

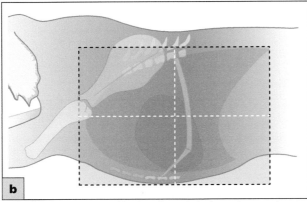

5.2 Patient positioning for a right lateral recumbent view of the thorax. **(a)** The forelimbs should be pulled well forward and the sternum elevated so that it lies at the same height as the spine. **(b)** The X-ray beam is centred at the caudal aspect of the scapula.

Dorsoventral view

The DV view is preferred for assessment of the cardiac silhouette, as on a VD view the cardiac silhouette rotates to one side, distorting its size and shape. It is also a useful view to lateralize lesions seen on a lateral view (e.g. allows lesions arising in the mediastinum to be distinguished from those involving the

lung). The DV view is safe for animals in respiratory distress, that may not tolerate being positioned in lateral recumbency. On a DV/VD view, the spine should be straight and the sternum superimposed on the spine. The forelimbs are extended cranially and the scapulae appear symmetrical.

- The animal is positioned in sternal recumbency with the elbows abducted and the forelimbs drawn forwards. The hindlimbs should remain in a normal 'crouching' position.
- The head and neck are gently extended and can be supported on a foam pad.
- In studies not performed under general anaesthesia, long sandbags are placed over the neck and hindquarters of the animal for restraint.
- A radiolucent trough or foam wedges (Figure 5.3) may be useful to support a deep-chested animal (pushing sandbags or other radiopaque structures too close to the ventral thoracic wall should be avoided as they may obscure some of the lung field).
- The thorax should be straight, so that the spine and sternum are superimposed.
- The X-ray beam is centred in the midline at the level of the caudal scapula, and collimated to include the thoracic inlet and the entire diaphragm. Lateral collimation is dependent upon the body condition and the reason for investigation. For suspected chest wall lesions, the X-ray beam is collimated to include the skin and superficial tissues. For the investigation of thoracic disease in thin animals, the X-ray beam is collimated to just inside the skin edges; in obese animals, the X-ray beam is collimated to the lateral extent of the ribs. A left or right marker should be included within the collimated area.

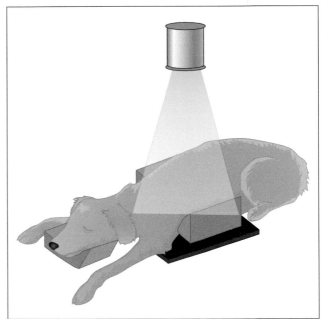

5.3 Patient positioning for a DV view of the thorax. The thorax should be straight with the sternum and spine superimposed. In deep-chested animals, a radiolucent plastic or foam trough can be used to stabilize the animal and avoid rotation. The X-ray beam should be centred to the caudal aspect of the scapula.

Ventrodorsal view

A VD view can be obtained as an alternative to the DV view and may be useful when lung pathology is suspected, as long as the animal is not in respiratory distress.

■ The animal is positioned in dorsal recumbency, supported in a radiolucent foam or plastic trough if necessary (Figure 5.4).
■ The forelimbs are drawn forwards. A sandbag around each leg may be used for restraint. The hindlimbs should remain in a neutral 'frog-legged' position. Sandbags may be used over the hindlimbs, if necessary, for restraint.
■ The thorax should be straight so that the spine and sternum are superimposed.
■ The abdomen and pelvis should be straight to avoid rotation of the caudal thorax.
■ The X-ray beam is centred in the midline at the level of the mid-sternum and collimated to include the thoracic inlet and the diaphragm. The collimation should extend laterally to include just the skin edges.
■ A left or right marker should be included within the collimated area.

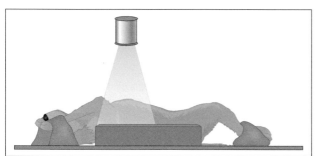

5.4 Patient positioning for a VD view of the thorax. The thorax should be straight with the sternum and spine superimposed. In deep-chested animals, a radiolucent plastic or foam trough can be used to stabilize the animal and avoid rotation. The X-ray beam is centred on the mid-sternum.

Additional views

Additional views of the thorax that may be obtained include oblique DV/VD views, erect lateral views and the lateral decubitus view. These views allow further assessment of known/suspected lesions or can be used for animals in respiratory distress when restraint is not tolerated. The erect lateral and lateral decubitus views involve using a horizontally directed X-ray beam, making radiation safety an important consideration (see Chapter 2). With some direct digital radiography (DR) systems, where the detector is fixed in the table, it may not be feasible to use a horizontally directed X-ray beam.

Lateral decubitus view

The lateral decubitus (horizontal beam DV/VD) view is useful for detecting small volumes of pleural fluid or air. The animal should be positioned in lateral recumbency with the cassette supported vertically against the spine or sternum (Figure 5.5). Centring and collimation are as for VD/DV views. As with the erect lateral view, due consideration should be given to personnel safety and the direction of the primary beam.

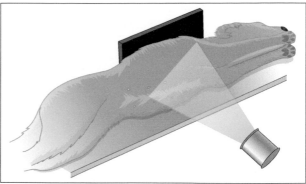

5.5 Patient positioning for a left lateral decubitus view of the thorax. When using a horizontal beam, radiation safety requires that the barrier at which the beam is directed is at least double brick thickness or lead lined to a thickness of 2 mm. The patient is positioned in lateral recumbency and the X-ray beam is collimated to the plate.

Erect lateral view

An erect lateral view may be obtained with the animal standing (Figure 5.6), in sternal recumbency or sitting. The horizontal beam lateral standing view may be useful in animals with severe respiratory compromise, where restraint in other positions is considered clinically unsafe. It can also be helpful in cases where a small pneumothorax is suspected or where gravity may alter the appearance of a lesion (e.g. allowing gas/fluid interfaces within a cyst or abscess to be recognized). Centring and collimation are as for the lateral

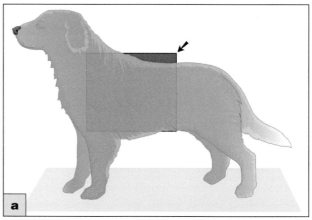

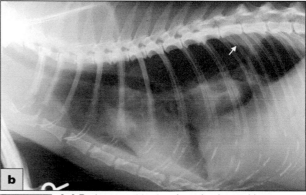

5.6 **(a)** Patient positioning for a horizontal beam lateral standing view of the thorax. The cassette (arrowed) is positioned vertically. Superimposition of the forelimbs and elbows over the cranioventral thorax will be greater than for the equivalent recumbent lateral view. **(b)** Recumbent lateral view of the thorax of a cat with an irregularly marginated, soft tissue opacity superimposed on the caudodorsal thorax (arrowed). (continues) ▶

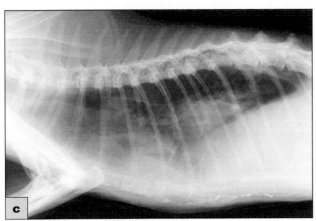

5.6 (continued) **(c)** The horizontal beam lateral radiograph demonstrates that this soft tissue opacity has moved and therefore represents fluid rather than a mass lesion.

view, although superimposition of the forelimbs over the cranial thorax is impossible to avoid if the animal is standing or sitting. The cassette must be supported against the thoracic wall; commercial cassette stands are available, but other options include suspending the cassette in a bag from a drip stand or propping it up with foam blocks and sandbags. Due consideration should be given to the direction of the primary beam to ensure that there is no risk of exposure to personnel.

Oblique ventrodorsal/dorsoventral views

These views are useful to 'skyline' thoracic wall lesions. From a standard VD/DV position, the animal is rotated in order to maximize the visibility of the lesion on the radiograph (Figure 5.7). If there is a palpable mass, the animal is rotated until the size of the shadow cast by the mass within the light of the light beam diaphragm is maximized. The X-ray beam is centred over the mass and the collimation reduced so that it only includes the area of interest; exposure factors usually need to be reduced compared with those for the entire thorax.

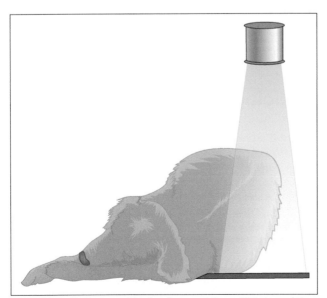

5.7 Patient positioning for an oblique DV view of the thorax. In most cases, this view is obtained in animals with a palpable thoracic wall mass. The thorax of the animal is rotated until the 'shadow' of the mass created by the light beam diaphragm is maximized.

Tangential craniocaudal view of the thoracic inlet

This view will 'skyline' the trachea at the thoracic inlet, but is difficult to achieve safely using non-manual restraint. To obtain the view, the animal is placed in sternal recumbency with the head and neck extended dorsally and caudally (Figure 5.8). The X-ray beam is directed caudoventrally and centred on the thoracic inlet. Other techniques such as fluoroscopy or endoscopy are usually preferred to image the trachea.

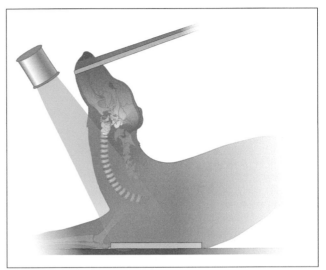

5.8 Patient positioning for a tangential craniocaudal view of the thoracic inlet. This view is very difficult to achieve without restraint by sedation or general anaesthesia, and has largely been superseded by endoscopy and CT. The endotracheal tube must be removed before the exposure is taken.

Film–screen combinations

For conventional X-ray film–screen combinations, there is a 'trade off' between exposure factors and image resolution. For imaging the thorax, a medium to fast speed film–screen combination is desirable in order to keep exposure times short. Large cassettes are preferable to enable the entire thorax to be included on one image. The thorax of most dogs can be fitted on to a 35 x 43 cm cassette/detector plate, although with some giant breeds this will require careful centring and positioning to avoid excluding the periphery of the lungs. For giant-breed or obese dogs, a grid must be used. For cats and small dogs, a detail film should be used and the grid may be dispensed with.

Radiographic exposure

The selection of exposure factors is focused on limiting the potential for movement blur by minimizing exposure time. The milliampere second (mAs) setting must therefore be relatively low. As the thorax is an area with inherently high contrast between the air-filled lungs and the adjacent soft tissue and skeletal structures, a high kilovoltage (kV) should be selected to maximize the greyscale of the image, which results in a 'wide' range of shades of grey. This produces a radiograph with low contrast, allowing small structures such as bronchial walls and vessels to be visualized (see Chapter 2). Exposure factors should be increased if the pathological changes present mean that there is less air in the thorax (e.g.

with pleural effusion or large masses). Conversely, exposure factors should be reduced if pneumothorax is suspected.

To evaluate whether the exposure factors are adequate, the relative opacity of the skeletal structures and the soft tissue surrounding the thorax should be assessed; lung opacity should not be relied upon alone. In a properly exposed thoracic radiograph, it should be possible to visualize the cranial thoracic vertebrae clearly whilst still being able to identify the fine pulmonary markings in the thinner parts of the lung. On the DV/VD view it should be possible to clearly visualize the intervertebral disc spaces superimposed on the cardiac silhouette. Underexposure may mimic an interstitial pattern as the lungs appear diffusely increased in opacity. Overexposure can mask pathological increases in opacity by artefactually making the lungs appear more lucent.

Inspiratory radiographs

In most cases, thoracic radiographs should be taken at maximal inspiration or, if the animal is under general anaesthesia, during manual inflation of the thorax. Sedation may help to reduce the respiratory rate and make it easier to obtain the exposure at peak inspiration. The X-ray tube should be 'prepped' as the thoracic wall rises and the exposure taken at peak inspiration. In an intubated animal under general anaesthesia, it may be possible to temporarily stop respiratory movement.

Expiratory radiographs

There are a few exceptions where expiratory radiographs may be desirable, either because intrathoracic pressure is increased or because contrast between gas-containing/radiolucent lesions and non-inflated lung is increased during expiration. These include:

- Detection of gas-filled structures (e.g. bullae)
- Confirmation of collapse of the intrathoracic trachea/mainstem bronchi
- Detection of hyperinflation and 'air trapping' (e.g. in feline asthma)
- Detection of a small pneumothorax.

Reducing motion artefacts

The strategies for reducing motion artefacts on chest radiographs include:

- Temporarily occluding the nares (personnel should observe radiation protection requirements)
- Distracting the patient (e.g. whistling)
- Increasing the kV to allow the mAs to be reduced
- Using a faster film–screen combination (analogue film)
- Dispensing with a grid
- Sedation or general anaesthesia.

Contrast studies

With the exception of the oesophagus (see Chapter 4), the thorax is not an area where contrast medium is widely used for radiographic studies. Angiocardiography is commonly performed using fluoroscopy for interventional cardiology procedures but is rarely used for diagnostic purposes.

Thoracic radiography *versus* ultrasonography and computed tomography

- Thoracic radiographs provide no information on cardiac function and have poor accuracy for diagnosing many cardiac diseases. Echocardiography is the imaging modality of choice for the evaluation of cardiac disease.
- Echocardiography does not allow assessment of the lungs or pulmonary vasculature, both of which can be easily assessed on radiographs. Staging of congestive heart failure and monitoring the response to therapy for cardiogenic pulmonary oedema are best done radiologically.
- Pleural effusion results in border effacement of normal thoracic structures and may mask significant pathology. Thoracic ultrasonography is facilitated by pleural fluid. Ultrasonography allows guided thoracocentesis for diagnostic and therapeutic purposes as well as biopsy of thoracic masses.
- Ultrasonography only provides a limited field of view and assessment of the entire thorax is difficult or impossible. Computed tomography (CT) allows assessment of the entire thorax with cross-sectional images.
- CT allows assessment of air-filled lung, which is not possible with ultrasonography (due to the almost complete reflection of sound at the soft tissue–air interface).
- CT provides cross-sectional images with greater contrast than radiographs and has a much higher sensitivity for lung nodules and other pathology. CT is of particular value for assessment of pleural space disease, surgical planning for thoracic masses, assessment of vascular malformations, staging of neoplasia and investigation of respiratory disease where radiographs have been inconclusive. Due to motion artefacts, CT offers little or no advantage over radiography for the investigation of cardiac disease unless high end machines are available.

Radiological interpretation

There are many potential pitfalls in the radiological interpretation of thoracic radiographs. Some factors that can complicate interpretation are unavoidable and include:

- Superimposition of structures lying along the path of the X-ray beam
- The wide range of normal anatomical and physiological variables encountered, especially in dogs
- The overlap in radiological appearance between some physiological and pathological changes.

Other potentially complicating factors, such as movement blur and lack of lung inflation, can be eliminated or at least much reduced by using good radiographic technique (see Chapter 2).

Normal anatomy

Considerable breed and age variation is encountered when reviewing thoracic radiographs, particularly in dogs. A good knowledge of normal variations and access to a collection of normal radiographs and/or a good radiographic anatomy textbook will be invaluable in many cases. Examples of normal thoracic radiographs can be seen in Figures 5.9 to 5.13. Examples of some of the conformational variations encountered are illustrated in Figures 5.14 and 5.15.

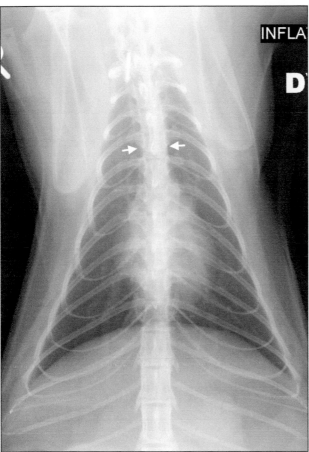

5.9 DV view of the thorax of a cat. The narrow cranial mediastinum (arrowed) should not exceed the width of the spine. Compare this with the dog in Figure 5.11 in which the normal mediastinum should not exceed twice the width of the spine.

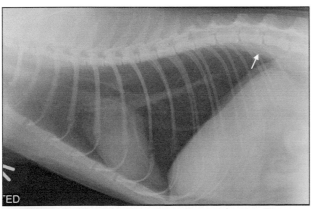

5.10 Right lateral view of the thorax of a cat. The small wedge of soft tissue between the spine and the tip of the caudodorsal lung (arrowed) is normal in the cat and is due to the increased visibility of the psoas minor muscle.

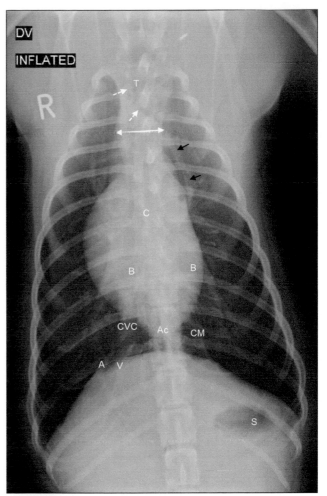

5.11 DV view of the thorax of a normal Springer Spaniel. A = caudal lobe pulmonary artery; Ac = cardiac apex; B = right and left caudal lobe bronchi; C = carina; CM = caudal mediastinal reflection; CVC = caudal vena cava; S = stomach; T = trachea; V = caudal lobe pulmonary vein; black arrows = cranioventral mediastinal reflection; dashed white arrows = lingula of the left cranial lung lobe; solid arrow = width of the craniodorsal mediastinum.

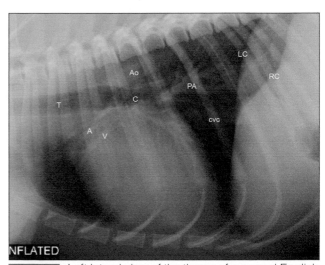

5.12 Left lateral view of the thorax of a normal English Springer Spaniel. A = cranial lobe pulmonary artery; Ao = descending aorta; C = carina; CVC = caudal vena cava; LC = left crus of the diaphragm; PA = caudal lobar pulmonary arteries and veins (superimposed); RC = right crus of the diaphragm; T = trachea; V = cranial lobe pulmonary vein.

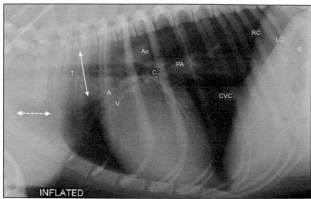

5.13 Right lateral view of the thorax of a normal English Springer Spaniel. A = cranial lobe pulmonary artery; Ao = descending aorta; C = carina; CVC = caudal vena cava; LC = left crus of the diaphragm; PA = caudal lobar pulmonary arteries and veins (superimposed); RC = right crus of the diaphragm; S = stomach; T = trachea; V = cranial lobe pulmonary vein; dashed arrow = lingula of the left cranial lung lobe; solid arrow = approximate height of the craniodorsal mediastinum.

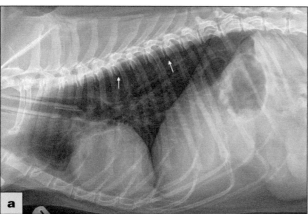

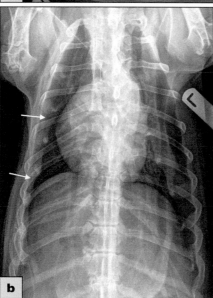

5.14 **(a)** Right lateral and **(b)** DV views of the thorax of a Bassett Hound. The thorax is broad and dorsoventrally flattened. On the lateral view this results in a lucent appearance to the mid-thoracic vertebral bodies (arrowed) which should not be mistaken for osteopenia. On the DV view the prominent costochondral junctions and skin folds should not be mistaken for retraction of the lung lobes and pleural effusion (arrowed). In this dog, the artefact is only recognized on the right side of the thorax because of axial rotation of the thorax.

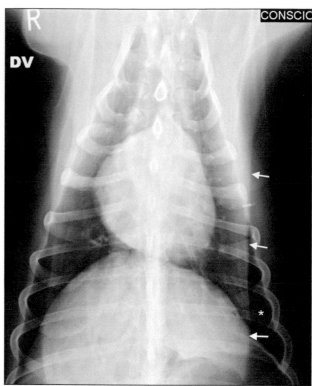

5.15 DV view of the thorax of a deep-chested dog. The skin folds (arrowed) are prominent and the lucent area (*) lateral to these lines should not be mistaken for pneumothorax. The distinction can be made by tracing the line of the skin fold beyond the thoracic wall, by recognizing that the change is symmetrical and that, using a bright light/adjusting contrast and brightness, vascular markings can be seen to extend to the periphery of the thorax.

Respiratory system

Trachea:

- The trachea is visible radiologically as a radiolucent tubular structure of even width.
- It extends from the larynx along the ventral neck, through the thoracic inlet to the base of the cardiac silhouette, ending caudally with a crest called the carina. Beyond this, the trachea branches into the two mainstem bronchi.
- The external tracheal wall is indistinguishable from the cervical and mediastinal soft tissue, unless there is adjacent air (pneumomediastinum or oesophageal air) or the tracheal rings are mineralized (a normal ageing feature).
- On a lateral radiograph, the trachea diverges from the cranial thoracic spine in most breeds and the carina is superimposed on the fourth or fifth intercostal space.
- On a DV/VD radiograph, the trachea is seen either superimposed over the spine or just to the right of the midline.
- The diameter of the trachea should not vary along its length. However, in some animals it may appear to be reduced in the region of the thoracic inlet due to ventral deviation of the dorsal tracheal wall, indenting the lumen. This has been erroneously termed 'pseudocollapse', although CT images have shown this to be a genuine (although clinically insignificant) luminal narrowing. This effect is exacerbated by head and neck extension.

- The position of the trachea is influenced by any rotation of the thorax and also by the position of the head and neck. Flexion of the neck can cause dorsal deviation of the trachea, usually at the thoracic inlet but sometimes more caudally.
- The origin of the left cranial lobe bronchus is usually seen as a radiolucent circle superimposed on the caudal trachea.

Lower airways:

- The two mainstem bronchi arise from the trachea at the level of the carina.
- The right bronchus divides into four lobar bronchi and the left bronchus divides into two lobar bronchi.
- The lobar bronchi subdivide further within each lobe.
  - Bronchial markings are normally only seen in the perihilar area, unless the bronchi have thickened or calcified walls.
  - Calcification (without thickening) of the bronchi is frequently seen as a normal ageing change (Figure 5.16).
  - Calcification can also result from hyperadrenocorticism or long-term corticosteroid administration.
- Bronchi are located between the pulmonary artery and vein, but may not necessarily occupy the entire space between the two vessels.
- The bronchial lumen should taper gradually towards the periphery of the lung field.
- On VD views, the angle of divergence of the mainstem bronchi is greater than on the DV view.

Pulmonary parenchyma:

- The right lung is divided into cranial, middle, caudal and accessory lobes.
- The left lung has two lobes: a cranial lobe, which is divided into cranial and caudal parts that unite dorsally, and a caudal lobe.
- The cranial lobes are not symmetrical. The left cranial lobe extends further forward than the right;

however, the right cranial lobe is wider, extending across the midline on the DV view.
  - The tip of the left lung lobe (known as the lingula of the left cranial lobe) extends slightly across the midline, resulting in a triangular to oval lucent area overlying the first two ribs on lateral views of the thorax. This apparent 'split' in the appearance of the cranioventral lung field should not be over-interpreted as pathology.
  - The cranioventral mediastinum is displaced to the left by the wider right cranial lobe. It appears as a curvilinear soft tissue opacity to the left of the midline, extending between the thoracic inlet and the cardiac silhouette. In obese animals, this reflection may be widened by fat and should not be mistaken for a cranial mediastinal mass.
- The accessory lobe lies caudal to the cardiac silhouette, extends across the midline to the left and appears larger on the VD view compared with the DV view.
- The division between two adjacent lung lobes is called an interlobar fissure (Figure 5.17).
- The branching soft tissue markings within normal lungs represent the pulmonary vasculature.
- The vessels should taper towards the periphery and are the only markings normally seen in the periphery of the lung.
- Blood vessels seen 'end-on' appear more radiopaque than those seen in long axis.
- The appearance of the lungs varies considerably between inspiration and expiration (Figure 5.18). Areas of increased opacity seen on expiratory radiographs should not be over-interpreted as they may appear normal following full inflation of the lung lobes.
- The alveolar walls and interstitium are not recognized as discrete structures.
- In older animals, multiple irregular calcified areas within the lungs and, occasionally, the pleura are termed pulmonary osteomas or pulmonary osseous metaplasia (Figure 5.19). These are incidental findings and their opacity, shape and size distinguishes them from most metastatic nodules.

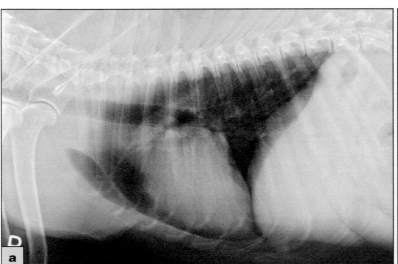
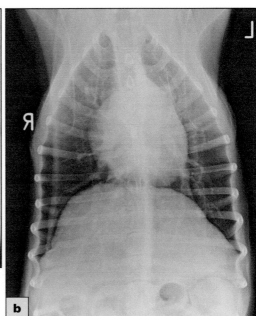

5.16 **(a)** Lateral and **(b)** DV views of the thorax of a clinically normal elderly dog. Note the increased visibility of the bronchial walls. This is a non-specific radiological finding in older animals. Changes due to chronic lower airway disease can appear similar.

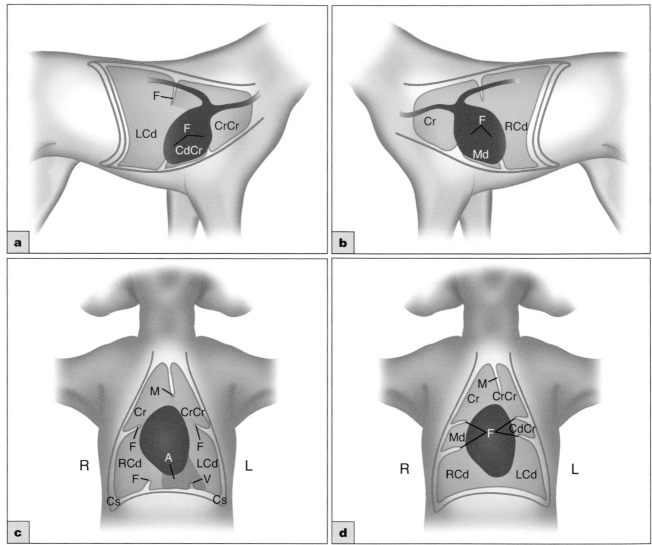

5.17 Location of lung lobes and fissures. Since only fluid-filled fissures that are tangential to the X-ray beam are visible, the volume of fluid and the position of the patient will determine the fissures that are seen. **(a)** Fissures of the lateral aspect of the left lung (looking right to left) are more likely to be seen when the patient is in left recumbency. **(b)** Fissures of the lateral aspect of the right lung (looking medial to lateral) are more likely to be seen when the patient is in right recumbency. **(c)** Fissures on the dorsal aspect of the lungs are more likely to be seen when the patient is in dorsal recumbency. **(d)** Fissures on the ventral aspect of the lungs are more likely to be seen when the patient is in ventral recumbency. A = accessory lobe; CdCr = caudal part of the left cranial lobe; Cr = right cranial lobe; CrCr = cranial part of the left cranial lobe; Cs = costodiaphragmatic recess; F = interlobar fissure; LCd = left caudal lobe; M = mediastinal reflection; Md = right middle lobe; RCd = right caudal lobe; V = caudoventral mediastinal reflection between the left caudal lobe and the accessory lobe (pleural fluid may accumulate adjacent to this reflection).

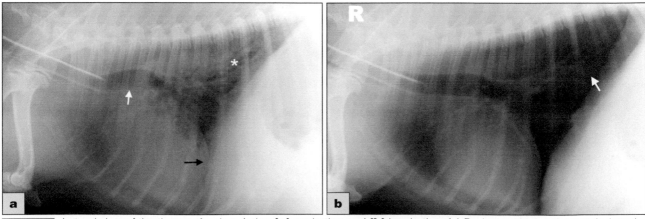

5.18 Lateral view of the thorax of a dog during **(a)** expiration and **(b)** inspiration. (a) During expiration the caudodorsal lung (*) is increased in opacity, which may be mistaken for a pathological infiltrate. The volume of the thorax is reduced with overlap of the cardiac silhouette and diaphragm (black arrow). Kinking of the terminal trachea (white arrow) should not be mistaken for a mass lesion at the heart base. (b) Following manual inflation. The lungs, although not maximally inflated, have a normal bronchovascular pattern (arrowed).

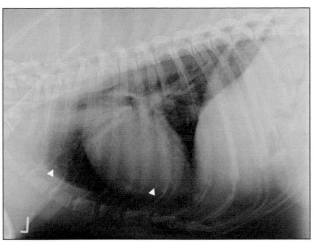

5.19 Lateral view of the thorax of a dog with pulmonary osteomas. These multiple scattered mineral opacities (arrowheads) are of no clinical significance. They appear more radiopaque than soft tissue nodules (e.g. metastases) of a similar size and are usually more irregular in shape.

Cardiovascular system

Heart:

- The cardiac silhouette seen on radiographs comprises the heart, pericardium, the contents of the pericardium (fat and a tiny amount of fluid) and the origin of the aorta and main pulmonary artery.
- The cardiac silhouette is roughly egg-shaped with the base dorsal and the apex ventral.
- The shape and size of the cardiac silhouette is usually assessed on the right lateral and DV views. On the VD view, the cardiac silhouette in dogs often has an elongated pointed apex.
- On the VD view, a focal bulge of the cardiac silhouette is present at the 1–2 o'clock position in approximately 25% of normal dogs and represents the main pulmonary artery.
- On the DV view, the apex of the cardiac silhouette usually lies to the left of the midline in dogs and on the midline in cats, although it can sometimes lie to the right of the midline in the absence of any abnormalities.
- The cardiac silhouette may be elevated by fat in some animals (Figure 5.20a) and this should not be confused with pleural fluid (which obscures the margins of the cardiac silhouette) or free air (which appears more radiolucent as it is of gas opacity).
- In cats, excessive fat can lead to an increase in opacity around the cardiac silhouette on both views. On the DV view, increased pericardial fat is recognized more focally to the right of the cardiac silhouette (Figure 5.20b).

Assessment of cardiac size: For assessment of overall cardiac size, three methods are commonly used:

- Subjective assessment based on the observer's experience of what is 'normal' for a certain species, breed and age of animal
- Evaluation of width in comparison with rib spaces and height relative to that of the thorax
- Vertebral heart score (VHS).

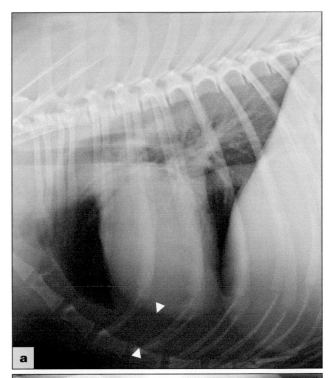

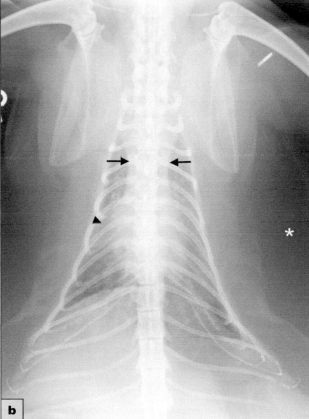

5.20 **(a)** Lateral view of the thorax of an obese dog. The cardiac silhouette is elevated by fat (arrowheads). Fat clearly outlines the cardiac silhouette, whereas pleural fluid or a ventrally located mass obscures it. When measuring the cardiac silhouette, any surrounding fat should not be included in the measurements. **(b)** DV view of the thorax of an obese cat. A large quantity of fat is present within the subcutis (*). Within the thorax, the cranial mediastinum is widened (arrowed) and fat is present within and adjacent to the pericardium (arrowhead). Fat surrounding the thorax will increase the overall opacity of the image, as well as increase scatter. The quality of the radiograph is degraded. In extreme cases, fat may also physically limit inspiratory movement.

Whichever method is used, it is important to make sure that the animal is optimally positioned for the radiograph; rotation will alter the projected size and shape of the cardiac silhouette, often leading to an apparent cardiomegaly. It is also important to ensure that the cardiac margins are clearly visible; if areas of alveolar infiltrate or pleural effusion lie adjacent to the cardiac silhouette, it will be impossible to obtain accurate measurements. If this is the case, it is sometimes possible to identify the pericardial fat as a radiolucent curvilinear area, which may allow an estimate of overall cardiac size to be made.

The normal width of the cardiac silhouette on lateral radiographs is 2.5–3.5 intercostal spaces in dogs and 2–2.5 intercostal spaces in cats. The normal height is approximately 65–70% that of the thorax. In dogs, if a line is drawn from the carina to the apex, approximately two-thirds of the cardiac silhouette should lie cranial to that line, and one-third caudal to the line. With age, particularly in cats, the cardiac axis tips forward; this is not clinically significant, but when measuring the cardiac silhouette, it is important to ensure that measurements of width are made perpendicular to the long axis of the cardiac silhouette rather than parallel with the long axis of the thorax.

On the DV view, in most dogs, the cardiac silhouette does not exceed two-thirds of the width of the thorax; this is a guide and may vary in normal animals with the cardiac silhouette appearing relatively wider on expiratory radiographs. The cardiac silhouette appears longer and narrower on a VD view compared with a DV view. In cats, the width of the cardiac silhouette on the DV view should not exceed 50% of the width of thorax. As an alternative measure in cats, the width of the cardiac silhouette should not exceed the length of four vertebral bodies. The width of the cardiac silhouette is measured on the DV view and then compared with the thoracic vertebrae on the lateral view, measured from the cranial aspect of the fourth thoracic vertebra (as per the VHS; see below).

An alternative objective measure of cardiac size, first described by Buchanan and Bücheler in 1995, is the VHS. This method measures the cardiac silhouette on the lateral radiograph in relation to the thoracic vertebral bodies, with the normal range being 8.5–10.6 for dogs and 7–8 for cats. There is considerable breed variation in the VHS of dogs (a number of breed-specific ranges have been established and of these the Boxer has one of the largest at 11.6 ± 0.6), whereas the VHS in cats is more consistent. One value of the VHS is that it limits the possible overestimation of cardiac size based on subjective assessment alone. An increased VHS is most likely to be seen with diseases that cause clinically significant cardiac remodelling, such as congenital or acquired valvular disease (which results in eccentric hypertrophy and volume overload), dilated cardiomyopathy and pericardial disease. The VHS is also useful as a means of demonstrating the progression of disease on radiographs of an animal repeated over a period of time. However, a normal VHS does not rule out cardiac disease, as some dogs with cardiac disease will have a value that falls within the normal range. The VHS does not provide information about the cardiac muscle *per se* and in cases of concentric hypertrophy may be normal. Since cardiac disease in cats often

causes concentric hypertrophy, the VHS is of questionable use in cases of feline heart disease.

Individual chamber enlargement may be assessed using the 'clock face' analogy, where the contour of the cardiac silhouette is compared with the numbers on a clock (Figures 5.21 to 5.24). This is probably most usefully applied to the DV view, but may also be used with the lateral view. The analogy helps to determine which chamber or major vessel is most likely to be responsible for any abnormal 'bulges' in the contour of the cardiac silhouette. Oblique positioning for a DV view may lead to artefactual 'bulging' mimicking individual chamber enlargement. It may also be possible in a normal animal to see a small bulge in the region of the main pulmonary artery on a DV view, if the radiograph was obtained during systole.

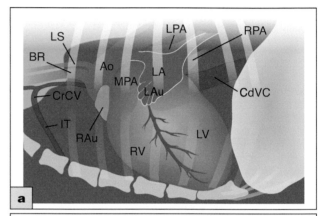

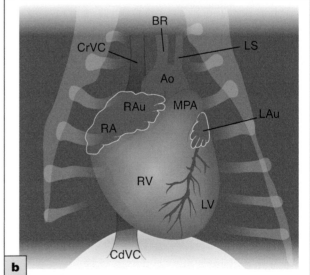

5.21 Location of the cardiac chambers in a dog. **(a)** Lateral view. **(b)** Ventral view. Note that on the ventral view, the ascending aorta, brachiocephalic trunk and left subclavian artery lie on the midline. The main pulmonary artery and left auricular appendage margins are superimposed on the centre of the cardiac silhouette. They are only visible individually when markedly enlarged and alter the margin of the cardiac silhouette. The left atrium (not shown) is superimposed on the centre of the cardiac silhouette (between the mainstem bronchi). Ao = aortic arch; BR = brachiocephalic trunk; CdVC = caudal vena cava; CrVC = cranial vena cava; IT = internal thoracic arteries and veins; LA = left atrium; LAu = left auricular appendage; LPA = left pulmonary artery; LS = left subclavian artery; LV = left ventricle; MPA = main pulmonary artery; RA = right atrium; RAu = right auricular appendage; RPA = right pulmonary artery; RV = right ventricle.

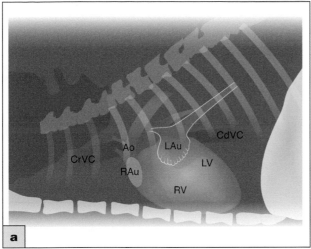

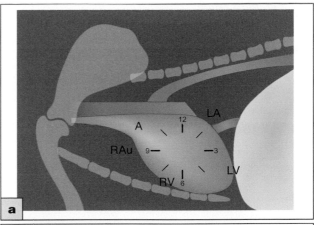

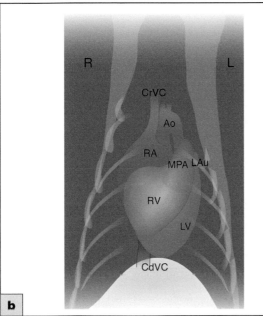

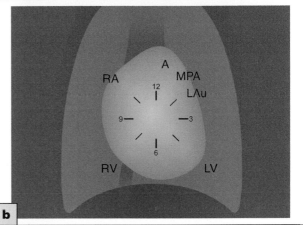

5.22 Location of the cardiac chambers in a cat. **(a)** Lateral view. **(b)** Ventral view. Note that on the ventral view, the main pulmonary artery and left auricular appendage margins are superimposed on the cardiac silhouette. They are only visible individually when markedly enlarged and alter the margin of the cardiac silhouette. The left atrium (not shown) is superimposed on the centre of the cardiac silhouette (between the mainstem bronchi). Ao = aortic arch; CdVC = caudal vena cava; CrVC = cranial vena cava; LAu = left auricular appendage; LV = left ventricle; MPA = main pulmonary artery; RA = right atrium; RAu = right auricular appendage; RV = right ventricle.

5.23 Location of the cardiac chambers using the 'clock face' analogy. **(a)** Lateral view. **(b)** DV view. A = aorta; LA = left atrium; LAu = left auricular appendage; LV = left ventricle; MPA = main pulmonary artery; RA = right atrium; RAu = right auricular appendage; RV = right ventricle.

'Time'	Lateral view	Dorsoventral view
12–01	Left atrium	Aortic arch
01–02	Left atrium	Main pulmonary artery
02–03	Left ventricle	Left auricular appendage
03–05	Left ventricle	Left ventricle
05–09	Right ventricle	Right ventricle
09–11	Right auricular appendage; aortic arch; main pulmonary artery	Right atrium
11–12	Aortic arch	Aortic arch

5.24 'Clock face' analogy for the location of the cardiac chambers.

Aorta:

Lateral view:

- The aortic arch is usually visible craniodorsal to the cardiac silhouette.
- In the absence of surrounding pathology, the descending aorta may be followed to the level of the diaphragm.
- On digital radiographs, in some obese animals (as fat provides additional contrast within the mediastinum) or if the oesophagus is distended with air, it may be possible to identify the brachiocephalic trunk and left subclavian artery exiting the aorta.

- The normal diameter of the aorta is similar to the height of a thoracic vertebral body.

Dorsoventral view:

- The aortic arch is visible cranial and to the left of the cardiac silhouette.
- On a well exposed radiograph, the left margin of the descending aorta is visible superimposed on the cardiac silhouette, just to the left of the midline.

In older cats, a focal bulge in the aorta may be seen at the junction of the ascending aorta with the aortic arch. This is an incidental finding.

Caudal vena cava:

- The caudal vena cava extends from the right crus of the diaphragm cranioventrally to merge with the caudal border of the cardiac silhouette.
- The caudal vena cava is most clearly seen on the VD and left lateral views.
- Usually the caudal vena cava is approximately the same width as the aorta, although the width varies with the cardiac cycle and intrathoracic pressure.
- The caudal vena cava is usually of even width, but can sometimes widen as it approaches the heart.

Pulmonary vessels: Radiological assessment of the pulmonary arteries and veins is an important part of evaluating a thoracic radiograph. Changes in their size can be indicative of congestive heart failure or other significant vascular pathology. Unlike the cardiac silhouette, pulmonary vessels cannot be assessed using echocardiography.

- Pulmonary veins lie ventral and central to the arteries (i.e. ventral to the corresponding artery on the lateral view and medial to the corresponding artery on the DV/VD view).
- On the lateral view, it is only possible to assess the cranial lobar vessels as the caudal lobar vessels are superimposed on each other.
  - The vessel pair seen best is that in the non-dependent lung. This vessel pair are more ventrally located and relatively magnified. The vessels can be measured where they cross the fourth rib; the artery and vein should be equal in size with a width not exceeding 1.2 times the diameter of the proximal third of the fourth rib.
  - The left lateral view may be preferable to the right lateral view for assessment of the cranial lobar vessels, as the right lobar vessels are less likely to be superimposed on the cranial mediastinum and may therefore be easier to visualize.
- On the DV/VD view, the caudal lobar vessels can be assessed and both the left and right pairs should be visible. The caudal lobar vessels are most clearly seen on the DV view. The artery and vein should be equal in size and should not exceed the width of the ninth rib at the point that they cross it.

Azygos vein:

- The azygos vein may be seen occasionally in breeds with a deep and narrow chest conformation as a linear soft tissue opacity immediately ventral to the caudal thoracic spine.
- In most animals, the azygos vein is only visible if there is free air in the mediastinum.

Pleural space

- The pleural space is the potential space between the parietal and visceral pleural membranes and is therefore not usually visible.
- In some instances, a pleural reflection between the lung lobes will be oriented tangentially to the primary X-ray beam and be seen as a thin radiopaque line extending laterally from the hilar area towards the thoracic wall or curving towards the cardiac silhouette from the thoracic wall.
  - In the absence of other radiographic changes, these pleural lines are likely to be incidental.
  - Pleural thickening or a tiny volume of pleural fluid cannot be distinguished from tangential pleural reflections as they all lead to a similar appearance.

Thoracic boundaries
Assessment of any thoracic radiograph should include the thoracic boundaries:

- Vertebrae
- Sternum
- Ribs (together with their associated areas of soft tissue)
- Diaphragm.

Structures on the thoracic wall may be superimposed on the lungs and care should be taken not to over-interpret nipples, skin nodules and ticks as pathological pulmonary nodules. Attention should be paid to the condition of the animal's coat and any surrounding bedding material. Mud on the coat will appear as radiopaque material, as will wet clumped hair or any ultrasound gel remaining on the coat.

Vertebrae:

- There are usually 13 thoracic vertebrae. The anticlinical vertebra is usually (but not always) T11.
- The thoracic spinous processes are tall and may not be fully visible on a well collimated thoracic radiograph.
- The vertebrae should be assessed for shape, margination, alignment and trabecular structure (see Chapter 9).
- Smooth new bone ventrally (spondylosis deformans) is a common but incidental finding.

Sternum:

- The sternum comprises eight bones. The manubrium is the most cranial sternebra and the xiphisternum is the most caudal sternebra.
- The sternum should be assessed for shape, margination, alignment and trabecular structure.
- Smooth new bone formation arising ventral to the endplates of the sternebrae (and occasionally bridging the gap between them) is a common but incidental finding.

Ribs:

- There are 13 pairs of ribs.
- The contour of the ribs should be smooth.
- The rib surface is relatively flat in dogs and rounder in cats.
- Costal cartilage is radiolucent in young animals but mineralizes with age.
- There may be considerable normal variation in the shape of the first rib in dogs.
- The ribs should be assessed for continuity, shape and trabecular structure.

Diaphragm:

- The thoracic surface of the diaphragm should be smooth and well defined due to contrast with the adjacent air-filled lung.
- The abdominal surface is not normally seen due to border effacement by the adjacent soft tissue of the liver and gastric wall.
- There is considerable variation in the appearance of the diaphragm, depending on:
  - Breed
  - Body condition score
  - Stage of respiration and degree of inspiration
  - Patient positioning
  - Centring and collimation of the X-ray beam.
  These factors lead to exceptions in the conventionally described appearance of structures on right *versus* left lateral recumbent and sternal *versus* dorsal recumbent radiographs.
- The right and left crura and the ventral dome or cupola can be distinguished on radiographs in the dog. The appearance of the diaphragm differs depending on whether the animal is positioned in right or left lateral recumbency, with the dependent diaphragmatic crus being displaced more cranially (see Figures 5.12 and 5.13).
- The caudal vena cava passes through the right crus of the diaphragm. On a left lateral view it can be seen to cross the most cranial crus of the diaphragm (left) and merge with the caudal (right) crus.
- The fundus of the stomach (often gas-filled) is visible immediately caudal to the left crus.
- The position of the diaphragm is helpful in determining the stage of the respiratory cycle at which the radiograph was obtained.
  - At full inspiration, the diaphragm is straighter and more caudally positioned, leading to separation caudoventrally between the cardiac silhouette and diaphragm.
  - During normal breathing, the diaphragm moves one-half to two vertebral lengths and the dorsal aspect of the diaphragm intersects the spine between T9 and L1, depending on the degree of inspiration.
- On a DV view of the thorax, the shape of the diaphragm is usually that of a single dome. On a VD view, three separate domed structures may be seen, representing the two crura and the cupola (Figure 5.25).

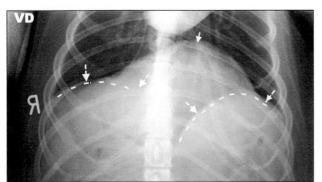

5.25 VD view of the thorax of a dog. The shape of the diaphragm differs compared with a DV view. Three 'domes' are created by the two crura (dashed arrows and lines) and the cupola (solid arrow) of the diaphragm.

Mediastinum

For radiological assessment, the mediastinum can be divided into three: the area cranial to the cardiac silhouette; the area of the cardiac silhouette; and the area caudal to the cardiac silhouette (Figure 5.26). The oesophagus extends within the mediastinum from the neck to the stomach.

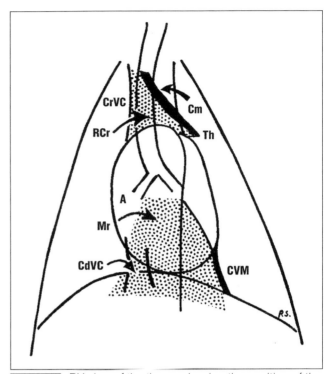

5.26 DV view of the thorax showing the position of the cranial, middle and caudal parts of the mediastinum, including the position of the thymus. A = accessory lobe of the right lung (seen as a dotted area); CdVC = caudal vena cava; Cm = cranial mediastinum; CrVC = cranial vena cava; CVM = caudoventral mediastinal reflection; Mr = mediastinal recess, which accommodates the accessory lobe of the right lung; RCr = right cranial lung lobe (seen as a dotted area); Th = position of the vestigial thymus. (Adapted from Suter (1984) with permission)

Oesophagus: The normal oesophagus is not normally visible on radiographs, although in animals under sedation or anaesthesia, mild to moderate dilatation may be present (seen more commonly in dogs than cats). This dilatation is usually recognized dorsal to the base of the cardiac silhouette. The oesophagus lies within the dorsal mediastinum, running dorsal and slightly to the left of the trachea and dorsal to the cardiac silhouette. On left lateral thoracic radiographs in normal dogs, the caudal oesophagus is occasionally visible as a soft tissue opacity band extending horizontally across the caudodorsal thorax, dorsal to the caudal vena cava and ventral to the aorta.

Cranial mediastinum:

- The cranial mediastinum (Figure 5.27) is thicker dorsally than it is ventrally as it includes the thoracic oesophagus, the large vascular structures supplying and draining the head, neck and forelimbs, the mediastinal lymph nodes and the vagosympathetic trunk.
- The normal craniodorsal mediastinum appears as a soft tissue band as, with the exception of the air

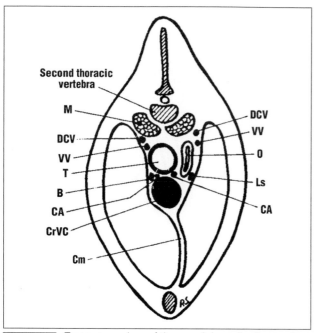

5.27 Transverse view of the cranial mediastinum at the level of the second thoracic vertebra. B = brachiocephalic artery; CA = right and left carotid arteries; Cm = cranial mediastinum; CrVC = cranial vena cava; DCV = right deep cranial vertebral vein and left deep cranial vertebral vein; Ls = left subclavian artery; M = longus colli muscle; O = oesophagus; T = trachea; VV = right and left vertebral veins. (Adapted from Suter (1984) with permission)

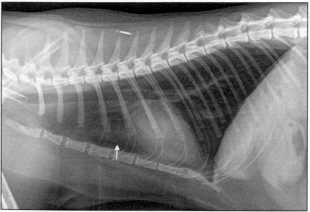

5.28 Lateral view of the thorax of a cat. The normal thymus is of soft tissue opacity and is approximately triangular in shape (arrowed). Caudally, it may efface the cranial border of the cardiac silhouette.

in the trachea, there is not enough contrast for the individual structures to be visualized. On a DV view, the craniodorsal mediastinum lies on the midline, cranial to the cardiac silhouette.

- A thinner cranioventral mediastinal reflection is present, which results from the displacement of the mediastinum across the midline by the right cranial lung lobe.
  - The reflection is seen on the lateral view as a curvilinear soft tissue opacity extending from the costochondral junction of the first rib to the sternum (see Figure 5.13).
  - On the lateral view, in dogs (primarily deep-chested breeds), the lucency of the lung seen cranial to this reflection is usually greater than that caudal, and this variation should not be over-interpreted as a bullous or cavitatory lung lesion.
  - On the DV view, in dogs, the cranioventral mediastinal reflection is seen extending obliquely on the left, cranial to the cardiac silhouette (see Figure 5.11). It is easiest to recognize when projected tangential to the X-ray beam or when widened by fat in obese animals.
- In young animals, the thymus may be seen (Figure 5.28). In dogs, it is usually best seen on the DV view as a triangular opacity extending from the midline towards the left ('thymic sail'). Occasionally, it may also be seen on the lateral view, cranial to the cardiac silhouette. In cats, it is best seen on the lateral view, in the cranioventral thorax, immediately adjacent to the cranial border of the cardiac silhouette.

Central mediastinum: The only mediastinal structures that can normally be identified in the central area of the thorax are the terminal trachea and the cardiac silhouette (see above).

Caudal mediastinum: Caudally there are two mediastinal reflections:

- Plica venae cavae – the reflection itself is not visible, but the caudal vena cava is consistently seen as a linear soft tissue opacity extending between the cardiac silhouette and the diaphragm, slightly to the right of the midline on the VD/DV view
- The caudoventral mediastinum (previously referred to as the 'cardiophrenic ligament') – this reflection is formed by the accessory lung lobe extending across the midline to the left. It is inconsistently recognized on the VD/DV view as a thin radiopaque soft tissue band extending between the apex of the cardiac silhouette and the diaphragm.

Röntgen signs

Size

- Assessment of size alterations is usually subjective. Objective size measurements are available for many thoracic structures, but often do not add to diagnostic certainty.
- Thoracic volume is influenced by abdominal contents. A large volume of abdominal fluid or mass lesions may cause cranial displacement of the diaphragm and reduce thoracic volume.
- Lung volume can change significantly. It can both increase and decrease under physiological and pathological conditions. It is important to assess critically lung volume as this has a considerable effect on the significance of any lung patterns.
- Physiological size variation may also be seen in the caudal vena cava, but is not usually evident in any other structures.
- Pathological changes in the size of the oesophagus, pulmonary vessels and trachea are often difficult to differentiate from normal as severe size alterations in these structures are relatively uncommon.

- A large increase in cardiac size generally reflects significant structural disease.
- The mediastinal width is influenced by the amount of fat deposited within it.

Shape

- Normal breed variation frequently mimics disease, especially cardiac disease.
- Shape changes associated with cardiac disease are more reliable than size changes.
- Apparent shape changes are often due to infiltrates or masses within the lungs and may alter the shape of the structures with which they efface.

Number

Variation in the number of thoracic structures is limited to the ribs, sternebrae and vertebrae (see Chapter 9). Alterations in the number of ribs are of no clinical significance. Changes in skeletal structure and conformation (shortened sternum, hemivertebral malformation) can alter chest conformation and size.

Opacity

- A general increase in opacity within the thorax indicates an accumulation of fluid or a cellular infiltrate within the pulmonary parenchyma, pleural space or mediastinum. Assessment of lung volume is critical in determining whether an increase in lung opacity is due to loss of air as a result of lung collapse (atelectasis) or replacement of air by cells/fluid (where lung volume is maintained). Loss of air from normal air-filled alveoli due to lung collapse results in an increased opacity and reduced lung volume.
- A reduced opacity within the thorax occurs due to the accumulation of air within the mediastinum, pleural space or lung. A decreased pulmonary opacity may also occur due to hypovolaemia, which reduces the relative proportion of soft tissue to air.
- Dystrophic mineralization is commonly recognized within the trachea, bronchi, aortic root and pulmonary parenchyma and is of no clinical significance, unless associated with soft tissue mass lesions. When mineralization is associated with soft tissue mass lesions or tracheobronchial lymphadenopathy, it is likely to indicate significant disease (neoplasia, granulomatous disease).
- Gas opacities in abnormal locations or of small volume are easily overlooked but may be significant (e.g. bullae or small volume pneumothorax).

Margination

- The structures of the thorax are recognized as separate from one another due to the presence of air in the alveoli or airways.
- Loss of visibility of the margins of structures within the thorax commonly results from border effacement with soft tissues or fluid.
- Changes in margination are usually associated with changes in shape and opacity.
- Changes in margination of the skeletal structures within the thorax are easily overlooked but may be significant (e.g. irregular periosteal reactions may be seen with aggressive bone lesions).

Location

- Retraction of the lung margins indicates pleural space disease.
- Loss of integrity of the diaphragm may result in the abnormal location of abdominal viscera within the thorax.
- The position of mediastinal structures is frequently used to assess disease and lung function.

Function

Oesophageal contrast studies allow some assessment to be made of function as well as anatomy.

Thoracic masses

Thoracic masses are common. The clinician should try to establish from which anatomical compartment (lung, thoracic wall or mediastinum) the mass arises as this determines the list of differential diagnoses. Many thoracic masses are readily identified as focal structures of soft tissue opacity; however, pleural effusion (where present) may mask the mass. The position of normal thoracic structures serves as important landmarks when assessing mass lesions within the thorax. The structures that should be assessed include:

- Mediastinum:
  - Displacement involving the cranial mediastinum, trachea, cardiac silhouette and, less commonly, the aorta and caudal vena cava.
- Diaphragmatic crura:
  - Cranial displacement within the hemithorax associated with a reduction in lung volume
  - Caudal displacement associated with an increase in lung and thoracic volume (usually air).
- Ribs:
  - Narrowing of the intercostal spaces due to loss of lung volume. Unilateral narrowing is easier to recognize than bilateral changes.
  - Widening of the intercostal spaces due to an increase in lung volume.

Mediastinal masses

- Mediastinal masses may be located anywhere within the mediastinum (Figure 5.29).
- Large craniodorsal masses displace the trachea ventrally on the lateral view (Figure 5.30). Small masses are easily overlooked as they cannot be distinguished from the longus colli muscles, which lie ventral to the vertebral bodies of T1–T5.
- Large cranioventral masses (see Figure 5.88) displace the trachea dorsally (and sometimes laterally and to the right). The cranial border of the cardiac silhouette may be effaced by the mass or the entire silhouette may be displaced caudally. Smaller masses dorsal to the sternum may be subtle, but as long as the forelimbs are adequately retracted from the cranioventral thorax, they can usually be recognized. The ventral margin of the lung is displaced dorsally by the mass.
- Large caudodorsal masses (Figure 5.31) are surrounded by the lungs and therefore are easily identified, but a DV/VD view is required to localize the mass to the midline. Smaller masses arising

dorsally and adjacent to the body wall may be overlooked, especially those within the dorsal costodiaphragmatic recesses as they are only bordered, not surrounded, by air-filled lung. These masses partially efface the diaphragmatic crura.

- Caudoventral mediastinal masses are uncommon and must be distinguished from diaphragmatic defects or rupture and accessory lung lobe pathology (Figure 5.32).
- Perihilar masses may arise from the heart base or lymph nodes. Heart base masses may result in focal dorsal displacement of the terminal trachea. Tracheobronchial lymph node enlargement can only be appreciated when moderate or marked. The enlarged lymph nodes result in a poorly circumscribed increase in perihilar soft tissue opacity. Displacement of the lobar bronchi is often best assessed on the VD view. Perihilar masses should be distinguished from post-stenotic enlargement of the aorta or pulmonary artery associated with congenital, and occasionally acquired, cardiac disease.

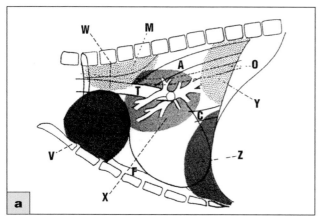

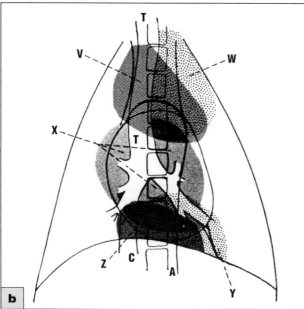

5.29 (a) Lateral and (b) DV views of the thorax illustrating the five main locations of mediastinal masses. A = descending thoracic aorta; C = caudal vena cava; F = fat in ventral mediastinum; M = shadow of intrathoracic part of the longus colli muscle; O = oesophagus; T = trachea; V = cranioventral masses; W = craniodorsal masses; X = hilar and perihilar masses; Y = caudodorsal masses; Z = caudoventral masses. (Reproduced from Suter (1984) with permission)

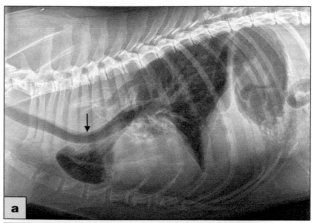

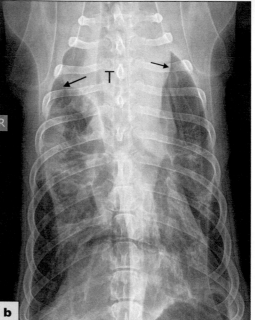

5.30 (a) Lateral and (b) DV views of the thorax of a dog with a craniodorsal mediastinal mass. (a) The large soft tissue mass ventral to T1–T6 results in ventral displacement (arrowed) of the intrathoracic trachea. The displaced cranial lung lobes are poorly inflated and extend only to the second rib. (b) On the DV view, the mass (arrowed) results in widening of the cranial mediastinum but does not cause significant lateral displacement of the trachea (T).

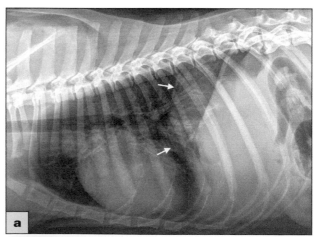

5.31 (a) Lateral view of the thorax of a dog with a large caudodorsal mediastinal mass. The mass (arrowed) is superimposed on the caudodorsal lung fields and dorsal two-thirds of the diaphragm. The mass obscures the caudal vena cava. (continues) ▶

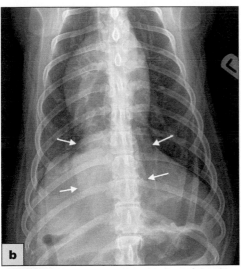

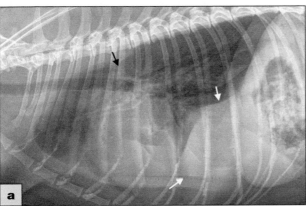

5.31 (continued) **(b)** DV view of the thorax of a dog with a large caudodorsal mediastinal mass. The mass (arrowed) is localized to the midline. The differential diagnoses include a neoplastic mass, granuloma or abscess arising from the mediastinum itself, or a mass lesion involving the caudal oesophagus.

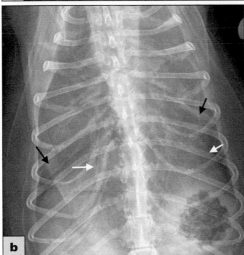

5.32 **(a)** Lateral and **(b)** DV views of the thorax of a dog with a caudoventral mediastinal mass.
(a) The mass (white arrows) effaces the caudoventral border of the cardiac silhouette and the cranioventral diaphragm. Pleural effusion is present with widening of the pleural fissures (black arrow). (b) The location of the mass (white arrows) is partially obscured by pleural fluid. Note the widened pleural fissures (black arrows). As the volume of pleural fluid is not large, the mass is suspected to arise on the midline and extend slightly to the left. Differential diagnoses include a caudoventral mediastinal mass, accessory lung lobe mass or a diaphragmatic defect.

Intrapulmonary masses

- May appear as single or multiple soft tissue nodular or mass lesions (nodule <3 cm; mass >3 cm).
- They are surrounded by air in most cases, but may present as lobar consolidation.
- An increase in lung lobe size or displacement of the mediastinum by a pulmonary mass is uncommon.
- Obstruction of a lobar bronchus by small lesions can result in loss of lung volume and a shift in the mediastinum towards the lesion.

Thoracic wall masses

- Even though frequently large at the time of presentation, thoracic wall masses are easily overlooked when viewed *en face* or are difficult to distinguish from intrapulmonary masses. When the margin of a mass is projected tangential to the X-ray beam it is more easily recognized. Masses in the costodiaphragmatic angle are easily overlooked. Masses which expand into the thorax displace the adjacent lung lobes. The broad angle of displacement between mass and lung is known as the 'extrapleural sign'.

Mass effect within the thorax

- Pleural fluid may displace the trachea dorsally and mimic a mass. Patient positioning (e.g. axial rotation or marked ventroflexion of the neck) may result in dorsal displacement of the trachea and mimic a thoracic mass lesion.
- A mass effect within the thorax or displacement of mediastinal structures is usually associated with soft tissue masses, but occasionally is due to the effect of air-filled structures. These changes are usually recognized as a shift in the mediastinum associated with an increase or decrease in lung volume.
  - With a loss of lung volume (due to general anaesthesia, positional atelectasis or bronchial obstruction) the mediastinal shift is towards the same side. The hemidiaphragm on the side of the volume loss is usually cranially positioned.
  - With an increase in lung volume (due to emphysematous changes caused by a 'ball valve' effect of mass lesions or due to a bronchogenic cyst) the mediastinal shift is away from the lesion. There is usually little change in the appearance of the diaphragm.

Trachea

Specific approach to interpretation

For a full evaluation of the trachea, it is necessary to obtain a lateral view of the neck as well as of the thorax. A DV or VD view may be helpful in some cases, but quite often these views add little information as the trachea is partially or fully superimposed on the spine. When assessing the cervical trachea, the endotracheal tube should be removed prior to obtaining the radiographs.

Size and shape

The diameter of the trachea should be approximately 20% that of the thoracic inlet, although this ratio is reduced in Bulldogs and other brachycephalic breeds, where it can be as small as 0.14. Slight variation in tracheal diameter with phase of respiration is normal, but there should not be significant narrowing. Differentiation of tracheal hypoplasia and collapse requires both inspiratory and expiratory radiographs to allow assessment of any dynamic component to the narrowing. The diameter of the trachea should be consistent along its length, from the caudal aspect of the larynx to the tracheal bifurcation. Focal narrowing may be due to intraluminal disease (e.g. submucosal haemorrhage due to anticoagulant toxicity), mass lesions, foreign bodies or stenosis (congenital or acquired). Focal narrowing of the trachea due to extraluminal disease is commonly seen with cranioventral mediastinal masses, especially in conjunction with tracheal displacement.

Opacity

The lumen of the trachea should always be air-filled. Intraluminal nodules, foreign bodies or large accumulations of discharge may all result in a focal increase in opacity within the tracheal lumen highlighted by air.

Margination

Only the internal surface of the trachea should be visible and should appear straight and smooth. The outer wall of the trachea is only seen if there is mediastinal free air, air in the oesophagus or the tracheal rings are calcified. A normal radiographic appearance does not exclude disease, as some conditions may be present without any detectable radiographic changes.

Location

Within the thorax the trachea usually diverges from the thoracic vertebrae, although in some barrel-chested breeds it may be parallel to the vertebral column. Tracheal position varies with that of the head and neck. The trachea may be displaced by cervical/mediastinal masses or cardiomegaly (Figure 5.33). The location of focal tracheal displacement in association with an increase in soft tissue opacity is an important radiological sign. Dorsal and rightward deviation of the trachea cranial to the carina may occur with heart base or cranioventral mediastinal masses. Elevation of the trachea at the carina often indicates left-sided cardiomegaly. Ventral displacement of the trachea cranial to the cardiac silhouette is often associated with oesophageal dilatation. In cases of tracheal displacement, the diameter of the trachea should be assessed as narrowing of the trachea indicates compression by an extrinsic mass.

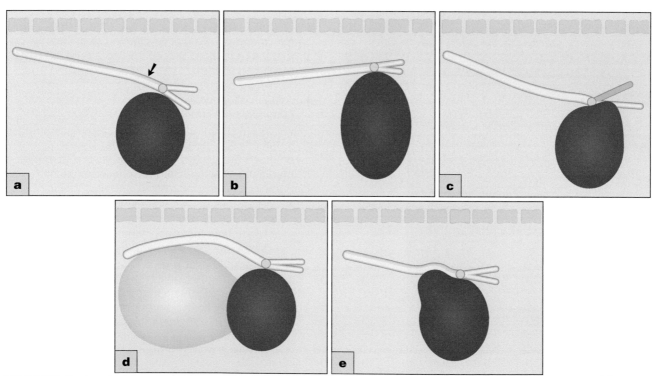

5.33 Basic principles of tracheal and bronchial displacement on the lateral thoracic radiograph. The position of the trachea and the mainstem bronchi can be used to assess for the presence of cardiac disease and mediastinal masses. **(a)** Normal. In most breeds, the trachea diverges gradually from the thoracic spine towards the base of the cardiac silhouette. In some breeds with a shallow conformation there may be no divergence, and in some deep-chested breeds the intrathoracic trachea may diverge even when significant cardiac enlargement is present. The distal trachea curves slightly ventrally cranial to the carina (arrowed). **(b)** Enlargement of the left ventricle results in elevation of the trachea along its length. The trachea no longer diverges but is almost parallel to the thoracic spine. **(c)** Enlargement of the left atrium results in dorsal displacement of the left mainstem bronchus (shown in dark blue). **(d)** Cranial mediastinal masses result in elevation of the trachea cranial to the cardiac silhouette. Depending on the size and location of the mass, the dorsal displacement may be focal or along the length of the trachea. Very large masses may compress and narrow the lumen of the trachea. **(e)** Heart base masses result in focal elevation of the trachea immediately cranial to the carina. This has been termed the 'bowler hat' sign. The terminal trachea is displaced to the right on the DV view. Note that the position of the terminal trachea is usually not altered on the lateral view in animals with tracheobronchial lymphadenopathy.

Common conditions

Tracheal collapse

This is a degenerative disease, which predominantly affects middle-aged to older toy and small-breed dogs. It is a dynamic condition and may be difficult to exclude on plain radiography, although obtaining radiographs during both inspiration and expiration increases the chance of detecting collapse. Inspiratory collapse typically involves the cervical region, whereas expiratory collapse involves the intrathoracic trachea. The condition can involve the entire trachea and in some cases may also involve the mainstem bronchi. Obstruction of the nasopharynx or larynx can lead to collapse of the cervical trachea and this should be considered as a cause, especially if tracheal collapse is seen in a cat.

Radiological features:

- Radiological features of tracheal collapse are best evaluated on the lateral view and include:
  - Narrowing of the caudal cervical trachea during inspiration
  - Narrowing of the thoracic trachea during expiration.
- The narrowing is unlikely to be consistent, so a normal appearance does not rule out collapse.
- If radiographs are taken using positive pressure ventilation (i.e. manual inflation under general anaesthesia), then the trachea may appear wider than normal on inspiration due to ballooning of the trachealis muscle.
- The ventral tracheal wall remains straight, but the dorsal wall may appear ill defined or irregular if there are inflammatory mucosal changes or uneven changes in the tracheal rings.
- CT (or a rostrocaudal tangential view; see Figure 5.8) demonstrates a change in the cross sectional area. The appearance of the trachea alters from round to an oval or 'C' shape.
- A dynamic assessment of the trachea using fluoroscopy or an endoscopic examination may be necessary for diagnosis (Figure 5.34).

Foreign bodies

Tracheal foreign bodies (Figure 5.35) are not common and may be harder to detect than oesophageal foreign bodies. Very radiopaque foreign bodies (e.g. stones or metallic objects) are usually obvious, but small radiolucent foreign bodies are normally not visible. Superimposition of airway secretions and, potentially, ribs may make foreign bodies hard to detect. Animals with tracheal foreign bodies are likely to present acutely with dyspnoea and respiratory noise compared with animals with bronchial foreign bodies, where coughing is a more common reason for clinical presentation. Tracheal foreign bodies typically lodge close to the tracheal bifurcation, appearing as masses within the lumen.

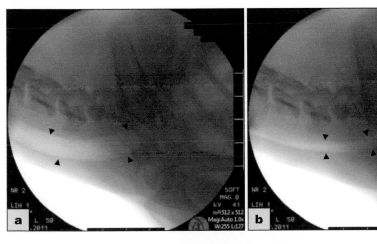

5.34 Lateral fluoroscopic images of the cervical trachea of a dog with tracheal collapse. On fluoroscopic images, the normal radiographic opacities are reversed (i.e. air appears white). **(a)** During expiration the tracheal diameter (arrowheads) is even throughout its length. **(b)** During inspiration, the air-filled lumen collapses (arrowheads). In a normal animal, the tracheal luminal diameter should not change significantly between inspiration and expiration.

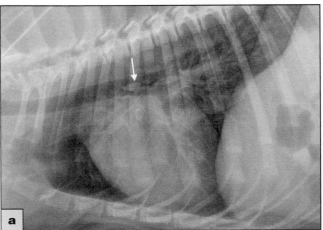
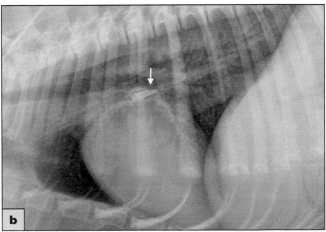

5.35 **(a)** Left lateral and **(b)** right lateral views of the thorax of a dog with a tracheal foreign body (arrowed) that has lodged in the left cranial lobar bronchus. (a) The foreign body (a canine tooth) is visible superimposed on the distal trachea. The margins are poorly defined due to atelectasis of the left cranial lobe. (b) The affected lobe is uppermost and well inflated and the tooth is surrounded by air making it clearly visible. (Courtesy of the University of Cambridge) (continues) ▶

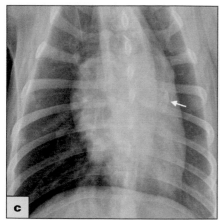

5.35 (continued) **(c)** DV view of the thorax of a dog with a tracheal foreign body (arrowed) that has lodged in the left cranial lobar bronchus. The tooth is difficult to recognize as it is superimposed on the cardiac silhouette. This study demonstrates the importance of obtaining both lateral views and an orthogonal view, as well as the selection of appropriate exposure factors, which allow the lesion to be localized on the DV view. Underexposure of the DV view would probably have prevented the tooth from being recognized. (Courtesy of the University of Cambridge)

Radiological features:

- Direct detection of the foreign body is possible if it is radiopaque (e.g. stone, tooth or small piece of bone). Two views should be taken for localization, although superimpostition of the spine may hinder interpretation of the DV/VD view.
- The geometric shape of some foreign bodies that are of soft tissue opacity (e.g. plastic or rubber) may aid their detection.
- Mucus surrounding a small radiolucent foreign body may lead to a focal increase in luminal opacity, which is not definitive, but would increase suspicion of a foreign body.

Hypoplasia

Tracheal hypoplasia is a congenital condition in some dog breeds (it is one component of brachycephalic airway obstruction syndrome), where the cross-sectional area of the trachea is reduced by at least 50% (Figure 5.36). Breeds commonly affected include English Bulldogs and small brachycephalic dogs; it is rare in cats.

Radiological features:

- Uniform narrowing of the trachea (compared with localized narrowing usually seen with tracheal collapse).
- Uniform thickening of the tracheal wall.
- Concurrent congenital abnormalities (such as megaoesophagus and pulmonic or aortic stenosis) may be present.

Stenosis

Tracheal stenosis is a focal narrowing of the trachea, which usually develops following a traumatic insult such as a bite wound, intubation injury or tracheal surgery. A stenotic lesion has to be relatively severe to result in clinical signs.

Radiological features:

- Focal, consistent tracheal narrowing (Figure 5.37).

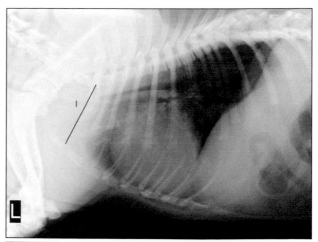

5.36 Lateral view of the thorax of a Bulldog with hypoplasia of the trachea. The ratio of the tracheal luminal diameter to the thoracic inlet is 0.09 (normal range for non-brachycephalic breeds is 0.21 ± 0.03 and for Bulldogs is 0.11 ± 0.03). The trachea is uniformly narrowed along its length.

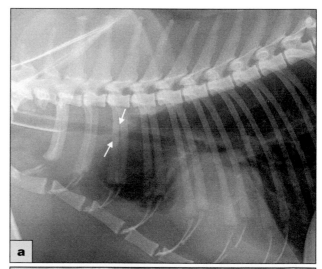

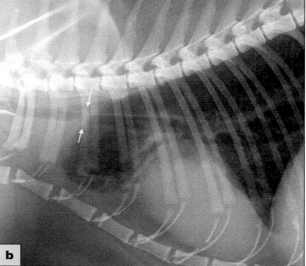

5.37 **(a)** Left and **(b)** right lateral views of the thorax of a cat with focal narrowing of the trachea (arrowed). The trachea should be of even diameter along its length. The narrowing is consistent on both views and was confirmed using endoscopy. Narrowing may be acquired following trauma associated with overinflation of the endotracheal tube cuff, foreign body trauma or inflammation.

Tracheal masses

Masses within the trachea are rare; they can sometimes occur due to neoplasia, granulomatous/parasitic lesions, polyps or focal haematomas.

Radiological features:

- Focal soft tissue opacity within the tracheal lumen (Figure 5.38). If the mass obstructs the whole trachea or a mainstem bronchus, underinflation of the lung may be seen.
- Extrinsic masses adjacent to the trachea may displace the trachea. Distortion of the lumen is unusual due to the rigidity of the tracheal rings.

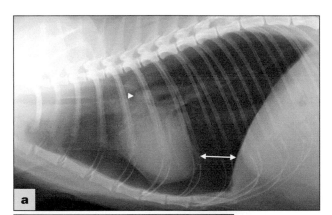

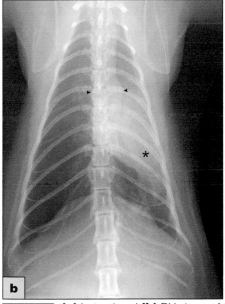

5.38 **(a)** Lateral and **(b)** DV views of the thorax of a cat with a tracheal mass at the level of the carina. (a) There is an increase in soft tissue opacity within the terminal trachea (arrowhead). The left cranial lobe bronchus is obstructed, resulting in a reduction in lung volume, and the right lung lobes consequently show compensatory overinflation (double-headed arrow). (b) The caudal sub-segment of the left cranial lung lobe is collapsed (*), resulting in a mediastinal shift to the same side (arrowheads). The trachea itself is not clearly seen as it is largely superimposed on the spine.

Submucosal thickening or infiltration

This may be seen following tracheal haemorrhage as a result of trauma or a coagulopathy (Figure 5.39). Diffuse neoplastic conditions such as lymphoma may, in theory, cause similar narrowing, but this is rarely seen.

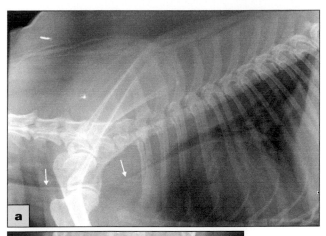

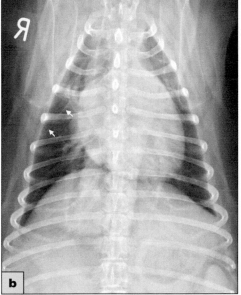

5.39 **(a)** Lateral and **(b)** DV views of the thorax of a dog with extensive luminal narrowing of the trachea due to submucosal haemorrhage. (a) The band-like thickening (arrowed) is most severe within the thoracic inlet, with sparing of the terminal trachea. (b) The trachea lies in a normal position. A pleural line (arrowed) is present in the right fourth to fifth intercostal spaces, which could represent pleural thickening/fluid or may be incidental.

Radiological features:

- Narrowing of the trachea either focally or diffusely.
- Wall thickening – if the tracheal rings are mineralized, they will be seen to maintain a normal diameter.
- The mediastinum may also be widened in cases of haemorrhage and there may be concurrent pulmonary changes.

Tracheal laceration or avulsion

Traumatic injuries such as bite wounds, road traffic accidents and iatrogenic injury following intubation can lead to tearing or complete avulsion of the trachea.

Radiological features:

- Alteration in the shape of the trachea with irregularity of the lumen.
- 'Pseudotrachea' in the case of complete rupture (a ballooned area of gas lucency where tracheal rings are not visible).
- Pneumomediastinum (see Figure 5.91).

Lungs

Specific approach to interpretation

When interpreting radiographs of the lungs, it is essential to appraise the technical factors of the radiograph first to assess the degree of inflation. When an animal is positioned in lateral recumbency, even for a very short period of time (and particularly under general anaesthesia), collapse occurs in the dependent lung lobes (see Figure 3.8). On a subsequent DV/VD view, some degree of collapse (full or partial) will usually be evident, unless the lungs are manually inflated or the animal is repositioned in sternal recumbency for some time prior to radiographic exposure, to permit re-inflation of the lung. Full or partial collapse leads to an increase in lung opacity, which may mask pathology. A mediastinal shift also occurs towards the side of the collapse. With digital radiography, the normal broncho-interstitial lung markings are often seen more clearly than on conventional analogue radiographs. The clinician should take care not to overdiagnose interstitial lung disease as isolated interstitial lung disease is relatively rare.

In normal animals:

- The division between the lung lobes is not usually evident, except when a pleural reflection lies tangentially to the X-ray beam and is projected as a thin radiopaque line
- Lung parenchyma is radiolucent due to the large proportion of air-filled alveoli
  - In older animals, some degree of fibrosis can develop, increasing the interstitial markings in the lung
- Pulmonary blood vessels are visible as linear soft tissue opacities and should be the only lung markings seen in the periphery of the thorax
  - Vessels should taper gradually towards the periphery of the lung
  - The artery and vein should be approximately equal in size
  - Blood vessels viewed end-on appear as circular radiopacities that are the same diameter as, but more radiopaque than, the vessel from which they arise
  - The radiopacity and diameter of end-on vessels are useful criteria to assess when attempting to distinguish vessels from metastatic or other nodules. End-on vessels appear more opaque than metastatic nodules of the same diameter as they represent a greater thickness or length of tissue. End-on vessels are of similar or equal diameter to the adjacent vessels from which they branch
- The airways contain air and therefore appear radiolucent
- Bronchial walls may be seen as thin radiopaque lines (or circles when viewed end-on) in the perihilar area, but should not normally be visible in the periphery of the thorax
- Bronchi are located between a pulmonary artery and vein. Where the walls of bronchi are not visible, their position may be inferred from that of the vessels
  - Walls may calcify with age and become more visible in some chondrodystrophic breeds, but should remain thin

- Hyperadrenocorticism and prolonged corticosteroid administration can also lead to bronchial calcification, but this is not common
- Bronchi should be oriented in relatively straight lines; their path may be altered if there are changes in adjacent structures (e.g. left atrium or lymph nodes)
- Bronchi should taper smoothly towards the periphery of the thorax.

Pulmonary parenchyma: normal variations

Age:

- Young animals often have more radiopaque lungs than adults, due to a higher water content of the interstitium.
- Older animals may also have an increased interstitial component due to fibrosis.
- Bronchial walls may calcify with age, making the bronchi more visible, but walls should not be thickened.
- Pulmonary osteomas/pleural plaques may be seen in older animals (see Figure 5.19). These are the result of heterotopic bone deposition, leading to scattered, often irregularly shaped, nodules of mineral opacity. Osteomas should not be mistaken for metastatic nodules.

Body condition: A large amount of subcutaneous fat increases the depth of the soft tissues around the thorax and hence leads to a generalized increase in lung opacity, which can mimic an interstitial infiltrate. In extreme cases, peripheral fat may also restrict the degree to which the lungs can inflate, which increases lung opacity even further.

Species:

- In cats, on a lateral radiograph, the caudodorsal lung margin is separated from the spine by the wedge-shaped soft tissue opacity of the psoas minor muscle. In dogs, the dorsal lung margins meet the vertebral column and any soft tissue opacity between is due to pathology (usually representing pleural fluid).
- The clavicles may be seen in cats if the collimated area extends to include the shoulders.
- The costochondral junctions in cats are typically more T-shaped than in dogs, with the costal cartilages being more evenly and smoothly mineralized.

Size

The size of the lung lobes varies physiologically with the phase of respiration and, due to variation in the relative proportion of air to soft tissue, there is usually concurrent alterations in lung opacity. Assessment of the size and shape of the lung lobes is important, especially when evaluating lungs that have an increased opacity, and allows differentiation between atelectasis, consolidation and pulmonary masses. A reduction in lung volume with a corresponding increase in opacity indicates atelectasis, whereas consolidation of the lung results in an increase in opacity and normal lung volume. Pathological increases in lung lobe size may occur with pulmonary masses (which are of soft tissue opacity) or emphysema/air-trapping (which results in a decrease in lung opacity). Demonstration of air-trapping requires radiographs to be taken during expiration to show that the affected lung remains inflated.

Alteration in lung lobe volume is best assessed on the DV view using the position of the mediastinal structures to infer lung volume. In normal animals, the mediastinal structures are midline with ventral lateralization to the left. The size of the lung lobes lateral to the cardiac silhouette on the DV view should be approximately equal. A unilateral reduction in lung volume results in displacement (shift) of the mediastinal structures *towards* the atelectatic lung. There may also be cranial displacement of the crus of the diaphragm on the affected side. In contrast, if there is lung pathology with no alteration in lung volume, the position of the mediastinal structures will be unaffected. Pathology that results in an increase in lung volume may result in a mediastinal shift *away* from the affected lung.

Shape

The lung lobes are normally roughly triangular in shape. A change in shape can be seen with pulmonary masses located peripherally within a lung lobe, as well as with chronic inflammatory/infectious pleural space disease, where fibrosis and thickening of the pleura leads to rounding/deformation of the adjacent lung. Focal atelectasis within a lung lobe can result in a depression in the margin of the lobe.

Opacity

When assessing the lungs, it is important to consider the radiographic and individual factors that can influence their appearance, before diagnosing a pathological change. Obesity, underexposure, expiration, atelectasis and pleural and chest wall diseases all result in an artefactual increase in lung opacity, and these need to be ruled out before attributing an increase in lung opacity to a pathological process. The opacity of the lung is predominately dependent upon the balance between the volume of air in the alveoli and the adjacent/overlying soft tissues. Put simply, a genuine increase in lung opacity occurs either due to a reduction in the volume of air within the lung (e.g. atelectasis) or an increase in soft tissue/fluid (e.g. pneumonia, oedema or mass), or a combination of the two processes. Assessment of shape and size of the affected lobe is important in determining which of these processes is occurring, and careful evaluation of the DV view for a mediastinal shift is important to determine lung volume. Most diseases result in an overall increase in lung opacity, either regional or diffuse. The distribution of any increase in lung opacity is important in prioritizing differential diagnoses as pulmonary diseases often have predilection sites within the lung lobes. It is less common for lungs to appear less opaque or hyperlucent.

Increased lung opacity: If the lungs have an increased opacity, the distribution and pattern of change are important for creating the differential diagnoses list. Four main lung patterns are recognized: bronchial (see page 144), alveolar, interstitial and vascular (see page 157). The interstitial pattern may be subdivided into nodular and unstructured/reticular/linear. In addition, focal changes such as mass lesions can lead to a regional increase in opacity. In many cases, an increase in opacity is due to a mixed lung pattern. In these cases, the predominant pattern is likely to be most important in deciding on the likely differential diagnoses. Originally, the lung patterns were described to correlate radiological findings with pathological findings. Despite the terms used for the patterns, pathological changes are often not confined to one compartment of the lung and there is much overlap in the radiological appearance of different diseases. Classification of pulmonary lung disease using lung patterns is generally most accurate if widespread areas of the lung are involved. In most cases of pulmonary pathology, additional tests such as bronchoscopy and airway cytology are required for a definitive diagnosis.

Alveolar lung patterns: An alveolar pattern is an important radiological finding and is almost always clinically significant. An alveolar pattern results from filling of the alveoli by:

- Oedema (cardiogenic or non-cardiogenic) (Figures 5.40 and 5.41)
- Exudate (pneumonia) (Figure 5.42)
- Blood (Figure 5.43)
- Neoplastic cells (Figure 5.44).

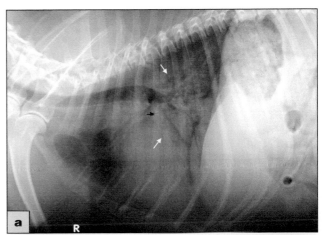
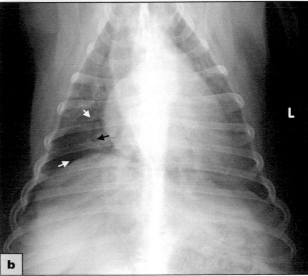

5.40 **(a)** Right lateral and **(b)** DV views of the thorax of a dog with an alveolar lung pattern (as a result of pulmonary oedema secondary to congestive cardiac failure). Note the tall heart and fluffy increase in opacity in the perihilar area, which obscures the caudodorsal margin of the cardiac silhouette (white arrows). Thickening of the bronchial wall is due to peribronchial oedema (black arrow). (continues) ▶

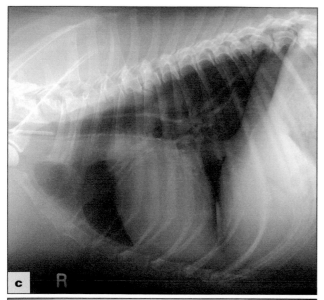

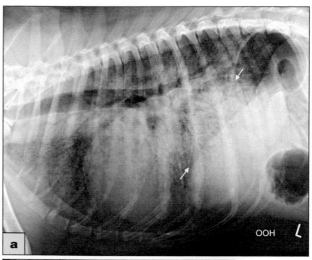

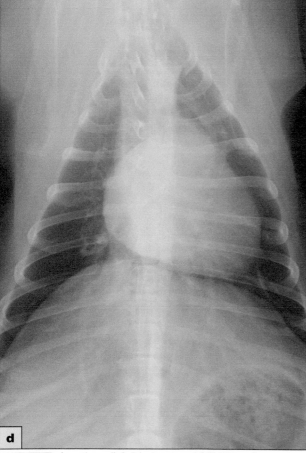

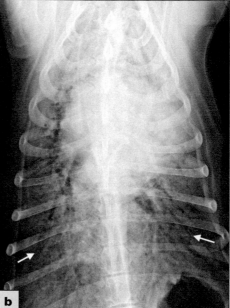

5.40   (continued) **(c)** Lateral and **(d)** DV radiographs of the same dog as in (a) and (b) following diuresis. The oedema has resolved and the cardiac outline is now clearly visible.

5.41   **(a)** Left lateral and **(b)** DV views of the thorax of a dog with an alveolar lung pattern (as a result of pulmonary oedema due to left-sided congestive heart failure). The widespread alveolar infiltrate is 'fluffy' and less confluent cranially and dorsally, but becomes more intense (consolidated) in the perihilar and caudodorsal lung regions (arrowed). Occasional air bronchograms are present. Factors that must be considered to confirm that the radiographic changes are due to cardiogenic pulmonary oedema include distribution of the changes, size of the cardiac chambers and pulmonary venous enlargement, as well as breed and clinical findings. In this dog, the lobar veins are difficult to assess due to the severity of the pulmonary changes, the left atrium is obscured on the lateral view and, as it is a deep-chested dog, assessment of cardiac size is more difficult. Hence, clinical findings and response to treatment are important considerations.

The classic features of an alveolar lung pattern include:

- An increase in lung opacity, which may be:
  - Patchy or homogeneous, depending on the extent of the alveolar filling
  - Focal, multifocal or diffuse, depending on the cause and severity.
- Obliteration of the margins of any soft tissue structures (border effacement) immediately adjacent to the area of alveolar filling (pulmonary vessels, heart, diaphragm)
- Air bronchograms, seen as branching radiolucent lines, due to air in bronchi within consolidated areas of lung. They are visible due to the contrast created between air and material of soft tissue opacity filling the surrounding alveoli. Air bronchograms are not visible in all cases of alveolar disease (e.g. if the bronchus is filled with fluid or cells, or if the alveolar disease is patchy or

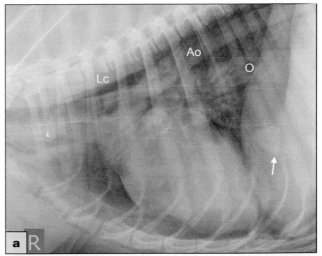

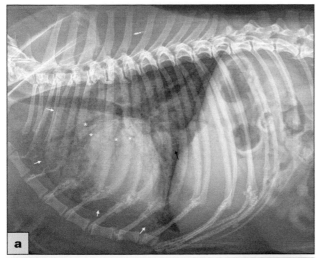

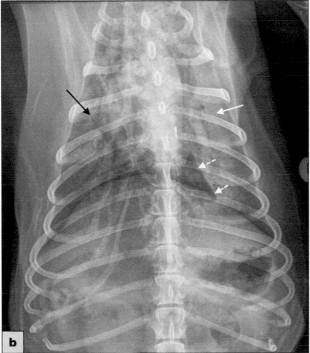

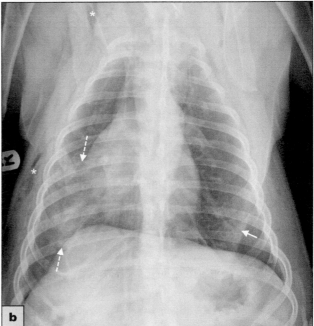

5.42 **(a)** Right lateral and **(b)** DV views of the thorax of an obese dog with an alveolar lung pattern (due to aspiration pneumonia). (a) Note the severe (but incomplete) consolidation of the cranioventral lung lobes, extending to the periphery of the lobes (white arrows). The margins of the consolidated lung lobes can be identified because of the large deposits of subpleural fat. Multiple air bronchograms (*) as well as peribronchial thickening (black arrow) are visible. (b) The lobar consolidation is bilateral, but appears worse on the left side (solid white arrow) compared with the right side (black arrow). Note the conspicuous lobar sign between the consolidated left lung lobes and the normally inflated accessory lobe of the right lung (dashed white arrows).

5.43 **(a)** Right lateral and **(b)** DV views of the thorax of a dog with an alveolar pattern (due to lung contusion/haemorrhage secondary to trauma). (a) Pneumomediastinum (*) is present, allowing the external margins of the aorta (Ao), caudal oesophagus (O) and longus colli muscles (Lc) to be seen. A poorly circumscribed focal area of consolidation (arrowed) is evident superimposed on the diaphragm between the seventh and eighth ribs. (b) A large area of consolidation (poorly circumscribed) is visible in the right lung adjacent to the cardiac silhouette (dashed arrows), in addition to the smaller focal area in the left caudal thorax (solid arrow) (as seen on the lateral view). Subcutaneous emphysema (*) is present. No rib fractures are visible. Haemorrhage following trauma usually presents as focal or multifocal areas of poorly circumscribed pulmonary consolidation.

not adjacent to a major airway)
- A bronchus outlined by a well delineated pulmonary artery and vein is a normal feature and should not be mistaken for an air bronchogram
- Increased visibility of the borders of individual lung lobes:
  - A 'lobar sign' is created when the alveolar pattern within an affected lung lobe extends to the lobar margin and lies adjacent to aerated lung. This allows the margin of the consolidated lung to be visualized
  - A 'wallpaper effect' represents a variation of the 'lobar sign', where the lobar boundaries are highlighted due to the difference in distribution and intensity of the alveolar pattern between lobes. This has been likened to the pattern created by slightly mismatched wallpaper stripes, where the mismatch highlights the adjoining edges.

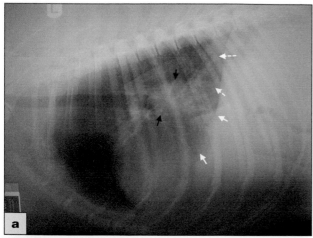

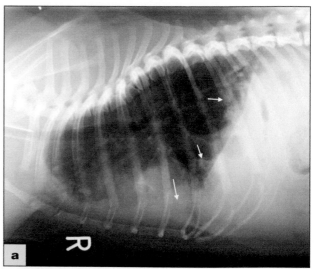

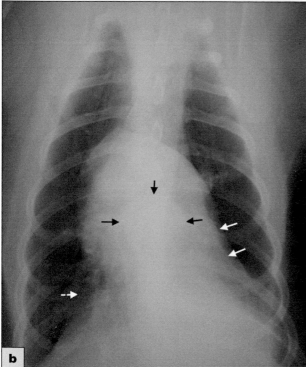

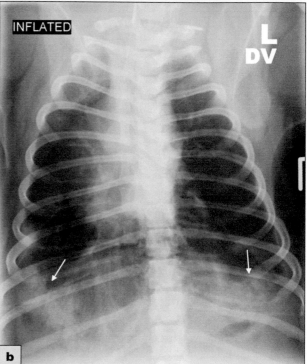

5.44 **(a)** Right lateral and **(b)** DV views of the thorax of a dog with an alveolar pattern as a result of neoplastic infiltration due to histiocytic sarcoma. The accessory lung lobe (solid white arrows) and areas of the caudodorsal lung lobes (dashed white arrows) are affected. The caudal aspect of the cardiac silhouette and the ventral aspect of the diaphragm are effaced by the consolidated lung. The middle tracheobronchial lymph node is enlarged and the caudal lobe bronchi are displaced laterally (black arrows).

5.45 **(a)** Right lateral and **(b)** DV views of the thorax of a dog with *Angiostrongylus vasorum* infection. The alveolar infiltrate is located predominantly at the periphery of the lung fields on both views (arrowed). This case shows a typical distribution pattern for *Angiostrongylus*-related pneumonia, although in other cases a patchier, diffuse or even nodular pattern may be present.

An alveolar pattern indicates significant pulmonary disease, but is a non-specific finding and can occur with a wide range of diseases. The distribution of the changes is an important feature when assessing an alveolar pattern, and in conjunction with the history and clinical findings may help to determine the most likely cause. Localization can include:

- Ventral (e.g. aspiration pneumonia)
- Perihilar (e.g. cardiogenic oedema)
- Lobar (e.g. lung lobe torsion)
- Caudodorsal (e.g. non-cardiogenic oedema)
- Peripheral (e.g. *Angiostrongylus* infection) (Figure 5.45).

Atelectasis can appear similar to alveolar filling, as it leads to a diffuse increase in opacity of the collapsed area or lobe. The main distinguishing feature is volume loss; a collapsed lung lobe occupies less space, leading to a mediastinal shift towards that side. Typical air bronchograms are also not seen with atelectasis, as the alveoli surrounding the bronchi are collapsed rather than filled with material of soft tissue opacity.

Interstitial lung patterns: Interstitial lung patterns can be subdivided into:

- Nodular patterns
- Unstructured/reticular/linear patterns.

Nodular pattern is the term used to describe a pattern of circular soft tissue opacities, which may be located anywhere within the lung field (Figure 5.46). Nodules must be distinguished from end-on blood vessels and superimposed skin structures (e.g. nipples, warts and ticks). Nodules are usually the result of metastatic neoplasia, but can be caused by primary neoplasia and granulomatous lesions. When screening for metastatic disease, both left and right lateral views should be taken to obtain a non-dependent and well inflated view of each lung. The best chance of detecting pulmonary nodules is when they are surrounded by well inflated lung, as the air provides contrast with the lesions. If only one or two small nodules are present, they will probably only be visible on one of the views.

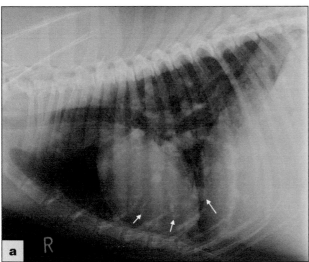

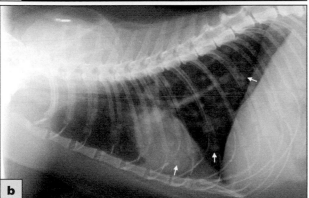

5.46 Lateral views of the thorax of **(a)** a dog and **(b)** a cat with pulmonary metastases. The multiple nodular soft tissue opacities (arrowed) are of variable size and irregular in shape. Many are indistinct.

Nodular patterns can be subdivided according to the characteristics of the nodules. Within aerated lung, a single nodule becomes radiologically visible when it reaches 3–5 mm in diameter. Smaller nodules may be seen if they are close together and become superimposed, creating a composite shadow (sometimes referred to as the 'bunch of grapes' effect).

■ 'Cannonball' pattern – this term is used to describe a small number of nodules that have grown to a relatively large size (Figure 5.47). They are usually homogeneous in opacity, but occasionally may appear cavitary (due to central

necrosis and communication with an airway). 'Cannonball' nodules are usually neoplastic in origin.
■ Miliary pattern – this pattern comprises multiple, small coalescing nodules. These nodules may be too small to be radiologically apparent individually, but are seen due to their composite effect (Figure 5.48). Differential diagnoses include:
• Metastatic neoplasia (most common)
• Pulmonary lymphosarcoma
• Pneumonia (fungal, haematogenous bacterial, mycobacterial)
• Disseminated intravascular coagulation.

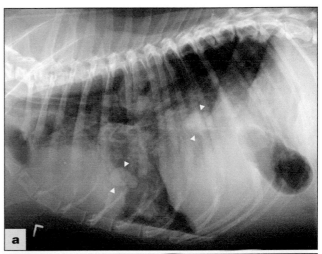

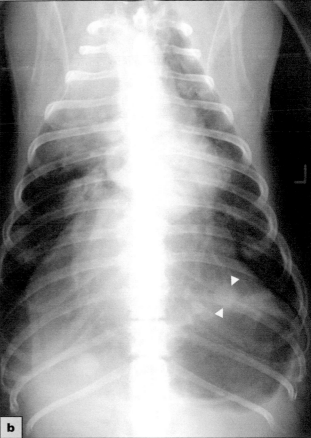

5.47 **(a)** Right lateral and **(b)** DV views of the thorax of a dog with a cranial thoracic mass and multiple large 'cannonball' metastases. The metastases (arrowheads) are most visible where they overlie the caudal border of the mass and the diaphragm.

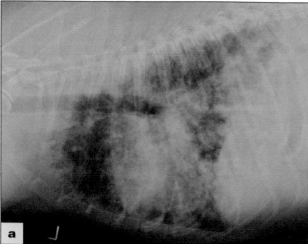

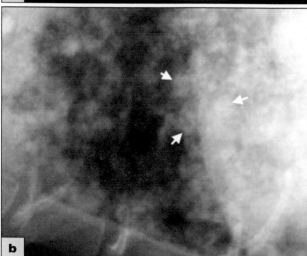

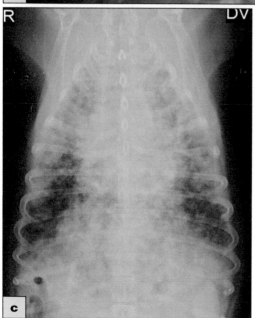

An unstructured/reticular/linear pattern results from a more diffuse swelling of the interstitial space. Although several descriptive terms are used, it is difficult to subdivide these patterns (unstructured, reticular or linear) accurately based on the radiographic appearance alone. An unstructured/reticular/linear pattern may be diagnosed if there is an increase in lung opacity, the pulmonary vessels are still visible, and bronchial/alveolar patterns have been excluded. It is the most difficult pattern to diagnose confidently, as artefacts created by the patient or exposure factors can mimic it. The differential diagnoses for an unstructured/reticular/linear interstitial pattern include:

- Interstitial oedema (usually early or resolving)
- Viral and protozoal pneumonia (Figure 5.49)
- Pulmonary fibrosis
- Diffuse neoplastic infiltration:
  - Lymphosarcoma (Figure 5.50)
  - Metastatic neoplasia (e.g. mammary gland carcinoma).
- Paraquat poisoning
- Haemorrhage (usually early or resolving).

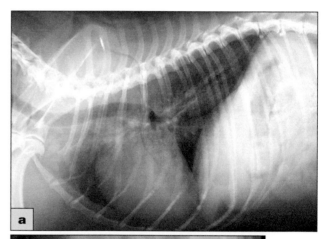

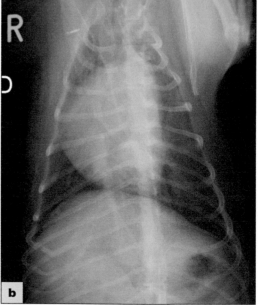

5.48 (a) Left lateral, (b) magnified left lateral and (c) DV views of the thorax of a dog with a diffuse miliary lung infiltrate. There are numerous small (miliary) nodules throughout all the lung lobes. In many cases, individual nodules are difficult to recognize (arrowed) and superimposition of multiple nodules results in large composite shadows which mimic alveolar disease. This pattern is more frequently due to neoplasia (metastatic or lymphosarcoma) but the differential diagnoses include rare forms of pneumonia (fungal, mycobacterial or haematogenous bacterial) and disseminated intravascular coagulation.

5.49 (a) Right lateral and (b) DV views of the thorax of a dog with *Pneumocystis carinii* pneumonia. The interstitial pattern appears as a diffuse, hazy increased opacity, which blurs the margins of the normal intrathoracic structures (cardiac silhouette, large lobar vascular structures and lobar bronchi). The DV view is rotated, which limits accurate assessment of the cardiac silhouette.

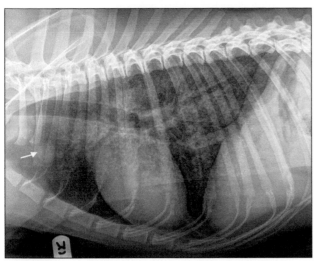

5.50 Right lateral view of the thorax of a dog with lymphoma. A diffuse, interstitial pulmonary infiltrate is present throughout the lungs. Although a degree of peribronchial thickening is present, the interstitial pattern predominates. There is mild enlargement of the presternal lymph node (arrowed) but the tracheobronchial lymph nodes are not visibly enlarged.

In addition, this pattern often forms part of a mixed lung pattern due to the close association between the interstitium and the peribronchial tissues and alveoli. Underinflation, underexposure and obesity may all be mistaken for an unstructured/reticular/linear interstitial pattern. Thus, body condition should be considered when interpreting lung opacity and an unstructured/reticular/linear interstitial pattern should only be diagnosed on a radiograph in which the thorax is:

- Inflated
- Well exposed
- Free from pathology that causes partial lung collapse (e.g. pleural effusion).

Radiological features of this type of pattern include:

- A mild-to-moderate increase in lung opacity (localized or, more commonly, diffuse)
  - Homogeneous
  - Linear
  - Reticular
  - Honeycomb
- Pulmonary blood vessels remain visible (in contrast with an alveolar pattern), although they may appear blurred and less well marginated than normal.

Mixed lung patterns: Mixed lung patterns are common. When interpreting radiographs where the lung pattern is mixed, it is helpful to try and identify the predominant pattern and base the most likely differential diagnoses around this. Many common diseases present with a mixed pattern (Figure 5.51).

Cavitary lesions: Cavitary lesions (Figure 5.52) are of mixed opacity with a soft tissue periphery and a gas-filled centre. Lesions that contain a mixture of fluid/soft tissue and gas appear more opaque than

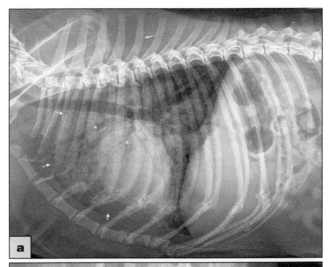

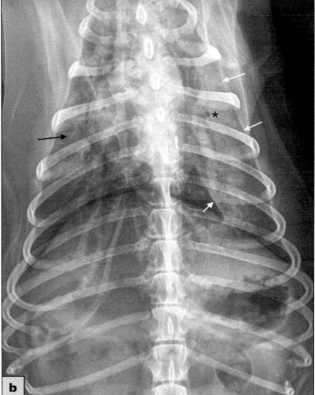

5.51 **(a)** Right lateral and **(b)** DV views of the thorax of a dog with a mixed lung pattern due to aspiration pneumonia. There is extensive consolidation (alveolar pattern) of the left cranial lung lobe with air bronchograms (∗) visible. The left border of the cardiac silhouette is effaced by the consolidated left lobe (white arrows). The changes within the left lung lobes caudal to the cardiac silhouette and within the right lung (interstitial pattern) are more patchy, blurring, but not effacing, normal thoracic structures (black arrows). Note the increased thickness of the bronchial walls (bronchial pattern) leading to the area of consolidated lung.

gas and less opaque than soft tissue, depending on the relative proportions of each. Unless a horizontal X-ray beam is used (not recommended), a fluid line will not be visible. With cavitary lesions, the thickness and margination of the wall is the key determining feature in differentiating cavitated nodules/masses from bullae/blebs. Abscesses, granulomas and neoplasms have thick irregular walls, whereas bullae and blebs are thin-walled.

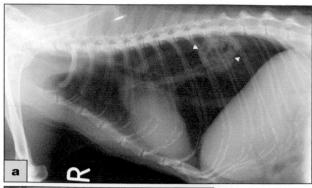

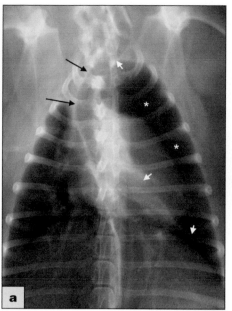

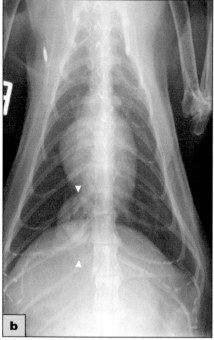

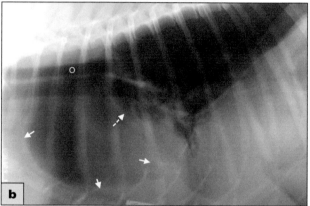

5.52	**(a)** Right lateral and **(b)** DV views of the thorax

of a cat with a cavitary mass (arrowheads) in the right caudal lung lobe. The wall of the mass is thick and irregular. Neoplasia (both primary and metastatic) is the most common cause of cavitary lesions. Abscesses and granulomas can occasionally present as cavitary mass lesions. Signalment, clinical findings and diagnostic sampling of the mass are required to confirm the diagnosis. The mass was aspirated under ultrasound guidance and although not conclusive, carcinoma was suspected.

Decreased lung opacity: Causes of hyperlucent lung fields include:

- Air-trapping – air can enter the alveoli during inspiration but cannot leave during expiration. Increased expiratory pressure leads to damage to the alveolar walls and subsequent formation of bullae. This may be seen with:
  - Allergic small airway disease (e.g. feline asthma)
  - Emphysema (congenital or acquired) (Figure 5.53)
  - Obstructive bronchial or tracheal masses (see Figure 3.5).
- Hypoperfusion (leading to hyperventilation):
  - Hypovolaemia
  - Right-to-left shunting lesions
  - Pulmonic stenosis
  - Right heart failure
  - Pulmonary thromboembolism.

5.53	**(a)** DV and **(b)** lateral views of the thorax of a

dog with hyperinflation of the left cranial lung lobe. (a) The left cranial lung lobe (white arrows) is hyperinflated with displacement of the trachea to the right (black arrows). The mediastinal shift is marked such that there is incomplete inflation of the right cranial lung lobe with the tip only reaching the third intercostal space. The hyperinflated lobe lacks lung and vascular markings (*), indicating emphysema. (b) The hyperinflated left cranial lobe (solid white arrows) and the cranial lobar vessels (dashed white arrow) are visible. The emphysematous changes were due to a 'ball valve' effect of chronic distortion and inflammation of the left cranial lobe bronchus. O = air-filled oesophagus.

If there is clinical or radiographic suspicion of pathology causing increased lucency of the lungs, thoracic radiographs taken during expiration may be helpful. During expiration, normal lung parenchyma is more opaque, providing better contrast with any air-containing lesions and making them more visible. If air-trapping is present, the usual variation in appearance between inspiration and expiration will be absent or less marked, with the diaphragm remaining flattened and caudally positioned and the lungs appearing consistently well aerated.

Radiological features may include:

- An overall decrease in lung opacity
- A caudally positioned, flattened diaphragm
- Small pulmonary vessels, if the lungs are hypoperfused

- A small cardiac silhouette
- The presence of bullae, seen as thin, curving radiopaque lines surrounding a radiolucent area.

Location

Abnormal location of the lung lobes most commonly occurs when the affected lobe is compressed or distorted by adjacent masses or pleural fluid. In cases of pleural fluid, there is commonly folding of parts of the lung (especially ventrally), which can result in bizarre shapes. Abnormal location of the lungs also occurs with lung lobe torsion (see below) and rarely with herniation outwith the chest wall. In animals that have undergone lung lobectomy, the remaining lobes enlarge to fill the potential space.

Common conditions

Pneumonia

Pneumonia is common in both cats and dogs, and in many cases the clinical signs (e.g. pyrexia) and findings are indicative of infectious airspace disease. The radiological features of pneumonia are non-specific and overlap with other causes of alveolar disease, although the distribution and temporal evolution of changes helps differentiate pneumonia from other diseases.

Pneumonia most commonly results in an alveolar pattern, but the extent varies depending upon the severity of the disease. In most cases, lung infection also involves the airways so a concurrent bronchial pattern is common. In cases of aspiration pneumonia, the ventral aspects of the lungs are typically the most severely affected (Figure 5.54). This is due to gravitational effects and orientation of the bronchi, which facilitates accumulation of infectious/irritant material ventrally. In cases of parasitic pneumonia (e.g. *Angiostrongylus vasorum*) changes are often seen in the caudodorsal lung fields. If the pneumonia is secondary to oesophageal disease, radiological signs reflecting this may be visible. Absence of cardiomegaly and pulmonary venous distension in conjunction with the distribution of the alveolar pattern helps differentiate pneumonia from cardiogenic pulmonary oedema.

Pulmonary oedema

Pulmonary oedema is radiologically divided into cardiogenic (due to left-sided congestive heart failure) and non-cardiogenic. Non-cardiogenic pulmonary oedema is uncommon and may occur due to a number of different causes, including:

- Upper airway obstruction
- Neurogenic (e.g. secondary to seizuring)
- Electrocution
- Near-drowning.

The diagnosis of non-cardiogenic oedema is normally based upon a known history in conjunction with acute onset respiratory signs. Non-cardiogenic oedema (Figure 5.55) results in changes in the alveoli and has a predilection for the caudodorsal lung lobes, often involving the right caudal lobe. There is no vascular enlargement or signs of left-sided cardiomegaly. Cardiogenic pulmonary oedema occurs secondary to an increase in left atrial pressure, and the

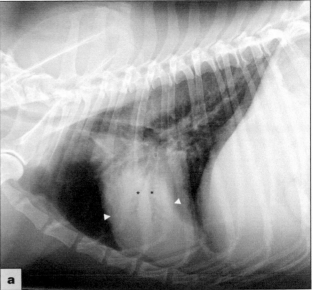
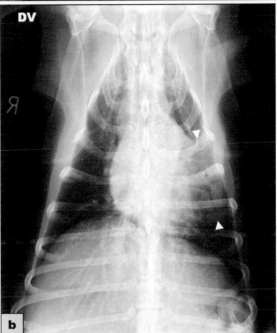

5.54 **(a)** Right lateral and **(b)** DV views of the thorax of a dog with aspiration pneumonia. The caudal part of the left cranial lung lobe is consolidated (arrowheads) and an alveolar pattern with air bronchograms (*) is visible on both views. It is important to take both right and left lateral views in cases of suspected aspiration pneumonia (as the changes are not so evident when in the dependent lung).

radiological changes of alveolar disease almost invariably occur in combination with evidence of left atrial enlargement and often pulmonary venous distension. Acute cardiogenic oedema may rarely occur without visible radiological signs of cardiomegaly (e.g. due to endocarditis).

Pulmonary haemorrhage

Pulmonary haemorrhage (see Figure 5.43) may be indistinguishable from other causes of alveolar disease, but there is often clinical evidence of haemorrhage elsewhere in the body. Coumarin (e.g. warfarin) intoxication may result in pleural and mediastinal haemorrhage; submucosal bleeding may also occur, leading to tracheal narrowing.

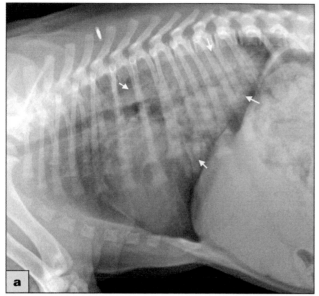

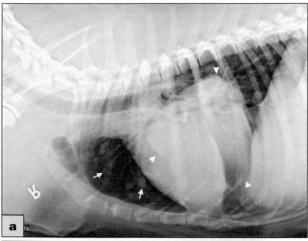

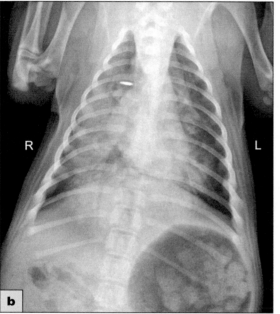

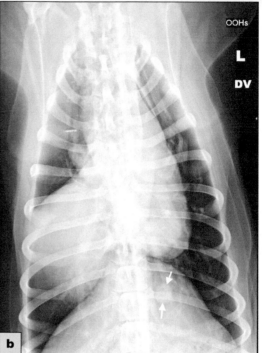

5.55 (a) Right lateral and (b) DV views of the thorax of a young dog with non-cardiogenic oedema. The lateral view shows the predominantly caudodorsal distribution (arrowed) of the alveolar infiltrate. On the DV view, the changes are bilateral but the right lung is more affected than the left lung. The thymus is visible cranial and to the left of the cardiac silhouette.

5.56 (a) Right lateral and (b) DV views of the thorax of a dog with a lung mass (histiocytic sarcoma). The well defined mass in the right caudal lung lobe (arrowheads) is in contact with the cardiac silhouette, resulting in border effacement. Several secondary nodules (arrowed) are visible in the cranial lung on the right lateral view, and on the DV view a nodule is visible overlying the left hemidiaphragm.

Pulmonary masses

Radiologically, a pulmonary mass appears as a discrete area of soft tissue (or less commonly, partly mineralized) opacity, replacing or compressing the surrounding aerated lung. The appearance of a mass can be similar to an area of alveolar infiltrate, but a mass is usually better marginated, more homogeneous and in most cases lacks air bronchograms (Figure 5.56). If air bronchograms are present, they are often narrowed or distorted. In some cases, a mass may appear cavitary due to central necrosis and gas accumulation (see Figure 5.52).

Lung masses usually have a peripheral location, whereas mediastinal masses tend to lie on or close to the midline. The exception to this is a mass lesion involving the accessory lung lobe, which lies caudally in the midline; accessory lung lobe lesions can be difficult to distinguish radiologically from mediastinal masses. If a mass lies in the periphery of the thorax or is in contact with the diaphragm, it is possible to examine it ultrasonographically. Radiographs are useful for the initial examination and localization of lesions and targeting of any subsequent ultrasonographic examination. Any aerated lung between a lesion and the chest wall precludes ultrasonographic examination as the sound waves are reflected by the air.

Most solitary masses are primary neoplasms. Differential diagnoses include granulomas, abscesses, cysts, haematomas and fluid-filled bullae or blebs. A solitary mass involving a single lobe could be excised surgically; if this is being considered, it is important to examine the rest of the lung carefully for any visible nodules that could represent metastatic lesions.

Radiological features:

- Single or multiple lesions within the lungs.
- Typically >3 cm in size (nodules are generally defined as <3 cm; masses are >3 cm).
- Usually round or oval in shape.
- Soft tissue opacity:
  - May have a cavitated centre due to necrosis
  - May contain areas of mineralization.
- Variable location.
- There may be secondary lymph node involvement (commonly seen with histiocytic sarcomas), seen as a focal perihilar increase in opacity.

Lung lobe torsion

Lung lobe torsion (Figures 5.57 and 5.58) can be spontaneous (especially in deep-chested breeds) or may occur secondary to underlying diseases that cause lobar collapse in conjunction with surrounding fluid or air, and hence allow increased mobility of the lobe. The right middle and left cranial lung lobes are most frequently affected. Torsion involves rotation of a lung lobe around its axis, leading to twisting and occlusion of the bronchi and pulmonary veins; arterial supply is usually preserved, at least initially. Pulmonary oedema develops, filling the alveoli, and there is sequestration of blood within the lobe. There may also be air-trapping due to bronchial occlusion. Alterations in interstitial pressure and decreased lymphatic drainage result in development of pleural effusion.

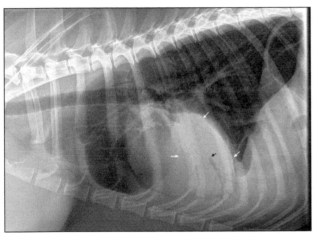

5.57 Left lateral thoracic view of a dog with torsion of the right middle lung lobe. The right middle lung lobe is consolidated (white arrows). The distal lobar bronchus appears as an air bronchogram but ends bluntly (black arrow) over the cardiac silhouette, and the proximal bronchus cannot be identified. A moderate volume of pleural effusion is present with retraction of the lung lobes, and fissure lines are also present. Blunt termination of a lobar bronchus, supported by other findings, indicates lung lobe torsion.

Radiological features:

- Initial increase in size of the affected lobe with rounding of the borders.
  - Lobe may decrease in size as necrosis develops.
- Increase in opacity of the affected lobe.
- Some air may still be present:
  - Small air bronchograms may be seen
  - A 'bubbly' vesicular gas pattern may

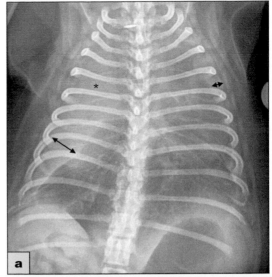

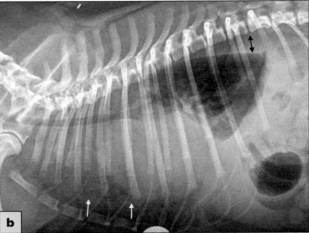

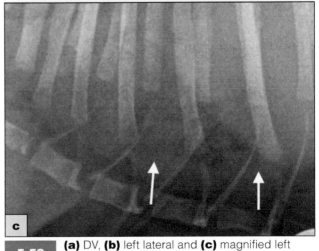

5.58 **(a)** DV, **(b)** left lateral and **(c)** magnified left lateral views of the thorax of a Pug with torsion of the right cranial and middle lung lobes. Pleural effusion (double-headed arrows) with retraction of the lung lobes is present on both the left and right sides. The volume of effusion is considerably larger on the right side, especially in the cranial thorax. The right cranial and middle lung lobes cannot be identified. They are consolidated and indistinguishable from the pleural fluid that has collected around the diseased lung lobe (*). On the left lateral view, the affected lobes have an indistinct vesicular or 'bubbly' appearance (white arrows). Asymmetrical pleural effusion, unequal collapse of the lung lobes within the ipsilateral hemithorax and a vesicular pattern are suggestive of lung lobe torsion. Although deep-chested breeds are typically associated with lung lobe torsion, chondrodystrophic small-breed dogs may also be affected.

occasionally be seen and, if present, this is strongly indicative of torsion.
- The lobar bronchus may end abruptly and/or may be traced in an abnormal direction (caudoventrally or dorsally).
- Pleural effusion is always present to some degree; it may be bilateral, asymmetrical or localized around the affected lobe.

Major airways

Pathology involving the major airways often results in coughing due to the location of the cough receptors within the trachea and mainstem bronchi. Pathology involving the bronchi can result in marked clinical signs with minimal radiological abnormalities, and high quality radiographs are required to visualize pathology confined to the bronchi.

Specific approach to interpretation

Bronchial disease, especially if acute, may be present without any detectable radiographic changes. Thus, a normal radiograph does not rule out disease. Conversely, in older animals, there may be radiographic changes within the airways in the absence of any clinical signs. The significance of any radiographic changes seen should always be assessed in conjunction with the clinical signs and the results of other diagnostic tests.

The abnormal appearance of the bronchi is called a *bronchial pattern* (Figure 5.59). This bronchial pattern may appear as increased linear markings (pairs of straight, slightly converging lines), which are often referred to as 'tramlines', or as ring-like markings ('doughnuts') when the bronchi are seen in cross section. These changes may be due to either thickening of the bronchial walls or peribronchial changes, resulting from cellular infiltrates in the surrounding interstitium. It is not possible to distinguish these two causes of increased visibility of bronchial markings on radiographs.

Size and shape

The major bronchi have a larger diameter than the adjacent pulmonary blood vessels. Unless the bronchial wall is mineralized or pathologically thickened, assessment of the diameter may not be possible (the space between the pulmonary artery and corresponding vein is larger than the bronchus). As the bronchi extend towards the periphery of the lungs, they should gradually reduce in diameter and each division should be smaller than the more proximal segment. Pathological dilatation of the bronchi (bronchiectasis) is commonly seen with bronchial disease and usually indicates chronic or severe disease (see below). Focal narrowing of the bronchial lumen is most commonly seen secondary to extrinsic compression (e.g. due to left atrial enlargement or pulmonary masses).

Opacity

Increased opacity of the bronchial walls is commonly due to either dystrophic mineralization or the result of increased soft tissue opacity caused by oedema or cellular infiltrates. Bronchial mineralization is, in most cases, an incidental finding.

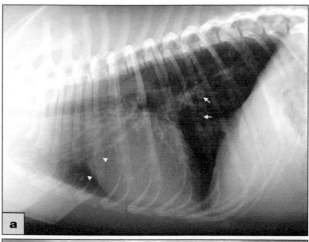
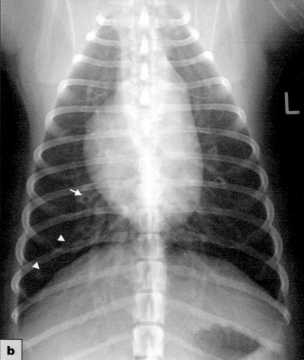

5.59 **(a)** Right lateral and **(b)** DV views of the thorax of a dog with a marked bronchial pattern. Note the thickened bronchial walls, seen as 'tramlines' (arrowheads) and 'doughnuts' (arrowed) that extend out to the periphery of the lungs.

Margination

Bronchial wall mineralization and age-related changes (if present) are normally sharply marginated. Indistinct margination is often present with peribronchial cuffing/oedema and often indicates significant bronchial disease.

Location

Abnormal orientation of the bronchi is rare but may be seen in conjunction with lung lobe torsion (see above) or due to displacement by masses.

Common conditions

Canine chronic bronchitis

Chronic bronchitis (Figure 5.60) is an inflammatory airway disease with many underlying causes, including infectious agents, allergies and parasites. It can be present in the absence of radiographic changes.

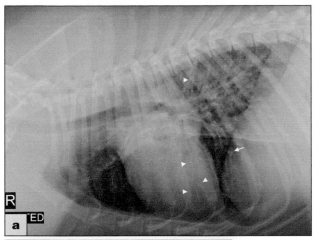

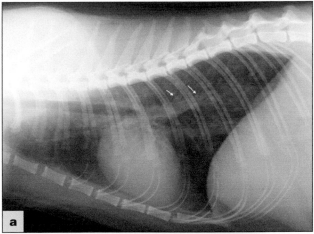

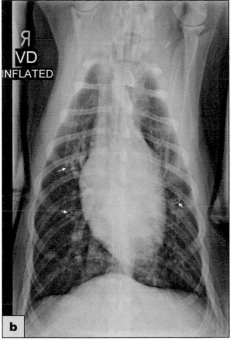

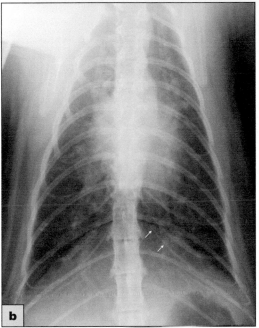

5.60 (a) Right lateral and (b) VD views of the thorax of a dog with chronic lower airway disease. There is a diffuse bronchial pattern with thickened bronchial walls, which appear as 'doughnuts' in cross-section (arrowed) and 'tramlines' in longitudinal sections (arrowheads). 'Doughnuts' are best recognized on the VD view and 'tramlines' on the lateral view.

5.61 (a) Right lateral and (b) DV views of the thorax of a cat with chronic allergic airway disease ('feline asthma'). Note the diffuse bronchial pattern, which in places appears nodular (arrowed) due to a combination of peribronchial thickening and the accumulation of mucus within the bronchial lumen. The margin of the cardiac silhouette is indistinct due to the large amount of pericardial fat.

Radiological features:

- Increased visibility of bronchial walls (increased number of bronchi are seen, especially in the periphery of the lung).
- Thickening of the bronchial walls and/or peribronchial infiltration.
- Mucus or exudate may accumulate in some bronchi. This increased soft tissue opacity within the bronchus may mimic pulmonary nodules.
- Pulmonary hypertension/cor pulmonale can occur, leading to right-sided cardiomegaly.

Feline chronic lower airway disease

This term includes 'feline asthma' (Figure 5.61) as well as non-allergic causes of small airway disease. A major feature of the condition is inflammatory changes leading to functional obstruction of the airways, resulting in air-trapping. Cats often present with severe dyspnoea and care should be taken when handling and positioning them for radiography. Normal radiographs do not exclude this condition.

Radiological features:

- Hyperinflation of the lungs, leading to a flat, caudally positioned diaphragm.
- Lung changes:
  - Most commonly a diffuse bronchial pattern due to peribronchial cuffing
  - In some cases there may be interstitial and/or alveolar pattern components.
- Mucus in the airways may result in a nodular appearance.
- Collapse of the right middle lung lobe is common due to airway obstruction.
  - Less commonly, collapse of the caudal part of the left cranial lobe may be seen.
- Rib fractures (acute or healing) may result from severe coughing/dyspnoea.

Bronchiectasis

Although discussed here as a distinct radiographic entity, bronchiectasis (Figure 5.62) is usually the result of chronic, severe lower airway disease. It is defined as irreversible bronchial dilatation and because it is irreversible, bronchiectasis is an important indicator in airway disease. If severe, bronchiectasis can result in recurrent pulmonary infections due to impaired muco-ciliary clearance.

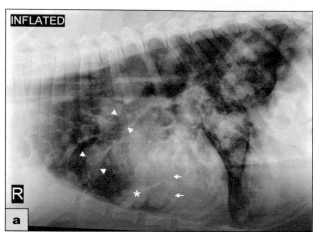

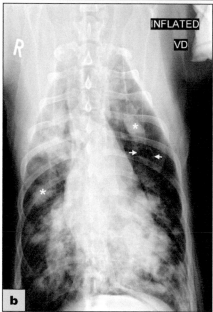

5.62 **(a)** Right lateral and **(b)** DV views of the thorax of a dog with bronchiectasis. The bronchial lumina appear widened (arrowheads) right out to the periphery of the lung. In places (e.g. over the cardiac silhouette) they have a sacculated or segmented appearance (arrowed). Areas of more homogeneous soft tissue opacity (✲) are likely to represent trapped or pooled secretions and areas of secondary bronchopneumonia. Emphysematous changes are recognized as coalescing areas with a soap-bubble appearance.

Radiological features:

- Cylindrical bronchiectasis – the bronchial lumen remains even but does not taper as usual as the bronchi divide.
- Saccular bronchiectasis – the bronchial lumen is uneven with round dilated areas within otherwise normal bronchi.
  - The dilatation, which is usually accompanied

by wall thickening, means that bronchi may be identified further into the periphery than normal.
- Generalized thickening of the bronchial walls.
- Increased opacity of the bronchial lumen, if there are areas of accumulated exudate.
- Secondary pathology may develop, including:
  - Localized abscesses developing from the coalition of saccules
  - Lung consolidation due to secondary pneumonia
  - Formation of bronchogenic cysts.

Bronchial foreign body

Inhaled foreign bodies are only visible if they are radio-paque; non-radiopaque foreign bodies are unlikely to be recognized in the acute stages if ventilation remains adequate.

Radiological features:

- Increased opacity within a bronchus (usually a caudal lobe mainstem bronchus) due to the foreign body and surrounding trapped secretions (Figure 5.63).
- Focal bronchopneumonia can develop, leading to:
  - Increased bronchial pattern within the affected lobe
  - Focal alveolar/interstitial pattern surrounding the affected bronchus.
- If untreated, this can progress to bronchiectasis and local abscessation.
- Atelectasis may be seen if the bronchus is occluded, with a corresponding mediastinal shift.

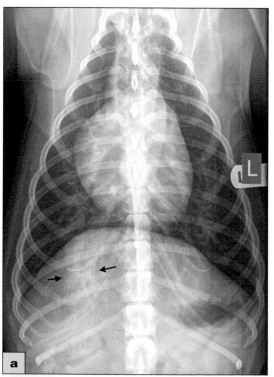

5.63 **(a)** DV thoracic radiograph of a dog with a bronchial foreign body. There is a poorly circumscribed infiltrate or increased soft tissue opacity (arrowed) surrounding the right caudal mainstem bronchus. Careful comparison with the left mainstem bronchus highlights the difference. (continues) ▶

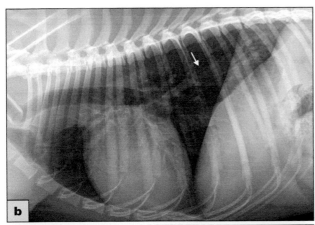

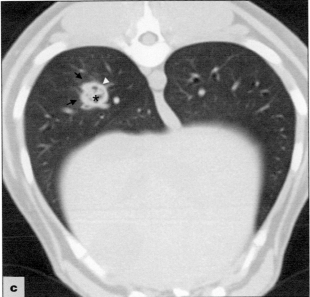

5.63 (continued) **(b)** Lateral thoracic radiograph and **(c)** CT image of a dog with a bronchial foreign body. (b) Little change, other than mild bronchial thickening (arrowed) is appreciated on this view. (c) Comparison with the CT image is helpful to understand the radiographic changes. Inhaled foreign bodies (*) tend to result in marked bronchial thickening (arrowhead), accumulation of discharge within the bronchus and a localized peribronchial interstitial infiltrate (arrowed). Lobar consolidation and pleural effusion are uncommon, although the foreign body may migrate caudally along the diaphragmatic crurae into the retroperitoneal space.

Bronchial neoplasia

Neoplasms, particularly carcinomas, can arise from the bronchi. It is not possible radiologically to distinguish neoplasia of bronchial origin from that arising from other tissues.

Radiological features: The radiographic pattern is variable, but usually involves nodular opacities or consolidation rather than a typical bronchial pattern.

Miscellaneous conditions

An increased bronchial pattern may be seen as a non-specific change, often in combination with other lung patterns, with some relatively rare conditions, including:

- Primary ciliary dyskinesia
- Bronchiolitis obliterans with organizing pneumonia.

Heart

Specific approach to interpretation

Radiologically, the heart cannot be distinguished from the pericardium and therefore the term cardiac silhouette is usually used to describe the composite shadow of the contents of the pericardial sac. Radiography can be useful for staging congestive heart failure, screening for metastases from cardiac masses and helping differentiate cardiac from non-cardiac causes of coughing. Many animals with cardiac disease (e.g. arrhythmias, hypertrophic cardiomyopathy or mild aortic stenosis) have a normal cardiac silhouette on radiographs; conversely, many animals with an abnormal cardiac silhouette have clinically silent disease. The diagnosis of congenital heart disease based on radiographs is often unreliable. Whilst specific patterns of alteration in cardiac shape are sometimes seen with congenital heart disease, in many cases these changes are non-specific.

Size

The overall size of the cardiac silhouette should be assessed subjectively and using one of the more objective methods for measurement (VHS (Figure 5.64) and height/width relative to the thorax). Consideration should also be given to the radiographic quality; rotation can lead to artefactual enlargement and the cardiac silhouette will look subjectively larger on an expiratory radiograph than on a well inflated view. There is also considerable breed variation in cardiac shape; reference to a normal radiograph of a particular breed can be helpful when trying to determine whether the cardiac silhouette is abnormal. It is also important to remember that not all cardiac diseases lead to cardiomegaly, and that with the relatively wide normal range (especially in dogs), an individual's cardiac silhouette may be enlarged and yet still fall within the normal reference range. The appearance of the cardiac silhouette varies considerably between cats and dogs; therefore, the radiological appearance of canine and feline cardiomegaly is discussed separately below.

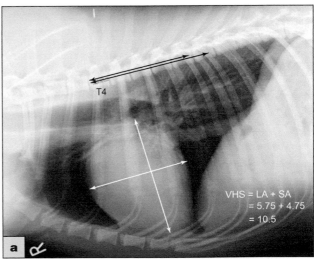

VHS = LA + SA
= 5.75 + 4.75
= 10.5

5.64 Lateral thoracic radiographs illustrating the vertebral heart score (VHS). **(a)** Normal heart. VHS = 5.75 (long axis) + 4.75 (short axis) = 10.5. (continues) ▶

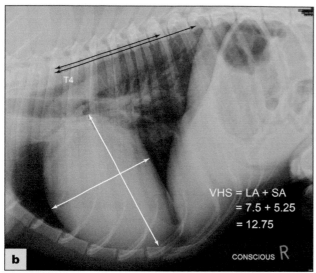

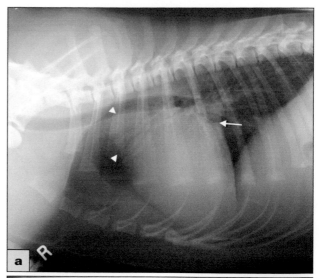

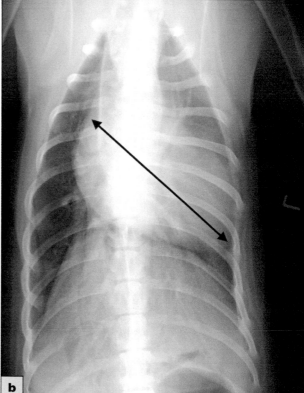

5.64 (continued) Lateral thoracic radiographs illustrating the vertebral heart score (VHS). **(b)** Cardiomegaly. VHS = 7.5 (long axis) + 5.25 (short axis) = 12.75. The long axis measurement is made from the ventral aspect of the left cranial lobe bronchus (note that although this is often referred to as the 'carina' or tracheal bifurcation, the carina can only be recognized on the DV view) to the apex. The short axis measurement is made by measuring the widest dimension of the cardiac silhouette, perpendicular to the long axis measurement.

Canine left-sided cardiomegaly: Causes of a predominately left-sided cardiomegaly in dogs include:

- Congenital:
  - Mitral valve dysplasia
  - Aortic stenosis (although in many cases the cardiac silhouette may be normal as left ventricular hypertrophy is concentric) (Figure 5.65)
  - Patent ductus arteriosus (Figure 5.66)
  - Ventricular septal defect.
- Acquired:
  - Endocardiosis (mitral valve degeneration)
  - Dilated cardiomyopathy
  - Bacterial endocarditis.

Radiological features:

- Lateral view (Figure 5.67a):
  - Increased height of the cardiac silhouette (>75% of the height of the thorax)
  - Elevation of the trachea at the carina
  - Elevation of the left caudal lobe bronchus (leading to 'splitting' of the mainstem bronchi)
  - Straightening of the caudal border
  - 'Tenting' (bulging) of the left atrium caudodorsally
  - Elevation of the caudal vena cava.
- DV view (Figure 5.67b):
  - Increased length of the cardiac silhouette
  - Bulge at the 2–3 o'clock position, representing enlargement of the left auricular appendage
  - Rounding of the margin of the left ventricle
  - Cardiac apex may be rounded and can be displaced to the right
  - With severe left atrial enlargement, the left atrium may be seen superimposed on the heart as a rounded soft tissue opacity lying between,

5.65 **(a)** Right lateral and **(b)** DV views of the thorax of a dog with left-sided cardiomegaly secondary to subaortic stenosis. The cardiac silhouette is tall on the lateral view with a bulge craniodorsally (arrowheads) in the region of the aortic arch, elevating the terminal trachea. The left atrium (arrowed) is enlarged, resulting in straightening of the caudal border of the cardiac silhouette. On the DV view, the cardiac silhouette is elongated (double-headed arrow). The typical enlargement of the aortic arch at the 11–1 o'clock position is not clearly seen in this case due to superimposition on the spine.

and leading to divergence of, the caudal mainstem bronchi. The differential diagnoses for this appearance include perihilar lymphadenopathy, which appears similar on the DV view, but does not cause the caudodorsal 'tenting' on the lateral view.

- Secondary features:
  - Pulmonary venous congestion (veins enlarged compared with the fourth rib on the lateral view

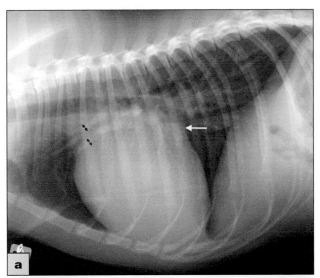

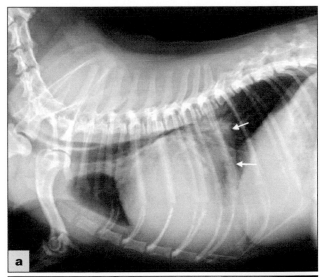

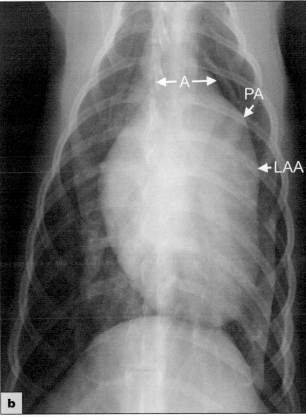

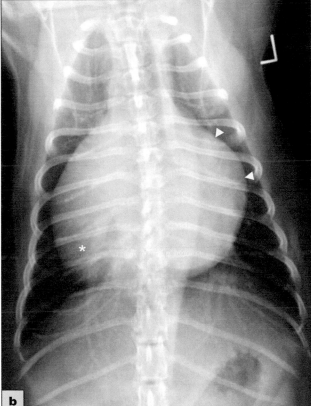

5.66 **(a)** Right lateral and **(b)** DV views of the thorax of a dog with cardiomegaly secondary to a patent ductus arteriosus. (a) The cardiac silhouette is wide and tall (generalized cardiomegaly). The caudal border is straightened due to left atrial enlargement (white arrow) and the cranial lobe pulmonary artery and vein are both enlarged (pulmonary overcirculation) (black double-headed arrows). (b) The cardiac silhouette is elongated. The enlargement of the aorta (A), pulmonary artery (PA) and left auricular appendage (LAA) ('three knuckles') is mild in this case.

5.67 **(a)** Right lateral and **(b)** DV views of the thorax of a dog with predominantly left-sided cardiomegaly due to degenerative mitral valve disease. On the lateral view, the caudal border of the cardiac silhouette is straightened, there is 'tenting' of the left atrium (arrowed) and the trachea is markedly elevated. On the DV view, there is a bulge on the left side of the cardiac silhouette in the region of the left auricular appendage (arrowheads) and rounding of the cardiac apex (*), which is displaced to the right.

and ninth rib on the DV, and larger than the corresponding artery)
- Alveolar filling due to pulmonary oedema:
  - Usually perihilar and patchy in the first instance
  - May be generalized and intense with acute cardiac failure.
- Aortic dilatation (post-stenotic) with aortic stenosis.

Canine right-sided cardiomegaly: Causes of a predominately right-sided cardiomegaly in dogs include:

- Congenital:
  - Tricuspid valve dysplasia
  - Pulmonic stenosis (Figure 5.68)
  - Atrial septal defects (although often do not lead to a detectable change on radiographs).

149

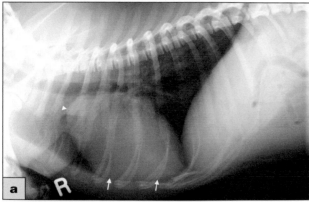

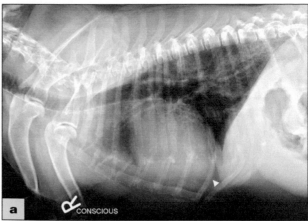

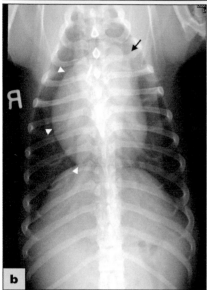

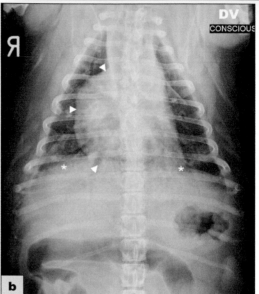

5.68   **(a)** Right lateral and **(b)** DV views of the thorax of a dog with right-sided cardiomegaly secondary to pulmonic stenosis. On the lateral view, the cardiac silhouette is wide and rounded craniodorsally (arrowhead) due to post-stenotic dilatation of the pulmonary artery. There is also increased sternal contact (arrowed). On the DV view, the cardiac silhouette has the characteristic 'reverse D' shape (arrowheads). Post-stenotic dilatation of the pulmonary artery has resulted in a bulge (arrowed) at the 1–2 o'clock position. In cases with less severe stenosis, the radiographic changes may be limited, with enlargement of the main pulmonary artery on the DV view being the only radiographic abnormality.

5.69   **(a)** Right lateral and **(b)** DV views of the thorax of a West Highland White Terrier with pulmonary fibrosis and predominantly right-sided cardiomegaly. On the lateral view, the cardiac silhouette is wide with the apex elevated from the sternum (arrowhead). On the DV view, the cardiac silhouette has a characteristic 'reverse D' shape due to right heart enlargement (arrowheads). The lung fields show a diffuse mixed interstitial and alveolar opacity (*) with some pleural lines visible between the lung lobes. The cranial mediastinum is widened on the DV view, probably due to fat.

■ Acquired:
  • Pulmonary hypertension – leads to right-sided cardiac enlargement secondary to increased pulmonary vascular resistance. Causes include:
    – Idiopathic pulmonary fibrosis (*cor pulmonale*)
    – Chronic pulmonary disease (*cor pulmonale*)
    – Parasites (*Angiostrongylus vasorum* and *Dirofilaria immitis*)
    – Primary pulmonary hypertension.
  • Endocardiosis (tricuspid valve degeneration).

Radiological changes:

■ Lateral view (Figure 5.69a):
  • Increased cranial component of the cardiac silhouette (greater than two-thirds of the cardiac silhouette lying cranial to a line drawn from the carina to the apex)
  • Increased width of the cardiac silhouette (greater than four intercostal spaces, although normal is breed dependent)
  • Elevation/rotation of the apex of the heart caudodorsally (a reliable feature if present)
  • Focal bulge craniodorsally if the right atrium is enlarged. The trachea may be elevated cranial to the carina by an enlarged right atrium
  • Sternal contact is breed dependent and not a reliable feature of enlargement.
■ DV view (Figure 5.69b):
  • Overall 'reverse D' shape with rounding of the right border and a relatively straight left border
  • Bulging at the 9–11 o'clock position, representing enlargement of the right atrium
  • Increase in the size of the cardiac silhouette on the right side, with a decreased distance between the cardiac silhouette and the right thoracic wall
  • Cardiac apex may be pushed further to the left.

- Secondary features:
  - Widening of the caudal vena cava (may be difficult to assess due to the normal physiological variation in width)
  - Pleural effusion
  - Hepatomegaly
  - Ascites
  - Pericardial effusion.

Canine generalized cardiomegaly: Some conditions cause generalized cardiomegaly from the outset (e.g. concurrent mitral and tricuspid valve disease); other conditions start by causing predominantly left- or right-sided enlargement, but by the time of clinical presentation will have progressed to cause more generalized changes. Causes of generalized cardiomegaly include:

- Congenital:
  - Patent ductus arteriosus
  - Ventricular septal defect.
- Acquired:
  - Concurrent mitral and tricuspid valve disease
  - Dilated cardiomyopathy
  - Pericardial effusion.

Radiological features:

- Lateral view (Figure 5.70a):
  - Increased height of the cardiac silhouette (>75% of the height of the thorax)
  - Increased width of the cardiac silhouette
  - Overall rounded appearance to the cardiac silhouette.
- DV view (Figure 5.70b):
  - Increased length of the cardiac silhouette
  - Increased width of the cardiac silhouette.
- Secondary features:
  - Signs of both left- and right-sided failure may be present.

Detecting 'mild' generalized cardiomegaly radiologically is difficult and unlikely to be accurate, even for an experienced observer, unless sequential radiographs from the same animal are available. However, even then, differences in the stage of respiration and cardiac cycle may make small differences hard to detect accurately. In cases where the cardiac silhouette is rounded in shape, pericardial disease remains a differential diagnosis for generalized cardiomegaly.

Feline cardiomegaly: In general, feline cardiac silhouettes are more consistent in shape and size on radiographs than canine cardiac silhouettes, making cardiomegaly easier to recognize. However, in many cases of feline heart disease (especially in the early stages) there is concentric left ventricular hypertrophy, which means that there is no radiologically apparent cardiomegaly. In cats, the left atrium is positioned more cranially, compared with dogs, and is therefore harder to identify on the lateral view. An enlarged feline cardiac silhouette may appear normal on the lateral view; however, with progressive enlargement, there may be an increase in the height of the cardiac silhouette, together with rounding of the cranial border and straightening/caudal angulation of the caudodorsal border. This results in the cardiac silhouette having a more 'kidney bean' rather than oval shape.

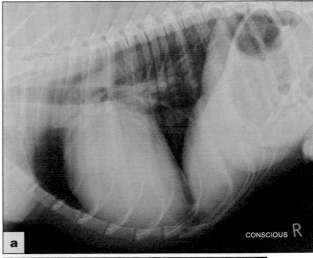

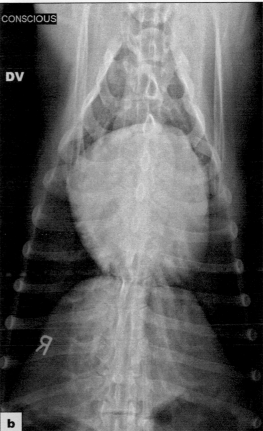

5.70 **(a)** Right lateral and **(b)** DV views of the thorax of a dog with generalized cardiomegaly. The cardiac silhouette is both wide and tall. Specific chamber enlargement is not visible. The vertebral heart score = 12.5. Differential diagnoses for this appearance include congenital heart disease, pericardial disease, dilated cardiomyopathy, degenerative valvular disease and secondary to chronic anaemia or bradycardia.

On the DV view, left atrial enlargement is seen at the left cranial border of the cardiac silhouette and the apex may shift to the right. The term 'valentine heart' has been used to describe biatrial enlargement in the cat and appears as widening of the cranial aspect of the cardiac silhouette on the DV view (Figure 5.71). Radiologically, it is difficult to distinguish between biatrial enlargement and marked left atrial enlargement, which can push the interatrial septum and right atrium across to the right.

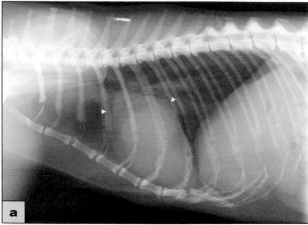

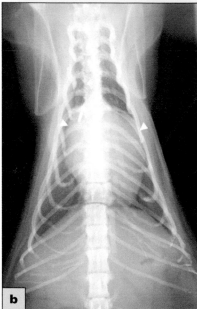

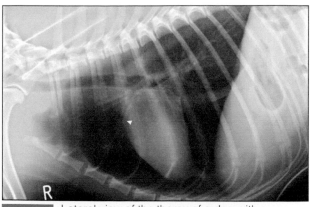

5.72 Lateral view of the thorax of a dog with microcardia as a result of hypoadrenocorticism. The cardiac silhouette is small and narrowed and displaced from the sternum by air-filled lung. The cranial lobar pulmonary vessels (arrowhead) are thin/thready and the lung parenchyma is generally more lucent in appearance due to hypovolaemia (undercirculation).

Radiological features:

■ The cardiac silhouette appears narrow and angular on both views.
■ The cardiac apex may be raised from the sternum.
■ Vascular changes may be present, including:
   • Narrowing of the caudal vena cava
   • Underperfusion of the lungs, leading to small, thread-like pulmonary arteries and veins, resulting in a hyperlucent appearance.

Shape

Shape is the most useful factor to determine whether cardiac enlargement is predominantly left-sided, right-sided or generalized. This helps narrow down the list of possible differential diagnoses. In dogs, left-sided enlargement leads to a tall cardiac silhouette with a straight caudal border and caudodorsal 'tenting' due to left atrial enlargement. Right-sided enlargement leads to a wide cardiac silhouette on the lateral view and a characteristic 'reverse D' shape (increased, rounded right cardiac border, normal left margin) on the DV view.

Margination

In a normal animal, the margins of the cardiac silhouette should be clearly delineated due to contrast with the surrounding air-filled lung. Some blurring occurs due to movement during the cardiac cycle, but this is usually minimal. Fat around the pericardium may also cause some blurring of the cardiac margins, which appears as a gradual transition in opacity (soft tissue of the cardiac silhouette–fat–air in the lung) rather than a more defined soft tissue–air interface. In cats, fat has more effect on the margins of the cardiac silhouette on the DV/VD view and may be seen as a focal triangular opacity on the right cranial margin of the cardiac silhouette.

Location

The position of the heart base is relatively fixed but the apex is free to move with gravity or can be displaced by an adjacent mass lesion. In lateral recumbency, the apex moves toward the dependent side due to physiological collapse of the dependent lung lobe. On a DV view, the cardiac apex usually lies to the left, but is

5.71 **(a)** Right lateral and **(b)** DV views of the thorax of a cat with cardiomegaly secondary to hypertrophic cardiomyopathy. The cardiac silhouette is enlarged and tall. The caudal vena cava is elevated and the dorsal third of the cardiac silhouette is widened (arrowheads). The increase in width is better appreciated on the DV view, where the cranial aspect of the cardiac silhouette occupies most of the width of the thoracic cavity.

Changes seen with right-sided enlargement in the cat are even less specific than those in the dog. The cardiac silhouette may appear rounder and increased in width on both views, but a 'reverse D' shape is not usually seen. It is important not to confuse the normal cranial rotation of the cardiac axis in older cats with clinically significant cardiomegaly. The axis of the cardiac silhouette changes, but the overall size should not; however, as a result of the rotation, the aortic arch may bulge into the cranial mediastinum, becoming more apparent (sometimes referred to as 'redundant aorta').

Microcardia: A decrease in cardiac size (Figure 5.72) can be caused by:

■ Hypovolaemia (shock and dehydration)
■ Hypoadrenocorticism (also known as Addison's disease)
■ Artefacts (e.g. deep-chested dogs, pneumothorax and overinflation of the lungs).

sometimes seen to the right of the dome of the diaphragm as a normal variant. Several congenital abnormalities, such as situs inversus (where the thoracic and abdominal organs are a 'mirror image' of normal), are also associated with a change in position of the heart.

Common conditions

Canine congenital heart disease

Clinical examination and echocardiography are the most reliable and accurate methods used to diagnose congenital heart disease in most dogs, but classic radiographic features are evident in few cases (Lamb et al., 2001). The limitations of radiography for diagnosing specific congenital diseases or specific chamber enlargement must therefore be recognized. Radiographs are obtained to provide a general assessment of cardiac size and shape and to assess for signs of decompensated cardiac disease, in particular pulmonary oedema in left heart failure. In right heart failure, hepatic congestion and ascites are better demonstrated using ultrasonography.

Aortic stenosis: Breeds commonly affected include Boxers, Golden Retrievers, Newfoundlands, German Shepherd Dogs, English Bull Terriers and some brachycephalic breeds such as the English Bulldog. Aortic stenosis results in concentric left ventricular hypertrophy.

Radiological features:

- Cardiac changes often unremarkable in mild to moderate cases.
- Left-sided cardiac enlargement (tall cardiac silhouette, tracheal elevation, straight caudal border, left atrial 'tenting') (see Figure 5.65).
- Post-stenotic dilatation of the aorta results in widening of the cranial mediastinum (11–1 o'clock position). The cardiac silhouette is elongated on both views, particularly the DV view.
- The appearance of the cardiac silhouette may be influenced by the presence of concurrent congenital disease (e.g. mitral valve disease).
- Signs of congestive heart failure (vascular congestion and/or pulmonary oedema) are uncommon, except in severe cases or with concurrent mitral valve disease.

Pulmonic stenosis: Breeds commonly affected include English Bulldogs, Boxers and terrier breeds. Pulmonic stenosis results in right ventricular hypertrophy.

Radiological features:

- Cardiac changes are often unremarkable or underestimated in mild to moderate cases.
- Enlargement of the main pulmonary artery segment (1–2 o'clock position) on the DV view tends to be a reliable finding in more severely affected cases (see Figure 5.68).
- Rounding and enlargement of the right border of the cardiac silhouette on the DV view (reverse D shape).
- Elevation of the cardiac apex from the sternum, widening of the cardiac silhouette on lateral views and a reduction in size of the pulmonary vasculature are less reliable findings.

- Signs of right-sided congestive failure (ascites, hepatic congestion, pleural effusion) are uncommon unless severe or associated with concurrent tricuspid dysplasia.

Patent ductus arteriosus: Small breeds (Miniature Poodle) are most commonly affected, but the condition can also be seen in other breeds (German Shepherd Dog). Shunting of blood from the aorta into the main pulmonary artery results in pulmonary overcirculation and volume overload of the left ventricle. Radiography is indicated to determine whether signs of left-sided cardiac failure are present (pulmonary oedema).

Radiological features:

- Small diameter shunts may result in no changes, but in most cases of patent ductus arteriosus changes are present.
- On the lateral view, signs of left-sided cardiac enlargement (tracheal elevation, straightening caudal cardiac border, tenting of the left atrium) are present. Severe changes result in global cardiac enlargement (see Figure 5.66).
- Enlargement of both the pulmonary arteries and veins indicates pulmonary overcirculation (but can also be seen with ventricular septal defects and severe left-sided heart failure with pulmonary hypertension).
- On the DV view, the cardiac silhouette is elongated and enlarged. Three bulges at the 11–1 o'clock (descending aorta), 1–2 o'clock (enlarged pulmonary artery) and 2–3 o'clock (left auricular appendage) positions results in the classic 'three knuckles' appearance, but this is not present in all cases.

Ventricular septal defects: This condition is commonly seen in the Keeshond. It is an intracardiac defect, leading to shunting of blood from the left ventricle into the right ventricular outflow tract and pulmonary overcirculation. The radiographic appearance is indistinguishable from patent ductus arteriosus.

Reverse patent ductus arteriosus: Reverse patent ductus arteriosus results in signs of cyanosis due to severe pulmonary hypertension.

Radiological features:

- The radiographic changes are similar to those associated with pulmonic stenosis.
- Enlarged right cardiac silhouette and main pulmonary artery on the DV view.

Mitral valve dysplasia: Breeds commonly affected include the Great Dane, English Bull Terrier and Golden Retriever.

Radiological features:

- Reflect left-sided cardiac enlargement (tall cardiac silhouette, elevation of the left mainstem bronchus, straight caudal border, left atrial 'tenting', widening of the tracheal bifurcation on the DV view).
- Radiographic changes are similar to those seen with acquired mitral valve disease, although age at presentation usually suggests congenital disease.
- The severity of the changes is related to the

volume of insufficiency. The changes seen with severe disease can be marked.

- Pulmonary oedema indicates left-sided congestive failure.

Tricuspid valve dysplasia: Larger breeds, especially Labrador Retrievers, are commonly affected.

Radiological features:

- Reflects right-sided heart enlargement (widening of the cardiac silhouette on the lateral view, rounding of the right side on the DV view). Changes are usually only recognized with moderate to marked disease.
- In severe disease, marked generalized cardiac enlargement may be present and must be distinguished from pericardial effusion.
- Right heart failure (enlargement of the caudal vena cava, ascites, hepatomegaly, occasionally pleural effusion).

Canine acquired heart disease

Degenerative atrioventricular valve disease: This condition most commonly affects small-breed dogs, but can also be seen in larger breeds.

Radiological features:

- Radiography is performed primarily to assess for signs of left- or right-sided congestive heart failure.
- Serial radiography demonstrating progressive cardiac enlargement is more reliable than any single evaluation. Previous radiographs should be compared with more recent studies.
- Mitral valve disease is more common than tricuspid valve disease. On the lateral view, signs of left-sided cardiac enlargement (elevation of the trachea and left mainstem bronchus, straightening of the caudal cardiac border, 'tenting' of the left atrium) are preset. On the DV view, widening of the tracheal bifurcation due to left atrial enlargement and a bulge at the 2–3 o'clock position due to enlargement of the left auricular appendage are present (see Figure 5.67).
- Severe left atrial enlargement can be spectacular, resulting in marked compression and displacement of the terminal trachea and lobar bronchi.
- Severe tricuspid valve disease, resulting in right-sided cardiac enlargement and right heart failure is less common.

Dilated cardiomyopathy: Breeds commonly affected include giant breeds (Dobermann, Deerhound, Great Dane) and spaniel breeds (Cocker Spaniel). Radiography is performed to evaluate for signs of congestive heart failure (predominantly left heart failure, but occasionally biventricular failure) and to distinguish dilated cardiomyopathy from other conditions that cause similar signs, as well as to assess the response to therapy.

Radiological features:

- Pre-symptomatic or occult disease is indistinguishable from breed-matched normal dogs, although left atrial enlargement may be present in dogs not showing clinical signs.

- Left-sided cardiac enlargement (tracheal elevation (less obvious is deep-chested breeds), straightening of the caudal cardiac border, 'tenting' of the left atrium) is present on the lateral view. On the DV view, the tracheal bifurcation is widened due to left atrial enlargement.
- In dogs with severe left-sided enlargement or biventricular involvement, the cardiac silhouette may have a globoid appearance, similar to that seen with pericardial effusion. However, left atrial enlargement and signs of left-sided congestive heart failure (pulmonary oedema) are not recognized with pericardial effusion.
- Pulmonary oedema indicates left-sided congestive failure.
- With biventricular failure, signs of right heart failure (enlargement of the caudal vena cava, ascites, hepatomegaly, occasionally pleural effusion) may also be present.

Canine pericardial disease

Pericardial disease can result from changes in the thickness and/or contents of the pericardial sac. Pericardial disease that does not lead to effusion (e.g. constrictive pericarditis) is unlikely to be recognized on radiographs. Causes of canine pericardial effusion include:

- Neoplasia:
  - Cardiac haemangiosarcoma
  - Heart base masses (e.g. aortic body tumours)
  - Mesothelioma.
- Idiopathic pericardial effusion:
  - Certain breeds are predisposed (e.g. Golden Retriever).
- Miscellaneous causes:
  - Right-sided congestive heart failure
  - Trauma
  - Coagulopathy
  - Uraemia
  - Left atrial rupture.

Radiological features:

- Enlargement of the cardiac silhouette in all dimensions.
- A rounded, globular appearance with no features of individual chamber enlargement.
- Sharply marginated cardiac silhouette as the pericardium does not move significantly during the cardiac cycle (in contrast to the myocardium).

Secondary features: Signs of right-sided failure usually occur due to cardiac tamponade and include:

- Wide caudal vena cava
- Pleural effusion
- Hepatomegaly
- Ascites.

Heart base masses

Heart base masses are rare and are nearly always neoplastic. They may cause little change to the outline of the cardiac silhouette unless the mass becomes large or causes secondary pericardial effusion (although effusion is more commonly seen secondary to right atrial or auricular masses than heart base tumours). Differential diagnoses of heart base tumours include aortic body tumours (chemodectomas) and ectopic thyroid or parathyroid tumours. Lymphadenopathy at the heart base (enlargement of the tracheobronchial lymph nodes) can also cause an increase in opacity in the perihilar area, but this usually manifests as increased opacity around and caudal to the tracheal bifurcation, whereas a heart base tumour usually lies mainly cranial to the bifurcation (Figure 5.73).

Radiological features:

- A soft tissue mass arising from the cranial or craniodorsal aspect of the heart.
- Elevation of the terminal trachea on the lateral view.
- Focal deviation of the terminal trachea to the right

on the VD/DV view.
- An enlarged, rounded cardiac silhouette if pericardial effusion is also present.

Feline congenital cardiac disease

The most common congenital cardiac defects in the cat include:

- Ventricular septal defect
- Mitral valve dysplasia
- Tricuspid valve dysplasia.

Other defects, including pulmonic and aortic stenosis, patent ductus arteriosus, atrial septal defects and Tetralogy of Fallot, are uncommon.

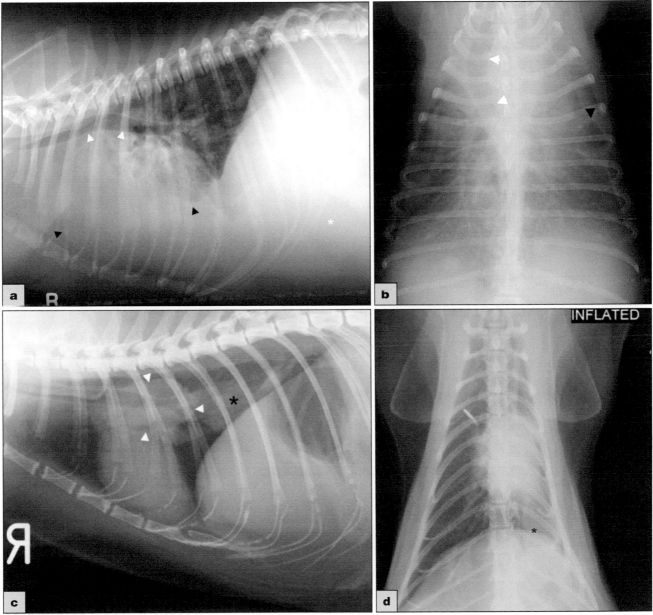

5.73 **(a)** Right lateral and **(b)** DV views of the thorax of a dog with a heart base mass. The terminal trachea (white arrowheads) is elevated dorsally on the lateral view and deviated to the right on the DV view. Retraction of the lung lobes from the thoracic wall (black arrowheads) by a soft tissue opacity and blurring of the margins of the cardiac silhouette indicate that pleural effusion is present. The ground glass appearance and distension of the cranioventral abdomen indicate ascites. For comparison, **(c)** and **(d)** are orthogonal views of a cat with a perihilar mass due to tracheobronchial lymphadenopathy as a result of a lung mass (*) in a caudal lobe. On the lateral view, the perihilar mass (arrowheads) is well marginated and is seen both ventral and dorsal to the terminal trachea and mainstem bronchi. There is no deviation of the terminal trachea. The DV view provides little information about the perihilar mass, but clearly shows severe volume loss and some consolidation of the left caudal lung lobe with a mediastinal shift and cranial positioning of the left hemidiaphragm.

Feline acquired cardiac disease

Cardiomyopathy is the most common acquired cardiac disease in the cat. The forms most commonly encountered are hypertrophic cardiomyopathy and restrictive cardiomyopathy. Dilated cardiomyopathy is now uncommon.

Hypertrophic cardiomyopathy: This is the most common form of feline myocardial disease. It is an acquired autosomal dominant trait characterized by concentric left ventricular hypertrophy, which can be focal or may involve the entire left ventricle. Left ventricular hypertrophy leads to diastolic dysfunction and subsequent atrial enlargement, which may be recognized on radiographs.

Radiological features:

- Left atrial enlargement, recognized as widening of the cranial aspect of the cardiac silhouette on the DV view.
- Increased height ± width of the cardiac silhouette on the lateral view.
- Secondary features:
  - Pulmonary venous distension
  - Pulmonary oedema – the appearance of cardiogenic oedema is more variable in cats than in dogs. It most commonly presents as a diffuse alveolar–interstitial infiltrate. The infiltrate is non-uniform in its distribution (there is no perihilar predisposition as seen in dogs). A bronchial component may be present in some cases, resulting in peribronchial cuffing
  - Pleural effusion
  - Pericardial effusion (usually small volume).

Restrictive cardiomyopathy: This form is characterized by a normal left ventricular wall thickness and chamber size, but reduced compliance of the ventricle leads to diastolic dysfunction and subsequent left atrial enlargement. It is not possible to distinguish the hypertrophic from the restrictive form of cardiomyopathy on radiographs as left ventricular wall thickness cannot be assessed. Radiographic assessment allows significant changes in size of the cardiac silhouette (principally due to atrial enlargement) to be identified and signs of congestive disease to be recognized.

Radiological features:

- Left atrial enlargement recognized as widening of the cranial aspect of the cardiac silhouette on a DV view.
- Increased height ± width of the cardiac silhouette on the lateral view.
- Secondary features:
  - Pulmonary venous distension
  - Pulmonary oedema seen as patchy alveolar, interstitial or mixed infiltrate
  - Pleural effusion
  - Pericardial effusion (usually small volume).

Thromboembolic disease is a common consequence of restrictive cardiomyopathy, due to the marked increase in left atrial size and the resultant haemodynamic changes. There are no specific radiographic features associated with thrombi, but they may be evident ultrasonographically, either within the left atrium or in the peripheral vasculature.

Dilated cardiomyopathy: This used to be a relatively common cause of cardiac failure in cats, but is now very rare following the introduction of routine taurine supplementation of feline diets. Other forms of feline myocardial disease may progress to dilatation (e.g. following myocardial ischaemia).

Radiological features:

- Generalized cardiomegaly with a rounded cardiac silhouette.
- Secondary signs of congestive heart failure, including pleural effusion.

Feline pericardial disease

Pericardial disease is less common in the cat than the dog. Differential diagnoses include:

- Congestive heart failure
- Pericardioperitoneal diaphragmatic hernia
- Feline coronavirus (the causative agent of feline infectious peritonitis, FIP)
- Lymphoma.

Radiological features: The radiological features in the cat are similar to those seen in the dog (i.e. a large rounded cardiac silhouette with sharp margins ± signs of right-sided failure) (Figure 5.74).

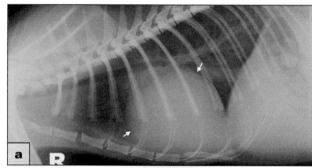

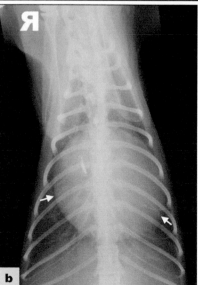

5.74 **(a)** Right lateral and **(b)** DV views of the thorax of a cat with pericardial effusion. The cardiac silhouette is large and rounded on both views with well defined margins (arrowed). Pericardial effusion in the cat occurs secondary to primary (myocardial) cardiac disease, neoplasia (lymphoma) or infectious disease (e.g. feline coronavirus (the causative agent of feline infectious peritonitis), feline leukaemia virus, feline immunodeficiency virus and toxoplasmosis).

Pulmonary vasculature and great vessels

Specific approach to interpretation

The degree of chest inflation and concurrent changes within the lungs have a considerable effect on the assessment of the pulmonary vasculature and great vessels. It is difficult to be confident about a significant change in pulmonary vascular size if radiographs are obtained during expiration, if there is motion blur, or if there is pulmonary infiltrate. Changes in the vasculature are generally associated with concurrent changes in the cardiac silhouette and lungs, and all should be assessed together. It is unusual for pulmonary vascular changes to be noted without recognizing concurrent cardiac changes. The cranial lobar vessels are visible on lateral views. A left lateral view may be preferable for assessment, as the right lung is better inflated and the right lobar vessels are less likely to be superimposed on the cranial mediastinum. The caudal lobar vessels are best seen on a DV or VD view.

Size

- The size of the cranial lobar pulmonary artery and vein can be compared with the diameter of the proximal third of the fourth rib on the lateral view. The normal range is 0.25–1.2 times the width or diameter of the rib at this level.
- The size of the caudal lobar vessels can be compared with the diameter of the ninth rib on the DV view. The normal range is 0.25–1 times the width or diameter of the rib.
- These ranges are quite wide, thus normal vessel size does not exclude disease. In addition, vascular disease may be present without radiographic signs of a change in vessel size.
- The paired lobar vessels (artery and vein) should be of similar diameter.
- The caudal vena cava appears smaller on the left lateral recumbent view of the thorax.
- The size of the caudal vena cava is influenced by the respiratory cycle as well as venous return.
- The diameter of the caudal vena cava is similar to that of the aorta.
- The diameter of the aorta is approximately the same as the height of the thoracic vertebral bodies bordering the vessel.
- The diameter of the aorta rarely reduces in size, whereas the diameter of the caudal vena cava changes readily depending on volume load.

Shape

- The margins of the lobar vessels should taper towards the periphery of the lungs.
- The diameter of the caudal vena cava increases slightly between the diaphragm and cardiac silhouette.

Opacity

- The lobar pulmonary vessels are of soft tissue opacity.

Margination

- Only the left margin of the descending aorta is visible on the DV/VD view. It defines the left side of the caudal mediastinum.
- The margins of the vessels should be smooth.

Location

- The left border of the descending aorta lies to the left of the midline.
- The caudal vena cava lies within the plica venae cavae to the right of the midline, between the accessory lung lobe and the right caudal lung lobe.
- The cranial lobar pulmonary arteries lie dorsal, and the caudal lobar pulmonary arteries lie lateral, to their companion lobar veins.

Vascular lung patterns

A vascular lung pattern refers to a change in the diameter (increase or decrease) or shape of the pulmonary arteries and/or veins.

Abnormal size

Increased vascular size: A vascular lung pattern commonly refers to an increase in the size of the pulmonary vessels. This may occur due to:

- Distension of the pulmonary arteries (Figure 5.75):
  - *Angiostrongylus vasorum/Dirofilaria immitis*
  - Pulmonary hypertension as a result of, for example, idiopathic pulmonary hypertension, right-to-left cardiac shunting or pulmonary thromboembolism.
- Distension of the pulmonary veins:
  - Congestive heart failure (left-sided).

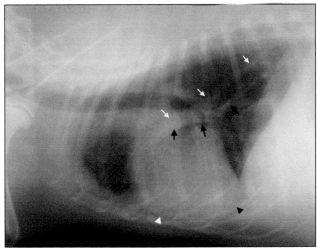

5.75 Vascular pattern: enlarged pulmonary arteries. Right lateral view of the thorax of a dog with pulmonary hypertension due to *Angiostrongylus vasorum* infection. The increased width of the cardiac silhouette and greater sternal contact (white arrowhead) indicate moderate enlargement of the right side of the heart. Elevation of the cardiac apex (black arrowhead) is suggestive of right ventricular (concentric) hypertrophy. The left (white arrows) and right (black arrows) caudal lobar pulmonary arteries are increased in size. There is a poorly circumscribed infiltrate in the periphery of the lung lobes. This pattern of vascular and cardiac enlargement may also occur with a reverse patent ductus arteriosus and pulmonary thromboembolism.

- Distension of both the pulmonary arteries and veins (Figure 5.76):
  - Most commonly due to left-sided heart failure associated with congenital or acquired mitral valve disease or myocardial failure (dilated cardiomyopathy) and, therefore, seen in conjunction with radiographic features of left-sided cardiac enlargement
  - Left-to-right cardiac shunts (Figure 5.77). These conditions lead to pulmonary overcirculation and volume overload of the heart (e.g. patent ductus arteriosus, ventricular septal defects and atrial septal defects). Pulmonary vessel enlargement may be difficult to assess if pulmonary oedema is present
  - Iatrogenic fluid overload.
- Enlargement of the caudal vena cava. This vessel is considered enlarged when its diameter is 1.5–2 times that of the aorta; however, the liver should be evaluated concurrently to assess for enlargement, congestion and ascites
- Enlargement of the aorta. This is uncommon, but significant when it does occur, and therefore is an important change to recognize. Aneurysmal dilatation is associated with damage to the wall due to *Spirocerca lupi* infection or rare conditions such as aortic coarctation.

The orientation, as well as the width, of the vessels should be assessed.

Decreased vascular size: A decrease in vessel size leads to an overall increase in the lucency of the lung fields. Decreased vascular size may be seen with:

- Hypovolaemia (shock, dehydration, haemorrhage) (see Figure 5.72).
- Right-to-left shunting lesions (Tetralogy of Fallot, reverse shunting patent ductus arteriosus)
- Severe pulmonic stenosis
- Pulmonary thromboembolism (Figure 5.78).

Abnormal shape

- Increased tortuosity of vessels has been described in diseases such as heartworm (*Dirofilaria immitis*). This is rare in the UK but should still be considered, particularly in any animal that has travelled under the pet passport scheme.

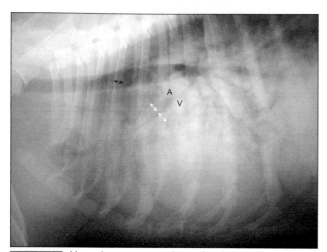

5.76 Vascular pattern: enlarged pulmonary arteries and veins. Lateral view of the thorax of a dog with severe pulmonary oedema due to left-sided congestive heart failure. The cranial lobar artery (A) and vein (V) are both enlarged (double-headed white arrows) compared with the diameter of the proximal third of the fourth rib (double-headed black arrow). The pulmonary vein is subjectively larger than the pulmonary artery. Assessment of the size of the pulmonary vessels is limited by the severity of the pulmonary oedema.

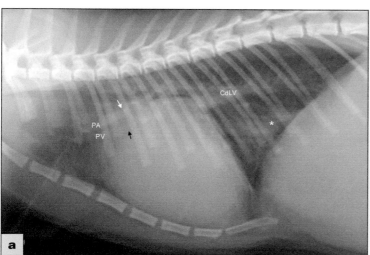

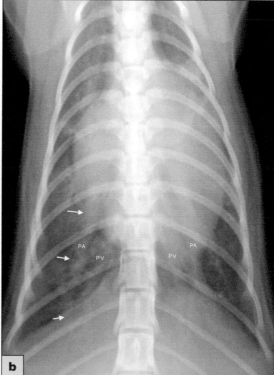

5.77 **(a)** Right lateral and **(b)** DV views of the thorax of a cat with pulmonary overcirculation secondary to a ventricular septal defect. There is generalized cardiomegaly, seen on both views as a tall, wide cardiac silhouette. The cranial and caudal lobar pulmonary arteries (PA; white arrows) and pulmonary veins (PV; black arrow) are enlarged, exceeding the size of the proximal fourth rib on the lateral view and the ninth rib on the DV view at the point at which they cross. The caudal lobar vessels (both arteries and veins (CdLV)) are superimposed on the lateral view. A patchy area (*) superimposed on the caudal vena cava on the lateral view is suggestive of pulmonary oedema.

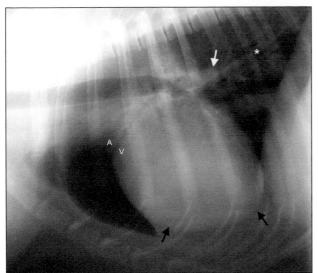

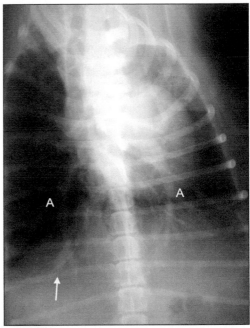

5.78 Vascular pattern: decreased vascular size. Lateral view of the thorax of a dog with a large thrombus occluding the main pulmonary artery and the left and right pulmonary artery branches. A soft tissue band (white arrow), consistent with an enlarged proximal left main pulmonary artery, narrows abruptly. The distal caudal lobe pulmonary arteries are thinned and indistinct (*). The lung fields generally appear hyperlucent (underperfused). One of the cranial lobe pulmonary arteries (A) is reduced in size compared with the companion vein (V). The cardiac apex is elevated (black arrows) due to right ventricular hypertrophy. Note that with pulmonary thromboembolism, the appearance of the lung is variable and can be normal, hyperlucent, consolidated or reduced in size due to atelectasis.

5.79 Vascular pattern: abnormal shape. DV view of the thorax of a dog with chronic pulmonary disease secondary to chronic *Angiostrongylus vasorum* infection (same dog as in Figure 5.75). The peripheral branches of the arteries (A) terminate abruptly (arrowed). The 'blunting' or 'pruning' of the arteries in this case is due to thromboembolism, inflammatory infiltrate and pulmonary fibrosis.

- The distal aorta may assume an undulating shape in aged cats. The cardiac silhouette may be cranially rotated ('lying down') with increased sternal contact, which has been anecdotally suggested to be associated with systemic hypertension.
- 'Pruning' (abrupt ending) refers to blunt termination of the lobar pulmonary arteries (Figure 5.79) and has been described in cases with heartworm as well as pulmonary thromboembolism. The abnormal shape is usually accompanied by right heart enlargement, which is typically only mild to moderate and easily overlooked.
- Focal widening of the distal descending aorta (aneurysmal dilatation) may occur with *Spirocerca lupi* infection (see Figure 5.106). Rarely, the proximal descending aorta may be focally narrowed (coarctation) at the level of the ductus arteriorsus and associated with aneurysmal dilatation distal to the coarctation.

Abnormal opacity

- Metastatic mineralization of the descending aorta is occasionally seen with chronic renal failure (secondary hyperparathyroidism).

Abnormal margination

- Rarely recognized as, even with a change in shape, the relatively small size of most vessels makes margination difficult to assess.
- The margins of the aorta are occasionally obscured by masses that arise within the caudodorsal mediastinum (Figure 5.80).

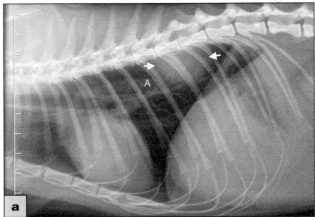

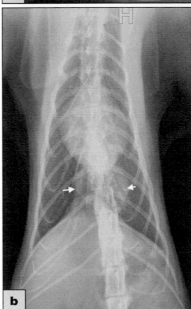

5.80 Vascular pattern: abnormal margination. **(a)** Lateral and **(b)** DV views of the thorax of a cat with an abscess in the caudodorsal mediastinum. An oval soft tissue mass (arrowed) lies dorsal to the aorta (A) on the midline. The aorta has been displaced ventrally by the mass. The margins of the aorta at the level of the mass cannot be recognized. (Courtesy of MyVet24/7)

Abnormal location

- In animals with a persistent right fourth aortic arch (resulting in signs of regurgitation and oesophageal dilatation), the left border of the aortic arch cannot be recognized. In addition, the distal trachea is displaced to the left by the persistent right aortic arch.
- The normal orientation of the pulmonary vessels may be altered by displacement of the lung lobes in the presence of pleural fluid or with lung lobe torsion (Figure 5.81).
- The location of the vessels may assist in localizing pathology (see Figure 5.80).

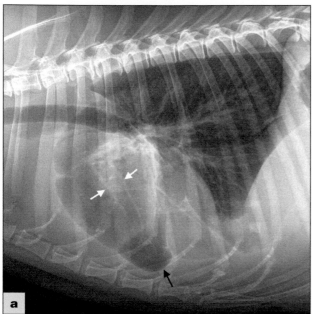

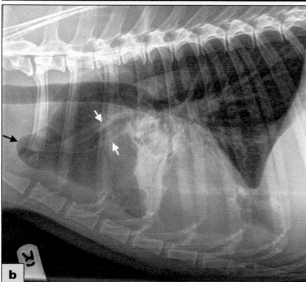

5.81 Vascular pattern: abnormal location. Lateral views of the thorax of a deep-chested dog with pleural effusion **(a)** before and **(b)** following drainage. (a) The lung lobes are retracted as a result of the pleural effusion. The left cranial lung lobe has rotated caudally such that the cranial tip of the lobe (black arrow) lies dorsal to the sixth sternebra. The cranial lobar vessels are kinked and redirected caudally (white arrows). There are no changes (consolidation, emphysema) within the lobe to suggest that torsion has occurred. (b) Following drainage, the lobe (black arrow) and lobar vessels (white arrows) have returned to their normal position and location.

Pleural space

Specific approach to interpretation

- In the normal thorax, the pleural space remains a potential space and is therefore not seen as a discrete structure.
- Occasionally, pleural reflections lie tangentially to the X-ray beam and are projected as thin, oblique, radiopaque lines on the radiograph. These are seen at anatomical locations corresponding to the divisions between the lung lobes (see Figure 5.17).
- Pleural thickening may also make pleural reflections more visible. However, it is not possible to distinguish pleural thickening from a normal pleural reflection on radiographs, unless the thickening also leads to cortication (thickening of the visceral pleura, leading to rounding of the lung lobe) and changes in lobar shape.
- An increase in opacity within the pleural space occurs due to fluid accumulation. The appearance of the fluid varies according to the location and volume, ranging from thin interlobar fissures to complete obliteration of thoracic detail.
- An increase in lucency within the pleural space is due to the presence of free air (pneumothorax). In these cases, in the absence of coexisting pathology, the diaphragm is clearly seen and the periphery of the thorax has an overall more lucent appearance with no visible pulmonary vasculature.

Common conditions

Pleural effusion

Bilateral effusion: Most pleural effusions in small animals are bilateral (Figure 5.82) as the mediastinum has fenestrations that allow communication between the two sides of the thorax. Radiographs help diagnose pleural fluid in most cases, but do not discriminate between the types of fluid that may be present. However, other radiographic changes may suggest the most likely reason for the presence of the fluid (e.g. right-sided cardiomegaly or evidence of trauma). The DV view is usually the most sensitive for detecting smaller effusions. The differential diagnoses for the different types of effusion include:

- Transudate – hypoproteinaemia
- Modified transudate – secondary to congestive heart failure, neoplasia or diaphragmatic rupture (particularly if the liver or spleen is incarcerated in the defect)
- Exudate:
  - Pyothorax (septic) – haematogenous spread of *Nocardia*, migrating foreign body or penetrating wound
  - Non-septic – FIP.
- Haemorrhage – coagulopathy or trauma
- Chylothorax – spontaneous or trauma.

Radiological features:

- Retraction of the lung lobe edges away from the thoracic wall by a band, region or area of homogeneous soft tissue opacity.

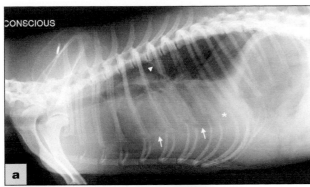

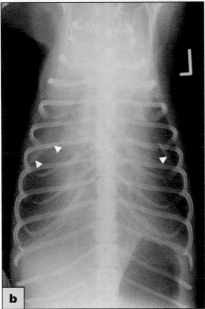

5.82 **(a)** Right lateral and **(b)** DV views of the thorax of a dog with bilateral pleural effusion. Note the elevation of the ventral borders of the lung lobes (arrowed), with 'scalloping' of the edges, on the lateral view. The ventral border of the diaphragm (∗) is obscured by fluid. The border of the cardiac silhouette is faintly visible as it is outlined by a thin strip of pericardial fat. There are classic fissure lines (arrowheads) visible bilaterally in the seventh intercostal spaces; these are seen more clearly on the DV view.

- Presence of interlobar fissures (soft tissue lines that are broad based at the periphery and taper towards the midline), particularly on the DV view.
- Rounding and separation of the lung lobe borders. The retracted lungs have a 'scalloped' appearance ventrally on the lateral view and on the DV view are rounded within the costophrenic angle.
- The borders of the cardiac silhouette and diaphragm in contact with the fluid are obscured as the normal contrast provided by adjacent air-filled lung is lost.
  - An estimate of cardiac size may still be made as the height can usually be inferred from the height of the carina and fat within the pericardium may outline the heart.
- Underlying pathology, such as mediastinal masses, may also be obscured by the fluid. To evaluate any concurrent pathology and search for a cause of the effusion, the radiographic study can be repeated following drainage, or thoracic ultrasonography can be performed.

- If the pleural effusion is long-standing (particularly with exudative effusions) pleuritis develops. This can lead to pleural thickening around the lung lobes. This appears as:
  - Irregular, undulating lung margins
  - Uneven retraction of the lung lobes from the thoracic wall, as adhesions may restrict the free distribution of fluid
  - Cortication (thickening of the visceral pleura on the surface of the lung lobe). Following drainage, the lungs fail to re-expand fully and thus retain a rounded outline with a radiopaque margin (Figure 5.83).

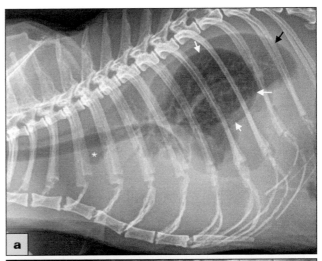

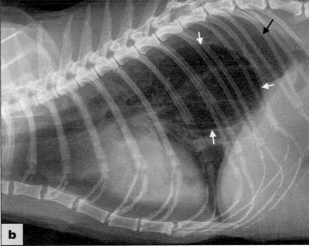

5.83 Right lateral views of the thorax of a cat **(a)** before and **(b)** following therapeutic thoracocentesis. (a) Note that despite the moderately large volume of pleural fluid, both caudal lung lobes are only partially collapsed and have a rounded appearance. One of the lobes (white arrows) is more markedly affected than the other (black arrow). A small volume of free air is present (∗) following previous thoracocentesis. (b) Following drainage, the shape and volume of the lung lobes is unchanged, indicating chronic pleural thickening or cortication.

Unilateral effusion: This can result when pleuritis and mediastinal thickening lead to closure of the normal fenestrations in the mediastinum. This is more likely to happen when the pleural fluid is thick or viscous (e.g. with pyothorax, chylothorax and FIP). The radiological appearance of unilateral *versus* bilateral effusions can be very different, and a DV view is likely to be more helpful than a lateral view in these cases.

Radiological features:

- Lateral view (fluid lying dependently within the thorax) – a homogeneous increase in opacity superimposed over the inflated upper lung, which may mimic a lung infiltrate.
- Lateral view (fluid uppermost) – increased soft tissue opacity dorsal to the sternum and rounding of the caudodorsal lung lobes.
- DV/VD view – soft tissue opacity in one hemithorax. The lung ipsilateral to the fluid will collapse.

Pneumothorax

The causes of pneumothorax include:

- Traumatic rupture of the lung parenchyma (or, rarely, a bronchus)
- Rupture of an air-containing lesion (bulla, abscess or cavitating neoplasm) (Figure 5.84)
- Perforating wounds to the thoracic wall
- Iatrogenic, following percutaneous thoracic drainage.

Radiological features: When assessing for pneumothorax with conventional radiography using a vertical beam, the DV view is preferred to the VD view. Alternatively, a decubitus VD view may be useful to detect a small pneumothorax.

- Radiolucent areas in the periphery of the thorax.
  - Lung markings are not present. These should not be confused with the more lucent areas lateral to a skin fold (see Figure 5.15).
  - Radiolucent areas are usually seen bilaterally on the DV view if the pneumothorax is bilateral.
- Retraction of the lungs from the thoracic wall.
- An increase in opacity of the lung due to collapse with sharp demarcation of individual lobes by air.
- Elevation of the cardiac silhouette (Figure 5.85) with a radiolucent area between the cardiac silhouette and sternum on the lateral view.
- In some cases, lung bullae may be seen. Animals

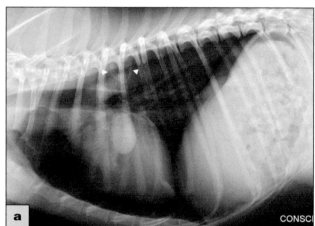

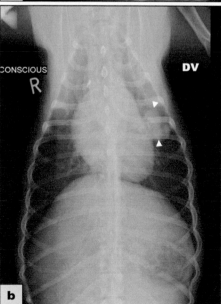

5.84 **(a)** Right lateral and **(b)** DV views of the thorax of a dog with pneumothorax secondary to a lung bulla. On the lateral view, the cardiac silhouette is elevated by a gas opacity. The wall of a bulla (arrowheads) is visible as a curvilinear opacity dorsal to the carina. The oval soft tissue opacity superimposed on the heart was thought to represent a fluid-filled bleb. On the DV view, the bleb (arrowheads) is clearly seen to the left of the cardiac silhouette, but the bulla is not visible.

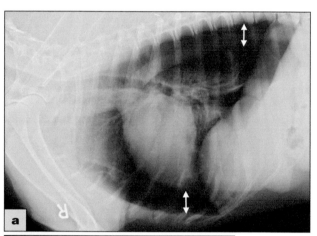

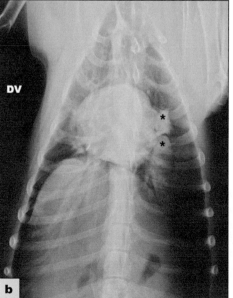

5.85 **(a)** Right lateral and **(b)** DV views of the thorax of a dog with spontaneous pneumothorax. On the lateral view, the heart is raised from the sternum by a gas opacity and there is free gas between the caudodorsal lung margins and the spine (double-headed arrows). The DV view allows the changes to be lateralized, and shows that the pneumothorax is worse on the left-hand side. The caudal part of the left cranial lobe and the left caudal lobe have both collapsed and are outlined by gas (*).

with changes confined to one lobe are potential surgical candidates. Lobectomy may prevent further leakage of air.

A *tension pneumothorax* (rare) occurs when air can enter the pleural space, but a valve-like effect is created preventing air from leaving with expiration, thus raising the pleural pressure above the atmospheric pressure. In these cases, additional radiological signs which may be seen include:

- Severe collapse of the lung lobes, which appear very radiopaque
- Flattening of the diaphragm
- The ribs lie perpendicular to the spine; the intercostal spaces are widened
- Rapid progression of clinical signs on serial radiographs (but ideally drainage should occur prior to repeat radiographs).

In very rare cases, the tension pneumothorax may be unilateral, in which case there is a mediastinal shift away from the affected side. In all cases, thoracocentesis is indicated to reduce the pleural pressure.

Pneumohydrothorax

Pneumohydrothorax is the term used when both free air and fluid are present within the pleural cavity. The radiological features are a mixture of those seen with pneumothorax and pleural effusion (Figure 5.86) and vary significantly according to the relative quantities and distribution of the fluid and air. Horizontal 'fluid lines' are only seen if a horizontal X-ray beam technique is used, and only then if there is no significant pleuritis (or other reason for the fluid to remain pocketed) so that the fluid is able to distribute freely within the pleural cavity.

Mediastinum

The mediastinum is the potential space between the two pleural sacs and contains the trachea, oesophagus, heart, thymus and major blood vessels. Many lymph nodes are also present within the mediastinum but are not recognized on radiographs unless enlarged. Other structures such as the thoracic duct and vagus and phrenic nerves are not usually seen at all on plain radiographs. The mediastinum communicates cranially with the fascial planes of the neck, and caudally with the retroperitoneal space.

Specific approach to interpretation

Assessment of the cranial mediastinum on the lateral view is largely subjective; the only structure that should always be clearly visible is the tracheal lumen. On a lateral view, the cranial mediastinum is seen as a soft tissue band running parallel to the trachea. On a DV view, the width of the cranial mediastinum in dogs should not exceed twice that of the vertebral column, and in cats should not exceed the width of the vertebral column. However, mediastinal width varies according to body condition (the width increases in obese animals) and breed (the cranial mediastinum is usually wider in brachycephalic breeds). The caudal mediastinum is

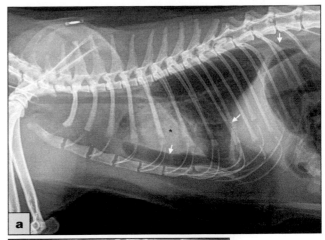

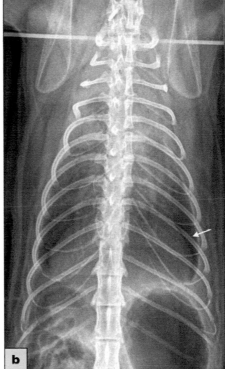

5.86 **(a)** Right lateral and **(b)** DV views of the thorax of a cat with pneumohydrothorax. The lateral view shows consolidation of a lung lobe (with a lobar sign) over the cardiac silhouette (∗) and a generalized increase in opacity within the thorax, indicative of pleural effusion. Several bubbles of free gas (arrowed) are visible caudoventrally over the cardiac apex and caudodorsally around the retracted lung lobes. On the DV view, the cardiac silhouette is effaced by the fluid and the free gas is more difficult to recognize, except focally on the left-hand side (arrowed). Classic 'fluid lines', demonstrating a fluid–gas interface, are only seen if a horizontal beam is used.

best assessed on a DV/VD view. The thin radiopaque line visible between the cardiac apex and the diaphragm represents the caudal mediastinal fold.

The cardiac silhouette, caudal vena cava and aorta should be well delineated on both lateral and DV views. Although a lateral view allows assessment of most of the normally visible mediastinal structures, a DV or VD view is essential to evaluate their position and determine whether any 'mediastinal shift' has occurred, as most mediastinal structures normally lie on or close to the midline (Figure 5.87).

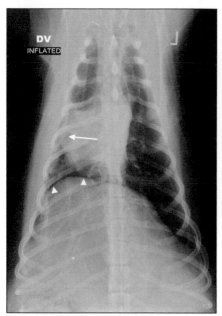

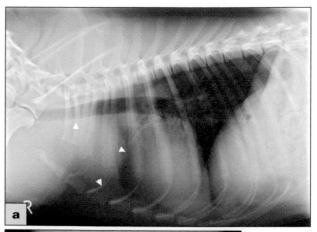

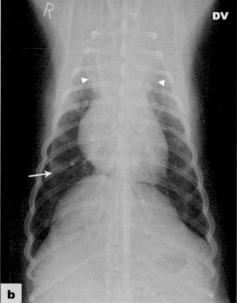

5.87 DV view of the thorax of a dog with a mediastinal shift to the right. The right middle lung lobe has collapsed and the cardiac silhouette is displaced to the right (arrowed). The right hemidiaphragm is cranially displaced (arrowheads). Although mediastinal shift is a physiological change, it prevents assessment of the collapsed area of lung and therefore repeat inspiratory radiographs should be obtained.

Common conditions

Mediastinal mass

Mediastinal masses usually lie close to the midline on a DV/VD view and are typically described according to their location within the thorax (cranial mediastinal masses are the most common).

Cranial mediastinal mass: The most common location for mediastinal masses is cranioventrally, with the mass lying ventral to the trachea and cranial to the cardiac silhouette.

Radiological features:

- A focal area of increased opacity (Figure 5.88), which on a DV/VD view lies close to the midline. A small mass may not be visible or just cause a change in the width or contour of the mediastinum. Masses may be sharply or poorly marginated.
- Caudal and/or lateral displacement of the lung ± partial collapse of the lung lobe(s).
- Displacement of adjacent mediastinal structures (e.g. dorsal displacement of the trachea and/or caudal displacement of the cardiac silhouette).
- Compression of the trachea cranial to the carina is commonly seen with large masses and is a valuable radiological sign. Displacement of the trachea due to other causes (e.g. large volume pleural effusion) does not result in tracheal narrowing.
- Loss of definition of any organ borders in contact with the mass (e.g. the cardiac silhouette).
- Detection of the mass in the presence of pleural or mediastinal fluid can be difficult.

Caudal mediastinal mass: Caudal mediastinal masses are rare compared with cranioventral masses.

5.88 **(a)** Right lateral and **(b)** DV views of the thorax of a dog with a cranial mediastinal mass. On the lateral view, the mass (arrowheads) lies in the cranioventral thorax and is of homogeneous soft tissue opacity. Note that the mass has elevated the trachea and displaced the cranial lung lobes caudally. On the DV view, the mass (arrowheads) lies on the midline resulting in widening of the cranial mediastinum. The prominent skin folds (arrowed) should not be overinterpreted as pneumothorax.

Differentiating caudal mediastinal masses from accessory lung lobe/axially located masses within the caudal lung lobes may be difficult as both may appear midline in location. In contrast to cranial mediastinal masses, which are commonly neoplastic, masses arising from the caudoventral mediastinum are often non-neoplastic.

Radiological features:

- Focal area of increased opacity caudally within the thorax, which on the DV/VD view lies in the midline (if dorsal) or slightly to the left of midline (if ventral).
- If masses contact the diaphragm, the diaphragm is not visualized due to border effacement.
- Caudodorsal masses most commonly arise from the oesophagus or perioesophageal tissues (Figure 5.89). Oesophageal contrast studies are often useful to determine if the mass involves the oesophagus.

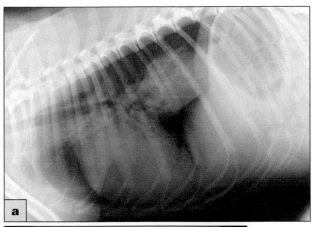

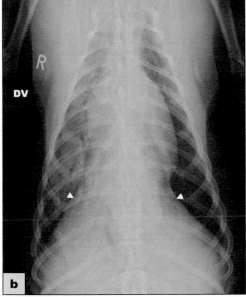

5.89 **(a)** Right lateral and **(b)** DV views of the thorax of a dog with a caudal mediastinal mass. On the lateral view, the mass is superimposed on the caudal lung, extending dorsally from the level of the caudal vena cava. The DV view localizes the mass (arrowheads) to the midline, making a caudal mediastinal location more likely. Accessory lung lobe masses can also have a midline location, but are usually positioned more ventrally. On ultrasound examination, the mass had a fluid-filled centre and a paraoesophageal mass was found at exploratory thoracotomy.

Perihilar mediastinal mass: Mediastinal masses within the perihilar region are most commonly due to tracheobronchial lymphadenopathy or heart base tumours (see above). Due to the lack of air or fat within the mediastinum, masses located in the perihilar region are poorly marginated. Recognizing displacement of the bronchi and trachea is key to differentiating perihilar masses from other causes of increased opacity (left atrial enlargement, cardiogenic pulmonary oedema) within the perihilar region.

Mediastinal lymphadenopathy
Lymph nodes within the mediastinum are only seen if enlarged, and are a differential diagnosis for both cranial and perihilar mediastinal masses. Enlargement of the cranial mediastinal lymph nodes results in a cranial mediastinal mass, which may cause elevation of the trachea and can distort the ventral contour of the cranial mediastinum on a lateral view. Enlargement of the sternal lymph nodes is seen as a focal increase in

opacity dorsal to the region of the second sternebra on the lateral view. They are usually less apparent on a DV/VD view, but are occasionally recognized as a midline soft tissue opacity distorting the contour of the cranial mediastinum. The main lymphatic drainage from the peritoneal cavity is via the sternal lymph nodes; therefore, enlargement of these nodes is commonly associated with inflammatory or neoplastic pathology within the peritoneal cavity. Other common causes of sternal lymphadenopathy include lymphosarcoma and malignant histiocystosis.

Enlargement of the tracheobronchial lymph nodes is also best seen on a lateral view, as an increase in the soft tissue opacity close to the carina (Figure 5.90). Radiography is very insensitive for demonstrating tracheobronchial lymphadenopathy, which has to

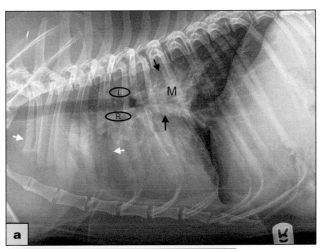

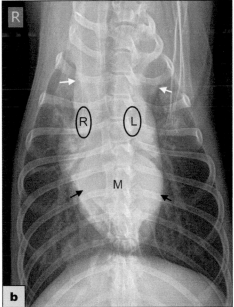

5.90 **(a)** Right lateral and **(b)** DV views of the thorax of a dog with marked mediastinal and tracheobronchial lymphadenopathy due to granulomatous lymphadenitis. The middle tracheobronchial lymph node (M) is markedly enlarged (black arrows). It appears as a large, indistinctly marginated, soft tissue opacity caudal to the carina on the lateral view. On the DV view, the lymphadenopathy has resulted in lateral displacement and compression of the mainstem bronchi. The location of the right (R) and left (L) tracheobronchial lymph nodes is shown. Note there is also marked enlargement of the cranial mediastinal/sternal lymph nodes (white arrows), but only slight tracheal elevation.

be severe to be reliably visualized. Depending on the location of the enlarged node(s), the tracheal bifurcation may be unaffected, raised or depressed. On a DV/VD view, enlargement can lead to increased divergence of the caudal lobar bronchi; left atrial enlargement results in a similar appearance, but enlargement of the cardiac silhouette on the lateral view should allow the distinction to be made. On the lateral view, enlargement of the middle bronchial lymph nodes results in ventral deviation of the mainstem bronchi; whereas, left atrial enlargement results in elevation of the bronchi. Calcification of the tracheobronchial lymph nodes can occur with mycotic pneumonia, in particular histoplasmosis, but this is very rare in the UK. Lymph nodes may also become opacified some time following inadvertent barium aspiration.

Pneumomediastinum

Pneumomediastinum (Figure 5.91) can result from extension of air from the neck (e.g. following a 'stick' injury) or (rarely) from cranial extension of pneumo-retroperitoneum. Extreme dyspnoea and rupture of the trachea or oesophagus can also lead to free mediastinal air. Pneumothorax can result from extension of pneumomediastinum, but pneumomediastinum cannot result from pneumothorax.

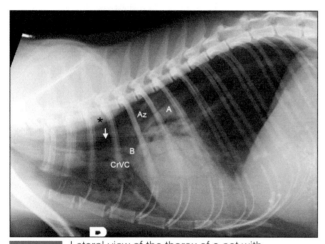

5.91 Lateral view of the thorax of a cat with pneumomediastinum secondary to dyspnoea (as a result of congestive heart failure). The heart is enlarged, although the pulmonary oedema has largely resolved. Note the heterogeneous appearance of the cranial mediastinum, with gas highlighting the longus colli muscles (*) and dorsal tracheal wall (arrowed), and extending ventral to the trachea to outline the brachiocephalic trunk (B) and cranial vena cava (CrVC). Note also the delineation of the right azygos vein (Az) cranial and dorsal to the aorta (A).

Radiological features:

- Loss of homogeneity of the cranial mediastinum on the lateral view.
- Delineation of structures not normally visible (e.g. cranial vena cava, external margin of the trachea and the azygos vein).
- On the lateral view, the cardiac silhouette may be elevated from the sternum by a gas lucency.
- The lung markings still extend to the periphery of the thorax on both views (unlike with pneumothorax).

Mediastinal fluid

Mediastinal fluid can occur alone or in association with pleural fluid. Fluid can be present due to haemorrhage (trauma/coagulopathy), infection (oesophageal rupture, FIP), hypoproteinaemia or congestive heart failure and in association with mediastinal masses.

Radiological features:

- Increased width of the mediastinum on a DV/VD view.
- Loss of definition of any soft tissue structures in contact with the fluid (e.g. cardiac margins and the diaphragm).
- Soft tissue 'fissure' lines extending from the midline out to the periphery. These are sometimes referred to as 'reverse fissures', as opposed to pleural fissure lines which have a broad base at the periphery. Reverse fissures are not specific for mediastinal fluid and may also be seen with localized pleural effusions.

Thoracic boundaries

The thorax is bordered dorsally by the vertebrae, laterally by the ribs, ventrally by the sternum and caudally by the diaphragm. The skeletal structures are associated with several types of soft tissue (muscles, fat, blood vessels, skin). At the thoracic inlet there is communication between the soft tissues of the neck and the mediastinum, so with some clinical presentations, especially traumatic injuries to the neck, it is important that the thorax is also assessed.

Specific approach to interpretation

Swelling and/or changes in opacity of the soft tissues surrounding the thorax may be seen on radiographs. One of the most common changes is subcutaneous emphysema following traumatic injury. Although not clinically significant in itself, it can complicate interpretation of a thoracic radiograph due to superimposed air (Figure 5.92).

Common conditions

Rib fractures

Rib fractures are a common finding following road traffic accidents, but fractures can also be the consequence of extreme dyspnoea. As with all fractures, it is important to establish that pre-existing pathology, such as an underlying neoplastic lesion (e.g. multiple myeloma), is not the reason for the fracture. Rib fractures are often multiple (Figure 5.93); they may also be segmental (two or more fractures of the same rib) and respiratory problems can arise in this instance if multiple adjacent ribs are affected. This is known as a 'flail chest' and is characterized by paradoxical respiratory movement of a section of the chest wall.

Radiological features:

- A lucent defect across the rib(s).
  - There may be displacement at the fracture site.
  - Fractures are usually transverse but can be oblique.
- May be seen incidentally during various stages of healing.

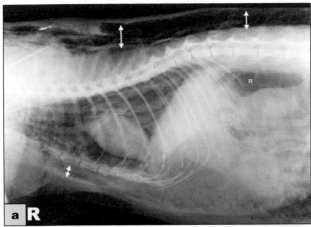

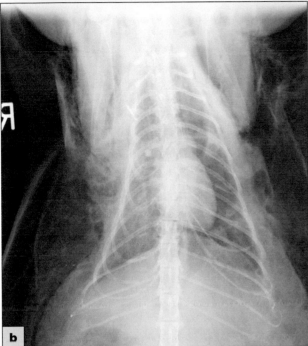

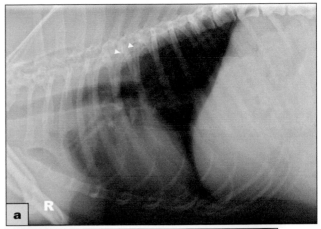

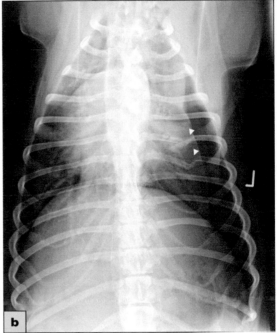

5.92 **(a)** Right lateral and **(b)** DV views of a cat with extensive subcutaneous emphysema, pneumomediastinum and pneumoretroperitoneum (R). The presence of subcutaneous air (double-headed arrows) complicates interpretation of thoracic radiographs as the gas lucencies are superimposed on the thorax.

5.93 **(a)** Right lateral and **(b)** DV views of the thorax of a dog with fractures of the sixth and seventh ribs (arrowheads) on the left-hand side and a unilateral pneumothorax. The fractures are easy to recognize on the DV view but are less obvious on the lateral view, due to a combination of the proximal location of the fracture and radiographic factors (rotation and some movement blur).

- Secondary features that may be present include:
  - Pneumothorax
  - Subcutaneous emphysema
  - Pulmonary contusion (seen as an alveolar infiltrate).

Conversely, if any of the above secondary features are seen on thoracic radiographs, it is important to look for evidence of trauma such as rib fractures.

Thoracic wall mass

Thoracic wall tumours may arise from bone (usually osteosarcoma or chondrosarcoma of a rib) (Figure 5.94) or the soft tissue structures of the thoracic wall. They are usually evident clinically as palpable swellings of the chest wall. Radiographs are helpful to ascertain the tissue of origin, the degree of involvement of other thoracic structures and the extent of the lesion. When assessing thoracic wall lesions, depending on the location of the mass, standard orthogonal views (especially the lateral view) may not be that helpful; oblique radiographic views are often more useful as it is possible to 'skyline' the lesion.

Radiological features:

- Expansion (widening) of the contour of the rib, often close to the costochondral junction.
- Thinning of the cortices and associated bone destruction.
- Periosteal reaction, both on the rib giving rise to the mass and often on the adjacent ribs as well.
- Soft tissue swelling.
- Mass effect. The adjacent lung margin is displaced medially, resulting in an 'extrapleural' sign. The mass effect may increase the distance between the affected rib and neighbouring ribs.
- Pleural fluid may be present, either localized to the area of the affected rib or more generalized.
- Masses arising from the soft tissues rather than the ribs are unlikely to cause any expansion of the contour of the rib.

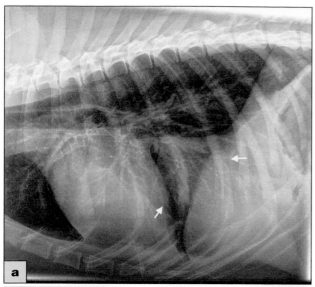

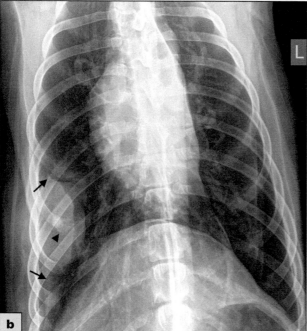

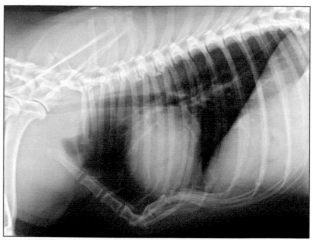

5.95 Left lateral view of the thorax of a dog with a congenital sternal anomaly. The fourth to sixth sternebrae are fused. The caudal sternum is angled dorsally and the costal arch is deformed.

5.94 **(a)** Right lateral and **(b)** DV views of the thorax of a dog with a rib tumour. The DV view is required to localize the large soft tissue mass (white arrows) seen on the lateral view. The mass has created an 'extrapleural' sign (i.e. the lung is pushed away by the mass, which has a broad base at the periphery of the thorax) (black arrows). The rib destruction and periosteal reaction (arrowhead) is easily overlooked on the lateral view.

Sternal deformity

Sternal deformities are common and include alterations in the number of sternebrae, the length of the sternebrae and their alignment (Figure 5.95).

Pectus excavatum: This is a congenital deformity seen in both cats and dogs, where the alignment of the sternum is abnormal. Pectus excavatum is usually an incidental finding but can be seen in association with other congenital abnormalities such as peritoneo-pericardial diaphragmatic hernia (PPDH). The presence of pectus excavatum can present a challenge when performing echocardiography as normal acoustic windows may need to be adjusted.

Radiological features:

- Dorsal displacement of the mid to caudal portion of the sternum. The angle of displacement is variable but can be marked.
- Abnormal curvature of the associated ribs and costal cartilages.
- The cardiac silhouette may be displaced dorsally and often laterally as well.

Sternal fractures

Sternal fractures are rare, but occasionally recognized following road traffic accidents or other trauma. Fractures of individual sternebrae may be identified, as well as changes in sternebral alignment.

Osteomyelitis

Sternal osteomyelitis is not common but can arise from contaminated wounds or migrating foreign bodies. A mixed lytic/productive reaction is seen, usually with associated soft tissue swelling.

Diaphragmatic rupture and hernia

The diaphragm should be assessed for shape, margination, position and integrity. The diaphragm may not be entirely visible if there is pathology in the thorax, including pleural and/or mediastinal fluid and caudal mediastinal or lung masses. The majority of diaphragmatic defects are caused by traumatic rupture (Figure 5.96). Congenital herniation is possible but rare.

Radiological features:

- Partial or complete loss of the diaphragmatic outline.
  - This is a non-specific finding as pleural fluid, lung consolidation or soft tissue masses adjacent to the diaphragm also lead to border effacement.
- Loss of definition/displacement of the normal thoracic contents, especially the cardiac silhouette, which may be dorsally displaced.

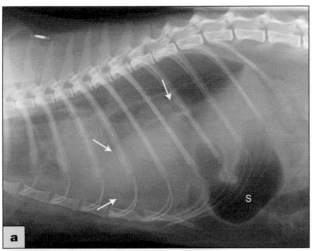

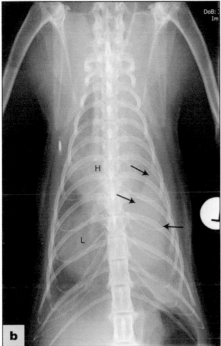

5.96 **(a)** Right lateral and **(b)** DV views of the thorax of a cat with a diaphragmatic rupture. (a) The position of the stomach (S) is abnormal. It is gas-filled and displaced cranially. The soft tissue opacity (arrowed) in the caudal thorax effaces the caudal border of the cardiac silhouette and the cranioventral diaphragm. It is lobulated in appearance, representing displaced liver and probably spleen as well. A small volume of pleural fluid can be seen elevating the cranial lung lobes. Subcutaneous emphysema is present ventral to the cranial sternum. (b) A triangular soft tissue opacity (arrowed), probably the spleen, lies between the left chest wall and the cardiac silhouette, with a rounded soft tissue opacity, probably the liver, present on the right. H = cardiac silhouette; L = liver.

- The presence of abdominal viscera within the thorax.
  - Easily recognized if ingesta and/or gas are present.
  - Less obvious if there is only a small tear with minimal displacement of abdominal structures (e.g. only mesentery or a single liver lobe).
  - The cranial abdominal viscera are usually displaced cranially or not identified within the abdomen.
- A mediastinal shift may be present on the DV/VD view.

- Pleural effusion (especially if the liver or spleen is incarcerated in the defect). This may hinder diagnosis in some cases, as the margins of the herniated organs are less well defined.
- Incidental evidence of trauma such as rib fractures may be seen.
- If a hernia (rather than a rupture) is present, it may appear more mass-like with containment of the abdominal viscera within a peritoneal sac.

If plain films are equivocal, a small amount of barium given orally followed by repeat radiographs may help to determine the position of the stomach and small intestine relative to the diaphragm (see Figure 3.23).

Peritoneo-pericardial diaphragmatic hernia

PPDH is a congenital defect that results in communication between the pericardial and peritoneal cavities. It may be present for years without causing clinical signs and is often an incidental finding. In some cases (e.g. where the stomach or intestine becomes incarcerated), PPDH becomes symptomatic leading to respiratory, cardiovascular or gastrointestinal problems.

Radiological features:

- Enlargement of the cardiac silhouette in all planes (Figure 5.97).
  - With an absence of any signs of congestive heart failure.
- Dorsal displacement of the trachea and caudal vena cava.
- Lack of definition of at least part of the cardiac silhouette as it 'merges' with the diaphragm.
- Mixed radiographic opacities within the cardiac silhouette (fat and frequently gas if intestine is displaced).
- Abnormal position of cranial abdominal organs.
- Concurrent sternal abnormalities are common (often a reduced number of sternebrae and absence or splitting of the xiphoid process).

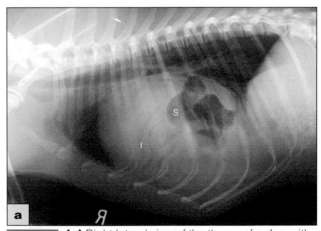

5.97 **(a)** Right lateral view of the thorax of a dog with a PPDH. The cardiac silhouette is markedly enlarged. Mixed opacities superimposed on the cardiac silhouette on both views localize these structures to within the pericardium. These opacities include areas of fat, linear gas opacities representing small intestinal loops (I) and a larger folded gas-filled viscus representing the stomach (S). The ventral diaphragmatic line is obscured, the sternum is shortened and the xiphisternum is absent. (continues) ▶

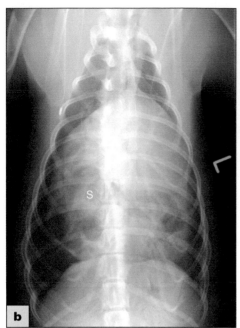

5.97 (continued) **(b)** DV view of the thorax of a dog with a PPDH. The cardiac silhouette is markedly enlarged. Mixed opacities superimposed on the cardiac silhouette on both views localize these structures to within the pericardium. These opacities include areas of fat, linear gas opacities representing small intestinal loops and a larger folded gas-filled viscus representing the stomach (S). The ventral diaphragmatic line is obscured, the sternum is shortened and the xiphisternum is absent.

- A persistent dorsal mesothelial remnant may be seen in cats as a soft tissue band between the cardiac silhouette and diaphragm, level with or just dorsal to the caudal vena cava.

Oesophagus

Specific approach to interpretation

The limitation of conventional film–screen radiography of the oesophagus is that it produces a static image of a dynamic structure. Fluoroscopy is the preferred technique as it allows oesophageal function to be assessed.

- The oesophagus is not radiologically visible in the normal dog and cat. However, small quantities of swallowed air may be seen in the cranial cervical and cranial thoracic oesophagus when dogs are restrained in lateral recumbency.
- Occasionally, left lateral thoracic radiographs of a normal animal show a linear, soft tissue opacity dorsal to the caudal vena cava. This finding usually represents a transient dilatation of the oesophagus due to gastric reflux into the caudal oesophagus.
- The oesophagus dilates following deep sedation or anaesthesia. It is not possible to differentiate oesophageal dilatation due to disease/dysfunction from that associated with anaesthesia on radiographs.
- Film radiography by convention evaluates the animal in lateral recumbency, which may limit recognition of, or underestimate, the volume of gas and fluid in a dilated oesophagus. A standing lateral view using a horizontal X-ray beam may

resolve the uncertainty by demonstrating a horizontal fluid level. A horizontal beam technique should only be used with due observation of radiation protection requirements. All horizontal beam exposures must be recorded.

- Survey films must always precede an oesophageal contrast study.
- Contrast radiography using barium sulphate is contraindicated when perforation is suspected.

Röntgen signs

- Size and location – oesophageal dilatation may be localized or generalized and involve the cervical region or be present cranial or caudal to the heart. This distinction helps determine the underlying cause. Focal dilatation occurs due to vascular ring anomaly, oesophagitis, a mass or a foreign body. Generalized dilatation occurs due to idiopathic megaoesophagus or neuromuscular disease. Dilatation cranial to the heart suggests a vascular ring anomaly. Foreign bodies usually lodge caudal to the heart.
- Opacity – this reflects the accumulation of gas, fluid or food material. Foreign bodies (even osseous foreign bodies) may only be recognized if surrounded by air.
- Shape – widening of the (usually caudal) oesophagus is associated with foreign bodies or large mass lesions.

Common conditions

Generalized dilatation

Generalized dilatation of the oesophagus (mega-oesophagus) has numerous causes.

Radiological features:

- On survey radiographs (Figure 5.98), the dilated oesophagus may be filled with air, fluid and/or food.
- With severe dilatation, the oesophagus causes ventral deviation of the thoracic trachea and heart base.

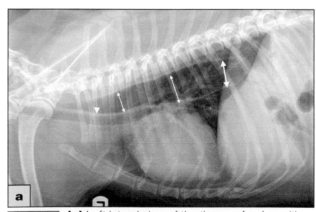

5.98 **(a)** Left lateral view of the thorax of a dog with signs of regurgitation and coughing. Generalized dilatation of the oesophagus is present (double-headed arrows). Caudally, the paired walls of the dilated oesophagus taper towards the diaphragm (lower oesophageal sphincter). The trachea is displaced slightly ventrally by the dilated oesophagus and the dorsal wall of the trachea (arrowhead) is recognized due to air in the oesophagus (tracheal stripe sign). Megaoesophagus is often more conspicuous on a left lateral view. (continues) ▶

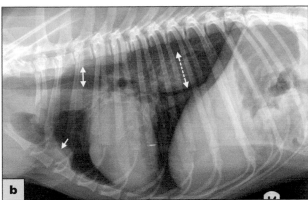

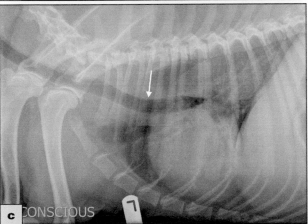

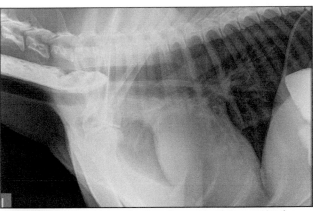

■ An impression of oesophageal motility can be gained from obtaining 'spot' radiographs following the oral administration of barium (Figure 5.100). For a complete and representative evaluation, a fluoroscopic examination should be performed (Figure 5.101).

5.100 Lateral (standing) radiograph of the neck of a dog with generalized megaoesophagus and oesophageal hypomotility. The ingested barium has not formed a discrete bolus. The barium is elongated with dilatation of the oesophagus aboral to the bolus. With normal oesophageal function, a tight bolus is formed as the oesophagus maintains a high pressure area in front and behind the bolus as it is propelled along the oesophagus.

5.98 (continued) **(b)** Right lateral view of a dog with generalized megaoesophagus, but in this patient the dilatation (white double-headed arrow) is less marked. Pooling of fluid in the caudal oesophagus is responsible for the soft tissue opacity band (white dashed headed arrow) in the caudal thorax. Note the sternal lymph node (arrowed) is enlarged. **(c)** Oesophageal dilatation results in ventral displacement (arrowed) of the intrathoracic trachea. The dilated oesophagus dorsal to the heart and within the caudal thorax is filled with fluid and gas.

■ The mediastinum usually appears widened on the VD view, and V-shaped tapering of the caudal mediastinum is usually present.
■ The extent of the oesophageal dilatation can be determined by contrast studies (Figure 5.99).

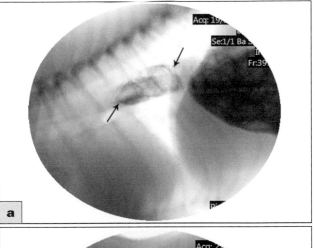

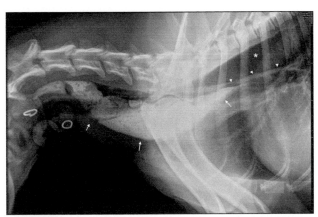

5.99 Lateral (standing) view of the neck of a dog with generalized megaoesophagus. A barium study has been performed (using semi-liquid food) and the contrast medium has pooled ventrally within the dilated cervical oesophagus (arrowed). Note the air dorsal to the barium (*) and the dilatation of the thoracic oesophagus. A tracheal stripe sign is evident (arrowheads).

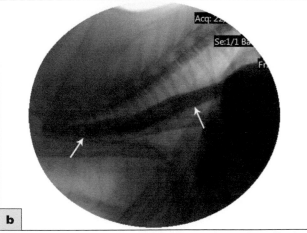

5.101 Fluoroscopic studies of oesophageal motility in **(a)** a normal dog and **(b)** a dog with oesophageal hypomotility. (a) A tight bolus (arrowed) has been propelled into the distal oesophagus. There is no oesophageal dilatation. (b) The bolus is elongated, indicating hypomotility (arrowed).

Localized dilatation

- Local dilatation may be due to segmental oesophageal hypomotility. This is not necessarily significant in young dogs.
- Localized oesophageal dilatation is recognized proximal to foreign bodies, strictures or mass lesions, which cause a degree of obstruction.
- Vascular ring anomalies (Figure 5.102) usually cause dilatation of the oesophagus in the cranial mediastinum.

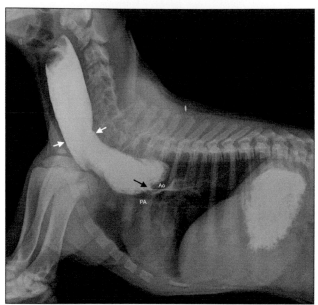

5.102 Lateral barium oesophagram of a dog with a vascular ring anomaly (persistent right aortic arch). The cervical and cranial thoracic oesophagus is markedly dilated with a barium/food mixture (white arrows). The dilated oesophagus narrows abruptly (black arrow) over the heart base. The approximate location of the ascending aorta (Ao) and main pulmonary artery (PA) are indicated.

- Oesophageal diverticula are uncommon and result in isolated areas of dilatation. Although diverticula can be congenital, acquired diverticula are more common. They are usually caused by protrusion of the mucosa through a weakened muscular wall. Diverticula can also be formed by constant tension on the oesophageal wall from adhesions or mass lesions located outside the oesophagus.
- In brachycephalic breeds, redundancy of the cranial oesophagus may mimic a diverticulum.
- Focal dilatation of the caudal oesophagus occurs with hiatal hernias and gastro-oesophageal intussusception.
  - A hiatal hernia (Figure 5.103) appears as an increased soft tissue opacity in the caudodorsal thorax effacing with the dorsal aspect of the diaphragm. Gas or rugal folds may be recognized in the portion of the stomach herniated into the caudal thorax. A positive-contrast gastrogram may show cranial displacement of the lower oesophageal sphincter and/or gastric rugal folds cranial to the hiatus. Fluoroscopy may be necessary to demonstrate intermittent herniation ('sliding hernia'). Hiatal herniation is occasionally seen as an incidental finding in sedated/anaesthetized cats.

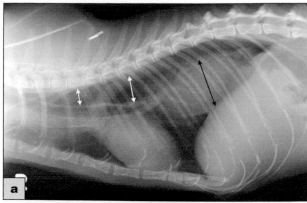

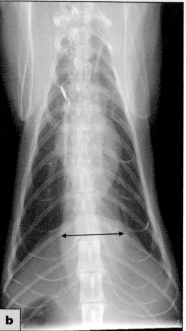

5.103 (a) Lateral and (b) DV views of the thorax of a cat with signs of recurrent regurgitation due to a hiatal hernia. There is a large midline soft tissue mass, consistent with herniated stomach (double-headed black arrow) in the caudodorsal thorax. The normal gas-filled stomach is not recognized. The oesophagus is dilated with air (double-headed white arrows), resulting in ventral displacement of the trachea.

- Gastro-oesophageal intussusception is uncommon. Megaoesophagus may be pre-existing, allowing invagination of the stomach into the thoracic oesophagus. The thoracic oesophagus is dilated, a fundic gas shadow in the abdomen is not visible or abnormal in appearance, and a well demarcated soft tissue opacity is present in the caudal oesophagus. A rugal pattern may be visible in the caudal oesophagus. Following barium administration, a partial or complete obstruction to the passage of contrast medium into the stomach is demonstrated. Aspiration pneumonia may be present.

Oesophagitis

Oesophagitis causes disruption in the normally smooth mucosal folds. Oesophagitis occurs due to ingestion of caustic substances or foreign bodies, infection or gastro-oesophageal reflux. The caudal third of the oesophagus is most commonly affected.

Radiological features:

- Survey radiographs are usually normal.
- An indistinct, funnel-shaped increase in soft tissue opacity may be recognized in the caudodorsal thorax if there is mild oesophageal dilatation.
- Following the administration of barium, the caudal oesophageal mucosa may be abnormal with 'smudging' and irregularity of the mucosal folds, adherence of barium to the mucosa and subsequent persistence of the barium after the bolus has been propelled into the stomach.

Oesophageal stricture

Stricture or stenosis results in localized dilatation cranial to the stenosis. Causes include spasm or stenosis of the lower oesophageal sphincter, vascular ring anomalies, extreme pressure from mediastinal and oesophageal masses, and cicatrix secondary to oesophageal trauma caused by a foreign body.

Radiological features:

- Consistently decreased diameter of a segment of the oesophagus on a contrast oesophagram.
- Dilatation of the oesophagus cranial to the stricture.

Oesophageal foreign body

Common oesophageal foreign bodies include bones, potatoes and apples, as well as non-food items. Common sites for obstruction include the thoracic inlet, heart base and the distal high pressure zone. Penetration or pressure necrosis may cause perforation of the oesophagus. Pressure at the level of the heart base may cause pulmonary thrombus formation. Any mucosal damage may progress to stricture formation.

Radiological features:

- On survey radiographs (Figure 5.104), oesophageal foreign bodies may be seen as soft tissue, mineral or metal opacities.
- Soft tissue foreign bodies may cause focal widening of the oesophagus.
- Localized dilatation of the oesophagus may be present cranial to the foreign body.
- Mediastinal widening, indicating mediastinal fluid, may be present if perforation has occurred.
- A contrast study is only required if the foreign body is radiolucent. Endoscopy should be considered instead of a contrast study.
- Barium and ionic iodinated contrast agents should not be used to assess the integrity of the oesophageal mucosa; endoscopy or the administration of a non-ionic iodinated contrast medium is indicated.

Oesophageal perforation

Oesophageal perforation (Figure 5.105) usually occurs secondary to a foreign body. It is a potentially life-threatening condition and should not be overlooked. If there is suspicion of oesophageal perforation, endoscopy or water-soluble non-ionic iodinated contrast media should be used.

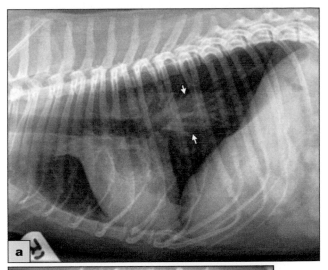

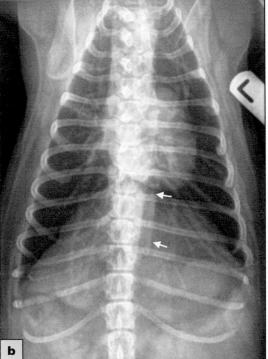

5.104 **(a)** Lateral and **(b)** DV views of the thorax of a dog with non-productive retching due to an oesophageal foreign body. The foreign body appears as a rounded soft tissue structure (arrowed) in the mid-dorsal thorax caudal to the cardiac silhouette. As the foreign body is not surrounded by gas, it cannot be distinguished from the walls of the oesophagus. On occasion, it may be difficult to recognize and distinguish mineralization of bone foreign bodies (e.g. knuckles or chop bones) from the surrounding soft tissue.

Radiological features:

- Both the cervical and thoracic oesophagus should be evaluated. On survey radiographs of the thorax, an increase in mediastinal widening may be present. Opaque food material and flocculation or free air may be recognized within the cervical soft tissues, superimposed on the cranial mediastinum or caudodorsal thorax.
- Radiopaque foreign bodies (e.g. bone) may be visible.
- An oesophagram may show leakage of contrast medium into the mediastinal space.

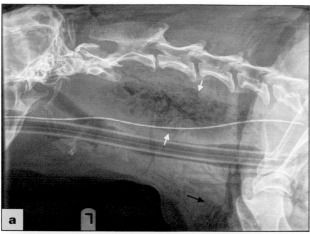

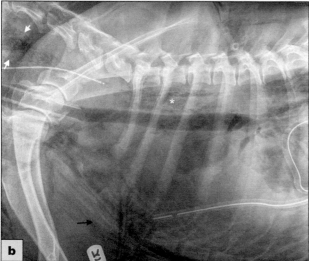

5.105 Lateral views of **(a)** the cervical region and **(b)** the thorax of a dog with perforation of the cervical oesophagus. A large area of mixed soft tissue–gas opacity (white arrows) is present ventral to the cervical vertebrae. This represents leaked gas and food material accumulated within the paraoesophageal fascia. The cervical trachea is displaced ventrally. Extensive subcutaneous emphysema (black arrows) and pneumomediastinum (*) are present. A large pleural effusion effaces the cardiac silhouette and chest drains have been placed.

Vascular ring anomaly

Vascular ring anomalies (see Figure 5.102) are caused by abnormalities in the embryological development of the aortic arches. The most common abnormality is persistence of the right fourth aortic arch.

Radiological features:

- The stricture is centred over the craniodorsal aspect of the heart base with severe dilatation of the cranial oesophagus.
- In severe cases, oesophageal dilatation may extend cranially the length of the neck.
- Ventral deviation of the trachea may be present when the cranial oesophagus is distended with fluid or ingesta.
- Dilatation of the caudal oesophagus may also be present.
- Contrast studies are necessary to confirm the site of the stricture.
- Concurrent aspiration pneumonia may be apparent.

Neoplasia

Oesophageal tumours are rare in the dog and cat, but appear to be more common in geographical areas where *Spirocerca lupi* is found. Fibrosarcoma and osteosarcoma develop from malignant transformation of oesophageal granulomas associated with *Spirocerca lupi* infection. Oesophageal carcinoma and leiomyosarcoma are the most common malignant oesophageal tumours in dogs. Squamous cell carcinoma is the most commonly diagnosed primary oesophageal tumour in the cat.

Radiological features:

- Survey thoracic radiographs (Figures 5.106 and 5.107) may be normal or reveal variable oesophageal dilatation.

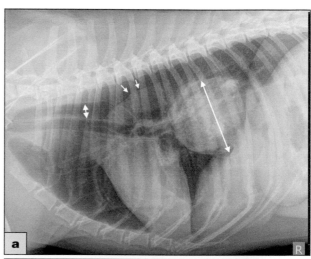

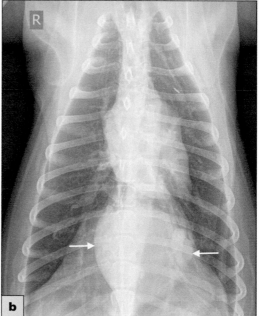

5.106 **(a)** Lateral and **(b)** DV views of a dog with signs of regurgitation. (a) A large rounded soft tissue mass is present in the caudodorsal thorax (long double-headed arrow). The mass has areas of indistinct mineralization of its caudodorsal and mid-ventral aspects. The oesophagus is mildly dilated cranial to the heart (short double-headed arrow). There is mild aneurysmal dilatation of the descending aorta dorsal to the carina (arrowed). The changes are due to a large mural mass associated with *Spirocerca* infection. (b) The DV view is important as it localizes the mass (arrowed) to the midline.

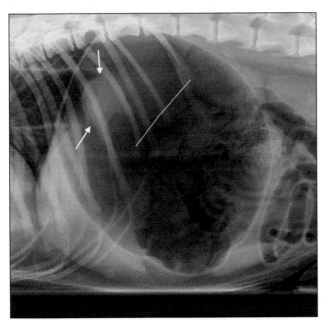

5.107 Lateral view of a dog with retching due to an oesophageal tumour. A discrete soft tissue mass (arrowed) is highlighted by gas in the moderately dilated terminal oesophagus. The stomach is also distended with gas. Note that the white linear structure overlying the stomach is a screen artefact. (Courtesy of MyVet24/7)

- A soft tissue midline mass or focal widening of the oesophagus may suggest the presence of a mass lesion.
- Oesophageal gas may define an intraluminal mass.
- Paraoesophageal lesions may displace the oesophagus.
- Aspiration pneumonia and/or a nodular lung pattern suggestive of pulmonary metastasis may be present.
- A barium oesophagram typically confirms the presence of an intraluminal mass or obstructive lesion, mucosal irregularity and ulceration.
- Concurrent radiological findings with *Spirocerca lupi* include spondylitis involving the caudal thoracic vertebrae, aneurysmal dilatation or mineralization of the aorta, and hypertrophic osteopathy.

Oesophageal fistula

Oesophageal fistula is a rare condition, which may be life-threatening. Fistulae may form between the oesophagus and the trachea, bronchi or lung paren-chyma. They may be congenital or acquired. In order to confirm the diagnosis of a fistula and determine its morphology and extent, contrast oesophagraphy should be performed using water-soluble, non-ionic iodinated contrast media.

Radiological features:

- Survey radiographs may be normal or show a focal pulmonary alveolar pattern, consistent with lobar pneumonia.
- Tracheobronchial lymphadenopathy may be present.
- Following oesophagraphy, contrast medium is seen entering the affected bronchus and lobe.

Cricopharyngeal achalasia

Cricopharyngeal achalasia is characterized by an inadequate relaxation of the cricopharyngeal muscle during swallowing. There are suggestions that this condition is more common in Springer and Cocker Spaniels, but it has been seen in a variety of breeds. Common clinical signs include difficulty swallowing, hypersalivation, gagging, exaggerated mandibular and head motion, and dropping of food from the mouth.

Radiological features:

- Survey radiographs reveal localized oesophageal dilatation in the cranial cervical region and possibly evidence of aspiration pneumonia.
- A plain radiograph following liquid barium administration may demonstrate misdirection/ aspiration of contrast material into the larynx and trachea.
- A barium swallow study with fluoroscopy is required to make a diagnosis.
- Animals with cricopharyngeal achalasia have the ability to generate a bolus of food in the pharynx (i.e. pharyngeal strength to push the food bolus into the oesophagus is adequate), but the cricopharyngeal sphincter remains closed. Misdirection may also occur due to incoordination of the swallowing reflex.

References and further reading

Baines SJ, Lewis S and White RA (2002) Primary thoracic wall tumours of mesenchymal origin in dogs: a retrospective study of 46 cases. *Veterinary Record* **150**, 335–339
Boag AK, Lamb CR, Chapman PS and Boswood A (2004) Radiographic findings in 16 dogs infected with *Angiostrongylus vasorum*. *Veterinary Record* **154**, 426–430
Bright RM, Sackman JE, DeNovo C and Toal C (1990) Hiatal hernia in the dog and cat: a retrospective study of 16 cases. *Journal of Small Animal Practice* **31**, 244–250
Buchanan JW (2004) Tracheal signs and associated vascular anomalies in dogs with persistent right aortic arch. *Journal of Veterinary Internal Medicine* **18(1)**, 510–514
Buchanan JW and Bücheler (1995) Vertebral scale system to measure canine heart size in radiographs. *Journal of the American Veterinary Medical Association* **206(2)**, 194–199
Corcoran BM, Cobb M, Martin MWS *et al.* (1999) Chronic pulmonary disease in West Highland White Terriers. *Veterinary Record* **144**, 611–616
Coulsen A and Lewis N (2008) *An Atlas of Interpretative Anatomy of the Dog and Cat, 2nd edn.* Blackwell Publications, Oxford
D'Anjou MA, Tidwell AS and Hecht S (2005) Radiographic diagnosis of lung lobe torsion. *Veterinary Radiology & Ultrasound* **46**, 478–484
Kirberger RM and Avner A (2006) The effect of positioning on the appearance of selected cranial thoracic structures in the dog. *Veterinary Radiology & Ultrasound* **47**, 61–68
Lamb CR, Boswood A, Volkman A and Connolly D (2001) Assessment of survey radiography as a method for diagnosis of congenital cardiac disease in dogs. *Journal of Small Animal Practice* **42**, 541–545
Lamb CR, Wikeley H, Boswood A and Pfeiffer DU (2001) Use of breed-specific ranges for the vertebral heart scale as an aid to the radiographic diagnosis of heart disease in dogs. *Veterinary Record* **148**, 707–711
Prather AB, Berry CA and Thrall DE (2005) Use of radiography in combination with computed tomography for assessment of non-cardiac thoracic disease in the dog and cat. *Veterinary Radiology & Ultrasound* **46**, 114–122
Schwarz T and Johnson VS (2008) *BSAVA Manual of Canine and Feline Thoracic Imaging.* BSAVA Publications, Gloucester
Sisson D and Thomas WP (1999) Pericardial disease and cardiac tumours. In: *Textbook of Canine and Feline Cardiology: Principles and Clinical Practice, 2nd edn,* ed. PR Fox *et al.*, pp. 569–701. WB Saunders, Philadelphia
Stickle RL and Love NE (1989) Radiographic diagnosis of esophageal diseases in dogs and cats. *Seminars in Veterinary Medicine and Surgery (Small Animal)* **4(3)**, 179–187
Suter PF and Lord PF (1984) *Thoracic Radiography: A Text Atlas of Thoracic Diseases of the Dog and Cat.* Suter, Wettswil, Switzerland

Radiology of the abdomen

Esther Barrett

Abdominal radiography is indicated for a wide variety of conditions, not only primary abdominal disease but also other disorders which may involve, or extend into, the abdomen. Radiography and ultrasonography are complementary imaging techniques and, if the equipment and funds are available, performing both will provide more information than a single modality alone. Abdominal radiography is best performed prior to ultrasonography, as it provides a better overview of the contents of the abdomen and helps to direct the ultrasonographic examination, whilst avoiding radiographic artefacts created by ultrasound gel remaining on the animal's coat.

The challenges associated with abdominal radiology of the dog and the cat include:

- Superimposition of the abdominal organs and viscera – the abdomen has greater superimposition of structures than most other body areas with the exception of the skull
- Relatively poor tissue contrast:
  - The interpretation of abdominal radiographs is hindered by the similar opacity of the majority of tissues within the abdomen
  - The inherently poor contrast is compounded by the greater amount of scatter created in the abdomen compared with other body areas.

Indications

- Gastrointestinal disease:
  - Vomiting
  - Suspected foreign body
  - Tenesmus, dyschezia and haematochezia
  - Diarrhoea.
- Urogenital disease:
  - Dysuria, stranguria and haematuria
  - Urinary incontinence
  - Anuria
  - Polyuria
  - Vaginal discharge
  - Pregnancy diagnosis and assessment.
- Non-specific disease:
  - Abdominal distension
  - Palpable abdominal masses or organomegaly

- Abdominal pain
- Pyrexia of unknown origin
- Weight loss
- Anorexia
- Jaundice
- Anaemia
- Investigation of hernias and abdominal wall swellings or masses
- Screening for primary or secondary neoplasia
- Screening for abdominal injury following trauma.

Restraint and patient preparation

Adequate patient preparation is important to obtain the maximum amount of information from an abdominal radiographic examination. The superimposition of ingesta and faecal material on the abdominal organs results in distracting artefacts. In addition, when the gastrointestinal tract and bladder are distended they occupy a significant amount of space within the abdomen, increasing superimposition of the other abdominal structures.

- Prior to elective abdominal radiography, it is recommended that food is withheld for 12 hours to ensure that the stomach and small intestine are relatively empty.
- The patient should be given the opportunity to defecate and urinate prior to abdominal radiography.
- If urinary tract studies are being performed, a cleansing, non-irritant enema (e.g. warm water) 2 hours before the examination ensures that the large intestine is empty of faecal material.
- Urogenital contrast studies should be performed under general anaesthesia, but for gastrointestinal contrast studies, general anaesthesia is contraindicated as it reduces gastrointestinal motility, making interpretation of transit time difficult, and poses a significant risk of aspiration of barium and gastrointestinal contents into the lung. If it is not possible to perform a gastrointestinal study in the conscious animal, light sedation using neuroleptanalgesia can be used as it has little effect on oesophageal or gastrointestinal motility.

Standard radiographic views

It is increasingly common practice that, if abdominal radiography is performed prior to abdominal ultrasonography, only a single lateral view of the abdomen is obtained. However, obtaining two orthogonal views (a lateral and a ventrodorsal (VD) view) remains the minimum recommendation for radiographic evaluation of the abdomen. If ultrasonography is not being performed, then two orthogonal views are required for interpretation. In cases of suspected gastrointestinal obstruction, it is often worthwhile taking both lateral views, in addition to the VD view, as this allows redistribution of gas and fluid within the intestine and stomach. The cause of mechanical obstruction may only be visible on one view due to the differing locations of fluid and gas on different views.

Laterolateral views

Either a left or right lateral recumbent view can be obtained. The radiographic appearance of the abdominal organs and viscera differ slightly between left and right lateral recumbency, due to the movement of gas and fluid within the gastrointestinal tract and the effect of gravity on the mobile viscera. Thus, whichever position is selected (either left or right recumbency), this should be used consistently to aid interpretation.

- The animal is positioned in lateral recumbency on the chosen side (i.e. on its right side for a right lateral view or on its left side for a left lateral view). The hindlimbs are drawn caudally and secured with ties/sandbags (Figure 6.1). Radiolucent foam wedges are placed under the sternum and between the femurs to help prevent rotation around the long axis.
- For cats and smaller dogs:
  - The X-ray beam is centred about two fingers' width caudal to the caudal-most part of the last rib, midway between the umbilicus and lumbar spine
  - The X-ray beam is collimated to include the diaphragm cranially (2–3 ribs cranial to the xiphisternum), the greater trochanter of the femur caudally, the vertebral bodies dorsally and the abdominal wall ventrally.
- For larger dogs (where the entire abdomen cannot be included on one cassette):
  - The X-ray beam is centred on the costal arch for images of the cranial abdomen and collimated to include the cranial limit of the diaphragm

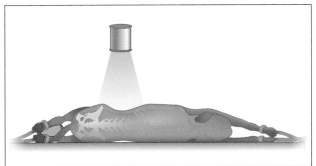

6.1 Patient positioning for a right lateral view of the abdomen.

- The X-ray beam is centred midway between the last rib and pelvic inlet for images of the caudal abdomen and collimated to include the greater trochanter of the femur caudally.
- For lower urinary tract studies:
  - The X-ray beam is centred on the bladder just cranial to the pelvic inlet. Collimation includes the perineum and penis (in male dogs) and perineum and vulva (in female dogs) to ensure that the entire urethra is included on the image
  - A separate film (with higher exposure factors) may be needed for the pelvic canal when using conventional radiography.

A lateral recumbent view with the hindlimbs drawn cranially is used to evaluate the lower urinary tract in male dogs as it allows assessment of the full length of the urethra without superimposition of the femurs.

- The patient is positioned as for a standard lateral view, but the hindlimbs are drawn cranially against the ventral body wall (Figure 6.2).
- The X-ray beam is centred at the level of the greater trochanter and collimated to include the entire perineal area.

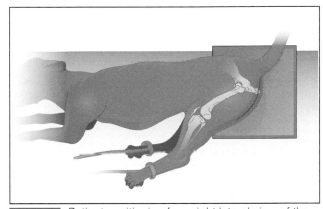

6.2 Patient positioning for a right lateral view of the abdomen with the hindlimbs pulled cranially to facilitate evaluation of the urethra in a male dog.

Ventrodorsal view

The VD view is preferred to the dorsoventral (DV) view as the abdominal contents tend to 'spread out' with the patient in dorsal recumbency. Thus, there is less superimposition of the abdominal structures and a reduction in soft tissue depth, resulting in less scatter.

- The patient is supported in dorsal recumbency using a radiolucent trough or foam wedges and sandbags (Figure 6.3).
- The lumbar and thoracic vertebrae are kept straight so that the sternebrae are superimposed on the vertebrae, avoiding axial rotation.
- The hindlimbs are, preferably, allowed to fall into a neutral ('frog-legged') position, which minimizes superimposition of skin folds on the caudal abdomen. Foam pads are placed to support the pelvis and prevent axial rotation in larger dogs.
- The X-ray beam is centred on the umbilicus and collimated to include the diaphragm cranially (2–3 ribs cranial to the xiphisternum), the greater trochanters of the femurs caudally and the skin edges laterally.

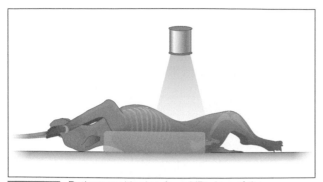

6.3 Patient positioning for a VD view of the abdomen.

Additional radiographic views

Occasionally, additional views may be of value for assessing the abdomen, particularly when evaluating the gastrointestinal and urinary tracts.

Dorsoventral view

The DV view may be useful for evaluating the gastro-intestinal tract, as the redistribution of gas and fluid may allow previously occult lesions to be identified. A DV view is most commonly obtained as part of a barium gastrogram.

- The animal is positioned in sternal recumbency with the forelimbs slightly abducted and the elbows flexed to stabilize the thorax. A radiolucent trough or foam wedges supported by sandbags may be necessary for narrow-chested patients.
- The hindlimbs are drawn caudally and laterally away from the abdomen (if possible) and secured using sandbags. If this is not possible (e.g. in a conscious or arthritic animal), the hindlimbs are flexed so that the animal is in a crouching position. The distal limbs are drawn slightly away from the abdominal wall to avoid superimposition on the abdomen.
- The lumbar and thoracic vertebrae should form a straight line and the vertebrae must be superimposed on the sternebrae.
- The X-ray beam is centred and collimated as for a VD view.

Lateral oblique views

The midline location of the bladder and urethra may limit assessment of the lower urinary tract on a stand-ard VD view due to superimposition of the pelvis on the caudal abdominal structures. Thus, right lateroventral–left laterodorsal oblique (RtLV-LeLDO) and left lateroventral–right laterodorsal oblique (LeLV-RtLDO) views are occasionally useful to evaluate the terminal ureters when performing intravenous uro-graphy. The right ureter is seen ventral to the vertebral column on a LeLV-RtLDO view, and the left ureter is visible ventral to the spine on a RtLV-LeLDO view.

- The animal is positioned in lateral recumbency (i.e. on its right side for a LeLV-RtLDO view and on its left side for a RtLV-LeLDO view). The sternum is elevated using a foam wedge so that the axis of the abdomen is rotated by 30–45 degrees.
- The uppermost hindlimb is abducted using a sandbag or tie.

- The X-ray beam is centred and collimated as for the standard lateral view.

Lesion-oriented oblique views

Lesion-oriented oblique views are also occasionally useful to highlight external swellings or masses.

Horizontal beam decubitus view

The main clinical indication for a horizontal beam decubitus view is to detect small volumes of free abdominal gas, which typically collects at the highest point of the abdomen beneath the non-dependent ribs with the animal positioned in lateral recumbency (Figure 6.4).

- A horizontal X-ray beam is used. Local Rules (see Chapter 2) must be reviewed to establish whether horizontal beam radiography is permitted. Extra care should be taken with regard to radiation safety to ensure that no personnel are exposed to the horizontally directed X-ray beam.
- The animal is positioned in left lateral recumbency.
- The cassette is supported against the patient's thoracolumbar spine, perpendicular to the horizontally directed X-ray beam, using sandbags or wedges.
- The X-ray beam is centred just caudal to the costal arch on the ventral midline of the abdomen and collimated to include the skin margins, and should include the highest point of the abdomen beneath the uppermost ribs, where the free gas is likely to collect.

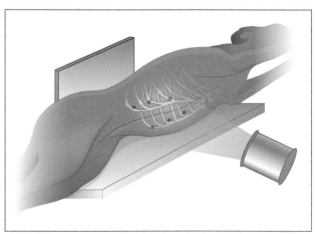

6.4 Patient positioning for a horizontal beam decubitus view of the abdomen with the animal in left lateral recumbency.

Film–screen combinations

For radiographic imaging of the abdomen, a medium speed film–screen combination is suitable for most animals. Large cassettes are preferable to enable the entire abdomen to be included on one image. The abdomen of most dogs can be included on a 35 x 43 cm cassette/detector plate, although for some giant breeds separate exposures may be required for the cranial and caudal abdomen.

Radiographic exposure

As the abdomen has inherently low contrast, a low kil-ovoltage (kV) and high milliampere second (mAs) technique should be used. The effect of scatter is minimized by using a grid for obese animals and where the depth of tissue to be imaged is >10 cm. With analogue film, it may not be possible to obtain a diagnostic exposure of the cranial and caudal abdomen on the same film if there are large differences in tissue thickness. Separate images are then required. Radiographs should be taken at the end of expiration, as the expiratory pause minimizes movement blur and the increased abdominal volume during expiration reduces superimposition of the abdominal viscera.

Value of radiography

Gastrointestinal disease

- Radiography is often of value for demonstrating suspected gastrointestinal obstruction, although the cause may not be apparent.
- It is useful for screening for gastrointestinal foreign bodies as almost all radiopaque, and many radiolucent, foreign bodies are visible on plain radiographs.
- It is the technique of choice when assessing for gastric dilatation and volvulus (GDV) as it allows volvulus to be differentiated from simple dilatation.
- It is the technique of choice for identifying free abdominal gas secondary to rupture of the gastrointestinal tract.
- It can be used to investigate the possible aetiology of tenesmus and dyschezia.
- It provides a screening assessment of the abdominal contents and landmarks prior to ultrasonography.
- It is useful for demonstrating gastrointestinal involvement in hernias and ruptures.
- It is often of limited value in the investigation of diarrhoea, unless the cause is related to an obstructive intestinal mass. Abdominal ultrasonography and/or endoscopy are more useful than radiography for evaluating patients with diarrhoea.
- Gastrointestinal contrast studies may be required to provide additional information on the location and wall thickness of gastrointestinal structures, and to demonstrate whether an obstruction is present as well the possible causes of any obstruction. However, gastrointestinal contrast studies have largely been replaced by ultrasonography.
- Contrast radiography is often of limited value for quantifying gastrointestinal function.

Urogenital disease

- Ultrasonography is the modality of choice for the initial investigation of most urogenital disorders (other than urethral disease) but plain radiography is useful for evaluating the number, size, shape and opacity of the kidneys and the size, shape, opacity and location of the urinary bladder. For many urogenital conditions, contrast studies are required (see Chapter 4).
- In animals that present with dysuria, stranguria and/or haematuria:
    - Plain radiography is relatively accurate for detecting radiopaque renal, ureteric, bladder and urethral calculi and allows assessment of the size, shape and number of calculi (more accurate than ultrasonography)
    - Contrast studies (e.g. pneumocystography, positive- and double-contrast cystography and positive-contrast retrograde urography) of the lower urinary tract are required to identify radiolucent bladder and urethral calculi, to evaluate the thickness and internal surface of the bladder wall, to identify any mural mass lesions, and to evaluate the appearance and location of the urethra. Ultrasonography of the bladder is a valuable technique; however, ultrasonographic evaluation of the intrapelvic urethra is precluded by the surrounding skeletal structures and positive-contrast retrograde urography is recommended as the initial imaging technique for urethral assessment
    - Plain radiography allows identification of prostatomegaly, but differentiation of the cause is often not possible. Ultrasonography is preferable in most cases as it provides further information about the internal prostatic architecture and can be used to guide fine-needle aspiration or biopsy, or a prostatic wash.
    - In animals where haematuria arises from the kidneys or ureters, intravenous urography and ultrasonography can both provide additional information about renal architecture. Intravenous urography, in particular, is valuable in demonstrating the size and location of the ureters.
- In animals that present with incontinence:
    - Plain radiography alone is rarely diagnostic and, in most cases, ultrasonography and/or contrast radiography is required to diagnose the cause of the incontinence
    - Intravenous urography, in combination with pneumocystography and retrograde urethrography, allows the ureters to be evaluated in animals where the ureter is suspected to terminate in an abnormal (ectopic) location. Lateral, VD and oblique (occasionally) views may be required to visualize ureteric terminations. Retrograde urethrography often demonstrates retrograde filling of ectopic ureters (see Figure 4.5). Ultrasonography is generally a more useful and less invasive technique for the evaluation of the kidneys and bladder lumen, and in experienced hands may also be used to identify ectopic ureters.
- In animals that present with anuria, an initial radiographic evaluation is important for identifying gross renal abnormalities, indirect signs of urinary tract rupture (abdominal or retroperitoneal effusion and loss of visualization of normal bladder/kidney) and some causes of lower urinary tract obstruction. The use of intravenous contrast media is contraindicated until acute anuric patients have been stabilized and rehydrated. Positive-contrast retrograde cystography is required to demonstrate bladder rupture.
- Polyuria is a non-specific clinical sign, and although abdominal radiography may be of limited diagnostic value, it allows animals to be assessed

for radiographic changes that could indicate a non-renal cause of the polyuria (such as pyometra). On occasion, it will provide valuable information.

- In animals that present with vaginal discharge, plain radiography can be useful to identify moderate to severe uterine enlargement.
- For the diagnosis of pregnancy:
  - Ultrasonography allows an earlier definitive diagnosis to be reached (by 28 days) and a better assessment of fetal viability to be made
  - Following fetal mineralization (from 35 days in the queen and from 41 days in the bitch), fetal numbers are more accurately predicted using radiography
  - Following parturition, radiography is a reliable technique to detect any retained fetuses.

Non-specific abdominal disease

- Radiography is valuable for differentiating a genuine mass lesion from normal structures (such as faecal material) and for determining the general location, and often the organ of origin, of a palpable mass.
- It is valuable for differentiating abdominal enlargement due to an abdominal mass, organomegaly or weak abdominal musculature from the presence of free fluid.
- It may allow the possible cause of a painful abdomen (e.g. acute intestinal obstruction, pancreatitis, peritonitis or trauma) to be characterized.
- It is used to screen the abdomen for abnormalities in animals presenting with vague clinical signs such as anorexia, weight loss and pyrexia, although the diagnostic yield is often low.
- It is useful for demonstrating disruption of the body wall or diaphragm and displacement of abdominal viscera in cases with suspected umbilical, inguinal, perineal or pericardioperitoneo-diaphragmatic hernias or with suspected diaphragmatic or body wall ruptures.
- It may help identify occult mass lesions in animals that are too large or too tense for accurate abdominal palpation.
- Although ultrasonography can provide valuable information about the internal architecture of an abdominal mass, radiography can provide an overview of the location of a mass and its relationship with the surrounding organs.
- The presence of a large volume of free abdominal fluid may make it impossible to differentiate between organs and viscera within the peritoneal cavity on radiography, although a mass effect may be appreciated by the displacement of gas-filled intestinal loops. In such cases, an ultrasonographic examination is recommended.
- The administration of contrast medium orally can be useful to demonstrate the position of the stomach and intestines. This may be important when inferring the position and shape of the liver in cases with suspected hepatomegaly, hepatic masses or jaundice, or when confirming the abnormal location of the gastrointestinal tract in cases with suspected diaphragmatic ruptures or hernias (see Figure 3.23).

Contrast studies

In the abdomen, there is limited or no contrast between the soft tissue organs. Thus, the fluid contents of the viscera of the gastrointestinal tract and urinary system cannot be distinguished from the soft tissue opacity of the surrounding walls. Contrast media are used to visualize and differentiate these soft tissues from one another (see Chapter 4).

Abdominal contrast studies that can be performed include:

- Gastrointestinal studies:
  - Barium swallow to evaluate the oesophagus (frequently used; best used in conjunction with fluoroscopy)
  - Positive- and negative-contrast gastrography (infrequently used)
  - Positive-contrast barium follow-through (increasingly infrequently used)
  - Positive- and negative-contrast colonography (rarely used).
- Urogenital studies:
  - Intravenous urography (frequently used)
  - Positive-, negative- and double-contrast cystography (frequently used)
  - Positive-contrast retrograde urethrography/vaginourethrography (frequently used).
- Miscellaneous studies:
  - Mesenteric portovenography (infrequently used).

Contrast studies of the abdomen, especially of the gastrointestinal tract, are often poorly performed which limits their diagnostic usefulness. Common problems encountered include:

- Administration of an insufficient volume of contrast media
- Insufficient number of radiographic views obtained
- Failure to obtain a 24-hour 'follow-up' lateral and/or VD radiograph after a barium follow-through study.

The increased availability of endoscopy and ultrasonography in general veterinary practice in recent years has significantly reduced the frequency with which radiographic contrast studies are performed.

Abdominal radiography *versus* ultrasonography – why use both?

- Intestinal foreign body – loops of gas-filled intestine are easily appreciated on radiographs, but can limit a thorough ultrasonographic examination. In cases of acute obstruction with multiple gas-filled intestinal loops or a radiopaque foreign body, a radiographic examination may well provide a rapid diagnosis without the need for ultrasonography.
- Diarrhoea – gastrointestinal wall thickening and abnormal motility in patients with diarrhoea cannot be assessed on survey radiographs but are readily evaluated using ultrasonography.
- Palpable abdominal mass – the general location of an abdominal mass is often easier to appreciate on a radiograph, but ▶

- determining the organ of origin may require ultrasonography.
- ■ Suspected abdominal fluid – free abdominal fluid results in loss of abdominal detail, limiting the information that can be derived from radiography. Free fluid allows excellent transmission of sound waves, generally facilitating ultrasonography.
- ■ Pregnancy diagnosis – pregnancy is detected earlier using ultrasonography and fetal viability can be assessed. Radiography provides a more accurate assessment of fetal numbers and can detect a retained fetus post-partum.
- ■ Neoplasia – any suspicion of neoplasia is an indication for thoracic radiography to assess for pulmonary metastases.
- ■ Guided biopsy – many lesions seen on radiography are non-specific and a definitive diagnosis requires histopathological or cytological evaluation. Image-guided biopsy of lesions is usually straightforward with ultrasonography.

Radiological interpretation

The interpretation of abdominal radiographs requires a logical approach and a good knowledge of normal, and variations in, radiographic anatomy. The order in which the different structures are evaluated is not critical, but a consistent and logical approach is important.

Normal anatomy

The abdomen is bounded by the diaphragm cranially, the muscles of the body wall ventrally and laterally, the pelvic inlet caudally, and the paraspinal muscles and spine dorsally (Figures 6.5 to 6.7). The main source of contrast within the abdomen is fat between the viscera. Other than the lumen of the gastrointestinal tract, the normal abdominal organs are of soft tissue or fluid opacity. There is quite marked variation in the normal abdominal radiological appearance due to age, breed, body condition, the effect of sedation and the diet of the animal. Conformational differences mainly affect the appearance of the liver and gastrointestinal tract. Deep-chested dogs (e.g. Dobermanns) have

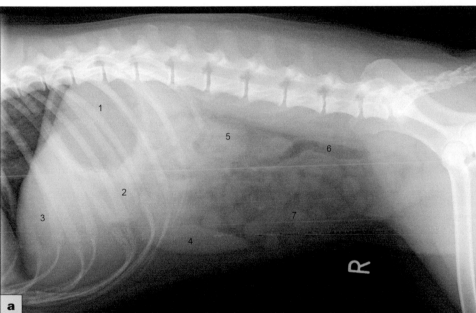

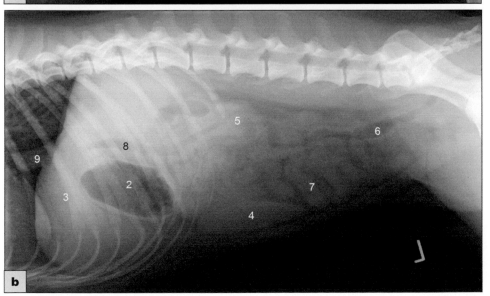

6.5 (a) Right and (b) left lateral views of the normal canine abdomen. 1 = gastric fundus and body of the stomach; 2 = pylorus (fluid-filled on right lateral view; gas-filled on left lateral view); 3 = liver; 4 = spleen (tail); 5 = left kidney (caudal pole); 6 = descending colon; 7 = small intestine; 8 = descending duodenum; 9 = caudal vena cava. (Courtesy of the University of Bristol)

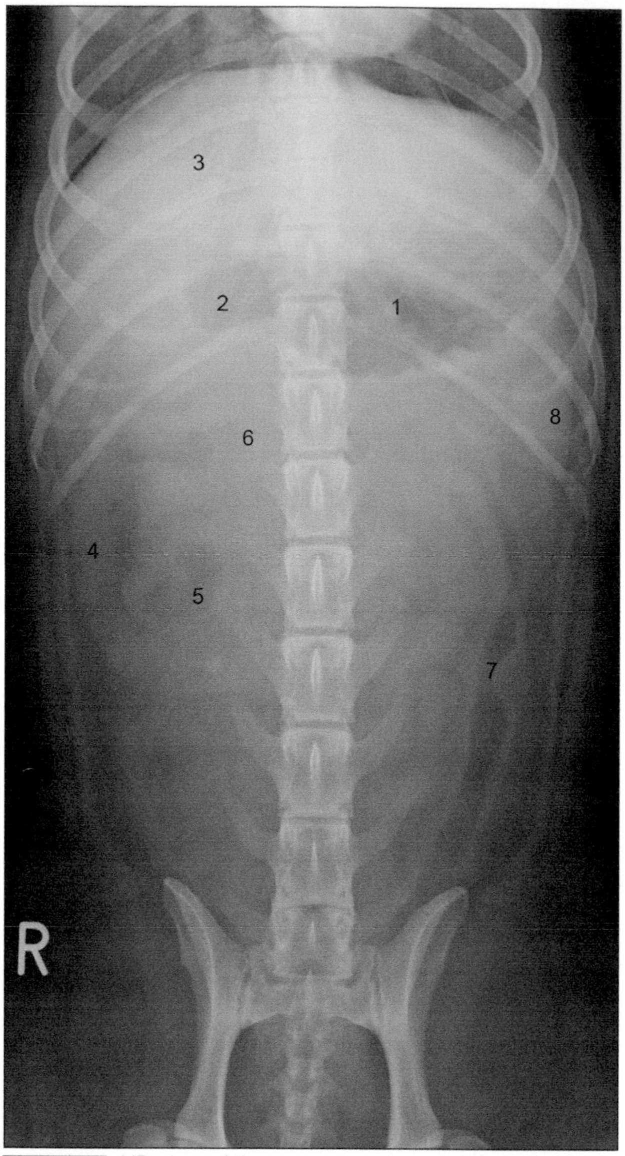

6.6 VD view of the normal canine abdomen (same patient as in Figure 6.5). 1 = body of the stomach; 2 = pylorus; 3 = liver; 4 = descending duodenum; 5 = caecum; 6 = transverse colon; 7 = descending colon; 8 = spleen (head). (Courtesy of the University of Bristol)

subjectively smaller livers compared with breeds of other body conformations because the liver is contained within the costal arch. In very young animals, and in patients where there is caudal displacement of the diaphragm (e.g. with a large volume of pleural fluid), the liver often appears subjectively large. The appearance of the solid parenchymal organs is relatively consistent (although haemodynamic factors may affect the size of the liver and spleen) but with the hollow viscera, normal physiological variation results in a range of different sizes and appearance. In obese cats, there are large focal deposits of fat within the falciform ligament, the inguinal region and the dorsal abdomen/retroperitoneum, and the small intestine may appear clumped in the mid-right side of the abdomen. In animals with little abdominal fat, serosal detail is reduced and should not be mistaken for ascites.

Gastrointestinal tract

The appearance of the gastrointestinal tract (size, shape and opacity) varies markedly due to normal physiological variations and the diet of the animal. The diet of the animal should also be considered when assessing the luminal contents, especially when determining the significance of mineralized material located within the gastrointestinal tract.

Stomach:

- The stomach is located in the cranial abdomen, immediately caudal to the liver and cranial to the transverse colon, and is usually contained within the margins of the ribcage.
- The oesophagus passes through the right crus of the diaphragm and enters the stomach at the level of the cardia.
- The largest part of the stomach comprises the fundus and body and lies to the left of the midline.
  - The fundus is a blind sac which is located dorsal to the cardia.
  - The body extends from the cardia to the ventral angle of the stomach.
  - In right lateral recumbency, gas typically rises to the highest point within the fundus and body.
  - In sternal recumbency, gas rises into the fundus.

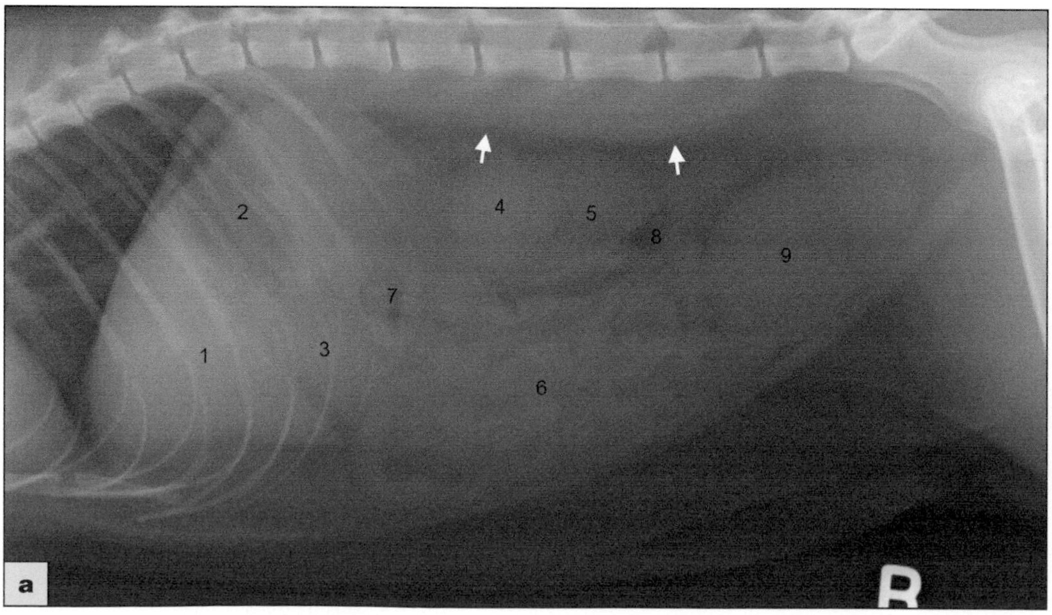

6.7 **(a)** Right lateral view of the normal feline abdomen. The large lumbar muscles in the cat are recognized as sharply defined soft tissue bands (arrowed) ventral to the vertebral column. 1 = liver; 2 = gastric fundus and body of the stomach; 3 = pylorus; 4 = right kidney; 5 = left kidney; 6 = small intestine; 7 = transverse colon; 8 = descending colon; 9 = bladder. (continues) ▶

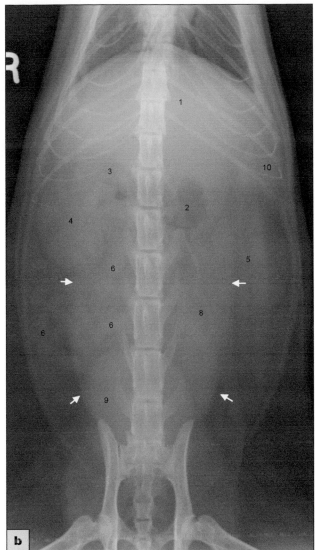

6.7 (continued) **(b)** VD view of the normal feline abdomen. The large lumbar muscles in the cat are recognized as sharply defined soft tissue bands (arrowed) on both sides of the vertebral column. 1 = liver; 2 = gastric fundus and body of the stomach; 3 = pylorus; 4 = right kidney; 5 = left kidney; 6 = small intestine; 7 = transverse colon; 8 = descending colon; 9 = bladder; 10 = spleen (head).

- The pylorus (consisting of the pyloric antrum and pyloric canal) is located ventrally, usually just cranial to the body, and to the right of the midline (dogs) or approximately on the midline (cats).
  - Typically, the pylorus contains gas when the animal is placed in dorsal or left lateral recumbency (see Figure 4.31).
  - When the animal is placed in right lateral recumbency, the pylorus is typically fluid-filled and appears as a round soft tissue opacity, which should not be mistaken for a mass or gastric foreign body.
  - The pylorus moves further to the right when the stomach is full (especially in the cat).
- The cardia is relatively fixed in position. The remainder of the stomach is attached cranially to the liver by the lesser omentum and caudally it is connected to the greater omentum, part of which is thickened to form the gastrosplenic ligament and attaches to the splenic head. The potential for displacement of the stomach is therefore fairly limited, but its location can be influenced by changes in the adjacent organs (liver, spleen, pancreas and diaphragm).
- The gastric axis is an imaginary line through the body and pylorus, recognized by gas in the lumen.
  - The axis is usually approximately parallel to the ribs on the lateral view and perpendicular to the spine on the VD view.
  - Where displacement is suspected, but the stomach lumen is not readily seen, a small amount of contrast medium can be administered to confirm the position of the stomach.
- The amount of fluid, ingesta and gas within the stomach lumen influences the size and shape of the normal stomach. In the majority of normal patients, after food has been withheld for 12 hours, the stomach should contain only a small volume of fluid and gas.
  - Occasionally, it may not be possible to identify a completely empty stomach.
  - An enlarged stomach may contain gas, solid food or liquid, and often a mixture of the three.
  - The enlarged gastric shadow is often rounded and bulges caudally beyond the costal arch.
  - Unless there is gastric torsion, the fundus and pylorus should retain their normal positions in the left dorsal (fundus) and right ventral (pylorus) aspects of the cranial abdomen.
- Rugal folds may be recognized as approximately parallel soft tissue ridges within the stomach lumen, highlighted by intraluminal gas.
- In obese cats, the presence of fat within the submucosal layer of the stomach wall may be seen radiographically as a linear area of relative lucency parallel to the luminal surface.

Small intestine:

- The small intestine comprises the duodenum, jejunum and ileum.
- It occupies most of the mid-ventral abdomen caudal to the stomach and cranial to the bladder, on a lateral radiograph.
- Intestinal loops appear as smoothly curving 'tubes' in long axis, and circular or ring-shaped opacities in cross-section. The loops should be evenly distributed and of roughly uniform diameter and are always narrower than the large bowel.
  - Dogs – the loops should be no greater than twice the width of the twelfth rib and no greater than the height of the body of the fifth lumbar vertebra.
  - Cats – the loops should be no greater than 12 mm.
  - No loop should be more than twice the diameter of any other loop.
- Peristaltic waves may be recognized on survey radiographs as transient segmental narrowing of the intestines.
- Small intestine gathered in the central abdomen of obese cats and some deep-chested dogs may mimic disease.
- The cranial duodenal flexure lies cranial and slightly dorsal to the pylorus.
- The descending duodenum extends caudodorsally from the pylorus, ventral to the mid-lumbar vertebrae and right kidney, and

adjacent to the right body wall, before curving medially at the caudal duodenal flexure.
- The jejunum and proximal ileum are radiologically indistinguishable from each other on survey radiographs.
- In the dog, the terminal ileum may be recognized at the ileocaecocolic junction by the caecum (normally gas-filled), which is located to the right of the midline at the level of L3–L4.
- In the fasted animal, the small intestine contains a mixture of fluid and gas, but in animals with aerophagia gas may be present throughout the gastrointestinal tract.
  - In the dog, intestinal contents are typically 30–60% gas.
  - In the cat, there is usually very little gas in the intestine.
- The serosal surface of the intestine is usually visible, provided there is sufficient abdominal fat.
- Small intestinal wall thickness cannot be assessed on plain radiographs because the soft tissue opacity of the wall is indistinguishable from fluid in the lumen.

Large intestine:

- The large intestine comprises the caecum, the ascending, transverse and descending colon, and the rectum.
- The caecum is located to the right of the midline at the level of L3–L4.
  - In the dog, the caecum usually contains gas.
  - In the cat, the caecum is small and usually not identifiable on radiographs.
- The ascending colon extends cranially in the mid-abdomen from the ileocaecocolic junction to the right of the midline and medial to the duodenum.
- The transverse colon crosses from right to left immediately caudal to the stomach.
- The descending colon extends caudally in the left mid-dorsal abdomen to the pelvic inlet.
- The colon beyond the pelvic inlet is termed the rectum.
- Although the large intestine is more consistent in position than the small intestine, some normal variations are recognized.
  - 'Redundant' colon, characterized by apparently excessive length and/or extra bends in the descending colon, can be a normal finding in large-breed dogs and obese cats. In this instance, the descending colon may have a more tortuous course or may be seen to the right of the midline.
- The colon and rectum are normally filled with varying amounts of heterogeneous faecal material and gas. Normal faecal material has a granular appearance of mixed gas, soft tissue and mineralized opacity.
- The normal size of the colon in dogs has been reported to be no greater than three times the small intestinal diameter, and not more than one and a half times the length of the seventh lumbar vertebra. In the cat, the normal colon diameter has been reported as less than 1.3 times the length of the L5 vertebra. However, it should be noted that colon size is variable and these objective measurements are rarely applied.

Liver

- The liver is recognized as a homogeneous soft tissue organ within the cranial abdomen. It merges with the caudal aspect of the diaphragm and gallbladder to create the hepatic silhouette.
- The hepatic silhouette lies almost entirely within the costal arch.
  - Cranially, the hepatic silhouette is demarcated by the line of the diaphragm.
  - Caudally, the hepatic silhouette is demarcated by the stomach.
  - The gastric axis should lie approximately parallel to the ribs on the lateral view and perpendicular to the spine on the VD view.
  - The ventral hepatic margin is usually defined by the adjacent falciform fat, especially in cats.
- On the lateral view, the caudoventral border should be well defined with a sharp angle.
  - The caudoventral border is completely contained within the costal arch in deep-chested dog breeds.
  - The caudoventral border protrudes slightly further caudally in barrel-chested dog breeds.
  - The liver appears relatively larger in young animals than in adults and may protrude beyond the costal arch.
  - The caudoventral angle of the liver also extends slightly further caudally when the patient is in right lateral recumbency compared with left lateral recumbency.
- On the VD view, the caudal margin is usually poorly demarcated.
- The liver consists of six lobes (left medial, left lateral, right medial, right lateral, quadrate and caudate lobes) and a gallbladder.
  - The liver lobes cannot usually be identified individually on radiographs, but in obese animals separation of the ventral aspect of the lobes may be seen on lateral views.
  - In cats, the gallbladder is occasionally recognized as a rounded soft tissue structure, extending ventrally beyond the liver margin.
- Assessment of liver size is subjective and often unreliable unless the increase or decrease in size is severe. Alterations in margination are often a more sensitive indicator of hepatic pathology than size alterations.

Spleen

- The spleen is recognized as a homogeneous soft tissue organ, which is relatively larger in the dog than in the cat. The normal spleen is of soft tissue opacity. As radiographic opacity is dependent on both the density and thickness of the structure being imaged, the opacity of the normal spleen may appear increased where it is folded (see Figure 3.27).
- The normal spleen is a smoothly marginated, elongated, tongue-shaped organ consisting of a head, body and tail.
- The head of the spleen is most reliably recognized on the VD view as a triangular soft tissue opacity adjacent to the left body wall, caudal to the fundus and craniolateral to the left kidney in both the dog and cat. It may lie within, or caudal to, the costal arch.

- The location of the head of the spleen should be consistent as it is anchored to the stomach by the gastrosplenic ligament.
- The splenic head can be difficult to identify on a lateral view, especially in dogs, as it silhouettes with the soft tissue opacities of the adjacent liver, stomach and left kidney.
- The body and tail of the spleen are relatively mobile. They usually extend ventrally along the left body wall and, depending on the size of the spleen, may extend across the mid-ventral abdomen to the right side. In the dog, the tail of the spleen is often recognized on the right lateral view as a triangular soft tissue opacity in the mid-ventral abdomen, extending along the ventral body wall. As its position is variable, the splenic tail may be located anywhere between the caudoventral margin of the liver and the apex of the urinary bladder. The splenic tail is not always seen on a left lateral view, and is less commonly seen in the cat. The position of the splenic tail is much more variable than that of the splenic head.
- The range of normal splenic size in the dog is wide, and the spleen is larger in sedated or anaesthetized animals. The spleen in German Shepherd Dogs and Greyhounds is especially large.
- Cats typically have more perirenal fat, making it easier to see the splenic head as a separate soft tissue opacity on the lateral view.

Pancreas

- The normal pancreas (Figure 6.8) comprises a left limb (which lies between the caudal aspect of the stomach and transverse colon), a body (which lies on the caudal aspect of the pyloroduodenal junction) and a right limb (which lies ventromedial to the descending duodenum).
- The normal pancreas is too small to be visible on radiography, so any displacement due to changes in adjacent organs will not be recognized.

Adrenal glands

- The normal adrenal glands are small retroperitoneal structures that lie either side of the aorta, craniomedial to the hilar area of their respective kidneys.
- The normal adrenal glands are <1 cm in cross-section in the dog, and usually <0.5 cm in the cat. Thus, they are too small to be seen radiographically, unless they are mineralized. Mineralization of the adrenal glands is an occasional incidental finding in older cats.

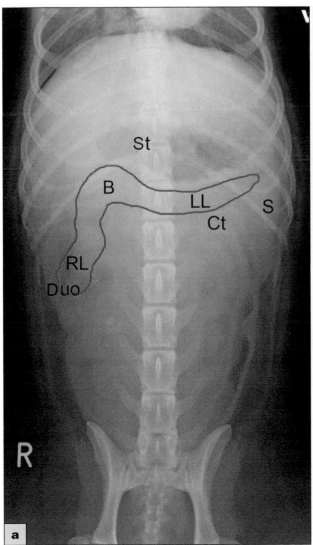

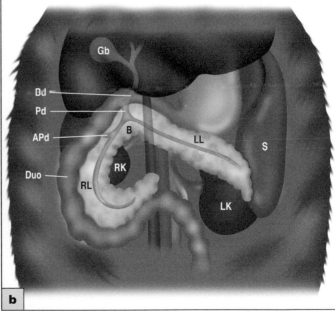

6.8 **(a–b)** The pancreas and its associated anatomical landmarks. The pancreas is V-shaped: the body (B) lies to the left of the pyloroduodenal angle with the left (LL) and right (RL) lobes extending caudal to the body of the stomach (St) and medial to the descending duodenum (Duo), respectively. The accessory pancreatic duct (APd) is the primary excretory duct in dogs and terminates at the minor duodenal papilla. The pancreatic duct (Pd) is the main excretory duct in cats and terminates at the major duodenal papilla together with the common bile duct (Bd). Gb = gallbladder; LK = left kidney; RK = right kidney; S = spleen.

Urinary tract

The appearance of the urinary tract is relatively consistent with little variation other than in bladder size.

Kidneys:

■ The kidneys are paired soft tissue retroperitoneal organs in the mid-dorsal abdomen, which are best assessed on the VD view.
■ The kidneys should be approximately equal in size.
■ Care must be taken not to mistake superimposition of the caudal pole of the right kidney and cranial pole of the left kidney for a single small kidney on the lateral view. Where the kidneys overlap, the increased depth of the superimposed soft tissues is seen as an increase in opacity.
■ On the VD view, superimposition of the nipples may appear as a focal area of increased opacity (especially in bitches) and should not be mistaken for a calculus.
■ In the dog:
  • Normal kidneys are smoothly marginated and bean-shaped with an indentation at the renal hilus on the VD view. On the lateral view, the dependent kidney is usually ellipsoid in shape with the non-dependent kidney appearing bean-shaped
  • Normal renal length is 2.5–3.5 times the length of L2 (assessed on the VD view)
  • The separation of the kidneys is more obvious on the right lateral rather than left lateral view
  • Right kidney:
    – Located at approximately the level of T12–L1
    – Cranially contacts the caudate lobe of the liver
    – Often poorly visualized due to its cranial location. Typically superimposed on the fundus of the stomach and head of the spleen on the lateral view
    – May not be seen as a separate structure on the VD view due to border effacement of the cranial pole with the liver.
  • Left kidney:
    – Usually located slightly more caudally and ventrally than the right kidney
    – May appear almost mid-abdomen in location in large dogs.
■ In the cat:
  • The kidneys tend to be more oval in shape and usually more clearly marginated than in dogs
  • The kidneys are superimposed more frequently and more caudally positioned than in dogs
  • Fat opacity within the renal pelvis is a normal finding and is most likely to be seen in obese cats on the VD view
  • The cranial pole of the right kidney is often separated from the liver by fat and is therefore easier to see than in the dog
  • Normal renal length (assessed on the VD view) (Figure 6.9):
    – Neutered cat: 1.9–2.6 times the length of L2
    – Entire cat: 2.1–3.2 times the length of L2.

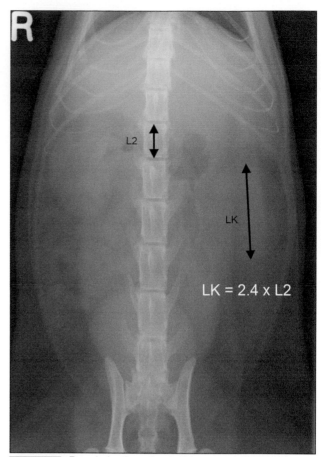

6.9 Renal size is estimated by comparing renal length with the length of L2 on the VD view. In the cat, normal renal length is 1.9–2.6 times the length of L2. In this case, the left kidney (LK) is 2.4 times the length of L2.

Ureters:

■ The ureters run caudally through the retroperitoneal space and terminate at the trigone of the bladder.
■ Ectopic ureters terminate in an abnormal location, most commonly the urethra, but occasionally the vagina or rectum.
■ Although the ureters are surrounded by retroperitoneal fat, they are too small to be visualized on plain radiographs unless they are markedly dilated.
■ In obese dogs, retroperitoneal fat outlining the fascial planes results in linear soft tissue opacities which should not be mistaken for the ureters.

Bladder:

■ The bladder is recognized as a homogeneous soft tissue opacity within the caudoventral abdomen. The trigone of the bladder and urethra are located within the retroperitoneum.
■ The bladder usually lies approximately on the midline on the VD view.
■ The only fixed point is at the bladder neck, hence the bladder is easily displaced by changes in adjacent structures.
■ In most cats, the entire bladder lies cranial to the pelvic inlet. The bladder neck is longer in cats than in dogs.

- In dogs, the bladder is typically an ovoid or pear shape and tends to lie slightly further caudally compared with the cat. In some dogs, especially bitches, the bladder neck may be intrapelvic.
- The size of the normal bladder varies markedly and a subjective assessment should be made, taking into account the opportunities for filling (availability of drinking water, intravenous fluids) and emptying the bladder at the time of radiography.
- In most dogs and cats, the serosal surface of the bladder is highlighted by fat within the surrounding mesentery and can be easily visualized.

Urethra:

- The urethra is not normally visible on survey radiographs.
- The urethra extends from the bladder neck to the external urethral orifice.
- In the dog:
  - The female urethra is typically fairly short and relatively wide, joining the vestibule just caudal to the vestibular–vaginal junction
  - The male urethra is much longer and consists of an intrapelvic, a perineal and a penile section.
- In the cat:
  - The anatomy of the female urethra is similar to that of the bitch
  - The tom cat has a perineal penis and a relatively narrow urethra.

Male reproductive tract

- The male genital system comprises a prostate gland, paired testicles and a penis.
- The canine penis is recognized by the presence of the os penis.
- The perineal penis of the cat is usually not visible on radiography.

Prostate gland:

- In the dog:
  - The prostate gland is located within the caudal retroperitoneum, caudal to the bladder neck, surrounding the proximal urethra and ventral to the descending colon/rectum
  - Depending on its size and the degree of bladder distension, the prostate gland may be seen within the abdomen just cranial to the pelvic brim, or may be intrapelvic and not radiographically visible. The prostate gland moves cranially as the bladder distends
  - In the entire dog, the prostate gland appears as a homogeneous, rounded, soft tissue opacity. The length and height of the prostate gland should occupy <70% of the diameter of the pelvic inlet on lateral radiographs
  - In neutered dogs, the prostate gland is smaller compared with entire dogs and often not radiographically visible.
- In the cat, the prostate gland is located more caudally and is smaller compared with the dog, and is not radiographically visible.

Testicles:

- The testicles are contained within the scrotum and are located outside the abdomen in the perineal region.
- The testicles of an entire male dog may be recognized caudal to the pelvis, as a bilobed, soft tissue opacity at the caudal periphery of the image or highlighted by scatter radiation.

Female reproductive tract

The normal non-gravid uterus and ovaries are not radiographically visible.

Other structures

The normal abdominal lymph nodes, lymphatic vessels and the portal vein are not radiographically visible.

Röntgen signs

Size

- Several organs can undergo considerable physiological distension, including the stomach, uterus and bladder (Figure 6.10).
- For other organs such as the liver and kidneys, a radiographically apparent increase or decrease in size may be a significant finding.
- Alterations in size (particularly of the liver and spleen) often need to be severe to be reliably detected.
- Changes in size may be recognized by:
  - Comparing the size of the organ to that of another structure (e.g. assessing renal size in relation to the length of the second lumbar vertebral body)
  - Assessing the extent of the organ in comparison with a relatively fixed landmark (e.g. assessing liver size by evaluating the location of the caudoventral hepatic margin relative to the costal arch)

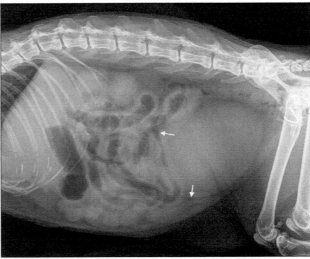

| 6.10 | Röntgen sign: size. Physiological distension of several organs, such as the stomach, bladder |

and uterus (due to pregnancy), can be substantial and should not be mistaken for disease. Pain may lead to delayed gastric emptying or reluctance to defecate or void urine. Physiological distension results in the displacement of other abdominal structures, especially small intestinal loops, as in this example of a dog with bladder distension (arrowed) due to urethral obstruction.

- Identifying changes in organ shape suggestive of enlargement (e.g. rounding of the caudoventral hepatic margin of an enlarged liver)
- Failing to identify structures that are normally visible, resulting in an 'empty' appearance to an area of the abdomen (e.g. displacement of the stomach into the thorax associated with a diaphragmatic or hiatal hernia) (Figure 6.11)
- Identifying the presence of a structure which is not normally radiographically visible (e.g. an enlarged uterus)
- Assessing the margins of the body wall, taking into account breed conformation and intra-abdominal fat deposits. Abdominal distension due to fluid (Figure 6.12a), masses or intra-abdominal fat results in a pendulous appearance to the ventral abdominal wall. A 'tucked up' appearance, by comparison, may be due to emaciation (Figure 6.12b), breed conformation (deep-chested breeds) or abdominal discomfort.

Shape

Alterations in the shape of an organ are frequently a more sensitive indicator of disease than alterations in size. A change in size often has to be marked to be reliably detected on radiographs. Changes in shape may occur due to:

- Physiological enlargement (e.g. as the stomach and uterus distend, they also change in shape)
- Pathological enlargement (e.g. rounding of the caudoventral hepatic margin in an enlarged liver or alteration of the renal margin with enlarged kidneys) (Figure 6.13)
- The presence of a mass lesion (e.g. rounding of the normally flattened triangular splenic tail due to a mass)
- Distortion by an adjacent organ (e.g. compression of the descending colon/rectum by an enlarged prostate gland)
- Fibrosis and scarring in chronic disease (e.g. small, irregularly marginated kidneys in patients with chronic renal disease).

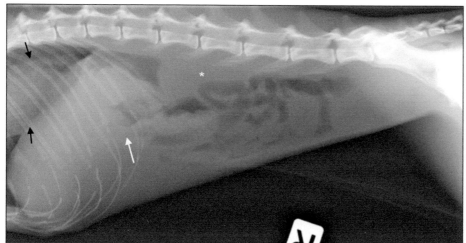

6.11 Röntgen sign: size. Lateral view of the abdomen of a cat with a hiatal hernia. The cranioventral abdomen (white arrow) appears 'empty' due to displacement of the stomach through the hernia (black arrows). In addition, the abdominal volume is small due to little, if any, abdominal and retroperitoneal fat (*), resulting in a 'tucked up' appearance and poor abdominal contrast.

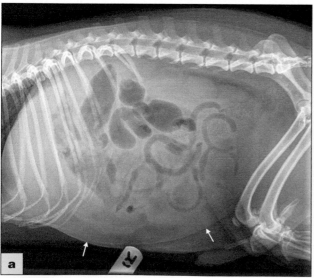
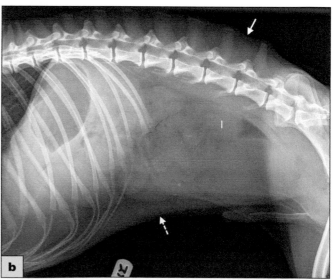

6.12 Röntgen sign: size. **(a)** Lateral view of the abdomen of a small-breed dog with ascites, resulting in abdominal distension. The ventral wall is pendulous (arrowed), the serosal margins, including that of the bladder, are blurred and the gas-filled intestinal loops have gathered or 'floated' centrally. **(b)** Lateral view of the abdomen of an emaciated dog with chronic diarrhoea and an intussusception (I). There is reduced muscle bulk (solid white arrow) dorsal to the spinous processes of the lumbar vertebrae, indicating emaciation. The abdomen has a 'tucked up' appearance (dashed white arrow) due to a combination of abdominal discomfort and emaciation.

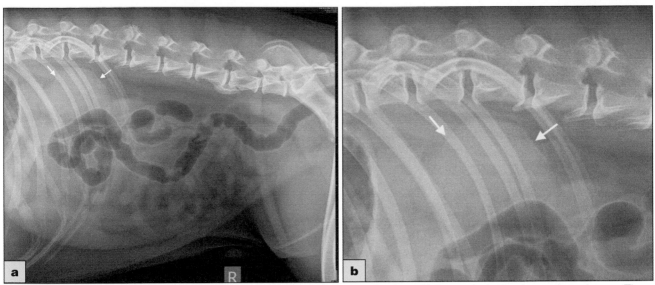

6.13 Röntgen sign: shape. **(a)** Right lateral view of the abdomen of a dog with haematuria due to renal carcinoma. The mid-dorsal margin of the right kidney (arrowed) has been expanded by a trapezoidal mass. **(b)** Magnified view.

Number

- The kidneys, adrenal glands, ovaries and ureters are normally paired structures. Of these, only the kidneys are usually radiographically visible.
- Failure to recognize an organ does not mean that it is absent (e.g. aplasia of one kidney), but is usually artefactual due to poor abdominal contrast or superimposition.
- Failure to recognize an organ can be a sign of disease and is usually associated with displacement of the missing structure. Examples include:
  - Herniation of viscera or organs through the abdominal wall or diaphragmatic defects (Figure 6.14)
  - Rupture of the viscera, particularly the bladder
  - Failure to recognize the normal caecum in a dog due to invagination into the colon as part of an intussusception (see Figure 6.12b).

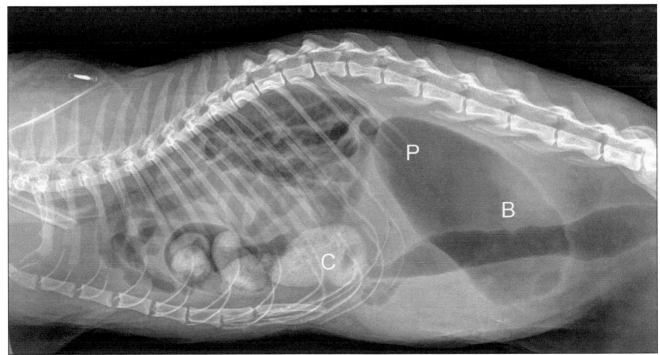

6.14 Röntgen sign: number. Lateral view of the thorax and abdomen of a Persian cat with dyspnoea. Ultrasonography was initially performed, but as a diaphragmatic defect and displacement of viscera was recognized during the study, radiography was requested. The radiographic study revealed a large diaphragmatic hernia. The small intestinal loops have herniated into the thorax *en masse* and the stomach is abnormally positioned with the pylorus (P) located craniodorsally and the body (B) located caudoventrally. The ascending colon (C) has also been displaced into the thorax. The location of the liver and spleen is uncertain, but herniation of all or part of these structures into the thorax is possible. This case emphasizes the value of radiography, as it provides a more comprehensive assessment of the displaced viscera than ultrasonography. (Courtesy of MyVet 24/7)

Opacity

- In the adult dog and cat, fat is less radiopaque than soft tissue. In very young patients, abdominal fat has a different composition ('brown fat') and appears radiographically more opaque than the fat opacity seen in adults. Fat deposits within the abdomen are usually due to physiological deposition within the connecting mesenteries and ligaments (falciform, transverse ligament of the bladder) and the retroperitoneal space. Occasionally, masses arising from fatty connective tissue (lipomas) originate within the abdominal or retroperitoneal spaces (Figure 6.15).
- Where two soft tissue structures overlap, the increased thickness of the superimposed tissues results in an area of increased opacity. This is commonly recognized where the kidneys overlap on a lateral view of the abdomen.
- A change in opacity is often an important radiological feature:
  - Increased soft tissue opacity due to the increased thickness of an abnormally enlarged soft tissue organ
  - Abnormal mineralized or metallic opacity within the gastrointestinal tract due to a foreign body
  - Mineralized opacities within the kidneys, ureters and bladder due to radiopaque calculi
  - Free abdominal gas in a patient with gastrointestinal perforation.

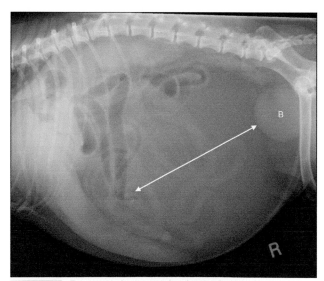

6.15 Röntgen sign: opacity. Lateral view of the abdomen of a dog with a large intra-abdominal lipoma. The lipoma displaces the small intestinal loops cranially (arrowed) and the bladder (B) caudally. However, as the mass is of fat opacity, it is more lucent than the adjacent soft tissue structures and their serosal margins remain visible. The mass is so large that it has resulted in a marked generalized enlargement of the abdomen.

Margination

- Abdominal organs are recognized as separate from each another due to the presence of mesenteric or retroperitoneal fat bordering the serosal margins of the organs or structures. This is termed serosal detail.
- Structures of the same opacity in contact with one another merge into one silhouette, so that separate borders are no longer radiographically apparent.
  - Free abdominal fluid results in loss of serosal detail because the fluid is in contact with the organs, and is of the same soft tissue opacity (Figure 6.16).
  - In very young patients, the increased opacity of 'brown fat' is similar to the soft tissue opacity of the adjacent organs, resulting in very poor serosal detail.
  - In emaciated patients, the lack of abdominal fat leads to the soft tissue organs coming into contact with each other, resulting in poor serosal detail.

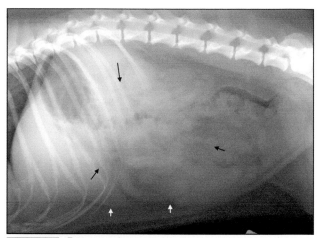

6.16 Röntgen sign: margination. Lateral view of the abdomen of a dog with localized peritonitis due to pancreatitis. There is a generalized increase in soft tissue opacity in the mid-cranial abdomen caudal to the stomach (black arrows). The serosal surfaces of the small intestine and cranial colon and the caudal margin of the stomach and liver are blurred. As the peritonitis and abdominal fluid are localized, the margins of other, unaffected, areas of the abdomen (e.g. the ventral margin of the liver and the ventrally located small intestinal loops) remain better defined (white arrows).

Position

Changes in the position of abdominal organs can be due to a change in the size and shape of adjacent structures, the presence of an abnormal structure, or the absence of a normal structure. The small intestinal loops are especially mobile and easily displaced, and the direction of displacement is useful in locating the abnormality.

- Splenomegaly may result in caudal, and often dorsal, displacement of the small intestines.
- A central abdominal mass (e.g. arising from a mesenteric lymph node) results in peripheral displacement of the small intestines.
- Disruption of the diaphragm (e.g. due to traumatic rupture) results in the displacement of the small intestines into the thoracic cavity (see Figure 6.14).

Function

Contrast studies may allow a very limited assessment to be made of the function of the abdominal organs.

Abdominal masses

The radiological differentiation of abdominal masses is challenging.

- A minimum of two orthogonal views should be obtained.
- In many cases the origin of the mass is obvious, but in others the organ of origin may be difficult or impossible to determine. Pedunculated masses, in particular, may appear remote from the organ of origin.
- In cases where the organ of origin cannot be easily identified, useful radiological features include the location of the mass and its effect on the adjacent organs (usually displacement and/or compression).
- Masses arising from a relatively fixed organ (such as the liver) or within a confined location (such as the kidneys within the retroperitoneal space) are also relatively fixed in position, with a more predictable effect on adjacent structures. Masses arising from more mobile organs (e.g. the intestines) or masses that are pedunculated are usually less fixed and their location may change with alterations in body position. Positional radiography can be used to evaluate the effect of gravity on the location of these masses.
- Displacement of adjacent organs is usually caused by a mass pushing the surrounding organs out of the way. Small intestinal loops are mobile and easily displaced by abdominal masses. The direction of displacement provides useful information about the location of the mass. Occasionally, a normal organ may be attached to the mass and pulled away from its normal location (e.g. ventral displacement of a normal kidney attached to an ovarian mass migrating ventrally within the abdomen)
- The general location of the mass within the abdomen can be used to create a list of the possible origins of the mass.
  - Craniodorsal – liver, adrenal glands, kidneys, ovaries, stomach or spleen (Figure 6.17).

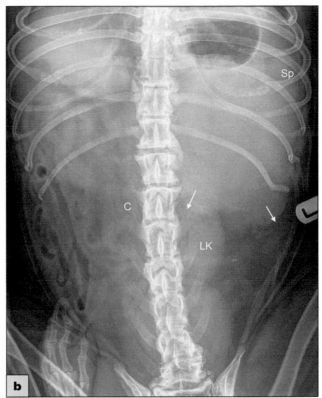

6.17 (continued) Röntgen sign: position. **(b)** VD view of the abdomen of a dog with a craniodorsal mass. As the mass (arrowed) arises in the left craniodorsal abdomen, the descending colon (C) has been displaced towards the right and the left kidney (LK) has been displaced slightly caudally. Masses in this location may arise within the left retroperitoneal space or from the left limb of the pancreas or stomach. The head of the spleen (Sp) is visible in this dog.

  - Cranioventral – liver, stomach or spleen (Figure 6.18).
  - Central – spleen, intestines, mesenteric lymph nodes, pancreas or ovaries (Figures 6.19 and 6.20).

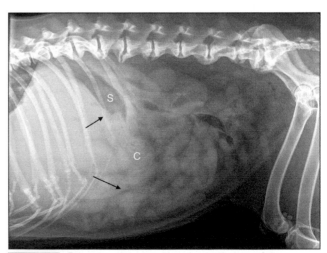

6.18 Röntgen sign: position. Lateral view of the abdomen of a dog with a cranioventral mass. A large soft tissue mass (arrowed) arising from the cranioventral abdomen (liver) has displaced the body of the stomach (S) caudally and dorsally. The transverse colon (C) is also displaced caudally, and the small intestines caudally and ventrally. Masses in this location may arise from the liver, spleen or stomach.

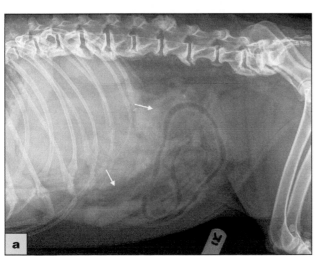

6.17 Röntgen sign: position. **(a)** Lateral view of the abdomen of a dog with a craniodorsal mass. The large soft tissue mass (arrowed) has displaced the small intestine ventrally and caudally. (continues) ▶

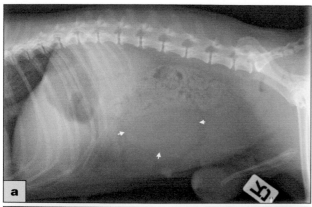

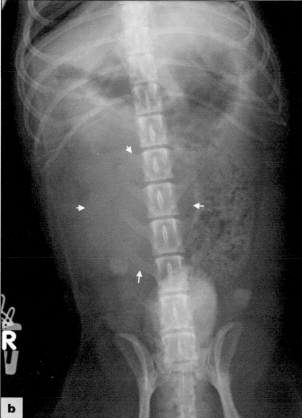

6.19 Röntgen sign: position. **(a)** Lateral and **(b)** VD views of the abdomen of a dog with a mid-abdominal mass. A large soft tissue mass (arrowed) lies within the centre of the abdomen and has displaced the small intestinal loops peripherally. On the VD view, the mass lies on the midline. There is no displacement of the descending colon, stomach, bladder or kidneys. Masses in this location may arise from the mesenteric lymph nodes, small intestine or, occasionally, the ovaries or a retained testicle.

- Caudodorsal – sublumbar lymph nodes, ureters or the terminal descending colon/rectum (Figure 6.21).
- Caudoventral – bladder, uterus, retained testicle or tail of the spleen (Figure 6.22).
- Mid-dorsal – retroperitoneal space or mesenteric root (see Figures 4.23 and 6.23).

■ Not all abdominal masses are neoplastic. Physiological organ enlargement, abnormal gastrointestinal distension, granulomatous infiltration (e.g. with feline infectious peritonitis), cysts (especially renal), reactive lymphadenopathy, abscesses and haematoma are important differential diagnoses.

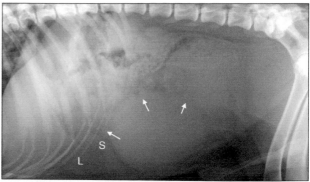

6.20 Röntgen sign: position. Lateral view of the abdomen of a dog with a mid-ventral mass. The large soft tissue mass (arrowed) has displaced the small intestines dorsally and cranially. The mass lies along the ventral abdominal wall. Caudal displacement of the small intestines is limited to some extent by moderate filling of the bladder. Masses in this location usually arise from the tail of the spleen or, occasionally, a peripheral small intestinal loop. L = liver; S = spleen.

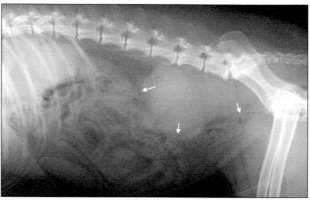

6.21 Röntgen sign: position. Lateral view of the abdomen of a dog with a caudodorsal mass. The large soft tissue mass (arrowed) has displaced the descending colon and bladder ventrally. Masses in this location arise from the caudodorsal retroperitoneal space and may be associated with lymphadenopathy as a result of lymphoma or other neoplasms arising within the pelvis, anal sac adenocarcinoma or prostatic carcinoma.

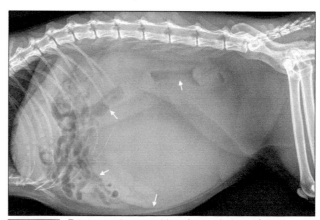

6.22 Röntgen sign: position. Lateral view of the abdomen of a cat with a caudal mass. The large soft tissue mass (arrowed) has displaced the small intestinal loops cranially and the descending colon dorsally. The bladder cannot be identified. The margin of the mass is sharply defined cranioventrally. Masses in this location can arise from the bladder, uterus, prostate gland or bladder wall. The size of the mass suggests that is not likely to be associated with physiological or pathological distension of the bladder. A cystic mass is an important consideration. (Courtesy of MyVet24/7)

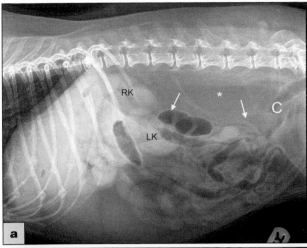

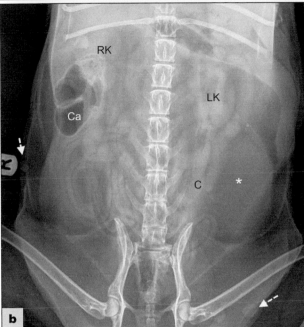

6.23 Röntgen sign: position. **(a)** Lateral and **(b)** VD views of a dog with a large mass (lipoma) arising in the mid-dorsal abdomen. The large mass (*) is of fat opacity and displaces the descending colon (C) and small intestines (solid arrows) ventrally on the lateral view and towards the midline on the VD view. The left kidney (LK) is displaced slightly cranially and ventrally by the mass. Masses in this location can arise from the retroperitoneal space or, occasionally, from the mesenteric root. Note the several small irregular rounded mineralized bodies (dashed arrows) within the subcutis, consistent with calcinosis cutis. Ca = caecum; RK = right kidney.

■ Ultrasonography is invaluable in providing additional information about the internal architecture of an enlarged organ or mass and, in the hands of an experienced operator, can be used to guide fine-needle or Tru-cut biopsy to obtain samples for cytological or histopathological evaluation.

Gastrointestinal tract

Radiological interpretation of the gastrointestinal tract can be challenging due to the normal physiological variation in size and contents. A careful clinical history should be taken in an attempt to distinguish between retching, regurgitation and true vomiting. For retching, pharyngeal radiography is indicated, whilst for regurgitation, thoracic radiography and oesophageal contrast studies are indicated (see Chapters 4 and 5). A critical part of the assessment of the gastrointestinal tract is to differentiate surgical from medical conditions, if possible.

Stomach

Specific approach to interpretation

In addition to assessment based on Röntgen signs (see below), the size and contents of the stomach should be evaluated with respect to the animal's diet and the time it last ate. As with the rest of the gastrointestinal tract, the wall thickness cannot be assessed reliably without the use of contrast media.

Size and shape: The normal stomach varies considerably in size depending on the amount of ingesta present. In the majority of normal patients, the stomach should contain only a small volume of fluid and gas after food has been withheld for 8–12 hours.

Gastric enlargement:

■ The stomach may be normal in position, normal or increasingly rounded in shape, and distended with mainly fluid and ingesta ± a small amount of gas. Causes include:
  • A recent meal
  • Delayed gastric emptying due to pyloric spasm, muscular hypertrophy, ileus secondary to peritonitis, pancreatitis, recent abdominal surgery or the nervous temperament of the patient
  • Pyloric outflow obstruction due to a foreign body, neoplasia and, occasionally, extramural inflammatory lesions (e.g. pancreatitis) or adhesions (see Figure 3.31). Chronic partial obstruction is often characterized by the accumulation of mineralized ingesta proximal to the obstruction ('gravel sign') (Figure 6.24).
■ The stomach may be normal in shape but distended with gas. Causes include:
  • Aerophagia secondary to dyspnoea, megaoesophagus or distress/anxiety
  • A motility disorder, possibly associated with megaoesophagus
  • Gastrointestinal ileus secondary to peritonitis, pancreatitis or recent abdominal surgery.
■ Marked distension of the stomach with gas and/or a small amount of ingesta is characteristic of gastric dilatation and often associated with gastric volvulus.

Stomach wall thickness: Gastric wall thickness can only be accurately assessed where the stomach is moderately distended and the wall is highlighted by gas or positive contrast media. Fluid within the stomach lumen can merge with the soft tissue opacity of the wall, resulting in a false impression of wall thickening. Ultrasonography is very useful for evaluating both the thickness and structure of the stomach wall. Thickening of the stomach may be seen due to:

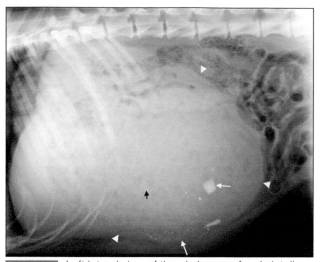

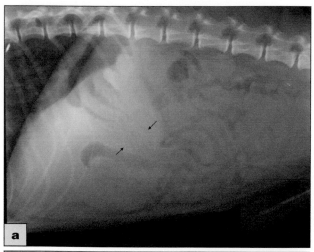

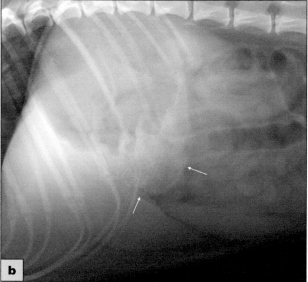

6.24 Left lateral view of the abdomen of a skeletally mature dog with a pyloric outflow obstruction. The stomach (arrowheads) is markedly distended and rounded and the small intestines are caudodorsally displaced. The generally homogeneous soft tissue opacity of the stomach suggests predominantly fluid content. Note the accumulation of particulate mineralized material (white arrows) within the ingesta in the pylorus consistent with a 'gravel sign', indicating chronic obstruction. A small volume of air in the non-dependent region of the stomach highlights thick sinuous rugal folds (black arrow).

- Muscular hypertrophy
- Chronic gastritis
- Eosinophilic infiltration
- Neoplasia
- Haemorrhage (e.g. due to coagulopathy).

Opacity: As well as varying in volume, the contents of the normal stomach also vary in opacity.

Mineralized or metallic opacity:

- The accumulation of small pieces of mineralized ingesta in the pylorus on a right lateral view of patients with chronic partial pyloric obstruction is referred to as a 'gravel sign'. Whilst the liquid component of the ingesta is able to pass the partial obstruction, the heavier, solid component is often held up and appears as a collection of mineralized opacities, similar in appearance to gravel (see Figures 6.24 and 6.30).
- The presence of foreign material (including metallic objects, stones and bones) is often an incidental finding in dogs. To determine the significance of this material, it should be considered in conjunction with the clinical presentation and indications for imaging.
- Retention of barium following a gastrointestinal contrast study may be significant in establishing the presence of a foreign body or lesion (ulceration/mass).
- Mineralization of the gastric folds may be seen with chronic renal failure (Figure 6.25).

Soft tissue or mixed soft tissue/gas opacity: A soft tissue (fluid) or mixed soft tissue/gas opacity within the stomach lumen is a normal finding following a recent meal or drink. In animals from which food has

6.25 **(a)** Lateral view of a dog with a cranial mediastinal mass and hypercalcaemia. Mineralization of the rugal folds is recognized as several linear opacities in the body of the stomach (arrowed). **(b)** Lateral view of a dog with chronic renal failure. The wall of the pylorus (arrowed) is mineralized.

been withheld for at least 12 hours, other causes of luminal contents with mixed opacity include:

- Foreign material of soft tissue opacity (e.g. material, hairballs)
- Delayed gastric emptying
- Pyloric obstruction
- A large gastric tumour or polyp.
  - The soft tissue opacity of the stomach wall, or any masses arising from the wall, merge with the soft tissue opacity of fluid and ingesta, making the two areas impossible to delineate.
  - Gastric ultrasonography or contrast radiography is indicated to assess for suspected gastric wall thickening or mass lesions.

Gas opacity:

- A small amount of gas within the stomach lumen is normal, both in fasted animals and those which have been recently fed.
- Gaseous distension of the stomach is abnormal.

Possible causes include:
- Aerophagia
- GDV (see Figures 3.15, 3.46 and 6.27).
■ Gas in the stomach wall (pneumatosis) is occasionally seen with ulceration and necrosis (e.g. secondary to GDV).

Margination: The entire serosal margin of the stomach is often not clearly defined and may only be appreciated ventrally, adjacent to the falciform fat. Cranially, the stomach merges within the soft tissue opacity of the liver, whilst caudodorsally it merges with the soft tissue opacity of the right kidney and splenic head and caudally with the pancreas (which is not radiographically apparent) and the cranial wall of the transverse colon.

■ Visualization of the serosal margins will be reduced further in emaciated or very young animals and by abdominal fluid (ascites).
■ Serosal margins are more easily visualized in the presence of free abdominal gas.

Position:

Cranial displacement: As the pylorus moves further cranially, the gastric axis appears more upright, or even angled from cranioventral to caudodorsal on the lateral view. Causes include:

■ Reduced liver size due to a congenital portosystemic shunt or hepatic fibrosis/cirrhosis
■ Cranial displacement of the liver (and/or abdominal viscera) through a diaphragmatic defect
■ Pressure from increased abdominal volume (e.g. due to advanced pregnancy or severe ascites)
■ An abdominal mass caudal to the stomach can cause cranial displacement, but is more likely to distort the shape or displace the stomach to the left (e.g. right-sided liver mass, pancreatic mass) or to the right (e.g. left-sided liver mass, splenic mass)
■ An apparently small liver and upright gastric axis can be a normal variation in deep-chested dogs.

Caudal displacement: The gastric axis is angled from craniodorsal to caudoventral on the lateral view, with caudal and dorsal displacement of the pylorus. The stomach may project beyond the last rib on both lateral and VD views. Causes include:

■ Hepatomegaly due to metabolic or steroid hepatopathy, hepatic lipidosis, diffuse or focal neoplasia, or venous congestion. Hepatomegaly usually also results in dorsal displacement of the stomach, recognized on the lateral view (see Figure 6.18).
■ Increased thoracic volume due to pleural effusion or pulmonary overinflation.

Common conditions

Gastric foreign bodies: Mineralized/metallic foreign bodies are easily identified, whereas radiolucent foreign bodies are harder to identify. A minimum of two orthogonal views are required to confirm the location and number of suspected foreign bodies (Figure 6.26). Obtaining four views (right and left lateral, VD and DV views) can redistribute gas and ingesta and help outline a foreign body.

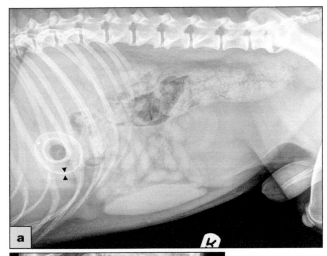
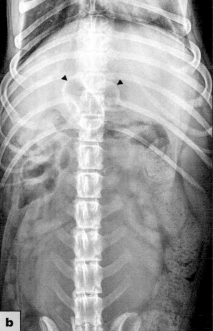

6.26 **(a)** Right lateral and **(b)** VD views of the abdomen of a dog with a gastric foreign body (a child's dummy). Although the stomach is empty the foreign body may still be responsible for causing obstruction as the dog may recently have vomited. The foreign body is easily recognized (especially on the lateral view) due to gas surrounding both the external and internal surfaces (arrowheads).

Radiological features:

■ Abnormal luminal contents, which are of mineral, metal or soft tissue opacity.
■ Gas may be trapped within radiolucent foreign bodies, resulting in bizarre or geometric gas patterns.
■ Although an obstructing foreign body can result in gastric distension, the stomach may appear empty in an acutely vomiting animal.
■ The presence of gastric distension with fluid/ingesta in an anorexic animal or in an animal that

has had no access to food/water for >12–15 hours is suggestive of ileus/delayed gastric emptying. Differentiating obstruction from functional causes can be difficult if the foreign body is radiolucent.

- In cases with possible partial obstruction, the stomach should be assessed for evidence of a 'gravel sign' (small accumulation of mineralized opacities in the pylorus/antrum).
- Contrast studies, ultrasonography and endoscopy may be necessary to identify gastric foreign bodies. On positive-contrast studies, a foreign body may be seen as a filling defect within the contrast medium pool.
- It should be considered that many gastric foreign bodies are incidental findings and unrelated to the clinical presentation.

Gastric dilatation and volvulus: Radiology is sensitive and specific for the diagnosis of GDV and is preferred to ultrasonography as the presence of gas hinders ultrasonographic evaluation. Significant gastric dilatation can occur due to aerophagia (e.g. due to respiratory disease, panting and anxiety) and in most cases, simple dilatation (unless very severe) of the stomach with gas is of no clinical significance. The diagnosis of volvulus is based upon visualization of the pylorus in an abnormal location. A right lateral recumbent radiograph (Figure 6.27) is the view of choice for demonstrating GDV, because with 180 degree torsion, the gas-filled pylorus can be seen lying dorsally to the fundus.

Radiological features:

- With GDV there is marked distension of the stomach by gas and/or a small amount of ingesta.
- Gastric volvulus is confirmed by recognizing rotation of the pylorus dorsally and to the left, with the fundus rotated ventrally and to the right. On a right lateral view, in cases of GDV, the pylorus is usually gas-filled and can be seen dorsal to the fundus. The pylorus can be differentiated from the fundus by the lack of rugal folds and visualizing the duodenum exiting the stomach. Although obtaining both right and left lateral recumbent views can help to establish the position of the pylorus, stabilization of the patient should be the priority in this emergency situation.
- Compartmentalization of the stomach, recognized as a soft tissue band crossing the stomach lumen, is very suggestive of volvulus.
- Concurrent torsion of the spleen may be recognized by enlargement and/or abnormal location and shape of the spleen.
- Linear gas lucencies within the stomach wall are suggestive of gastric necrosis and reflect a grave prognosis.
- Small intestinal ileus is commonly seen in conjunction with GDV.
- Oesophageal dilatation and hypovolaemia due to circulatory shock (i.e. small cardiac silhouette and pulmonary vessels) may be recognized in the caudal thorax.

Gastric neoplasia:

- The diagnosis of gastric neoplasia is often challenging on survey radiographs as most tumours are not visible. Contrast (ideally double-contrast) studies are usually necessary to confirm the presence of a lesion (see Figures 4.33 and 6.28). Ultrasonography is highly valuable and may allow guided fine-needle aspiration and/or biopsy.
- Differential diagnoses include:
  - Adenocarcinoma – most common in dogs and typically focal
  - Lymphoma – most common in cats and can be focal or diffuse
  - Leiomyoma/leiomyosarcoma (which can be quite large at the time of diagnosis and are often extraluminal) or mast cell tumours are seen less commonly.

Radiological features: Contrast studies may show:

- Localized or diffuse wall thickening (only reliably detected if the mass is large)
- Intraluminal filling defect consistent with a mass
- Persistence of the barium due to gastric ulceration after the stomach has emptied
- Delayed gastric emptying due to complete or partial obstruction of the pylorus.

Gastritis: This is very common, but the radiological diagnosis is usually presumptive based on ruling out a foreign body or other gross lesion. It is not generally possible to differentiate gastritis from chronic pancreatitis radiologically. In extremely rare cases, gastritis may result in gross thickening of the stomach wall and can resemble gastric neoplasia.

Radiological features:

- Survey radiographs are usually unremarkable, even though delayed gastric emptying or gastric distension may be present.

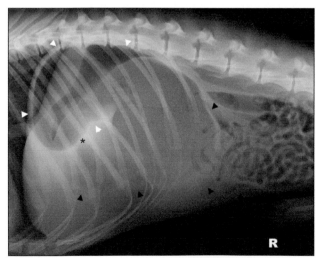

6.27 Right lateral view of the abdomen of a dog with GDV. The pylorus (white arrowheads) is rotated dorsally and is markedly dilated (mainly with air). The body and fundus of the stomach (black arrowheads) are also dilated and rotated ventrally and contain a mixture of gas and fluid. Rotation of the stomach has resulted in a soft tissue opacity (∗) partially dividing the dilated gastric lumen cranially. Although occasionally referred to as 'compartmentalization', this in truth just represents a fold in the gastric wall. Loops of gas-filled small intestine are caudally displaced. The spleen cannot be clearly identified. (Courtesy of the University of Bristol)

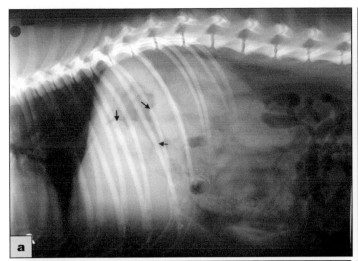

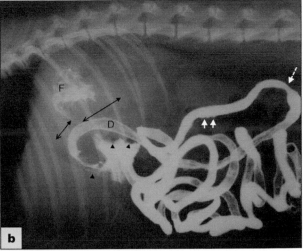

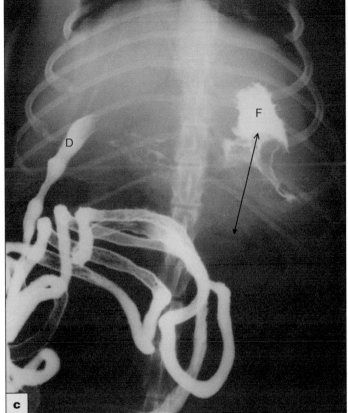

6.28 **(a)** Right lateral survey radiograph and **(b)** lateral and **(c)** VD positive-contrast gastrograms of a dog with a gastric tumour. (a) Gastric wall thickening or a gastric soft tissue mass (arrowed) is suspected, but the extent of the changes cannot be distinguished from the luminal fluid. (b–c) The extent of the marked irregular thickening of the wall of the body due to the gastric mass can be recognized (double-headed arrows). The mass appears as a large soft tissue filling defect on both the cranial and caudal margins of the stomach. There is no filling or distension of the lumen of the body of the stomach. The changes extend into the pylorus and proximal duodenum, where smaller filling defects (arrowheads) are visible. Note the focal narrowing of the segment of small intestine in the caudal abdomen in (b) due to a peristaltic wave (dashed white arrow) as well as the Peyer's patches (solid white arrows) on the anti-mesenteric border of the descending duodenum (D). F = fundus. (Courtesy of the University of Bristol)

■ Contrast studies may show:
  • Stomach wall thickening in chronic cases
  • The persistence of barium after the stomach has emptied due to gastric ulceration.

Pyloric stenosis, dysmotility and chronic outflow obstruction: This is a syndrome of delayed gastric emptying due to a variety of underlying causes (congenital, inflammatory disease, polyps, masses, adhesions) and typically presents with chronic vomiting. It is most common in young adult small-breed dogs (particularly brachycephalic breeds) with circumferential hypertrophy of the mucosa. Siamese cats are reported to be predisposed.

Radiological features:

■ Enlarged stomach filled mostly with fluid/ingesta within the lumen (see Figures 3.31 and 6.24).

■ 'Gravel sign' in the antrum/pylorus is common.
■ Focal dilatation of the antrum/pylorus is seen in some cases.
■ Barium studies show delayed gastric emptying with a 'beak' sign, which is a focal triangular area of contrast medium extending into the distal pylorus due to circumferential wall thickening.

Gastric perforation:

■ Stomach perforation/rupture typically results in a large amount of free gas and/or fluid within the abdomen.
■ On a right lateral view, free gas may be recognized collecting caudal to the diaphragmatic crura (usually the left crus), around the fundus of the stomach or colon. Both the internal and external aspects of the stomach or colon wall can be visualized. The free gas may be recognized as a

single, large, extra-intestinal gas bubble (especially if the patient has been recumbent for any length of time) or as multiple, variably sized, small gas opacities beyond the margins of the small intestinal loops (see Figure 3.25).

■ A left lateral decubitus view, using a horizontal beam, may be useful for demonstrating smaller amounts of free gas that have collected at the highest point of the abdomen, usually between the right liver lobes and body wall (see Figure 6.97).

■ Free abdominal fluid secondary to gastric perforation/rupture results in loss of serosal detail due to both the fluid itself and, if present, localized or generalized peritonitis.

Small intestine

Specific approach to interpretation

When evaluating the small intestine, it is vital to determine whether there is ileus and, if so, to differentiate mechanical ileus from functional causes. The size and opacity of the small intestine should be assessed critically. The volume of gas within the intestine is variable, and alterations in the shape of the gas shadows within the lumen are often more specific and sensitive radiological signs of a foreign body or mass. Differentiating the large intestine from the small intestine can be difficult in some animals and is critical when determining whether the small bowel is dilated. This distinction can usually be made by tracing the colon cranially from the pelvic inlet.

Size: The loops of the small intestine should be approximately even in diameter, although peristaltic waves may cause transient narrowing.

Ileus:

■ Ileus (intestinal dilatation) is an abnormal increase in the diameter of the small intestine and may be due to functional (Figure 6.29) or mechanical causes. Criteria cited for pathological dilatation include intestinal dilatation greater than four times the width of the last rib or greater than twice the height of the body of the fifth lumbar vertebra. Mild dilatation of the small intestine (e.g. where the bowel is between two and three rib widths) is often of uncertain significance as this can be seen in some apparently normal animals. At least two orthogonal views are required to localize the gas-filled loops and help differentiate dilated gas-filled small intestine from normal large intestine.

■ Obstructive (or mechanical) ileus occurs secondary to a small intestinal foreign body, an intestinal mass, an intussusception, entrapment through a hernia or adhesions. In obstructive disease, the severity of the luminal distension is related to the completeness of the obstruction. The greater the degree of dilatation, the greater the confidence that there is a mechanical obstruction. Most cases of mechanical obstruction result in focal dilatation (unless the obstruction is very distal), which helps differentiate this from functional causes where the dilatation is typically generalized. Assessment of

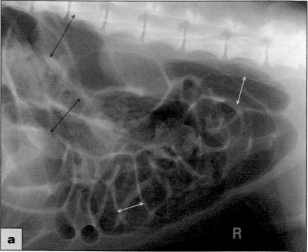

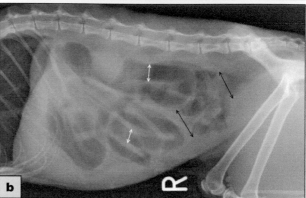

6.29 Functional ileus of the small intestine in **(a)** a dog and **(b)** a cat. Distended gas-filled loops occupy the entire abdomen. It is important to distinguish the large intestine (black double-headed arrows) from the small intestine (white double-headed arrows) based on the appearance of the intestinal contents and location. Large intestinal content is usually granular. The transverse colon can form a prominent loop in the craniodorsal abdomen caudal to the stomach. (b, Courtesy of the University of Bristol)

whether there are one or two 'populations' of small intestinal loops based on intestinal diameter can be helpful; where two 'populations' are identified, this should increase the suspicion that an intestinal obstruction is present.

■ Functional (or paralytic) ileus can occur secondary to hypokalaemia, peritonitis (chemical or inflammatory) or inflammation (enteritis), as well as following surgery. Dilatation of the small intestine with functional causes is usually only mild and is generalized. In severe cases of functional ileus, the bowel is strikingly uniform in diameter due to the absence of peristalsis.

■ Dilated loops may contain fluid, gas or a mixture of both. With obstructive disease, the dilated loops are often gas-filled in the early stages but become increasingly filled with fluid over time.

■ A 'sentinel' loop is a loop of bowel which consistently appears abnormally dilated and suggests localized disease or obstruction.

■ The number of dilated loops should be assessed:
  • A few dilated loops suggests a relatively proximal obstruction or a localized functional ileus (e.g. secondary to localized peritonitis, pancreatitis or recent surgery)

- Generalized dilatation of the intestinal loops is seen with generalized functional ileus, distal intestinal obstruction and mesenteric torsion (plus abnormal shape and location with volvulus).

Shape:

■ The small intestinal loops should have a gently curving tubular shape and be uniform in diameter. As the intestinal loops increase in diameter, the curves tend to change in shape and are more likely to be seen stacked up in the abdomen with sharper 'hairpin-like' curves.
■ Focal widening can be associated with intestinal mass lesions or intestinal foreign bodies.
■ Corrugation of the small intestine can be recognized occasionally on survey radiographs, but is appreciated better on ultrasonography or contrast studies. Causes include:
  - Enteritis
  - Plication of the intestinal loops along a linear foreign body
  - Peritonitis – including localized peritonitis due to pancreatitis, non-septic peritonitis due to bladder rupture and septic peritonitis due to gastrointestinal tract perforation (see Figure 3.20c)
  - Neoplasia – diffuse small intestinal lymphoma, carcinomatosis disseminated throughout the mesentery or pancreatic neoplasia.

Opacity: The normal small intestinal opacity is either that of soft tissue or gas, or a mixture of both.

Soft tissue opacity:

■ As fluid and soft tissue appear identical radiologically, it is not possible to distinguish fluid-filled intestinal loops from wall thickening on survey radiographs.
■ Dilated fluid-filled loops can be seen with obstructive or functional ileus.
■ Uterine enlargement appears as a soft tissue tubular opacity within the mid-ventral abdomen and should not be mistaken for dilated small intestinal loops. Normally, an enlarged uterus can be followed caudally into the pelvic canal, ventral to the colon.

Gas opacity: Gas-filled small intestinal loops, without intestinal dilatation, may be caused by:

■ Aerophagia secondary to dyspnoea, gastric torsion, hypokalaemia or early peritonitis
■ Enteritis.

Intestinal gas usually follows the shape of the intestinal loops. Consistent abnormalities in the shape of the intestinal gas can indicate disease and include:

■ Crescent-shaped gas opacity trapped between the intussuscipiens and the intussusceptum
■ Small tear-shaped bubbles associated with plicated small intestine due to a linear foreign body (see Figure 3.13)

■ Geometric shapes, created by a combination of trapped gas and soft tissue opacity, within the structure or folds of foreign bodies such as corn on the cob, fruit stones and foam or plastic toys.

Mineralized or metallic opacity: In the absence of intestinal dilatation, mineralized or metallic material may be an incidental finding, especially in dogs. Diet can influence the appearance of intestinal contents on radiography. However, where there is also evidence of dilated intestinal loops, such material may represent:

■ Foreign body obstruction
■ A 'gravel sign' due to the accumulation of small particles of mineralized ingesta proximal to a chronic partial obstruction (Figure 6.30)
■ Normal faecal material within the large intestine.

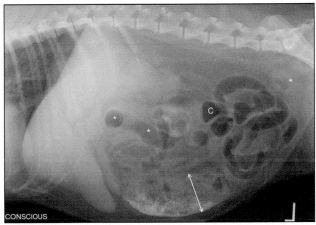

6.30 Right lateral view of the abdomen of a dog with chronic partial obstruction of the small intestine. A loop of small intestine in the mid-ventral abdomen is dilated by a large accumulation of mineralized material (double-headed arrow). The appearance is typical of a 'gravel sign'. It can be distinguished from mineral in normal faeces based on the ventral location of the loop within the abdomen and recognizing the appearance and location of the normal colon (*). C = caecum. (Courtesy of the University of Bristol)

Margination:

■ Serosal detail may be reduced or not visualized for the following reasons:
  - 'Brown fat' with a higher water content in very young animals
  - Emaciation
  - Abdominal fluid (ascites) including haemorrhage
  - Peritonitis
  - Carcinomatosis.
■ Serosal detail can be enhanced in animals with abundant mesenteric fat or in the presence of free abdominal air.
■ Corrugation of the serosal surface can be recognized in association with enteritis, plication caused by a linear foreign body, peritonitis or neoplasia.

Position:

■ The small intestine is very mobile and its position within the abdomen may be influenced by a variety of factors, including changes to the body wall, body condition, increased or decreased size of the adjacent organs and the presence of a linear foreign body or adhesions.

- Displacement of the small intestine outside the abdominal cavity may occur due to defects in the body wall or diaphragm. Depending on the number of loops displaced, the abdominal cavity can appear abnormally empty.
- Cranial displacement into the thoracic cavity indicates diaphragmatic rupture or peritoneal–pericardial diaphragmatic hernia.
- Displacement of the intestinal loops outside the body wall indicates disruption of the body wall with herniation in paracostal, umbilical or inguinal locations.
- Central bunching of the small intestinal loops may occur within the abdominal cavity. Pathological causes include:
  - Gathering of the loops along a linear foreign body
  - Adhesions between the loops or to other organs following previous abdominal surgery, intestinal perforation, peritonitis or neoplasia.
- In obese normal patients, especially the cat, the small intestinal loops can 'gather' centrally in the middle of the abdomen.
- Ventral displacement within the abdominal cavity is usually due to retroperitoneal disease, such as renomegaly, adrenomegaly, retroperitoneal effusion or mass lesions. Marked unilateral renal or adrenal gland enlargement also results in displacement of the small intestine to the left or right.
- Caudal displacement within the abdominal cavity can indicate hepatomegaly, gastric distension or splenomegaly (often together with dorsal displacement). An empty, ruptured or retroflexed bladder can result in caudal displacement of the intestinal loops into the area normally occupied by the bladder.
- Cranial displacement within the abdominal cavity may occur for a number of reasons:
  - Cranially located small intestinal loops approximating the diaphragm may be normal in some deep-chested dogs
  - A small liver, or herniation of the liver cranially through a diaphragmatic defect results in cranial displacement of the stomach and intestinal loops
  - A distended urinary bladder, gravid uterus, pyometra, marked prostatomegaly and paraprostatic cysts displace intestinal loops cranially.

Common conditions

Obstruction: The appearance of obstructive small intestinal disease depends on the location and duration of the obstruction and whether the obstruction is partial or complete. Variable amounts of gas and/or fluid may dilate the intestine proximal to the site of the obstruction.

The differential diagnoses for obstruction include:

- Foreign body
- Intussusception

- Intestinal tumour/mass
- Intestinal volvulus (very rare)
- Intestinal stricture secondary to adhesions (unusual)
- Intestinal strangulation in a hernia or mesenteric tear (unusual).

Radiological features:

- A proximal duodenal obstruction may not result in any intestinal dilatation.
- A proximal jejunal obstruction typically results in a few dilated intestinal loops.
- A distal jejunal obstruction typically results in many dilated intestinal loops.
- An acute obstruction typically results in markedly distended gas-filled loops, which may become increasingly fluid-filled over time.
- A 'gravel sign' may be recognized in cases of chronic partial obstruction.
- The descending colon may appear empty (but faeces in the colon do not rule out obstruction).

If the diagnosis cannot be reached with survey radiography, ultrasonography or contrast studies can provide further information.

Foreign body: Ingested foreign bodies are common in dogs, but uncommon in the cat.

- Foreign bodies may be mineralized or metallic and easily recognizable; however, they are more often of soft tissue opacity, which makes them more challenging to identify (Figure 6.31).
- Evidence of intestinal dilatation and odd gas patterns may focus attention to the site of a suspected foreign body.
- The presence of a 'gravel sign' is suggestive of a chronic foreign body causing partial obstruction.
- Positional radiography should be used to redistribute gas and fluid within the small intestine.
- Contrast studies can demonstrate dilatation of the intestine proximal to the obstruction and may highlight a luminal filling defect representing a foreign body.
- Linear foreign bodies typically cause intestinal plication (Figure 6.32) with crescentic or teardrop-shaped gas bubbles and bunching of the intestine.

Intussusception: This condition is seen most commonly in young dogs and cats, but occasionally occurs in older animals, usually in association with underlying pathology such as neoplasia. Although any segment of the intestine can be involved, the most common site is the ileocolic junction. An intussusception is often palpable as a 'sausage-shaped' mass, especially in young animals.

- There is dilatation of the proximal intestine with soft tissue opacity within the lumen at the site of the intussusception.
- A crescent-shaped gas opacity may be seen trapped between the intussuscipiens (the outer bowel segment) and the intussusceptum (the invaginated inner bowel segment).

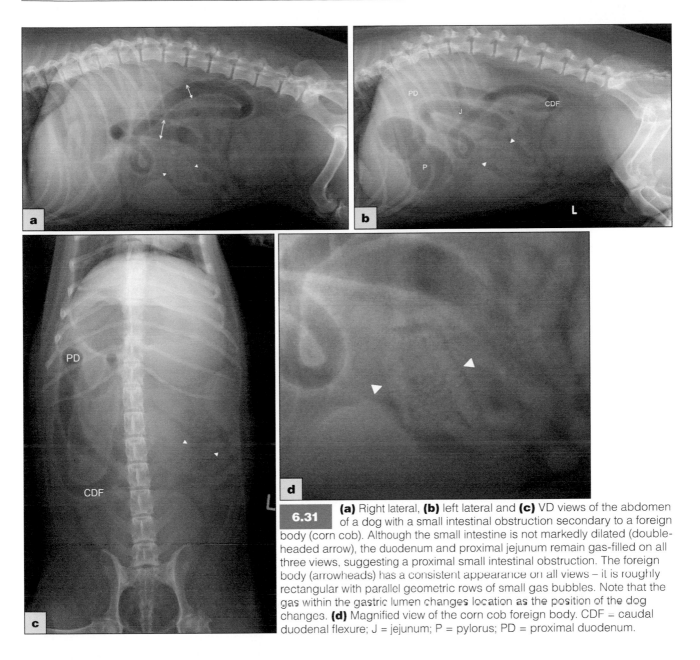

6.31 (a) Right lateral, (b) left lateral and (c) VD views of the abdomen of a dog with a small intestinal obstruction secondary to a foreign body (corn cob). Although the small intestine is not markedly dilated (double-headed arrow), the duodenum and proximal jejunum remain gas-filled on all three views, suggesting a proximal small intestinal obstruction. The foreign body (arrowheads) has a consistent appearance on all views – it is roughly rectangular with parallel geometric rows of small gas bubbles. Note that the gas within the gastric lumen changes location as the position of the dog changes. (d) Magnified view of the corn cob foreign body. CDF = caudal duodenal flexure; J = jejunum; P = pylorus; PD = proximal duodenum.

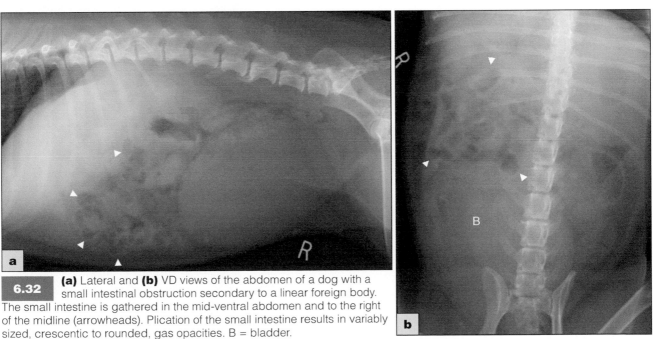

6.32 (a) Lateral and (b) VD views of the abdomen of a dog with a small intestinal obstruction secondary to a linear foreign body. The small intestine is gathered in the mid-ventral abdomen and to the right of the midline (arrowheads). Plication of the small intestine results in variably sized, crescentic to rounded, gas opacities. B = bladder.

- The normal caecal gas shadow may be absent in dogs with caecal involution and ileocaecocolic intussusception (Figure 6.33).
- The colon may be shortened in cases with ileocolic intussusception.
- A localized homogeneous soft tissue mass opacity may be seen within the colon in cases of ileocolic intussusception (see Figure 6.12b).
- Contrast studies typically reveal dilatation of the proximal intestine with narrowing of the contrast medium column within the intussusception. On the distal side of the intussusception, the contrast medium may highlight the invaginated loop as an intraluminal filling defect.

Intestinal tumours and masses: Intestinal tumours and masses occur most frequently in older dogs and cats. The mass itself cannot be differentiated radiologically from normal small intestinal loops unless it is twice the diameter of the small intestine (Figure 6.34). Masses can cause partial or complete intestinal obstruction. There is often involvement of the mesenteric lymph nodes; these nodes can be much larger than the intestinal mass. Most intestinal masses are neoplastic, although benign lesions do occur, but it is not possible to differentiate between them on radiography. The most common tumours are adenocarcinoma (usually focal) and lymphoma (focal or diffuse). Mast cell tumours and leiomyomas/leiomyosarcomas may also be seen.

- Large small intestinal masses are recognized as focal soft tissue masses, usually located within the mid-abdomen. It may not be possible to determine the origin of the mass without contrast studies or ultrasonography.
- If the tumour does not result in obstruction, plain radiographs may appear unremarkable.
- Dystrophic mineralization of some intestinal tumours or associated lymph nodes can be recognized as areas of irregular mineralization (see Figure 3.29).
- Localized enlargement of the intestine may be seen with focal masses. The serosal surface of the mass may be irregular and gas opacities within the intestinal lumen can be irregularly shaped.
- If wall thickening is severe, this may be visible on radiographs; however, care should be taken not to over-interpret this finding as it may be an artefact created by the intestinal contents of soft tissue opacity silhouetting with the intestinal wall.
- If small intestinal obstruction is present, contrast studies can demonstrate dilatation of the intestine proximal to the mass and an irregular filling defect at the location of the obstructing mass, with thickening of the wall and an irregular luminal surface.
- If the mass causes partial intestinal obstruction a 'gravel sign' may be seen.

Perforation: Intestinal perforation (see Figures 3.20 and 6.35) can be caused by a penetrating foreign body, ulceration (usually in the duodenum), bowel infarction or bowel dehiscence following enterotomy/enterectomy. Perforation results in intestinal contents leaking into the abdominal cavity.

Radiological features:

- Leakage of intestinal contents or perforation results in free gas within the abdomen and usually signs of peritonitis (localized loss of serosal detail and often corrugation of the small intestine). A small volume of abdominal fluid can be difficult to recognize, particularly in obese patients.

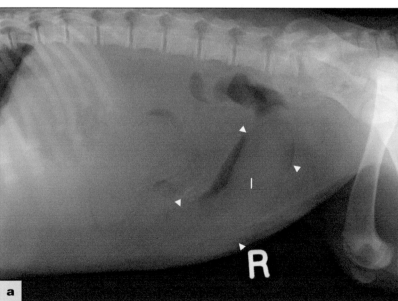
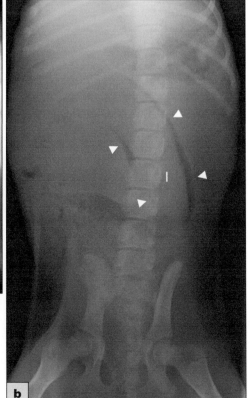

6.33 **(a)** Lateral and **(b)** VD views of the abdomen of an immature bitch with an ileocolic junction intussusception. The intussusceptum (invaginating loop) appears as a homogeneous tubular soft tissue opacity (I), highlighted by gas within the surrounding intussuscipiens (arrowheads = receiving loop). The poor serosal detail is typical of a young animal and does not necessarily indicate the presence of free abdominal fluid.

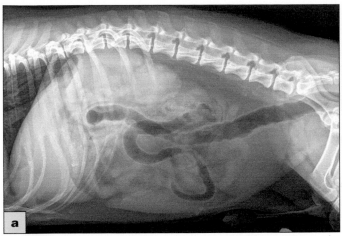
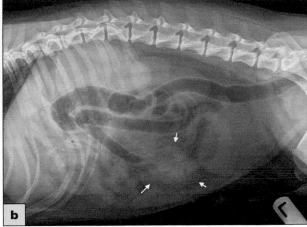

6.34 **(a)** Right and **(b)** left lateral views of the abdomen of a dog with an intestinal mass. The irregularly shaped soft tissue mass lies in the caudoventral abdomen, just cranial to the bladder (arrowed). The small intestinal loops are of normal diameter (not obstructed). The mass is surrounded by small intestinal loops, indicating that it probably lies within the mesentery. Note that abnormal structures (masses, lymph nodes, cysts) can only be recognized when they exceed the diameter of the adjacent small intestinal loops by two to three times. The mass is not visible on the right lateral view.

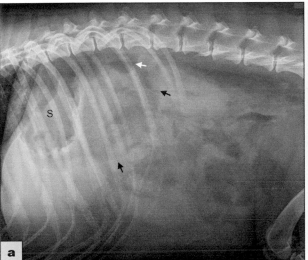
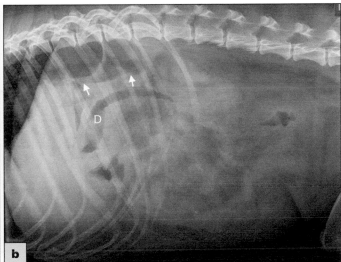

6.35 **(a)** Right and **(b)** left lateral views of the abdomen of a dog with intestinal perforation secondary to duodenal ulceration. Serosal detail is poor due to a relatively large volume of free abdominal fluid. (a) A large pocket of gas (black arrows) is evident in the craniodorsal abdomen caudal to the stomach (S). Smaller gas bubbles (white arrow) are more difficult to distinguish from gas within the intestinal loops. (b) The large gas pocket (arrowed) is located more cranially and highlights the caudal aspect of the left crus of the diaphragm. The duodenum (D) contains gas and has a corrugated appearance (due to spasm of the intestinal smooth muscle) (see also Figure 6.97).

- Free gas can be demonstrated by obtaining a VD view of the abdomen with the animal in lateral (usually left) recumbency using a horizontal beam (see Figures 6.4 and 6.97). Free gas, if present, collects beneath the costal arch.
- The use of barium as a contrast agent is contraindicated if there is suspicion of intestinal perforation. Alternative methods (ultrasonography, computed tomography (CT) or abdominocentesis) should be used to confirm whether an intestinal perforation is present. If a contrast study is considered necessary, iodine should be used instead. Leakage of iodine outside the gastrointestinal tract confirms perforation.

Enteritis: Survey radiographs are frequently unrewarding in patients with suspected enteritis and in the majority of cases are normal.

Radiological features:

- The small and large intestines may be empty of food material and formed faecal material, respectively, and may contain fluid and small air bubbles instead.
- In more severe cases, functional ileus ± intestinal corrugation can be seen.
- Contrast studies may demonstrate rapid intestinal transit time.

Infiltrative disease: Survey radiographs are usually unremarkable.

Radiological features: Diffuse intestinal wall thickening secondary to neoplastic (typically lymphoma) or inflammatory infiltration may be identified with contrast studies or ultrasonography.

Large intestine

Specific approach to interpretation

The large intestine is relatively consistent in appearance and radiological abnormalities are uncommon compared with other parts of the gastrointestinal tract. When evaluating the large intestine it is important to obtain radiographs of the entire rectum and pelvic canal. Due to the inherently poor contrast within the pelvic canal, lesions involving the rectum are often not visible radiographically. Focal ventral displacement of the large intestine in conjunction with narrowing is often seen with extramural or retroperitoneal masses and is an important radiological sign of retroperitoneal disease. In dogs, a 'redundant' colon is not uncommon and is the result of the colon being longer than normal; consequently, the redundant loop lies further cranial or ventral than normal. Care should be taken not to mistake a redundant loop of colon for displacement by a mass (which also results in a focal increase in soft tissue opacity adjacent to the displaced loop of colon).

Size: As with other storage viscera, the normal size of the colon is variable due to the animal's diet and time since it last defecated. Objective measures of normal size, although reported, rarely aid radiological interpretation. An increase in colonic diameter can be recognized with:

- Constipation or faecal retention due to pain on defecation or neurological abnormalities
- Obstipation (more severe faecal retention with mechanical obstruction to defecation). Possible causes include colonic stricture, narrowing of the pelvic canal due to malunion of an earlier fracture, prostatomegaly, neoplasia and perineal hernia
- Megacolon (hypomotility and dilatation of the colon). Possible causes include constipation, metabolic disease (hypokalaemia, hypothyroidism) and neurological disease (dysautonomia, sacrococcygeal agenesis in Manx cats), or it may be idiopathic (especially in the cat).

Shape:

- Although the normal colon is tubular in shape, variations in diameter may be recognized due to discrete faecal balls.
- Colonic peristalsis in normal animals is occasionally recognized as transient corrugation of the large intestine.
- Focal mass lesions are often difficult to recognize on survey radiographs, but a change in luminal shape may be recognized if an intraluminal mass lesion is surrounded by gas.

Opacity:

Soft tissue opacity:

- The empty colon is seen as a tubular soft tissue opacity.
- A homogeneous soft tissue opacity in association with a normal or increased large intestinal diameter suggests an increase in luminal fluid content. This may be due to diarrhoea. Intraluminal mass lesions, radiolucent foreign bodies and intussusceptions may also appear as homogeneous soft tissue opacities.

Gas opacity:

- This may be normal/diet-related or due to colitis.

Mineralized or metallic opacity:

- Chronic constipation, obstipation and megacolon are associated with increased opacity of the faecal content. Dehydrated faeces are typically of predominantly mineralized opacity.
- Small pieces of bone, small stones and small metallic objects are commonly identified, especially in the dog, and are usually incidental findings.

Margination:

- Serosal detail may be reduced or lost in emaciated animals or in very young dogs and cats, and with abdominal fluid, peritonitis or carcinomatosis.
- Serosal detail may be enhanced in animals with abundant mesenteric fat or in the presence of free abdominal gas.
- Corrugation of the serosal surface may be seen due to transient waves of peristalsis, peritonitis or severe colitis.
- Colonic or caecal perforation may result in abdominal leakage, leading to peritonitis and free abdominal gas, and if the rectum/caudal colon are involved, retroperitoneal inflammation with loss of detail and free retroperitoneal gas may also be present.

Position:

Ascending colon: Displacement of the ascending colon towards the midline may be due to an enlarged right kidney, enlargement of the right limb of the pancreas, dilatation of the duodenum or right-sided hepatomegaly.

Transverse colon: Caudal displacement and separation of the transverse colon from the stomach may be due to enlargement of the left limb of the pancreas.

Descending colon: The descending colon is the longest section of the colon and thus has the greatest potential for displacement.

- Displacement towards the midline or across to the right may be normal in large-breed dogs with a 'redundant' colon, but may also be due to enlargement of the left kidney, head or body of the spleen, or left-sided hepatomegaly.
- Ventral displacement of the proximal descending colon may be due to enlargement of the left kidney.
- Ventral displacement of the distal descending colon may be due to enlargement of the sublumbar lymph nodes or enlargement of the retroperitoneal space due to haemorrhage, urine leakage or mass lesions.

- Dorsal displacement of the distal descending colon may be due to prostatomegaly, uterine enlargement (pyometra, pregnancy) or a distended urinary bladder.
- Caudal displacement of the distal descending colon may be due to a perineal hernia or rupture, or rectal prolapse.

Rectum:

- Dorsal displacement of the rectum may be due to prostatomegaly, a vaginal, urethral or other pelvic mass, or distention of the urinary bladder.
- Ventral displacement of the rectum may be due to a dorsal pelvic mass.

Common conditions

Constipation, obstipation and megacolon: Obstipation is more severe than constipation; however, these conditions are not readily differentiated on radiographs. Radiographic evidence of a mechanical obstruction should be sought. Possible causes include:

- Atresia recti/atresia ani (severe narrowing of an imperforate rectum or anus) in very young patients
- Pelvic narrowing due to previous pelvic trauma (Figure 6.36)
- Perineal hernia
- Prostatomegaly
- Sublumbar lymphadenopathy
- Colonic or pelvic mass lesions
- Foreign body obstruction (rare).

Radiological features:

- Typically recognized as large intestinal dilatation with increasingly opaque faecal material.
- In cases of dysautonomia, dilatation of the stomach, small intestine and bladder, as well as megaoesophagus, may be seen.

Perineal hernia: Perineal hernias (Figure 6.37) are most commonly recognized in older entire male dogs. Rectal palpation of a suspected defect and identification of a perineal mass lesion on clinical examination carry a high index of clinical suspicion for a perineal hernia.

Radiological features:

- Survey radiographs may appear normal if there is no retroflexion of the bladder or prostate gland, or displacement of the colon or rectum into the hernia.
- Retroflexion of the bladder and prostate gland into the hernia is recognized as a soft tissue swelling at the tail base, together with an absence of the bladder and prostate gland from their normal location within the caudal abdomen.
- Displacement of the colon and rectum into the hernia is recognized as a mixed, partly mineralized opacity within the hernia and is often seen in association with radiographic evidence of constipation.

Mass lesions: Depending on their size, masses arising from the large intestine (Figure 6.38) may not be recognized on survey radiography unless bordered by gas. Pedunculated masses may be surrounded by intraluminal gas.

Radiological features:

- If the lesion results in large intestinal obstruction or stricture, then abnormal dilatation of the colon due to retained faeces may be present.
- Although ultrasonography is often useful, gas or shadowing faecal material may obscure the lesion.
- Positive- or double-contrast studies may highlight the mass as a luminal filling defect or as a region of localized wall thickening. The mucosal surface may be irregular and the affected segments may fail to distend compared with adjacent segments.

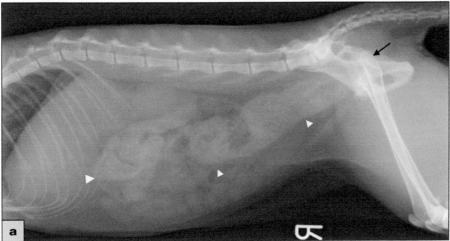
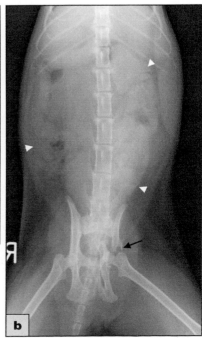

6.36 **(a)** Lateral and **(b)** VD views of the abdomen of a cat with constipation, secondary to a fracture, which has resulted in narrowing of the pelvis. The diameter of the colon is markedly increased. The lumen is filled with dense, partially mineralized faecal material. Almost the entire length of the colon is affected (arrowheads). The distension of the colon stops abruptly at the pelvis. The rectum does not contain any faecal material. A comminuted left ilium fracture (non-union) with medial displacement of the caudal fragment is the cause of the narrowing of the pelvis (arrowed).

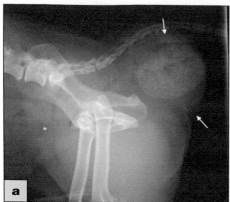
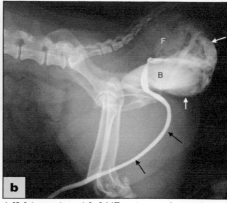
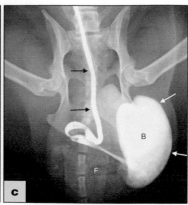

6.37 **(a)** Lateral survey radiograph and **(b)** lateral and **(c)** VD retrograde urethrograms of an intact male dog with dysuria due to a perineal hernia. (a) A large swelling (arrowed) extends dorsally from the caudal pelvis, elevating the tail. The swelling is of soft tissue opacity and there is a large faecal ball containing finely mineralized material superimposed on the centre of the swelling. The caudal abdomen has an empty appearance. The bladder is not recognized and the small intestinal loops (*) extend further caudally than normal to the pubis. (b–c) Retrograde urethrography has been performed. The bladder (B) has retroflexed (white arrows) into the perineal hernia and is partially filled with contrast medium on the lateral view. On the VD view, the large volume of faeces (F) within the right side of the hernia has displaced the bladder to the left. The urethra is denoted by the black arrows.

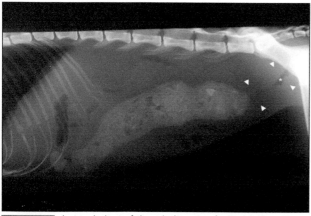

6.38 Lateral view of the abdomen of an elderly cat with carcinoma of the distal descending colon. The descending colon is distended with dense faecal material but tapers abruptly at the level of L7. The annular soft tissue mass (arrowheads) surrounds the narrow and irregular lumen of the colon (*). Ultrasonography or barium contrast studies would provide further information about the lesion. The lack of serosal detail in this case is due to the poor body condition of the cat and the lack of mesenteric or retroperitoneal fat. As a result, the outer margins of the mass cannot be recognized. (Courtesy of the University of Bristol)

- The most common large intestinal masses are polyps (focal, often with a narrow-based attachment), adenocarcinoma (usually focal, often annular) and lymphoma (focal or diffuse). Leiomyomas/leiomyosarcomas may also be seen.

Colitis: Survey radiographs may demonstrate a dilated, fluid-filled large intestine, but are frequently unremarkable.

Radiological features:

- Positive- or double-contrast studies may demonstrate diffuse wall thickening and/or mucosal irregularity.
- Colonoscopy and, in some cases, ultrasonography are preferred techniques to contrast studies to evaluate patients with colitis.

Perforation: Perforation of the colon or rectum can occur secondary to ulceration, perforating foreign bodies, neoplasia and trauma, or following colonic surgery.

Radiological features: Depending on the site of perforation, large intestinal contents may leak into:

- The peritoneal space – causing peritonitis, loss of serosal detail and free abdominal gas
- The retroperitoneal space – causing retroperitoneal inflammation, loss of serosal detail and free retroperitoneal gas.

Intussusception: The ileocolic junction is the most common site for an intussusception. Occasionally, caecocolic (caecal inversion), ileocaecal and colocolic (Figure 6.39) intussusceptions occur.

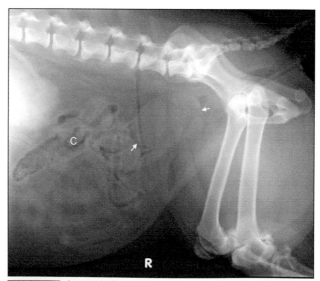

6.39 Lateral view of the abdomen of a dog with a colocolic intussusception. The intussusceptum appears as a soft tissue mass within the caudal descending colon. The cranial and caudal borders of the intussusceptum are bordered by gas (arrowed), creating the impression of a convex 'meniscus'. The colon (C) orad to the intussusception is filled with faecal material. Note that a catheter has been placed within the rectum to inflate the colon with air, providing better contrast (pneumocolon).

Radiological features:

- Small intestinal dilatation may be seen with an ileocolic intussusception. Characteristic crescent-shaped gas opacities may be present between the intussuscipiens and the intussusceptum.
- Caecal inversion may be suspected from the presence of a conical structure of soft tissue opacity in the right mid-abdomen, together with the loss of the normally gas-filled caecum.
- Colocolic intussusceptions vary in appearance and are difficult to identify on plain radiography.
- Following a pneumocolon or barium contrast study:
  - The proximal aspect of the intussuscipiens may be highlighted as a concave filling defect bulging into the lumen of the colon
  - Barium may track proximally between the intussusceptum and the intussuscipiens, resulting in the appearance of a 'coiled spring'.

Liver

Specific approach to interpretation

Assessment of liver size is subjective and evaluation of the margin is often unreliable as the majority of the liver surface is not visible due to border effacement by the stomach, diaphragm and right kidney. There is often poor correlation between radiological changes associated with liver disease and biochemical tests of liver function and enzymes.

Size

Alterations in the size of the hepatic silhouette are recognized by assessing the orientation of the gastric axis, which is an imaginary line extending from the centre of the fundus to the pyloric antrum. The normal gastric axis is approximately parallel to the ribs on a lateral view.

Generalized hepatomegaly:

- Caudal displacement of the pylorus on a lateral view results in increased craniodorsal–caudoventral angulation and anticlockwise rotation of the gastric axis.
- There is extension, and often rounding, of the caudoventral hepatic angle or lobe apices beyond the costal margin. With severe hepatomegaly, the apices can extend beyond the umbilicus.
- Hepatomegaly is a non-specific finding. Differential diagnoses include metabolic hepatopathy (e.g. secondary to hyperadrenocorticism, hypothyroidism or diabetes mellitus; Figure 6.40), venous congestion, nodular hyperplasia, diffuse primary or secondary neoplasia (e.g. lymphoma, mast cell tumour, malignant histiocytosis, widespread metastases) and acute hepatitis, as well as hepatic lipidosis, lymphocytic cholangitis and feline infectious peritonitis and toxoplasmosis in cats.

Localized hepatomegaly:

- Localized hepatomegaly (Figure 6.41) can be difficult to differentiate from more generalized enlargement.

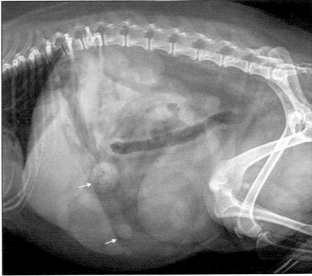

6.40 Lateral view of the abdomen of a bitch with generalized hepatomegaly due to diabetes mellitus. The caudoventral margin of the liver extends well beyond the margins of the costal arch (arrowed), and the pylorus is displaced caudally and lies partially outside the costal margin. Note that the pendulous appearance of the abdomen (probably due to the accumulation of fat within the abdomen, stretching the hepatic ligaments and weakening the ventral abdominal wall muscles) allows the enlarged liver to extend more ventrally.

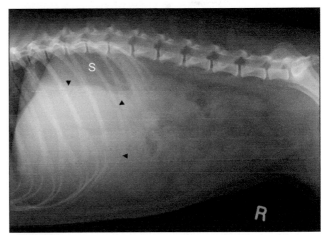

6.41 Lateral view of the abdomen of a bitch with localized hepatomegaly due to a focal hepatic mass (arrowheads). The localized area of hepatic enlargement in the mid-cranial abdomen has distorted the body of the stomach (S) and displaced it caudodorsally. Note that the pylorus is curved around the caudoventral aspect of the focal liver enlargement.

- A large left-sided lesion can cause caudal displacement of the stomach and spleen.
- A large right-sided lesion may cause caudal displacement of the right kidney, pylorus and proximal duodenum (less easy to appreciate on the lateral view) with displacement of the stomach to the left on the VD view.
- Differential diagnoses include focal neoplasia (especially hepatocellular carcinoma and biliary duct carcinoma), cystic changes (including biliary cystadenoma in cats), localized nodular hyperplasia, abscess, haematoma, granuloma and liver lobe torsion.

Microhepatica:

- On the lateral view, microhepatica (Figure 6.42) appears as cranial displacement of the stomach, resulting in an upright or caudodorsal–cranioventral angled gastric axis with clockwise rotation.
- Differential diagnoses include normal variation (especially in deep-chested dogs), cranial displacement of the liver (e.g. due to a diaphragmatic defect), congenital portosystemic shunts (typically seen in young animals), hepatic cirrhosis and idiopathic hepatic fibrosis (particularly in young German Shepherd Dogs).
- Hepatic cirrhosis and fibrosis are often accompanied by ascites.

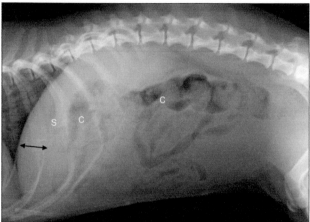

6.42 Lateral view of the abdomen of an adult chondro-dystrophic bitch with microhepatica. The liver (double-headed arrow) is a narrow, homogeneous, soft tissue band immediately caudal to the diaphragm. The stomach (S) is difficult to recognize and the gastric axis is rotated cranially. The colon (C) is filled with a large volume of semi-formed faecal material. (Courtesy of the University of Bristol)

Shape

- On the lateral view, the normal liver is approximately triangular in shape with a sharply angled caudoventral margin.
- Rounding of the caudoventral margin occurs in association with hepatomegaly.
- Distortion and irregularity of the normal hepatic silhouette is the result of focal hepatic enlargement or hepatic mass lesions bulging from the liver surface. A cirrhotic liver has an irregular nodular appearance.

Opacity

The normal liver should be of homogeneous soft tissue opacity.

Mineralized opacity:

- Amorphous mineralization throughout the hepatic parenchyma is usually due to dystrophic mineralization associated with hepatic neoplasia, chronic abscessation, granuloma, haematoma, nodular hyperplasia and, occasionally, parasitic migration or parasitic cysts.
- Cholelithiasis (Figures 6.43 and 6.44) can be recognized as multiple mineralized opacities superimposed on the right cranioventral liver in the

region of the gallbladder. It is frequently incidental, although chronic inflammatory disease of the biliary tract and biliary obstruction should be considered.
- Mineralization within the common bile duct is known as choledocholithiasis. It is identified as a single or multiple small mineralized bodies superimposed on the liver, extending craniodorsally from cranial to the pylorus to the region ventral to the right kidney.
- Dystrophic mineralization of the gallbladder wall can occur with chronic cholecystitis or (rarely) gallbladder neoplasia.
- Mineralization of the intrahepatic biliary tract is visible as branching linear mineralized structures and is usually associated with chronic cholangitis, but can also be recognized occasionally as an apparently incidental finding in older terrier breeds and Cavalier King Charles Spaniels.
- Penetrating metallic foreign bodies (e.g. swallowed needles and wires) are occasionally recognized within the liver parenchyma and are usually incidental findings.

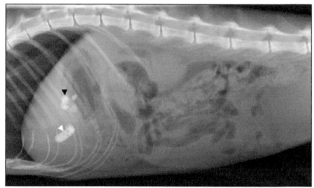

6.43 Lateral view of the abdomen of a cat with jaundice due to cholangiohepatitis. The large granular mineralized body (white arrowhead) superimposed over the ventral liver is consistent with a cholelith in the gallbladder. The collection of smaller choleliths (black arrowhead) cranial to the stomach are located within the terminal common bile duct.

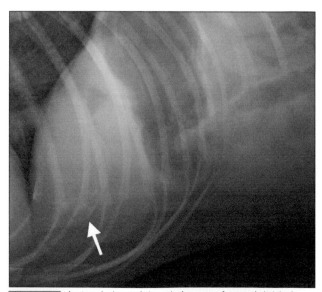

6.44 Lateral view of the abdomen of an adult bitch with fine mineralization of the gallbladder wall. The fine, curvilinear mineralization (arrowed) involves the ventral wall and is associated with irregularly mineralized choleliths within the gallbladder lumen.

Gas opacity:

- Hepatic gas opacity is an uncommon finding.
- Streaks or patches of gas within the hepatic parenchyma or gallbladder can be recognized with necrotizing hepatitis, emphysematous cholecystitis (Figure 6.45) and hepatic abscessation.
- Branching gas opacities may be identified due to:
  - Gas within the biliary tract (e.g. secondary to duodenal reflux into the common bile duct, chronic biliary obstruction or emphysematous cholecystitis)
  - Gas within the portal venous system (e.g. secondary to necrotizing gastroenteritis, gastric volvulus, clostridial infection, functional ileus or air embolism).

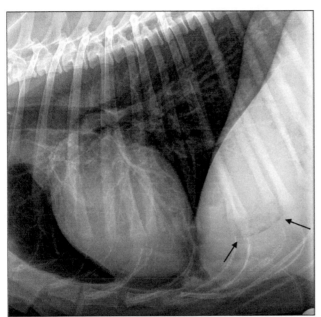

6.45 Left lateral view of the thorax of a dog with signs of acute abdominal pain. A curvilinear gas opacity (arrowed) is superimposed over the ventral liver in the region of the ventral aspect of the gallbladder. The changes are consistent with gas within the wall of the gallbladder (emphysematous cholecystitis) associated with a gallbladder mucocele (a form of necrotizing cholecystitis).

Margination

- The normal liver merges cranially with the diaphragm, caudally with the stomach, ventrally with the gallbladder and, in the absence of perirenal fat, on the right dorsal aspect with the cranial pole of the right kidney.
- The location of the cranial hepatic margin is inferred by the position of the diaphragm. This recognizable interface may be lost due to the presence of pleural fluid, a caudal thoracic mass lesion or a diaphragmatic defect.
- The caudal hepatic margin is inferred from the location of the gastric axis and is difficult to recognize when the stomach is empty.
- The ventral margin is most consistently recognized in cats due to the large volume of falciform fat. This margin is lost in emaciated or very young patients, or those with free abdominal fluid.

Position

- Cranial displacement of the hepatic silhouette may be seen with diaphragmatic rupture, peritoneoperi-cardial–diaphragmatic hernia or an increased abdominal volume due to advanced pregnancy, a large volume of ascites or a large abdominal mass.
- Caudal displacement of the hepatic silhouette may be seen with an increased thoracic volume due to hyperinflation of the lungs, pleural effusion or a large intrathoracic mass.

Common conditions

Abnormalities of the liver recognized radiologically are rarely specific for a single disease condition.

Neoplasia

Hepatic neoplasia (Figure 6.46) can result in localized or generalized hepatomegaly and, occasionally, a cranio-ventral abdominal mass which may not be obviously connected to the liver. Oral administration of barium can be used to define the location of the gastric axis and confirm suspicion of localized or generalized hepato-megaly, although ultrasonography is the preferred tech-nique to assess suspected hepatic mass lesions.

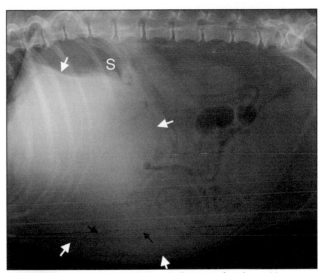

6.46 Lateral view of the abdomen of a dog with a hepatic mass. The large, rounded, soft tissue opacity mass (white arrows) in the cranial mid- and ventral abdomen has caused marked caudal and dorsal displacement of the stomach (S). The kidneys and intestines are also caudally displaced. There is stippled mineralization within the cranioventral liver (black arrows). The spleen is not visible on this view. (Courtesy of the University of Bristol)

Radiological features:

- Diffuse neoplastic infiltration may not be recognized on radiographs unless it results in generalized enlargement.
- Focal neoplastic hepatic masses that do not distort the hepatic margins or result in an increase in size cannot be detected on radiographs.
- The change in shape (expansion, rounding or widening) of the liver lobe margin is more easily appreciated with masses located ventrally within the liver lobes compared with those masses located dorsally. Masses located dorsally within the liver are usually identified based on displacement of adjacent structures.

Congenital portosystemic shunts

Congenital portosystemic shunts (Figure 6.47) are most commonly diagnosed in young animals (see also Figures 4.36 to 4.38).

Radiological features:

- Microhepatica.
- Renomegaly (dogs).
- Urate bladder calculi (usually radiolucent); calculi of mixed composition can be mineralized.
- Vertebral physitis (occasionally).
- Careful abdominal ultrasonography, mesenteric portovenography, computed tomography angiography (CTA) or magnetic resonance angiography (MRA) are required to confirm the diagnosis.

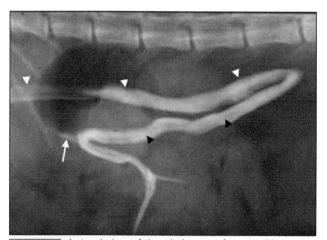

6.47 Lateral view of the abdomen of a cat with an extrahepatic shunt following mesenteric portovenography. A large anomalous vessel (black arrowheads) filled with contrast medium loops caudally to join the caudal vena cava ventral to L5 (white arrowheads). There is slight retrograde filling of the proximal portal vein (arrowed), which is reduced in diameter compared with the shunting vessel. (Courtesy of the University of Bristol)

Metabolic hepatopathy

Radiological features:

- Metabolic hepatopathy typically results in generalized hepatomegaly (Figure 6.48).
- With hyperadrenocorticism concurrent abnormalities can include a pot-bellied appearance to the abdomen, calcinosis cutis (see Figure 6.23) and bladder calculi. In cases of adrenal-dependent hyperadrenocorticism, an adrenal gland mass may occasionally be identified in the mid-dorsal abdomen.

Cirrhosis

Radiological features:

- Hepatic cirrhosis typically results in microhepatica with clockwise rotation of the gastric axis.
- Concurrent ascites secondary to portal hypertension is a common finding (Figure 6.49). The size of the liver is usually inferred from the angle of the gastric axis.
- In the absence of ascites, irregular margination of the hepatic surface may be recognized.

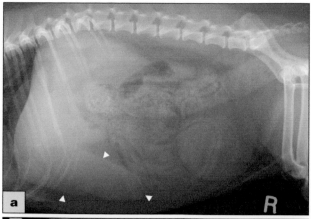

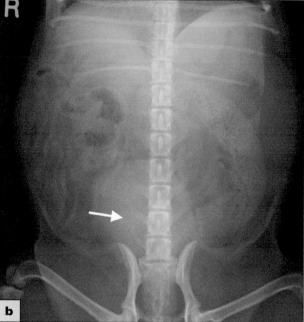

6.48 **(a)** Lateral and **(b)** VD views of the abdomen of a dog with hyperadrenocorticism. There is marked generalized hepatomegaly. The rounded caudoventral hepatic margin (arrowheads) extends well beyond the costal arch. Abdominal distension secondary to hepatomegaly and muscle weakness results in a 'pot-bellied' appearance to the abdomen. Radiopaque calculi are present within the urinary bladder (arrowed). (Courtesy of the University of Bristol)

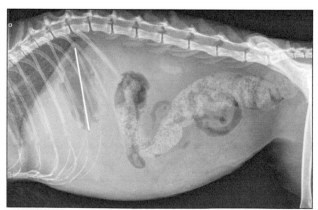

6.49 Lateral view of the abdomen of a cat with a large volume of abdominal fluid. The abdomen has a pendulous appearance. The serosal surfaces of the abdominal organs and viscera are almost completely effaced by the fluid. However, assessment of the angle of the gastric axis (white line) allows hepatic size to be estimated. (Courtesy of the University of Cambridge)

Spleen

Specific approach to interpretation

Size

There is wide variation in the size of the normal canine spleen, which makes an abnormally small spleen or splenomegaly difficult to identify unless accompanied by a change in splenic shape. The feline spleen is smaller and more consistent in size. Visualization of the splenic tail on a lateral radiograph of a cat is suggestive of splenomegaly.

Generalized splenomegaly:

- On the right lateral view, the spleen is thicker and longer with blunting of the normal triangular shape.
- Causes of generalized splenomegaly (Figures 6.50 and 6.51) include:
  - Normal breed variation (German Shepherd Dogs and Greyhounds, in particular, have large spleens)
  - Vascular congestion (common following the administration of acepromazine or barbiturates)
  - Diffuse, usually infiltrative, neoplasia (most commonly lymphoma, mast cell infiltration and malignant histiocytosis)
  - Extramedullary haemopoiesis
  - Splenic hyperplasia (e.g. secondary to chronic anaemia, chronic infection or nodular lymphoid hyperplasia).
- Severe enlargement of the spleen with rounding of the splenic margins may be seen following splenic torsion.

Localized splenomegaly:

- Given the mobility of the body and tail of the spleen, a splenic mass may be highly variable in position.
- Enlargement of the splenic body or tail is more likely to be identified on a lateral view as a variably sized, rounded, soft tissue mass in the mid-ventral abdomen causing displacement of the small intestines caudally and dorsally. On a VD view, the location of a mass in the body or tail is variable and can be seen in the left, mid- or right abdomen.

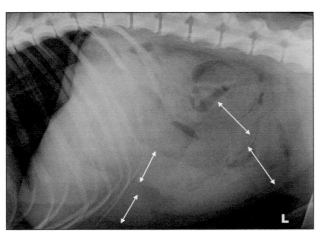

6.50 Lateral view of the abdomen of a male dog with marked generalized splenomegaly. The enlarged spleen (double-headed arrows) curves caudally and then folds and extends cranially, with the tip of the spleen located caudal to the costal arch. (Courtesy of the University of Bristol)

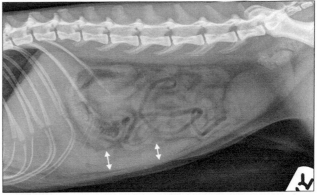

6.51 Lateral view of an adult cat with splenomegaly (double-headed arrows). In the normal cat, the spleen is usually not visible on a right lateral view.

- Enlargement of the splenic head typically results in displacement of the descending colon and small intestine towards the midline and caudal displacement of the left kidney.
- Causes of localized splenomegaly include:
  - Neoplasia (most commonly haemangioma, haemangiosarcoma and histiocytic tumours)
  - Extramedullary haemopoiesis
  - Nodular hyperplasia
  - Haematoma
  - Abscess.

Microsplenia:

- Microsplenia is unusual but is most commonly seen with splenic contraction following an acute bleed.
- When the spleen cannot be recognized, the possibility of prior surgical removal should be considered.

Opacity

A markedly enlarged spleen or a splenic mass has an increased soft tissue opacity compared with the normal, thinner spleen.

Mineralized opacity: Mineralization of the spleen is occasionally seen due to dystrophic mineralization associated with neoplasia, chronic abscess or haematoma.

Gas opacity: Gas opacity within the spleen is rare but can occur due to splenic abscess (Figure 6.52) or the proliferation of gas-forming organisms following splenic torsion.

Shape

- Splenic torsion can be recognized as a large C-shaped soft tissue opacity in the mid-ventral abdomen. This may occur as an isolated condition or in conjunction with gastric volvulus.
- Generalized splenic enlargement results in increased thickness and/or length of the spleen with blunting of the triangle and an increasingly ovoid cross-sectional shape.
- Localized splenomegaly usually presents as a variably sized, rounded, soft tissue mass in the mid-ventral abdomen.
- Irregularity of the normally smooth splenic surface is occasionally recognized and is due to splenic fibrosis (e.g. secondary to peripheral infarction or trauma).

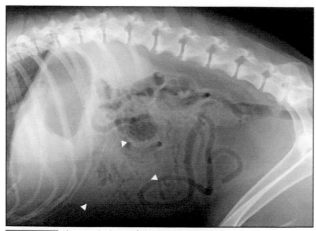

6.52 Lateral view of the abdomen of a dog with a splenic abscess. The abscess appears as a poorly marginated, soft tissue mass (arrowheads) in the mid-ventral abdomen, within which is an area of mottled gas opacity. (Courtesy of the University of Bristol)

Margination

- Loss of the normally visible splenic margins may be due to:
  - Emaciation
  - Free abdominal fluid, including haemorrhage from a bleeding splenic mass or peritoneal effusion in association with splenic torsion.
- Margins may not be visible in young animals.
- Caudal and dorsal displacement of the intestines may be a useful indication of a splenic mass where the splenic margins cannot be seen.
- Splenic margins may be more clearly seen due to:
  - Free abdominal gas
  - A large volume of mesenteric and retroperitoneal fat.
- Irregularity of the splenic margins may be due to localized areas of fibrosis (e.g. secondary to infarction or trauma).

Position

- Cranial displacement of the splenic head occurs with:
  - Microhepatica
  - Diaphragmatic rupture/peritoneopericardial–diaphragmatic hernia
- Cranial displacement of the splenic tail can occur with:
  - Normal variation in deep-chested dogs
  - Microhepatica
  - Diaphragmatic rupture/peritoneopericardial–diaphragmatic hernia
  - A large caudal abdominal mass or advanced pregnancy.
- Caudal displacement of the spleen may be seen due to:
  - Left-sided or generalized hepatomegaly
  - Gastric enlargement or distension.
- Ventral displacement of the spleen may be seen due to:
  - Splenic torsion
  - Ventral body wall rupture.
- Displacement of the spleen to the right side of the abdomen can occur with splenic torsion.

Common conditions

Splenomegaly is a common and non-specific radiological finding. Radiography cannot distinguish between malignant and benign causes of splenic masses, but is used to localize the mass as of probable splenic origin and to evaluate for free abdominal fluid and pulmonary metastases.

Splenic masses

Splenic masses are common in the dog and haemo-abdomen due to rupture of a splenic mass is not uncommon. The radiological appearance of haemo-abdomen depends on the volume of free blood present within the abdominal cavity. A small volume of haemorrhage causes localized blurring of the serosal surfaces, but with increasing volume serosal detail may be completely lost and the splenic margins more difficult to identify. The presence of a splenic mass with free abdominal fluid is highly suggestive of haemangiosarcoma. Benign masses of the spleen are not uncommon, but do not typically result in free abdominal fluid.

Radiological features:

- A mass arising from the splenic body (Figure 6.53) or tail typically has the appearance on a lateral view of a variably sized, rounded, soft tissue mass in the mid-ventral abdomen with caudal and dorsal displacement of the small intestines. The appearance is more variable on the VD view, lying anywhere across the width of the cranial abdomen, with caudal (and possibly right or left) displacement of the small intestines.
- A mass arising from the head of the spleen (Figure 6.54) is usually easier to identify on the VD view, where it is seen as a soft tissue mass in the left craniodorsal abdomen, causing displacement of the descending colon and small intestine towards the midline and caudal displacement of the left kidney.
- Dystrophic mineralization of a splenic mass is occasionally present.
- There may be localized or complete loss of serosal detail due to haemorrhage from a bleeding splenic mass.
- The most common neoplastic masses are haemangioma and haemangiosarcoma.
- Non-neoplastic masses include extramedullary haemopoiesis, haematoma, abscess and nodular hyperplasia.

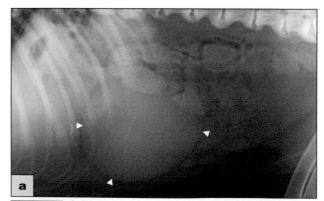

6.53 **(a)** Lateral view of the abdomen of a dog with a mass arising from the body of the spleen. The rounded soft tissue mass (arrowheads) in the mid-ventral abdomen has displaced the small intestines caudally. (continues) ▶

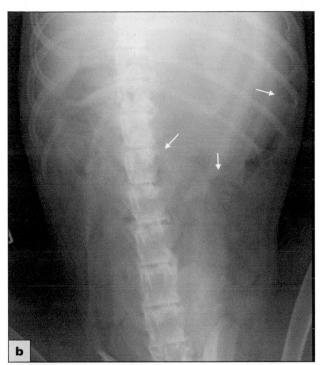

6.53 (continued) **(b)** VD view of the abdomen of a dog with a mass arising from the body of the spleen. The mass (arrowed) has displaced the large intestine caudally and towards the midline.

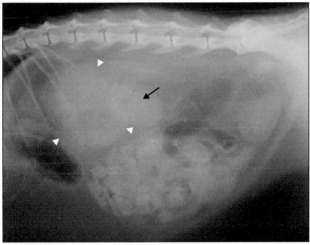

6.54 Lateral view of the abdomen of a cat with a mass arising from the head of the spleen (arrowheads). The stomach has been displaced cranially and the kidneys have been displaced caudoventrally (arrowed). (Courtesy of N Hayward)

Splenic torsion

Splenic torsion occurs when the spleen rotates around its hilus. It is most commonly seen in large, deep-chested dogs. It presents as an isolated condition or in conjunction with gastric volvulus.

Radiological features:

- The spleen appears as a large C-shaped soft tissue mass in the mid-abdomen on the lateral view with caudal displacement of the small intestines. On the VD view, it is seen as a large soft tissue mass in the right cranial abdomen with displacement of the duodenum and small intestines to the left.

- The splenic head is not recognized in its normal left cranial position on the VD view.
- A localized or generalized loss of serosal detail may be present due to peritoneal effusion.
- Rarely, small gas bubbles can be recognized in the splenic parenchyma due to the proliferation of gas-forming bacteria.
- Gastric volvulus may be a concurrent finding with gas distension of the stomach lumen and displacement of the pylorus to the left dorsal abdomen.

Pancreas

Although abdominal radiography is an important part of the diagnostic assessment of the vomiting patient, unless a large pancreatic mass is present, it is an insensitive technique for the diagnosis of pancreatic disease. Ultrasonography is a useful technique in conjunction with species-specific pancreatic lipase immunoreactivity (PLI) testing.

Specific approach to interpretation

Size

Depending on the severity of the pancreatic enlargement, displacement of adjacent structures may be visible radiographically.

- Enlargement of the left limb can result in caudal displacement of the transverse colon.
- Enlargement of the body and right limb can result in right lateral displacement of the descending duodenum.
- Pancreatic enlargement recognized radiographically may be due to:
  - Pancreatitis – although the pancreas itself may be only mildly enlarged, concurrent inflammation of the peripancreatic mesentery can create a more apparent mass effect
  - Pancreatic neoplasia
  - Cavitatory or cystic pancreatic lesions.

Opacity

- An enlarged pancreas is usually of soft tissue opacity.
- Acute pancreatitis may result in a localized area of increased soft tissue opacity due to focal peritonitis and localized loss of the normal mesenteric fat opacity.
- Dystrophic mineralization is rare but may be identified with chronic pancreatitis, pancreatic neoplasia or necrosis of the peripancreatic fat.
- Rarely, mineralized pancreatic calculi or inspissated secretions may be recognized.

Shape and margination

Pancreatitis may be recognized as an ill defined area of poor serosal detail in the craniodorsal abdomen, and is best seen on a VD view. Pancreatic neoplasia has a similar appearance to pancreatitis or may appear as a variably shaped and sized soft tissue mass with less localized loss of serosal detail compared with pancreatitis. However, this differentiation is not always possible. Changes in the margin of the pancreas itself cannot be easily recognized; however, the possibility of pancreatic disease may be inferred from changes to adjacent structures. Ileus and corrugation of the descending duodenum or transverse colon may be noted, and the serosal surface detail of adjacent structures may be reduced or lost.

Position

The normal pancreas is not visible on radiography, so any displacement due to changes in adjacent organs will not be recognized.

Common conditions

Pancreatitis

Radiography is an insensitive technique for the diagnosis of pancreatitis.

Radiological features:

- Increased soft tissue opacity may be present in the right craniodorsal to mid-abdomen, together with a localized loss of serosal detail due to peripancreatic inflammation (Figure 6.55).
- Lateral displacement of the duodenum and, occasionally, caudal displacement of the colon (Figure 6.56) may be recognized due to inflammation of the pancreas and peripancreatic mesentery.
- Functional ileus of the duodenum can be recognized as a mild gas-filled dilatation of the descending duodenum.

Pancreatic neoplasia

Pancreatic masses (Figure 6.57) cannot be differentiated radiologically from pancreatitis and the two conditions may exist concurrently. Small exocrine pancreatic tumours and insulinomas are not visible radiographically.

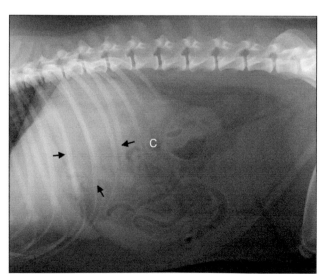

6.55 Lateral view of the abdomen of a dog with pancreatitis. The localized loss of serosal detail in the mid- and craniodorsal abdomen is secondary to pancreatic inflammation and localized peritonitis (arrowed). The transverse colon (C) no longer lies adjacent to the caudal aspect of the stomach.

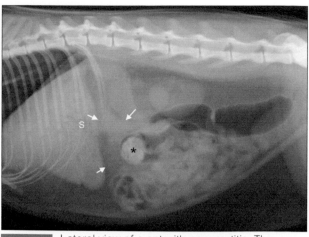

6.56 Lateral view of a cat with pancreatitis. The transverse colon (*) is displaced caudally away from the stomach (S) by a soft tissue opacity with poorly circumscribed, hazy margins (arrowed) consistent with an enlarged left limb of the pancreas. (Courtesy of N Hayward)

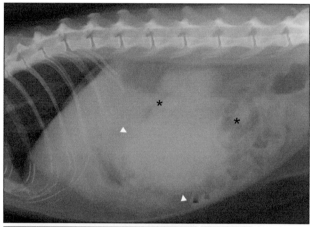

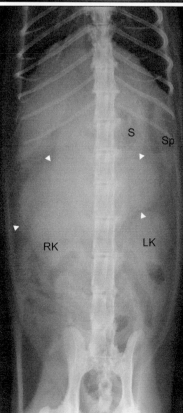

6.57

(a) Lateral and **(b)** VD views of the abdomen of a cat with a pancreatic mass. The mass (arrowheads) in the mid-ventral abdomen is large and irregularly rounded and displaces the colon (*) caudally and dorsally.
LK = left kidney;
RK = right kidney;
S = stomach;
Sp = spleen.
(Courtesy of N Hayward)

Adrenal glands

The location of the adrenal glands in the craniodorsal abdomen means that even quite large lesions may be missed on abdominal radiography as they are usually of soft tissue opacity and may silhouette with the soft tissue opacities of the adjacent kidneys, spleen, liver and stomach. Abdominal ultrasonography is therefore a more sensitive technique for evaluating the size and shape of the adrenal glands. The adrenal glands are relatively fixed in location and are very rarely (if ever) displaced by adjacent structures.

Specific approach to interpretation

Size
An adrenal gland mass is unlikely to be radiographically apparent unless it is at least 2 cm in diameter.

Opacity

- Normal adrenal glands are of soft tissue opacity. However, incidental mineralization of the adrenal glands in older cats (Figure 6.58) is occasionally recognized as a focal area of mineralized opacity craniomedial to one or both kidneys.
- In dogs, irregular mineralization, especially in conjunction with a soft tissue mass, is more likely to be associated with adrenal gland neoplasia.
- In dogs, mineralization of the adrenal glands with no enlargement or soft tissue mass is seen rarely in cases of hypoadrenocorticism (especially in Cocker Spaniels).

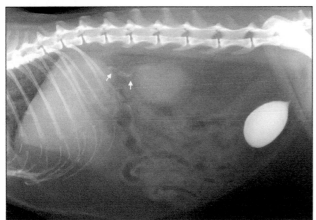

6.58 Lateral view of the abdomen of a cat with mineralized adrenal glands (arrowed). Incidental mineralization in older cats should be distinguished from other causes of abdominal mineralization which may be of clinical significance (e.g. ureteric calculi). (Courtesy of N Hayward)

Common conditions

Adrenal gland neoplasia
Small adrenal gland masses are not apparent radiographically. Surprisingly large adrenal gland masses may also go unrecognized on radiography, especially in dogs where the mass may be located within the ribcage/costal arch and can silhouette with the soft tissue opacities of the adjacent kidney, liver and stomach. The primary differential diagnoses are adenoma, adenocarcinoma, phaeochromocytoma and myelolipoma. A functional aldosterone-secreting adenoma or adenocarcinoma is a possible differential diagnosis in older cats presenting with hypokalaemia; such masses may be recognized on radiography if large enough.

Radiological features:

- The retroperitoneal location of the adrenal glands means that, even when dramatically enlarged, they remain within the dorsal abdomen and can cause caudal and/or lateral displacement of the adjacent kidney and ventral displacement of the peritoneal organs.
- Adrenal gland neoplasia may be seen as a soft tissue mass, sometimes with areas of mineralization (Figure 6.59).
- Pulmonary metastases are rare.

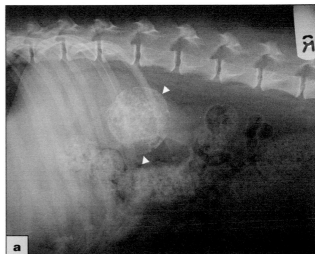
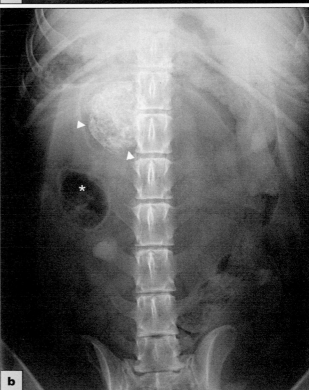

6.59 **(a)** Lateral and **(b)** VD views of the abdomen of a dog with a mineralized right adrenal gland mass. The mass (arrowheads) in the right craniodorsal abdomen is densely mineralized. The right kidney is not well visualized on either view. The caecum is denoted by the asterisk. (Courtesy of G Hammond, University of Glasgow)

Hyperadrenocorticism

Although commonly diagnosed in the dog, hyperadrenocorticism is an uncommon condition in the cat. Adrenal gland enlargement is rarely radiographically apparent, even in patients with the adrenal-dependent hyperadrenocorticism. In experienced hands, ultrasonography is a valuable technique for the evaluation of adrenal gland size and the identification of adrenal gland mass lesions.

Radiological features:

- Hepatomegaly may be seen with caudal displacement of the gastric axis and rounding of the caudoventral hepatic margin. Cats do not show steroid-related hepatopathy, but hepatomegaly is commonly seen secondary to concurrent diabetes mellitus.
- Distension of the urinary bladder may be seen secondary to polydipsia and eventual bladder atony.
- Opaque calcium phosphate or calcium oxalate calculi can occasionally be identified.
- A 'pot-bellied' abdominal contour may be recognized due to a combination of muscle weakness, hepatomegaly and urinary bladder distension.
- Dystrophic soft tissue mineralization may be recognized as calcinosis cutis and occasionally as interstitial pulmonary mineralization.

Urinary tract

Kidneys and ureters

Specific approach to interpretation

Survey radiography is limited to the assessment of renal size, shape and opacity. Normal ureters cannot be seen on survey radiographs. Ultrasonography is useful in evaluating the internal architecture of the kidneys, but normal ureters cannot be seen. Intravenous urography is therefore an important complementary technique to identify and assess the renal pelves and ureters (Figure 6.60). Survey radiographs provide no information on renal function and there is often poor correlation between renal size as assessed on radiography and biochemical tests of renal function. Changes in renal size are specific but relatively insensitive indicators of renal disease. Changes in renal shape are often more sensitive indicators of renal pathology and careful attention should be paid to evaluating the margins and shape of the kidneys.

Size: The normal renal length in the dog is 2.5–3.5 times the length of L2 (when assessed on a VD view). The normal renal length in a neutered cat is 1.9–2.6 times the length of L2 and in an entire cat is 2.1–3.2 times the length of L2 (when assessed on a VD view).

- Marked enlargement of the right kidney results in ventral deviation of the duodenum and displacement of the ascending colon towards the midline.
- Marked enlargement of the left kidney results in displacement of the descending colon ventrally and towards the midline.

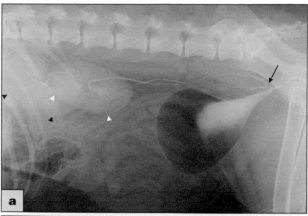

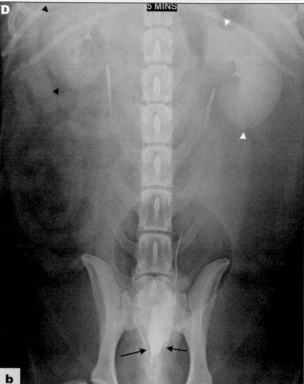

6.60 **(a)** Lateral and **(b)** VD intravenous urograms in a normal neutered male dog. The ureters (arrowed) terminate normally at the trigone of the bladder. These images were taken approximately 5 minutes after the intravenous administration of contrast medium. The renal parenchyma (right kidney = black arrowheads; left kidney = white arrowheads), renal pelves and ureters are opacified and contrast medium is seen entering the bladder. A pneumocystogram has been performed to facilitate identification of the ureteric terminations. (Courtesy of the University of Bristol)

- Mild to moderate renal enlargement may be due to:
  - Acute nephritis or pyelonephritis (unilateral or bilateral)
  - Congenital portosystemic shunt in the dog (bilateral)
  - Compensatory hypertrophy (unilateral with the contralateral kidney small or absent).
- Moderate to marked enlargement (Figure 6.61) may be due to:
  - Hydronephrosis (unilateral or bilateral)
  - Infiltrative neoplasia (e.g. lymphoma; unilateral or bilateral)
  - Focal or multifocal primary or metastatic neoplasia (usually unilateral, may be bilateral)

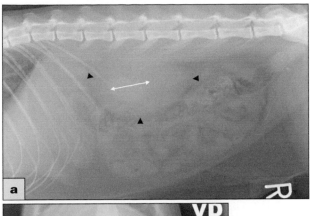

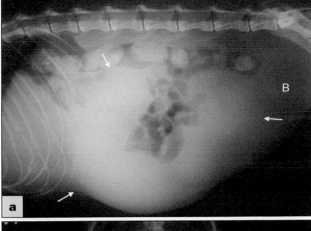

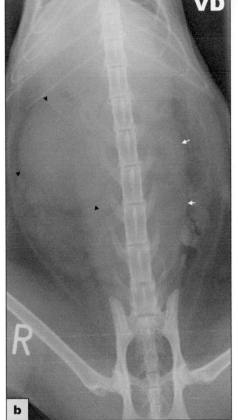

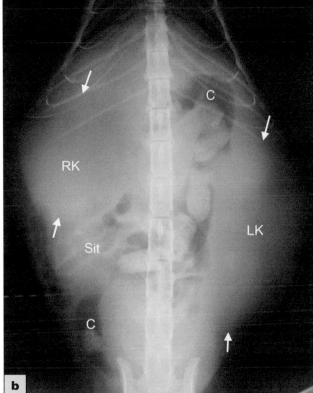

6.61 **(a)** Lateral and **(b)** VD views of the abdomen of a cat with unilateral renomegaly. The enlarged right kidney (arrowheads) is superimposed on the smaller left kidney (double-headed arrow) on the lateral view. On the VD view, the left kidney is difficult to define due to the bulk of the sublumbar muscles (arrowed). The differential diagnoses for unilateral renomegaly with smooth margins and a homogeneous appearance include severe hydronephrosis (obstructive), compensatory hypertrophy, perirenal pseudocyst or unilateral neoplasia. (Courtesy of the University of Bristol)

6.62 **(a)** Lateral and **(b)** VD views of the abdomen of a cat with bilateral perirenal pseudocysts. Both kidneys are markedly enlarged (arrowed). On the lateral view, the kidneys are so large that they silhouette with each other and with the liver cranially and the bladder (B) caudally. On the VD view, the left kidney (LK) appears more markedly enlarged than the right kidney (RK). Note that the small intestines (Sit) are displaced centrally and to the right by the left kidney, and caudally by the right kidney. C = colon.

- Feline infectious peritonitis (usually bilateral)
- Perirenal pseudocysts (typically seen in older male cats; unilateral or bilateral) (Figure 6.62)
- Polycystic kidney disease (especially Persian cats; usually bilateral)
- Renal haematoma, abscess or granuloma (usually unilateral).
- Reduced kidney size (Figure 6.63) may be due to:
  - Renal hypoplasia or dysplasia (unilateral or bilateral)
  - Chronic renal disease (unilateral or bilateral).

Normal canine and feline ureters are too small to be seen on plain radiographs. However, dramatic dilatation of the ureters can occur, usually secondary to ureteric obstruction, and may be recognized as a band-like, tortuous soft tissue opacity within the retroperitoneal space.

Number: Unilateral renal agenesis is rare. Renal ultrasonography and/or intravenous urography are usually indicated to confirm the presence of only one kidney. Failure to visualize the right kidney is common due to border effacement with the liver.

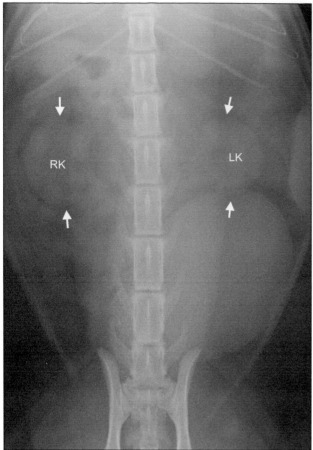

6.63 VD view of the abdomen of a cat with bilaterally small and irregular kidneys (arrowed). LK = left kidney; RK = right kidney. (Courtesy of the University of Bristol)

Opacity:

Mineralized opacity:

- Renal calculi:
  - Often difficult or impossible to differentiate from dystrophic mineralization
  - Recognized as small focal mineralized opacities located within the renal diverticula or 'staghorn' mineralized opacities within the renal pelvis
  - May be an incidental finding.
- Ureteric calculi:
  - Small mineralized opacities superimposed on the retroperitoneal space anywhere along the length of the ureter
  - Superimposed mineralized faecal material should not be mistaken for ureteric calculi.
- Nephrocalcinosis:
  - Diffuse increased opacity of the renal parenchyma secondary to hypercalcaemia
  - Underlying causes include chronic renal failure, hyperparathyroidism, hyperadrenocorticism, hypervitaminosis D and ethylene glycol poisoning.
- Dystrophic mineralization may be seen with chronic lesions such as neoplasia, haematoma, abscess, granuloma or chronic infarction.
- Incidental mineralization of the adrenal glands in cats may be mistaken for renal mineralization, and dystrophic mineralization at the sites of ovariohysterectomy may be mistaken for ureteric calculi.

Gas opacity:

- Most commonly iatrogenic due to ureteral reflux of gas following pneumocystography.
- Pyelonephritis with gas-forming bacteria (rare).
- In cats with a large amount of fat within the renal pelvis, the relative lucency may be mistaken for gas.

Shape:

- In many conditions, enlarged kidneys retain their smooth outline but become increasingly rounded in shape.
- Irregularly marginated kidneys, normal or enlarged in size, may be seen due to:
  - Polycystic kidney disease
  - Focal or multifocal primary or metastatic renal neoplasia
  - Renal haematoma, abscess or granuloma.
- Abnormally small kidneys may be smooth or irregular in outline.
- Hypoplastic kidneys tend to be smoothly marginated.
- Kidneys with chronic end-stage disease tend to have an irregular appearance.
- An unusually large and tortuous ureter may be seen as an undulating soft tissue band within the retroperitoneal space in cases with dramatic ureteral dilatation.

Margination:

- Partial or complete loss of clear renal margination may be due to:
  - The normal cranial location of the right kidney (exaggerated in deep-chested dogs)
  - Little or no retroperitoneal fat in emaciated or very young animals
  - Retroperitoneal effusion
  - Congenital absence of one kidney/previous nephrectomy.
- Enhanced visualization of the renal margins may be due to:
  - Increased retroperitoneal fat in obese animals
  - Free gas in the retroperitoneal space.

Position: Due to their retroperitoneal position, significant ventral displacement is uncommon, even with dramatically enlarged kidneys. Displacement of the kidneys in the absence of an adjacent mass is almost invariably of no clinical significance. Renal ectopia occurs rarely and may result in cranial displacement of the kidneys (into the thorax in some extreme cases). The left kidney is relatively mobile and in large-breed dogs it may appear to be displaced ventrally, where it can be mistaken for a mid-abdominal mass. Ectopic ureters terminate in an abnormal location: most commonly the urethra, but occasionally the vagina or rectum. Unless markedly dilated, the location of the ureters cannot be seen on plain radiography.

Common conditions

Chronic renal disease: The changes associated with chronic renal disease are non-specific. In addition, there is poor correlation between the changes observed and renal function.

Radiological features:

- Kidneys are usually small and may be either smoothly or irregularly marginated.
- Irregular areas of renal mineralization can be seen and may represent calculi or dystrophic mineralization.
- Changes may be unilateral or bilateral.
- In cases of renal dysplasia, signs of renal secondary hyperparathyroidism may be seen (see Chapter 8).
- Mineralization of the gastric mucosa, pulmonary vessels and myocardium is a rare feature of chronic renal disease.

Renal and ureteral calculi: Most renal and ureteral calculi are radiopaque and recognized as mineralized opacities on survey radiographs (Figures 6.64 and 6.65).

Radiological features:

- Calculi may vary in size and shape and may be unilateral or bilateral and single or multiple.
- Renal calculi are typically identified within the renal diverticula or renal pelves.

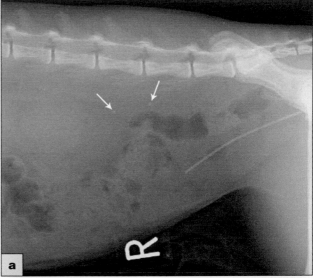

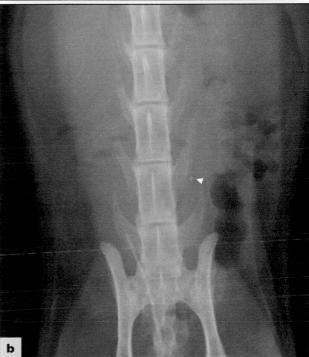

6.65 **(a)** Lateral and **(b)** VD views of the abdomen of a cat with ureteric calculi. Although two small mineralized calculi (arrowed) are visible dorsal to the colon on the lateral view, only one, within the left ureter (arrowhead), can be seen on the VD view. The second is obscured by the lumbar vertebrae. The tip of a urinary catheter lies within the bladder and a small gas bubble is superimposed. (Courtesy of the University of Bristol)

- Ureteral calculi may be recognized anywhere along the length of the ureter. A dilated and tortuous ureter is consistent with ureteral obstruction.
- Bladder calculi may also be present.
- Superimposed faecal material may mimic renal or ureteral calculi.
- Ultrasonography and/or contrast studies may be useful for confirming the presence of calculi.
  - Calculi appear as filling defects within the renal pelves or ureters.
  - Renal pelvic or ureteral dilatation may be present secondary to complete or partial obstruction.

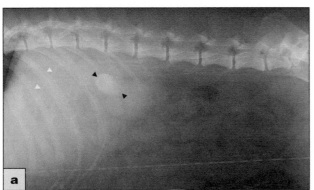

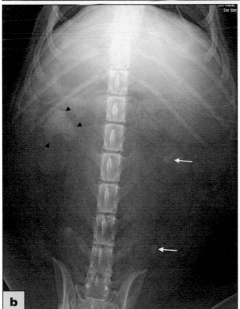

6.64 **(a)** Lateral and **(b)** VD views of the abdomen of a dog with a large 'staghorn' calculus within the right renal pelvis (black arrowheads). An additional finding associated with the chronic azotaemia is faint mineralization of the gastric mucosa (white arrowheads). This patient has very prominent nipples (arrowed) which shouldn't be mistaken for additional areas of mineralization.

Pyelonephritis or acute nephritis: Although mild renal enlargement may occasionally be recognized, survey radiographs are usually unremarkable.

Radiological features:

- Dilatation or distortion of the renal pelvis may be seen on intravenous urography in cases of pyelonephritis (Figure 6.66).
- Laboratory findings are more useful for the diagnosis of acute nephritis, which cannot be recognized from intravenous urography and has a non-specific appearance on ultrasonography.

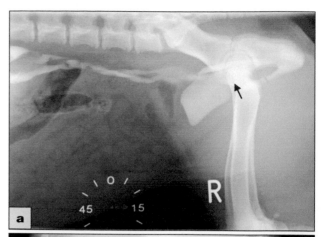

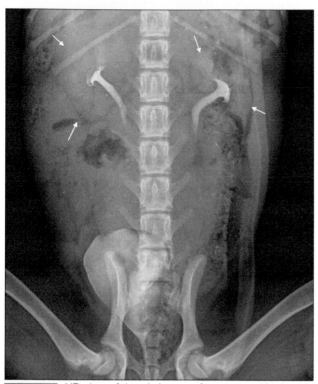

6.66 VD view of the abdomen of a puppy with chronic pyelonephritis secondary to chronic cystitis associated with a bladder diverticulum and calculi. There is reduced serosal detail associated with the age of the dog and the large volume of faecal material. However, it is possible to recognize that the renal margins (arrowed) are irregular, consistent with chronic disease. The renal pelves and ureters are irregularly dilated with indistinct filling defects due to debris (pyonephrosis).

Hydronephrosis: Without the use of ultrasonography or intravenous urography (Figure 6.67), it is impossible to differentiate the soft tissue opacity of a fluid-filled renal pelvis from the soft tissue of the surrounding kidney parenchyma. Hence, on survey radiography hydronephrosis cannot be differentiated from the normal kidney or, if renal enlargement is present, from renal neoplasia, perinephric pseudocysts, abscesses or granulomas.

Radiological features:

- Hydronephrosis may be unilateral or bilateral.
- Intravenous urography may demonstrate:
  - Mild renal pelvic dilatation with the overall size of the kidneys appearing normal on survey radiographs (e.g. due to pyelonephritis, ectopic ureters or early ureteral obstruction)

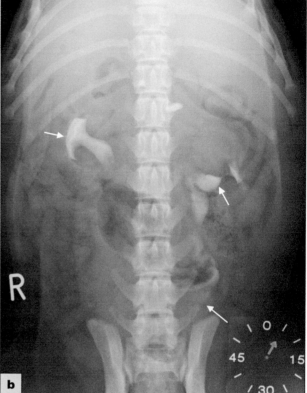

6.67 Intravenous urography. **(a)** Lateral (taken after 15 minutes) and **(b)** VD (taken after 5 minutes) views of the abdomen of a dog following intravenous administration of contrast medium. Both renal pelves and ureters (white arrows) are moderately dilated, consistent with hydronephrosis and hydroureter, respectively. The caudal location of the bladder neck (black arrow) obscures the ureteric terminations; however, the presence of contrast medium in the bladder suggests that at least one ureter terminates in the normal location. There is no spillage of contrast medium around the perineum, which would be expected with an ectopic ureter. To rule out an ectopic ureter, intravenous urography should be followed by a retrograde study. (Courtesy of the University of Bristol)

- Increasingly dramatic renal pelvic dilatation, resulting in significant renomegaly on survey radiographs. Dramatic dilatation is more likely with pelvic or ureteral obstruction (e.g. due to ureteral calculi, neoplasia or stricture, including accidental ligation during ovariohysterectomy, which is more common in the cat)
- Concurrent ureteral dilatation.

Ectopic ureters: It is rare to make a definitive diag nosis of ectopic ureters from plain radiographs.

Radiological features:

- Kidneys may be large and megaureter recognized.
- The bladder is usually small if both ureters are ectopic.
- With experience it may be possible to identify an ectopic ureter on ultrasonography. However, in most cases intravenous contrast studies are indicated to demonstrate the exact termination of the ureter (Figure 6.68).

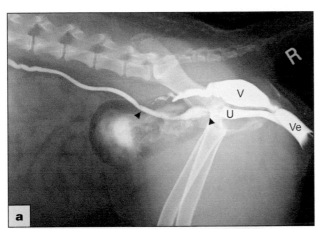

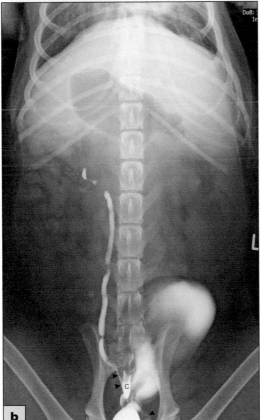

6.68 **(a)** Lateral and **(b)** VD views of the abdomen of an entire bitch with an ectopic ureter. Retrograde vaginourethrography has been performed. The right ureter is ectopic. It is moderately dilated and terminates abnormally within the proximal urethra (arrowheads). Note that a pneumocystogram has been performed to improve visualization of the termination of the ureters and that there is good distension of the vestibule (Ve), vagina (V) and urethra (U). C = cervix.

- Abnormalities recognized on an intravenous urogram include:
  - Abnormal termination of the ureter(s), usually within the urethra, but occasionally the uterus, vagina or rectum
  - Dilatation of the abnormal ureter(s).
- A retrograde urethrogram can be used to confirm the termination of an abnormal ureter within the urethra and should be performed as part of intravenous urography when assessing for ectopic ureters.
- Reflux of air into the ureters or renal pelves may be present following pneumocystography.

Renal neoplasia: Renal neoplasia (Figure 6.69; see also Figure 4.9) can only be recognized on survey radio- graphy when it results in an obvious change in renal size or shape.

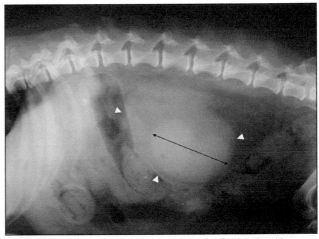

6.69 Lateral view of the abdomen of a bitch with unilateral renal carcinoma. The normal sized left kidney (double-headed arrow) is superimposed on the ventral aspect of the markedly enlarged and irregularly shaped right kidney (arrowheads) in the craniodorsal abdomen. (Courtesy of P Mahoney)

Radiological features:

- Diffuse infiltrative neoplasia, most commonly lymphoma, usually results in generalized renomegaly and is often bilateral.
- Focal neoplastic lesions are more likely to cause irregular distortion of the renal margins as well as an increase in renal size.
  - Primary renal neoplasia is usually unilateral, although occasionally both kidneys can be affected. Causes include renal cell carcinoma, transitional cell carcinoma and nephroblastoma.
  - Metastatic renal neoplasia may be unilateral or bilateral. Causes include haemangiosarcoma, histiocytic sarcoma, lymphoma and metastasis from a primary tumour in the contralateral kidney.
- Intravenous urography may demonstrate:
  - Enlarged, often abnormally shaped, kidneys
  - Patchy renal parenchymal enhancement and/or filling defects caused by the abnormal neoplastic tissue.
- Ultrasonography is likely to be more useful.

Renal cysts: Polycystic kidney disease is a hereditary condition recognized most frequently in Persian cats and characterized by cystic lesions throughout the kidneys. Renal cysts are occasionally identified in the dog (Figure 6.70) and are usually incidental findings.

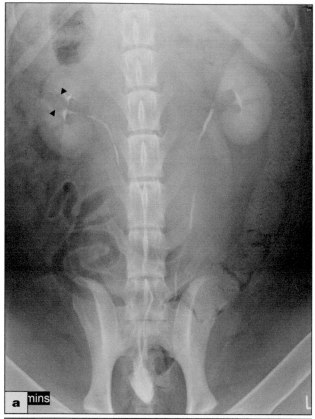

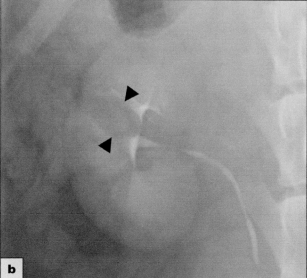

6.70 Intravenous urography in a dog with a cyst in the right kidney. **(a)** VD view of the abdomen obtained 5 minutes following the intravenous administration of an iodinated contrast medium. The renal cyst appears as a smoothly marginated, ovoid filling defect in the lateral cortex of the right kidney (arrowheads). The cyst distorts the renal pelvis focally, resulting in a small filling defect. The renal cyst was demonstrated on ultrasonography. Although other differential diagnoses for a focal filling defect include neoplasia, granuloma and abscess, the smooth margins are more suggestive of a benign lesion. **(b)** Magnified view. (Courtesy of the University of Bristol)

Radiological features:

- Small cysts may be completely contained within the renal parenchyma; thus, the kidneys may appear normal on survey radiographs.
- Larger cysts often bulge from the renal surface, resulting in irregular renal enlargement.
- Polycystic kidney disease is usually bilateral, although the radiographic changes may appear unilateral.
- Following the administration of intravenous contrast medium, the cystic areas will not enhance and appear as filling defects within the enhanced surrounding renal parenchyma. In complex cystic lesions, the cysts are so numerous and variable in size that discrete filling defects can be difficult to recognize.
- Renal ultrasonography is a very sensitive technique for identifying renal cysts.

Renal or ureteral rupture: Renal or ureteral rupture is most commonly caused by severe abdominal trauma, and results in the leakage of urine and blood into the retroperitoneal space. Rupture is usually unilateral although, rarely, patients may present with bilateral injury.

Radiological features:

- Loss of retroperitoneal detail (streaky, wispy appearance). The appearance is indistinguishable from retroperitoneal haemorrhage (see Figure 6.104).
- Retroperitoneal enlargement with ventral bulging of the retroperitoneal space and ventral displacement of the abdominal organs.
- The thorax, abdomen and skeleton must be assessed for evidence of concurrent injuries (e.g. pelvic fracture).
- Intravenous urography demonstrates leakage of contrast medium from the ruptured kidney or ureter into the retroperitoneal space.

Bladder and urethra

Survey radiography is useful to evaluate the location, size and shape of the urinary bladder in the dog and cat, but does not allow the luminal surface of the bladder wall to be visualized or radiolucent cystic calculi to be recognized. The normal urethra is not radiographically visible.

Specific approach to interpretation

Size:

Bladder: The size of the normal bladder varies markedly and a subjective assessment should be made, taking into account the opportunities for filling (availability of drinking water and intravenous fluids) and emptying the bladder at the time of radiography. The normal urethra is too small to be seen.

- Distended bladder – this may be a normal finding in an animal that has not recently urinated. Alternative causes include:
  - Polyuria/polydipsia
  - Bladder atony (e.g. in patients with hyperadrenocorticism)

- Non-obstructive urinary retention (neurogenic, psychogenic, painful)
- Obstructive urinary retention (urethral calculi, prostatomegaly, urethral/bladder neck neoplasia, urethral stricture) (Figure 6.71).
- Small bladder – causes include:
  - Recent urination
  - Anuria
  - Bladder or ureteral rupture (an assessment for loss of abdominal and/or retroperitoneal detail due to leakage of urine should be made)
  - Bilateral ectopic ureters and bladder hypoplasia
  - Non-distensible bladder (e.g. due to chronic cystitis and neoplasia).

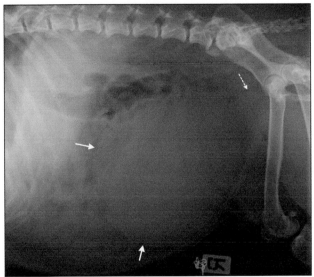

6.71 Lateral view of the abdomen of a male dog with marked bladder distension secondary to a urethral tumour. The distended bladder (solid arrows) displaces the small intestinal loops cranially and the ventral abdominal wall ventrally. The proximal urethra (dashed arrow) is subjectively increased in diameter. Pathological bladder distension must be distinguished from physiological distension secondary to polydipsia, reluctance to void during hospitalization or pain. The pelvic urethra in bitches, and the pelvic and penile urethra in male dogs, should be evaluated for a cause of the obstruction (particularly calculi).

Urethra: Urethral neoplasia may be associated with significant urethral enlargement, recognized as a soft tissue mass, most commonly within the pelvis where it may cause displacement of the adjacent rectum.

Shape:

Bladder: Changes in bladder shape may be seen due to compression by adjacent organs, most commonly an enlarged colon, uterus or prostate gland. An irregularly marginated bladder may be seen due to:

- Bladder diverticula and other malformations
- Extensive bladder rupture and partial collapse of the bladder (with a small rupture, the bladder may appear normal in shape)
- Extensive bladder neoplasia with transmural extension.

Urethra: Changes in the shape of the urethra cannot be recognized without retrograde urethrography or vaginourethrography.

Opacity: The normal canine and feline bladder and urethra are soft tissue structures.

Mineralized opacity:

- Small foci of mineralized opacity seen within the bladder lumen or along the length of the urethra are usually due to calculi. The opacity of the calculi varies with mineral content:
  - Struvite, calcium oxalate, calcium phosphate and silicate calculi are usually radiopaque
  - Cystine and urate calculi are usually radiolucent and therefore cannot be seen on survey radiographs.
- A small mineralized opacity may occasionally be seen in the area of the distal urethra due to a vestigial os penis in a tom cat or a hermaphrodite patient.
- Foreign material (most commonly air gun pellets) is occasionally recognized in the bladder lumen.
- Dystrophic mineralization of bladder neoplasms may be seen, most commonly in the trigone area.
- Fine mineralization of the bladder wall may be present with chronic cystitis (Figure 6.72).

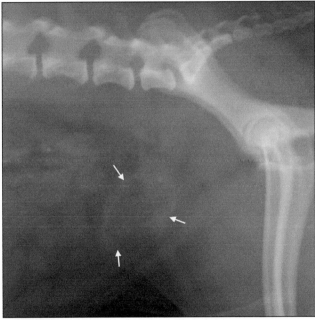

6.72 Lateral view of the abdomen of a dog with chronic cystitis. The bladder is small with fine, irregular, diffuse dystrophic mineralization of the mucosa (arrowed). Note that although the bladder wall appears thickened, it is not possible to assess the thickness without the bladder being adequately distended.

Gas opacity:

- Iatrogenic gas opacity due to previous cystocentesis or urethral catheterization is common.
- Iatrogenic emphysematous cystitis may occur following pneumocystography in a bladder that is poorly distensible due to severe inflammation or neoplasia.
- Emphysematous cystitis appears as a gas opacity, tracking through the bladder wall and within the bladder lumen (Figure 6.73). This is uncommon but is more likely to be seen in patients with concurrent diabetes mellitus.

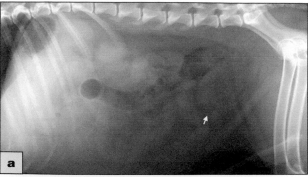

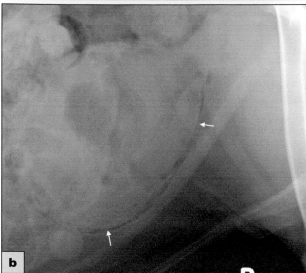

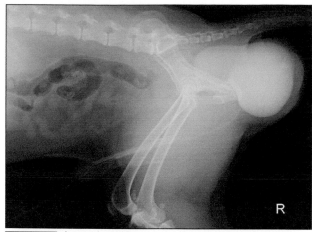

6.74 Lateral positive-contrast cystogram of a male dog with retroflexion of the bladder into a perineal hernia. Small intestinal loops extend caudally to the pubis as a result of the absence of the bladder. (Courtesy of the University of Bristol)

6.73 Lateral radiographs of the caudal abdomen of two dogs with emphysematous cystitis. **(a)** The gas (arrowed) within the bladder wall is more difficult to recognize as it is predominantly projected *en face*. **(b)** Some of the gas is projected in profile along the ventral bladder wall and the intramural location (arrowed) is more easily recognized. Further large gas shadows are superimposed on the bladder. Intramural gas must be distinguished from overlying gas-filled small intestinal loops, subcutaneous emphysema and free abdominal gas.

- Ventral displacement of the bladder:
  - Within the abdomen – can be caused by sublumbar lymphadenopathy, constipation and uterine enlargement
  - Ventral to the body wall – can be caused by an inguinal hernia or ventral body wall rupture.

Common conditions

Cystitis: Survey radiography is usually unremarkable, although the bladder may appear small due to the increased frequency of urination (Figure 6.75).

Radiological features:

- Double-contrast retrograde studies provide excellent luminal mucosal detail.
  - Often unremarkable with acute cystitis.
  - With chronic cystitis, bladder wall thickening and mucosal irregularity are frequently present, especially cranioventrally.
- Similar findings are recognized on ultrasonography, which is a more sensitive technique.
- Emphysematous cystitis is an uncommon condition, recognized by the presence of intramural and often intraluminal gas.

Margination: Difficulty or failure to recognize the margin of the bladder may indicate:

- Emaciated or very young animal
- Empty bladder
- Bladder not in a normal location (e.g. due to retroflexion into a perineal hernia; see Figure 6.74)
- Free abdominal fluid (including urine due to bladder rupture).

Position:

Bladder:

- Cranial displacement of the bladder may be due to:
  - Cranial migration of a very full bladder
  - Prostatic enlargement in male dogs
  - Obesity in cats.
- Caudal displacement of the urinary bladder may be due to:
  - An unusually short urethra (especially in bitches)
  - Retroflexion of the bladder into a perineal hernia (usually in entire male dogs) (Figure 6.74).

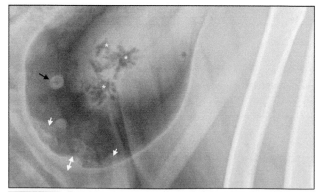

6.75 Double-contrast cystogram in a bitch with chronic cystitis. The vertex of the bladder is thickened (double-headed arrow). Polypoid thickening of the mucosa surrounded by gas is recognized in profile (white arrows) as well as *en face* (black arrow). Calculi within the central pool of contrast medium appear as stellate filling defects (*). (Courtesy of the University of Cambridge)

Bladder and urethral calculi: The opacity of bladder and urethral calculi varies with mineral content. Radiolucent calculi cannot be seen on survey radiography, and ultrasonography or bladder contrast studies are required for identification.

Radiological features:

- Struvite, calcium oxalate, calcium phosphate and silicate calculi are usually radiopaque (Figure 6.76).
- Cystine and urate calculi are usually radiolucent and therefore cannot be seen on survey radiographs.
- Although most calculi are small, large bladder stones may occasionally be >5 cm in diameter.
- The entire urethra should be assessed critically, especially in male cats and dogs, for the possible presence of calculi.
  - In the male dog, a lateral view centred on the caudal abdomen, with the hindlimbs secured cranially to avoid superimposition, is used to assess the urethra. The fabellae, in particular, may mimic a calculus.

- The kidneys and ureters should also be evaluated for calculi.
- Urethral obstruction by a calculus results in marked distension of the bladder.
- Double-contrast studies of the bladder may demonstrate:
  - A collection of calculi settled dependently within the centre of the bladder, which appear as filling defects within the contrast medium pool. Filling defects may also be seen with:
    - Air bubbles, which are usually perfectly round in shape and tend to migrate to the periphery of the contrast medium pool (Figure 6.77)
    - Blood clots, which are usually irregular in shape and may be located anywhere within the pool of contrast medium.
- A positive-contrast retrograde urethrogram is useful to identify urethral calculi, which appear as filling defects.
  - Calculi should not be mistaken for air bubbles, which are commonly introduced into the urethra during the procedure. Air bubbles should be perfectly round and easily move position when further contrast medium is introduced.

Bladder and urethral neoplasia: Bladder tumours are most frequently identified in the trigone area and can extend caudally to involve the urethra. The urethra can also be the primary site of the tumour. Unless the tumour is large enough to distort the shape of the bladder, survey radiographs may appear unremarkable.

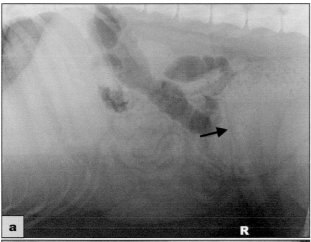

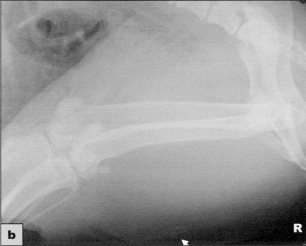

6.76 Lateral views of **(a)** the cranial abdomen and **(b)** the pelvis of a male dog with a radiopaque cystic (black arrow) and urethral (white arrow) calculi. The large size of the dog necessitates at least two views for a complete assessment: a view of the cranial abdomen to include the kidneys and bladder; and a view of the caudal abdomen to include the pelvis and urethra. The hindlegs have been pulled forward to avoid superimposition of the fabellae on the os penis, which may be mistaken for calculi. (Courtesy of the University of Bristol)

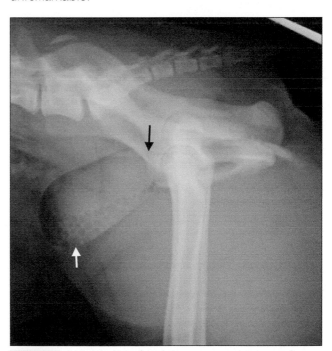

6.77 Lateral view of an intravenous urogram and pneumocystogram in a young bitch. Multiple radiolucent filling defects (white arrow) are highlighted by the pool of contrast medium within the bladder. The peripheral, rather than central, location and very rounded appearance of the filling defects are consistent with air bubbles rather than radiopaque calculi. The bladder neck in this animal is caudally located and one of the ureters (ectopic) is mildly dilated (black arrow). (Courtesy of the University of Bristol)

Radiological features:

- If a urethral tumour is large enough, it can cause recognizable displacement of adjacent structures, such as the rectum.
- Bladder distension may be present if the tumour causes urethral obstruction (see Figure 6.71).
- Dystrophic mineralization of a mass is occasionally recognized on survey radiographs.
- The caudal retroperitoneal area should be examined for evidence of sublumbar lymphadenopathy.
- Ultrasonography is useful for the evaluation of the bladder, proximal urethra and sublumbar lymph nodes, but cannot be used for assessment of the intrapelvic urethra due to the bony pelvis.
- Contrast studies are useful to identify bladder tumours and are the technique of choice for evaluation of the urethra.
  - Bladder tumours (Figure 6.78) should be highlighted on a contrast study, either by air or positive-contrast medium.
    - Most likely to be located at the bladder trigone.
    - Usually seen as a focal, irregular intraluminal mass with a broad-based attachment to the bladder wall.

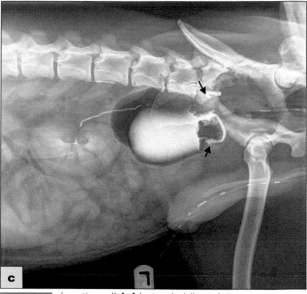

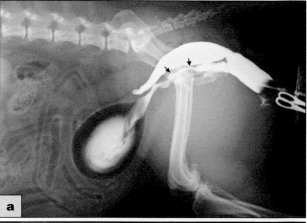

6.78 (continued) **(c)** Lateral oblique intravenous urogram and retrograde urethrogram of a male dog with haematuria due to a bladder tumour. (b–c) The terminations of both ureters (arrowed) are surrounded by the mass but not obstructed.

- On positive-contrast retrograde urethrography, urethral tumours (Figure 6.79) appear as abnormal irregular margination of the luminal contrast medium column due to ulceration and thickening of the urethral wall.
  - There may be concurrent irregular leakage of contrast medium, especially into the prostate gland of the male dog.

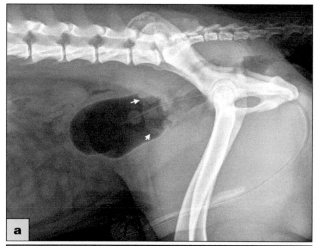

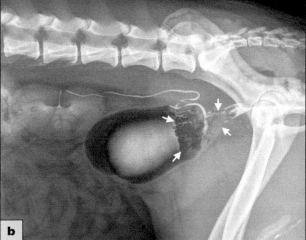

6.78 **(a)** Lateral pneumocystogram and **(b)** lateral intravenous urogram and retrograde urethrogram of a male dog with haematuria due to a bladder tumour. (a) A large, lobulated, soft tissue mass opacity (arrowed) results in a filling defect in the trigone and proximal urethra. (b–c) The terminations of both ureters (arrowed) are surrounded by the mass but not obstructed. (continues) ▶

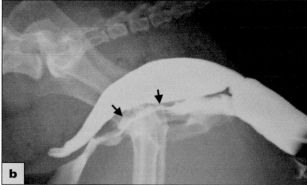

6.79 **(a)** Lateral double-contrast cystogram and retrograde vaginourethrogram in a bitch with urethral neoplasia. The intrapelvic urethra (arrowed) is of variable diameter, irregularly marginated and poorly filled with contrast medium. **(b)** Magnified view.

Bladder and urethral rupture: With a small bladder rupture, survey radiographs may be unremarkable.

Radiological features:

- A more extensive bladder rupture can result in an irregular appearance to the bladder. Free abdominal fluid may be present and serosal detail lost (Figure 6.80).
- Urethral rupture is rarely recognized on survey radiographs.
- Positive-contrast retrograde cystography/ urethrography is the technique of choice to identify a ruptured bladder or urethra.
  - Contrast material may be recognized leaking into the abdomen or around the urethra.
- Concurrent injuries, especially of the pelvis, may be present.

- The bladder may have an elongated or tethered appearance (to the region of the umbilicus) when empty.
- Traumatic diverticula may occur due to partial thickness rupture of the bladder wall at any site. On plain radiographs, they can appear as focal soft tissue bulges from the bladder margin.
- Both congenital and traumatic diverticula are more easily recognized with contrast radiography, where they are seen as contrast medium-filled outpouchings of the bladder lumen.
  - Congenital diverticula are cranioventral.
  - Traumatic diverticula can occur at any point along the bladder margin.
  - Thickening of the bladder wall and irregularity of the mucosa indicates concurrent chronic cystitis.

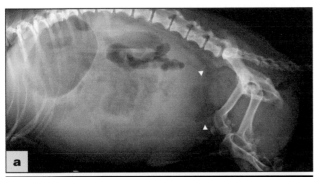

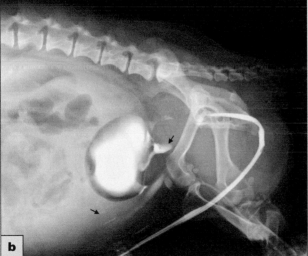

6.80 **(a)** Lateral survey radiograph of the abdomen and **(b)** positive-contrast retrograde cystogram of a male dog with rupture of the urinary bladder. (a) The margins of the bladder cannot be identified (arrowheads). The abdomen has a pendulous appearance and generalized blurring of serosal detail throughout due to free abdominal fluid. (b) Contrast medium (arrowed) appears as a streak, demonstrating leakage into the abdominal cavity.

Bladder diverticula: Congenital bladder diverticula result in outpouching of the bladder apex at the site of attachment between the bladder and urachus in the fetus (Figure 6.81).

Radiological features:

- On survey radiography, congenital (urachal) diverticula may appear as smooth cranioventral soft tissue bulges at the bladder apex.

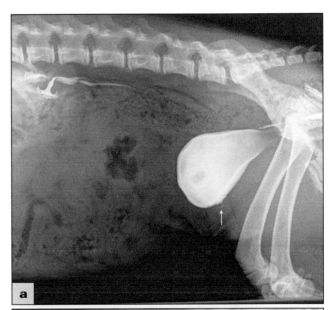

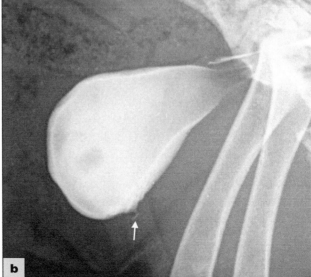

6.81 Lateral views of the abdomen of two young dogs with bladder (urachal) diverticula.
(a) Excretory urography and retrograde vaginourethrography have been performed (same dog as in Figure 6.66). The bladder is moderately distended with contrast medium. The ventral bladder wall is thickened and irregular, consistent with chronic cystitis. Contrast medium has also filled the diverticulum at the bladder vertex (arrowed). **(b)** Magnified view. (continues) ▶

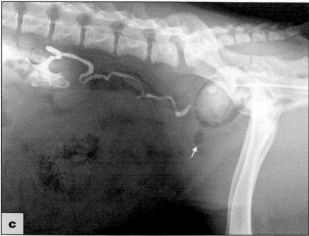

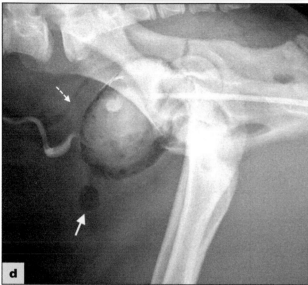

6.81 (continued) Lateral views of the abdomen of two young dogs with bladder (urachal) diverticula. **(c–d)** Excretory urography and pneumocystography have been performed. The renal pelves are dilated and the ureters are dilated and tortuous (one ureter contains air (dashed arrow) and the other contains contrast medium). The bladder is small and the neck is intrapelvic. A large, irregularly marginated, elliptical diverticulum (solid arrow) at the vertex of the bladder is filled with gas.

Male reproductive tract

Specific approach to interpretation

Survey radiography is useful for providing information about the size and location of the canine prostate gland (Figure 6.82). The feline prostate gland is not visible radiographically, and prostatic disease is rare in the cat. Radiographic assessment of the testicles is rarely of value, unless looking for evidence of an intra-abdominal testicle in a cryptorchid patient. Radiography is useful for identifying penile urethral calculi and is occasionally indicated for assessing other diseases of the os penis. Ultrasonography is a very valuable technique for assessing the prostate gland and testicles, whilst positive-contrast retrograde urethrography is useful for the evaluation of prostatic disease, and in particular for confirming the location of the prostate gland, assessing prostatic asymmetry and evaluating urethral integrity.

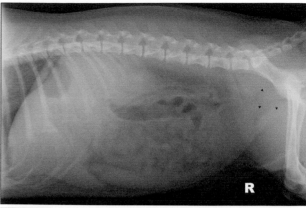

6.82 Normal prostate gland in a young, entire male dog. The cranial aspect (arrowheads) is defined by the small amount of fat between the prostate gland and the bladder neck, body wall and descending colon. (Courtesy of the University of Bristol)

Size

The size of the normal prostate gland is best assessed on a lateral radiograph. A useful 'rule of thumb' is that the diameter of the prostate gland should not exceed 70% of the diameter of the pelvic inlet (i.e. from the pubis to the ventral sacrum) in a normal entire male dog. A decrease in size results in the prostate gland becoming intrapelvic and radiographically invisible.

- Prostatic enlargement may cause cranial and ventral displacement of the bladder and dorsal displacement ± compression of the rectum.
- Causes of prostatic enlargement include:
  - Normal variation in Scottish Terriers, which are reported to have larger prostate glands than other similar sized breeds
  - Benign prostatic hyperplasia
  - Paraprostatic cysts – enlargement can be quite dramatic, with the cyst appearing similar in size to the urinary bladder.
  - Prostatic enlargement may also be seen with prostatic neoplasia and prostatitis, but is not usually dramatic.
- Causes of a decrease in size of the prostate gland include neutering, degenerative atrophy and the effect of oestrogens.

Shape

The normal prostate gland is ovoid/rounded in shape. Prostatic symmetry cannot be assessed with plain radiography, but requires delineation of the urethra with positive-contrast medium.

- Irregularity of the prostate gland outline may be seen with prostatic neoplasia and prostatitis.
- Paraprostatic cysts may be single or multiple and, although usually connected to the prostate gland by a stalk, are seen as additional, sometimes multilobed, soft tissue opacities, mimicking additional bladder shadows.

Opacity

The normal prostate gland is of soft tissue opacity. On a VD view, the superimposition of the prepuce approximately midline on the caudal abdomen appears as an area of increased soft tissue opacity and should not be mistaken for a mass lesion.

Mineralized opacity: Causes of prostatic mineralization may include:

- Dystrophic mineralization of prostatic neoplasia
- Dystrophic mineralization of severe, chronic prostatitis/abscessation
- Dystrophic mineralization of a paraprostatic cyst (fine 'eggshell' mineralization is sometimes observed around the periphery of paraprostatic cysts)
- Calculi within the prostatic urethra.

Gas opacity:

- A prostatic gas opacity is most commonly iatrogenic due to the reflux of air following a pneumocystogram.
- It is occasionally seen due to the presence of gas-forming bacteria in cases of prostatitis or prostatic abscessation.

Margination

Visualization of the margins of the prostate gland depends on it being located cranial to the pelvic brim and highlighted by fat within the adjacent mesentery. Non-visualization of the prostate gland may be due to:

- Normal intrapelvic location of a small prostate gland
- Lack of abdominal fat in an emaciated animal
- Abnormal caudal location of a prostate gland displaced into a perineal hernia.

Poorly defined prostatic margins may be seen due to inflammation or infiltration of the surrounding tissues. Causes include prostatic neoplasia and prostatitis.

Position

Caudal displacement of the prostate gland may occur with a perineal hernia.

Common conditions

Benign prostatic hyperplasia

Benign prostatic hyperplasia (Figure 6.83) occurs in entire male dogs.

Radiological features:

- Smoothly defined prostatic enlargement.
- Cranial displacement of the bladder.
- Dorsal displacement ± compression of the descending colon and rectum.
- A contrast retrograde urethrogram usually shows approximately symmetrical enlargement of the prostate gland about the urethra.

Prostatitis

Radiological features:

- The prostate gland may be normal in size or may be mildly to moderately enlarged.
- The prostate gland may be irregular in shape.
- Ill defined prostatic margins are sometimes apparent due to inflammation of the surrounding tissues.

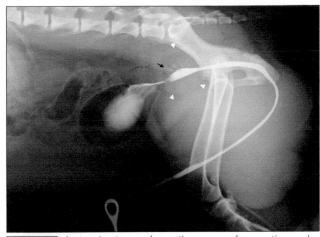

6.83 Lateral retrograde urethrogram of an entire male dog with benign prostatic hyperplasia. The enlarged prostate gland (arrowheads) is smoothly marginated and symmetrical about the urethra. The margins of the urethra are smooth. There is retrograde filling of the prostatic ducts (arrowed), which is smooth and well defined.

- Dystrophic mineralization is occasionally seen in cases of severe, chronic prostatitis.
- A contrast retrograde urethrogram may show asymmetrical enlargement of the prostate gland.

Prostatic neoplasia

Prostatic neoplasia (Figure 6.84) occurs in both entire and neutered male dogs.

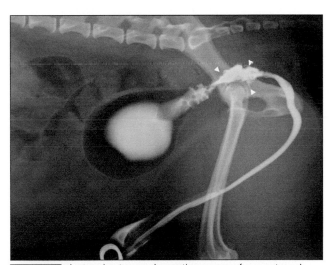

6.84 Lateral retrograde urethrogram of a neutered male dog with prostatic neoplasia. Although the prostate gland is not dramatically enlarged, it is larger than would be expected for a neutered dog. The prostatic urethra (arrowheads) is markedly irregular with reflux around the urethra into the prostate gland. There is no evidence of sublumbar lymphadenopathy or reactive new bone formation along the ventral aspect of the lumbar vertebral bodies in this case.

Radiological features:

- Prostatic enlargement is variable and often not dramatic.
- The prostate gland is often irregular in outline and the margins may be ill defined.
- Dystrophic mineralization of the tumour may be seen.

- Concurrent radiographic changes suggestive of neoplasia include:
  - Reactive new bone formation along the ventral aspect of the lumbosacral spine and pelvis
  - Sublumbar lymphadenopathy
  - Occasionally, local loss of serosal detail due to inflammation.
- A contrast retrograde urethrogram may show:
  - Asymmetrical enlargement of the prostate gland
  - Irregular extravasation of contrast medium due to neoplastic invasion and loss of urethral integrity.

Paraprostatic cysts

Radiological features:

- Large cysts appear as homogeneous soft tissue opacities and may mimic additional bladder shadows.
- A peripheral rim of 'eggshell' mineralization is sometimes seen around the cyst (Figure 6.85).
- Contrast retrograde studies may be required to differentiate the bladder from the adjacent cystic structures.

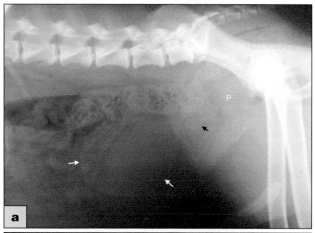

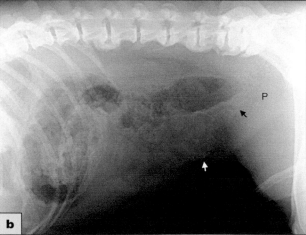

6.85 Lateral views of the abdomen of two entire male dogs with paraprostatic cysts. **(a)** The cyst is large with fine 'eggshell' peripheral mineralization (white arrows). A narrow stalk (black arrow) connects the cyst to the prostate gland (P). The bladder is empty. **(b–c)** The cyst is small with peripheral mineralization (white arrow) but the stalk (black arrow) connecting the cyst to the prostate gland (P) is long. (a, Courtesy of P Mahoney; b, Courtesy of Vetcall Veterinary Surgery) (continues) ▶

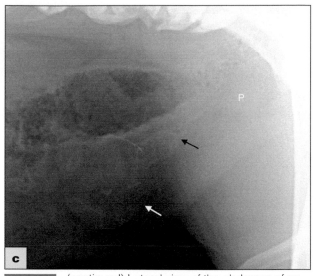

6.85 (continued) Lateral view of the abdomen of an entire male dog with a paraprostatic cyst. **(b–c)** The cyst is small with peripheral mineralization (white arrow) but the stalk (black arrow) connecting the cyst to the prostate gland (P) is long. (Courtesy of Vetcall Veterinary Surgery)

Cryptorchidism

Cryptorchidism is seen in both dogs and cats and may be inherited. One or both testicles fail to descend normally through the inguinal canal into the scrotum, and may be located anywhere between the inguinal region and the ipsilateral kidney. Testicles retained within the abdomen are more likely to become neoplastic.

Radiological features:

- A normal sized inguinal or abdominal testicle is unlikely to be recognized on abdominal radiographs.
- A neoplastic intra-abdominal testicle may be recognized as an abdominal mass lesion anywhere within the mid-caudal abdomen (Figure 6.86).

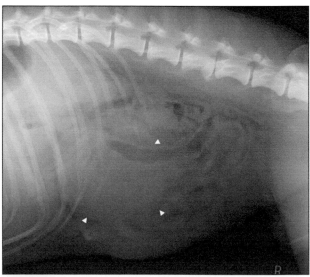

6.86 Lateral view of the abdomen of a male dog with a neoplastic retained testicle. The retained testicle appears as a mid-abdominal mass (arrowheads) with peripheral displacement of the small intestine.

Female reproductive tract

Specific approach to interpretation

The normal ovaries and uterus are not usually visible on plain radiographs of the non-pregnant dog or cat. Although radiography may be used for the diagnosis and assessment of pregnancy, ultrasonography can provide additional information about the viability of the fetuses. A plain abdominal radiograph can be very useful in determining whether a palpable mass present when whelping/kittening has apparently finished represents a remaining fetus.

Size and shape

Ovaries:

- Unlike the kidneys and adrenal glands, the ovaries are intraperitoneal structures and when enlarged they tend to migrate ventrally into the abdomen and, if large and heavy enough, may end up being located ventral to the small intestine along the ventral abdominal wall.
- Causes of ovarian enlargement include ovarian neoplasia, ovarian cysts and haematoma.
- Ovarian enlargement may be recognized on a lateral view as a mid-abdominal mass lesion.
- On a VD view, the mass is usually lateralized.
  - A right ovarian mass may displace the ascending colon and small intestine towards the midline or across to the left.
  - A left ovarian mass may displace the descending colon and small intestine towards the midline or across to the right.

Uterus:

- The uterus is usually indistinguishable from normal small intestine until it is at least 2–3 times the diameter of the small intestine (Figure 6.87).

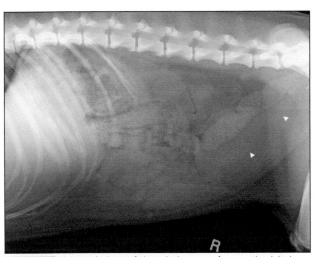

6.87 Lateral view of the abdomen of an entire bitch with uterine enlargement. The uterine horns (arrowheads) can be recognized due to the large volume of intra-abdominal fat and by their orientation and location, extending obliquely cranioventral over the bladder. The uterus can only be distinguished from small intestinal loops when it is 2–3 times the diameter of the small intestinal loops. (Courtesy of the University of Bristol)

- Generalized enlargement:
  - Causes include pyometra, mucometra/hydrometra, early pregnancy (usually <35 days) and a post-partum uterus (for up to 7 days following parturition)
  - Enlargement of the uterine body is recognized as a tubular soft tissue opacity between the colon and bladder, displacing the descending colon dorsally
  - Distension of the uterine horns is seen as a tortuous tubular soft tissue opacity superimposed on, and often extending cranial to, the bladder, displacing the small intestines cranially and medially.
- Segmented uterine enlargement is seen as multiple soft tissue masses along the length of the uterine horns:
  - Most likely due to pregnancy
  - May also be due to loculated pyometra, mucometra or hydrometra.
- Focal enlargement:
  - Causes include neoplasia, focal or stump pyometra, or a small litter
  - Focal enlargement of the uterine body causes dorsal deviation ± compression of the descending colon (and possibly rectum) and ventral displacement ± dorsal indentation of the urinary bladder (seen radiographically as separation of the colon and bladder)
  - Focal enlargement of one of the uterine horns is seen as a non-specific, mid-caudal abdominal mass, usually causing cranial and medial displacement of the small intestines.

Cervix and vagina: Enlargement of the intrapelvic cervix or vagina due to the presence of a cervical or vaginal mass may displace and compress the rectum dorsally.

Opacity

Ovaries:

- Ovarian masses are usually of soft tissue opacity and may be due to ovarian neoplasia, ovarian cysts or haematomas.
- Mineralization of an ovarian mass is occasionally seen:
  - Ovarian teratomas (or teratocarcinomas) are germ cell tumours, which may contain mineralized skeletal structures or even teeth
  - Unstructured or sometimes peripheral dystrophic mineralization may be seen in an ovarian mass.

Uterus:

- An enlarged uterus of soft tissue opacity may be seen due to pyometra, mucometra, hydrometra, early pregnancy or uterine neoplasia.
- Intra-uterine gas opacity is rare and may potentially be confused with the normal gas-filled small intestine. It may be seen with:
  - Emphysematous pyometra
  - Fetal death (see Figure 6.90).
- Mineralization of the uterus:

- Most commonly seen due to normal mineralization of fetal skeletons (from day 41 in the bitch and from day 35 in the queen)
- Occasionally due to dystrophic mineralization of a uterine mass.

Cervix and vagina: Masses arising from the cervix and vagina are normally of soft tissue opacity, but may occasionally be mineralized.

Margination

As with other abdominal organs and mass lesions, visualization of the serosal surface of enlarged ovaries or an enlarged uterus depends on the presence of sufficient abdominal fat.

- Although not typically visible, occasionally a normal non-gravid uterus may be seen highlighted by fat between the bladder and descending colon in an obese bitch or queen.
- Indistinct margination of an ovarian mass or enlarged uterus may be seen due to:
  - Lack of abdominal fat in an emaciated patient
  - Free abdominal fluid
  - Diffuse or localized peritonitis (e.g. due to leakage of purulent material from a pyometra).

Position

The ovaries are located in the mid-dorsal abdomen, just caudal to the ipsilateral kidneys. The normal ovaries are too small to be visible radiographically. The uterus lies between the descending colon and bladder with the cervix usually located just cranial to the pelvic brim. The vagina extends caudally from the cervix, through the pelvic canal to join the vestibule, which opens at the vulva. Although not visible on plain radiography, the vestibule and vagina, and sometimes the uterus and uterine horns, are demonstrated on a contrast retrograde study (Figure 6.88).

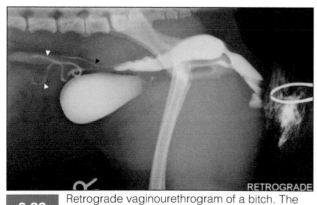

6.88 Retrograde vaginourethrogram of a bitch. The normal uterine body and horns (white arrowheads) have filled with contrast medium. An ectopic ureter is visible (black arrowhead) entering the vagina. (Courtesy of the University of Bristol)

Common conditions

Pregnancy

In experienced hands, abdominal palpation and ultrasonography are sensitive techniques and can be used to diagnose pregnancy before it becomes radiographically apparent. The use of radiography during pregnancy does present a radiation hazard to the fetuses (this risk diminishes in the final third of the pregnancy).

Radiological features:

- Pregnancy is not radiographically visible until about 25–30 days.
- It is initially seen as a non-specific soft tissue enlargement of the uterus.
- From 30–40 days, the uterus takes on a segmented appearance as the individual fetal sacs enlarge.
- In the queen, fetal mineralization may be seen from 35 days.
- In the bitch, fetal mineralization may be seen from 41 days.
- Normal fetuses typically lie in a slightly curved position.
- Radiography is more accurate than ultrasonography for the assessment of fetal numbers (best achieved by counting fetal heads) (Figure 6.89).

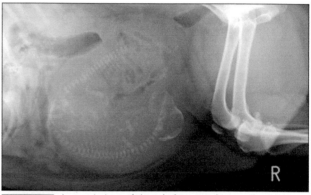

6.89 Lateral view of the abdomen of an entire bitch during late pregnancy. Two fetuses can be identified. (Courtesy of the University of Bristol)

Problems associated with pregnancy and parturition

Ultrasonography is a more accurate technique for the assessment of fetal viability, as real-time imaging allows detection of the fetal heartbeats. Radiological assessment of the fetuses is usually not possible until they have mineralized.

Radiological features:

- Fetal death may be recognized as:
  - Loss of normal curvature of the fetal spine, with the fetus often appearing hyperextended
  - Malalignment of the fetal skeleton with collapse and overlap of the skull bones (Spalding sign)
  - Fetal disintegration and demineralization
  - Mummification (seen as a compacted, tightly coiled fetus of increased opacity)
  - A gas opacity within or around the fetal sacs (can be confused with overlying intestinal gas) (Figure 6.90).
- Ectopic fetus:
  - Fetus located outside the tubular uterine shadow
  - Often tightly curled
  - May be concurrent peritoneal effusion.
- Dystocia:
  - Radiography can be a very useful technique in the evaluation of dystocia

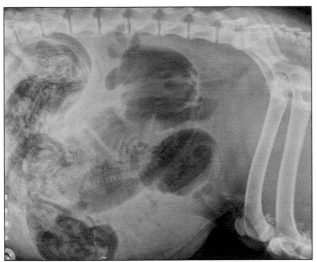

6.90 Lateral view of the abdomen of a bitch revealing a gas opacity within and around the fetal sacs, consistent with fetal death. Gas associated with fetal death must be distinguished from overlying gas-filled intestinal loops. (Courtesy of Mandeville Veterinary Hospital)

- Problems which may be identified radiographically include:
  - Fetal malpresentation (e.g. a fetus seen at the pelvic inlet with the head or limb in the incorrect position for delivery)
  - Oversized fetuses
  - Physical obstruction (e.g. maternal pelvic fracture).
- Post-partum:
  - Radiography is a quick and sensitive technique for confirming the presence of a retained fetus.

Pyometra

Radiological features:

- Characterized by fluid distension of the uterus.
- Enlargement of the uterine body is recognized as a tubular soft tissue opacity between the colon and bladder, displacing the descending colon dorsally.
- On the lateral view, distension of the uterine horns is seen as a convoluted soft tissue opacity, extending cranially into the mid-abdomen and displacing the small intestinal loops further cranially (Figure 6.91).
- On the VD view, the distended horns usually lie close to the body wall, displacing the small intestine and descending colon towards the midline.
- Mildly distended uterine horns can be mistaken for normal fluid-filled small intestinal loops.
- A stump pyometra may be seen as a focal soft tissue enlargement of the uterine body, causing dorsal deviation and compression of the descending colon and rectum.
- Rarely, a loculated pyometra may be identified as segmented enlargement of one or both uterine horns.
- Indistinct margination of the enlarged uterus may be seen if there is peritonitis due to leakage of the uterine contents.

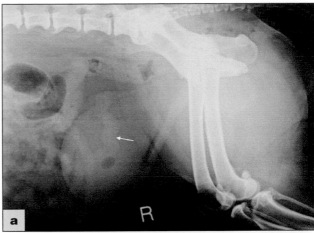

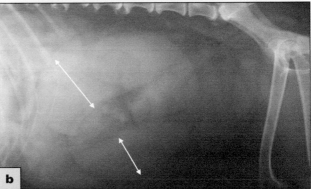

6.91 Lateral views of the abdomen of two entire bitches with pyometra. **(a)** There is mild uterine enlargement (arrowed). **(b)** A large pyometra with large, sinuous, homogeneous soft tissue loops (double-headed arrows) fill the mid- and caudal abdomen and should not be mistaken for dilated small intestinal loops, which have been displaced cranially.

Ovarian neoplasia

Small ovarian tumours may not be visible radiographically.

Radiological features:

- Providing they are of sufficient size, ovarian neoplasms are usually seen as non-specific, mid-abdominal mass lesions (Figure 6.92).
  - As the ovaries are intraperitoneal structures, an ovarian mass can migrate ventrally to lie on the ventral abdominal wall.
  - On the VD view, an ovarian mass is likely to be lateralized, displacing the adjacent descending or ascending colon and small intestines towards the middle of the abdomen.
- Causes include granulosa cell tumours, adenocarcinomas and teratomas.
- Most ovarian tumours are of soft tissue opacity.
  - Mineralized skeletal elements and/or teeth may be recognized within a teratoma or teratocarcinoma.
  - Dystrophic mineralization of ovarian neoplasms is occasionally seen.

Uterine neoplasia

Uterine neoplasia is uncommon.

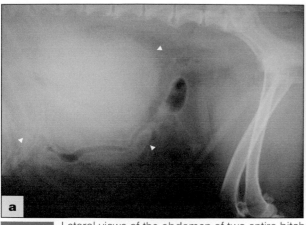
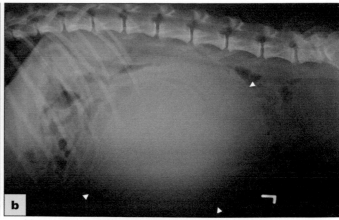

6.92 Lateral views of the abdomen of two entire bitches with ovarian neoplasia. **(a)** The mass (arrowheads) lies within the mid-dorsal abdomen and has displaced the small intestine ventrally and peripherally. Ovarian masses should be differentiated from those masses arising from the small intestine or within the mesentery (in particular, lymphadenopathy). **(b)** The mass (arrowheads) is extremely large and homogeneous, filling the mid-ventral abdomen and displacing the majority of the small intestinal loops cranially. Such a large mass must be distinguished from splenic masses, pedunculated hepatic masses, cystic masses within the mesentery and focal masses within the uterus. (a, Courtesy of G Hammond, University of Glasgow; b, Courtesy of R Hagen)

Radiological features:

- Uterine neoplasia is typically seen as a soft tissue mass arising from the uterine body or either of the uterine horns.
- A mass arising from the uterine body causes dorsal deviation ± compression of the descending colon (and possibly the rectum) and cranioventral displacement ± dorsal indentation of the urinary bladder.
- Neoplasia of the uterine horns appears as a non-specific, mid-caudal abdominal mass.
- Dystrophic mineralization of uterine neoplasms may occasionally be seen.
- Contrast retrograde studies are valuable in determining the origin of the mass.
- Mesenchymal uterine tumours (leiomyomas, leiomyosarcomas) are most frequently identified in the dog.
- Uterine adenocarcinoma is most frequently identified in the cat.

Cervical masses
The normal cervix is not radiographically visible unless highlighted by contrast medium.

Radiological features:

- A large cervical mass may be seen as a soft tissue opacity between the bladder and descending colon/rectum.
  - It may cause dorsal displacement and compression of the colon/rectum.
  - It may cause cranioventral displacement of the bladder.
  - Compression of the bladder neck/intrapelvic urethra can cause an obstruction, resulting in distension of the urinary bladder.
- Contrast retrograde studies are valuable in determining the origin of the mass, which may be highlighted as a filling defect.
  - Possible causes include neoplasia (most commonly leiomyosarcoma), abscess and granuloma.

Vaginal masses
A vaginal mass is often better evaluated by palpation and direct inspection. Depending on its size and location, a vaginal mass may have a variety of radiological appearances.

Radiological features:

- A soft tissue mass displacing and compressing the rectum and/or descending colon dorsally.
- Distension of the urinary bladder due to compression and obstruction of the urethra.
- A contrast retrograde study of the vagina is helpful in highlighting the size and shape of the mass, which appears as a filling defect within the vagina (Figures 6.93 and 6.94).
- Causes include vaginal polyps, prolapse, neoplasia (usually benign, such as leiomyoma, fibroma and adenoma), abscesses, haematomas, granulomas and cysts.

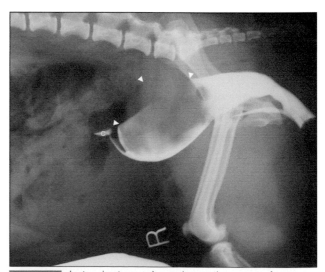

6.93 Lateral retrograde vaginourethrogram of an entire bitch with a vaginal mass. The positive contrast medium outlines the ventral aspect of a large soft tissue filling defect, consistent with a cranial vaginal mass (arrowheads). The cervix (C) is cranially displaced.

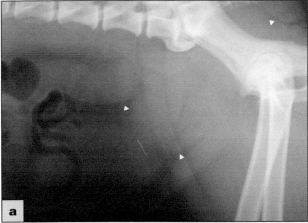

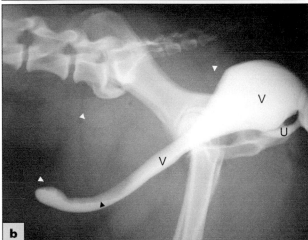

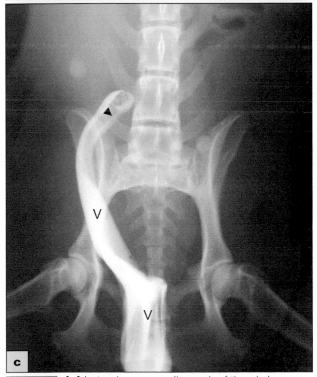

6.94 **(a)** Lateral survey radiograph of the abdomen and **(b)** lateral and **(c)** VD retrograde vaginourethrograms of an entire bitch with a large vaginal mass. (a) The soft tissue mass (arrowheads) extends cranial to the pelvic brim, displacing the bladder further cranially. (b–c) The mass (white arrowheads) lies to the left and dorsal to the vagina. Indentation and displacement of the vagina by the mass results in a broad but shallow, smoothly marginated filling defect (black arrowhead). U = urethra; V = vagina. (Courtesy of P Mahoney)

The abdominal space and body wall

Specific approach to interpretation

Size, shape and position

Peritoneal cavity: The peritoneal cavity is the space between and around the major organs and intestines, which is lined by peritoneum and limited cranially by the diaphragm, ventrally and laterally by the body wall, caudally by the pelvic inlet and dorsally by the retro-peritoneum. The mesenteric lymph nodes lie fairly centrally within the peritoneal cavity, flanking the course of the mesenteric vessels. Changes in the size, shape and position of the peritoneal cavity include:

- Distension of the abdominal cavity:
  - Recognized initially as a pot-bellied appearance with the abdomen becoming increasingly round with further distension
  - Causes include obesity, organomegaly, muscle weakness, free abdominal fluid and marked pneumoperitoneum.
- Decreased volume of the abdominal cavity:
  - Recognized as a 'tucked up' appearance with inward displacement of the abdominal wall
  - Causes include emaciation and displacement of the viscera outside the abdominal cavity due to a hernia or rupture.
- Disruption of the abdominal wall:
  - Usually recognized as the abnormal displacement of the abdominal organs outside the peritoneal cavity (Figure 6.95)
  - Causes include umbilical, inguinal, perineal and pericardio-peritoneo-diaphragmatic hernias, and body wall and diaphragmatic ruptures.
- Focal changes in the shape of the abdominal wall may be seen due to:
  - Mammary gland development, which may be normal or neoplastic
  - Abdominal wall masses:
    - Lipomas are common
    - Other causes include other neoplasms, seromas (especially post-surgical), abscesses and haematomas.

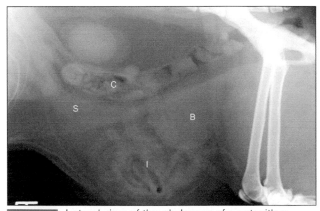

6.95 Lateral view of the abdomen of a cat with a ventral body wall rupture. The bladder and the majority of the small intestinal loops are displaced ventrally through the defect and lie within the inguinal region. The peritoneal cavity appears 'empty' with only the liver, spleen (S), stomach and colon (C) remaining. B = bladder. (Courtesy of the University of Bristol)

■ Mesenteric lymphadenopathy:
  • Marked enlargement of the mesenteric lymph nodes may be seen as ill defined, mid-abdominal masses causing peripheral displacement of the intestines.

Retroperitoneal space: The retroperitoneal space forms the dorsal aspect of the abdomen and is limited dorsally by the sublumbar muscles and spine, laterally by the body wall, caudally by the pelvic inlet and ventrally by the peritoneum. Cranially, the retroperitoneal space is continuous with the mediastinum via the aortic hiatus in the diaphragm. Normal retroperitoneal structures include the kidneys, adrenal glands, ureters, abdominal aorta, caudal vena cava, sublumbar lymph nodes, bladder neck and prostate gland. The sublumbar lymph nodes are located in the retroperitoneal space ventral to the lumbar spine at the level of L6–L7.

Enlargement of the retroperitoneal space is recognized on a lateral view as ventral displacement of the small and large intestines:

■ Diffuse retroperitoneal enlargement may be seen with obesity (especially in cats), retroperitoneal effusion (usually haemorrhage or urine), diffuse inflammation/abscessation (e.g. due to a migrating foreign body) and extensive ureteric dilatation
■ Focal retroperitoneal enlargement may be seen due to:
  • Retroperitoneal neoplasia arising from the kidneys, adrenal glands or sublumbar muscles
  • Sublumbar lymphadenopathy
  • Retroperitoneal abscess.

Opacity and margination

Peritoneal cavity:

■ The normal peritoneal cavity contains varying amounts of mesenteric fat, which provides abdominal detail by highlighting the serosal surfaces of the surrounding organs.
■ Increasing soft tissue opacity of the peritoneal space results in the normal fat opacity being obscured and the normal serosal detail becoming lost.
  • A mottled, patchy increase in peritoneal opacity results in blurring but not complete loss of serosal detail.
    – Changes may be generalized or localized.
    – Causes include a wet or dirty hair coat, small volumes of free peritoneal fluid, peritonitis, pancreatitis, moderate mesenteric lymphadenopathy, diffuse neoplastic infiltration of the mesentery (carcinomatosis) and steatitis.
  • A generalized, homogeneous 'ground-glass' soft tissue opacity may be seen in emaciated or very young patients, or patients with free abdominal fluid.
■ Mineralization of the peritoneal cavity can be difficult to differentiate from mineralized material within the gastrointestinal tract or mineralization of the abdominal organs. Possible causes include:
  • Dystrophic mineralization of abnormal peritoneal soft tissues (e.g. due to carcinomatosis, a foreign body reaction, chronic abscess, haematoma or mesenteric cyst)

• Gastrointestinal leakage of barium or iodine contrast media from a previous contrast study.
■ Peritoneal fat opacity.
  • The presence of relatively radiolucent fat throughout the abdominal mesentery, highlighting the serosal surfaces of the soft tissue organs is a normal finding.
    – Some very obese cats may have sufficient intra-abdominal fat to displace organs to one side (may be seen on a VD view) subsequent to lateral recumbency.
  • Occasionally, an intra-abdominal lipoma may be recognized as an abdominal mass which is of fat opacity.
■ Peritoneal gas opacity.
  • A large amount of free gas within the abdominal cavity is recognized as collections of gas outside the gastrointestinal cavity, most easily seen where it highlights the caudal aspect of the diaphragm and enhances visualization of the serosal surface of the gastrointestinal tract and the margins of the other abdominal organs (Figure 6.96).

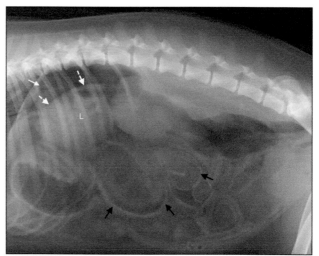

6.96   Lateral survey radiograph of the abdomen of a dog with pneumoperitoneum. A large volume of free abdominal gas, best appreciated in the craniodorsal abdomen, highlights the caudal aspect of the diaphragm (solid white arrow) and the serosal surfaces of the abdominal organs (L = liver; dashed white arrows = cranial serosal surface of liver) and viscera (black arrows = colon and caecum).

  • Smaller volumes of free gas are more challenging to identify. A useful technique is to position the patient in left lateral recumbency, which allows the gas to rise to the highest point, usually under the right costal arch. A left lateral decubitus view using a horizontal beam can then be used to identify this gas (Figure 6.97).
    – Before carrying out these studies, the Local Rules should be reviewed to see whether horizontal beam radiography is permitted within the practice. Extra attention to radiation safety is required.
  • Causes of free abdominal gas include:
    – Post-laparotomy – it is normal to see free gas within the abdominal cavity for up to 10 days following abdominal surgery

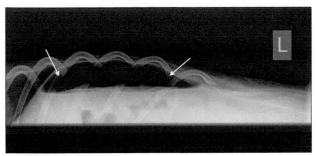

6.97 Left lateral decubitus view used to detect free abdominal gas. The gas has collected in the uppermost part of the abdomen (arrowed) and a fluid line (fluid–gas interface) is present.

- Perforation of a hollow viscus – most commonly the stomach or intestines, but possibly the bladder or uterus
- A penetrating wound through the abdominal wall.

Retroperitoneal space:

- Fat within the normal retroperitoneal cavity outlines the margins of the kidneys, the ventral aspect of the sublumbar muscles and very occasionally highlights the aorta, vena cava and ureters as they run through the retroperitoneal space.
- Increased soft tissue opacity within the retroperitoneal space obscures the normal renal silhouettes and the ventral aspect of the sublumbar muscles.
  - Causes of a generalized increase in soft tissue opacity throughout the retroperitoneal space include:
    - A very young or emaciated patient with little retroperitoneal fat
    - Retroperitoneal fluid (most commonly urine or haemorrhage).
  - A more localized increase in soft tissue opacity may be seen due to:
    - A retroperitoneal or sublumbar tumour, abscess or haematoma
    - Sublumbar lymphadenopathy.
- Mineralization of the retroperitoneal space must be differentiated from mineralization within the overlying intestines.
  - Mineralization superimposed on the retroperitoneal space may also be seen due to mineralization of the kidneys and adrenal glands, or due to ureteric calculi.
  - Occasionally, mineralization of a retroperitoneal tumour, abscess or haematoma may be seen.
- Increased fat opacity within the retroperitoneal space may be seen due to:
  - Excessive fat in an obese patient (especially cats)
  - Retroperitoneal lipoma.
- Free gas within the retroperitoneal space enhances the margination of the retroperitoneal organs, highlighting structures such as the aorta, caudal vena cava and ureters which are not normally visible radiographically (Figure 6.98). Causes of free retroperitoneal gas include:
  - Extension of a pneumomediastinum through the aortic hiatus
  - Penetrating wound.

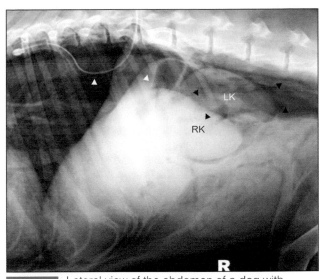

6.98 Lateral view of the abdomen of a dog with pneumoretroperitoneum. There is extension of a pneumomediastinum into the retroperitoneal space. The margins of the cranial abdominal aorta (white arrowheads) and caudal vena cava (black arrowheads), which are not usually visible, can be seen as they are surrounded by gas. The triangular gas opacity in the retroperitoneum surrounds and highlights the left (LK) and right (RK) kidneys. (Courtesy of the University of Bristol)

Common conditions

Abdominal effusion

Although abdominal radiography may be useful for confirming the presence of abdominal effusion in a patient with a distended abdomen, the abdominal organs will be obscured by the fluid, limiting the radiographic evaluation of any gas-filled structures. Abdominocentesis and abdominal ultrasonography are much more useful than radiography in the evaluation of patients with abdominal fluid.

Radiological features:

- With a small volume of free fluid, there is blurring of the serosal margins to give a mottled and patchy appearance of the abdomen (Figure 6.99).

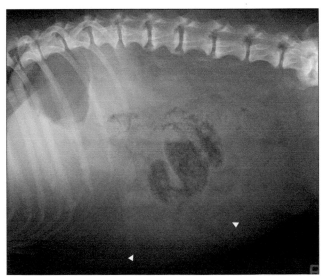

6.99 Lateral view of the abdomen of a dog with a small volume of free abdominal fluid. The serosal detail of the abdominal organs (liver) and viscera (small intestine) is blurred (arrowheads).

- With larger volumes of fluid, complete loss of serosal detail with a homogeneous 'ground-glass' soft tissue opacity is seen throughout the peritoneal space (Figure 6.100).
  - Unless there is concurrent retroperitoneal effusion, the renal silhouettes and retroperitoneal fat opacity often remain evident in the dorsal abdomen.
  - Evidence of abdominal distension can be used to differentiate a large volume of abdominal fluid from loss of detail due to emaciation (where the abdominal contour is likely to be 'tucked up') (Figure 6.101).
  - Fluid types include:
    - Transudate/modified transudate (e.g. secondary to hypoproteinaemia, right-sided heart failure, portal hypertension, obstruction of the caudal vena cava or lymphatic fluid)
    - Haemorrhage (e.g. due to a bleeding tumour, trauma or coagulopathy)

- Urine (due to urinary bladder rupture)
- Bile (due to gallbladder rupture)
- Exudate (e.g. secondary to peritonitis or feline infectious peritonitis).

Peritonitis

Radiological features:

- Blurring of serosal detail (Figure 6.102) may be seen due to peritoneal inflammation and/or small volumes of free fluid.
- Complete loss of serosal detail may be seen where there is a large volume of free fluid.
- If peritonitis is due to gastrointestinal rupture, varying amounts of free abdominal gas may be present.
  - Smaller volumes of free air may be difficult to differentiate from gas within the gastrointestinal tract. Where permitted, a left lateral decubitus view using a horizontal beam may be useful.
  - Larger volumes of free air enhance the serosal details, as well as highlight structures not usually seen, such as the caudal aspect of the diaphragm and the individual lobes of the liver.
- Dilated and/or corrugated loops of intestine may be recognized due to secondary ileus, intestinal inflammation and/or adhesions in more chronic cases.

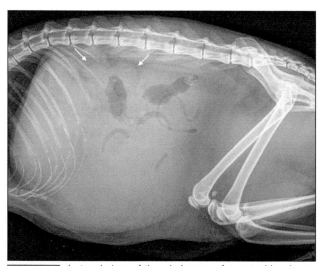

6.100 Lateral view of the abdomen of a cat with a large volume of abdominal fluid. This has resulted in a pendulous appearance to the abdomen and effacement of the margins of all the soft tissue structures. Loops of gas-containing small intestine have floated to the central (upper) part of the abdomen. The retroperitoneal space is not affected and the dorsal margin of one of the kidneys (arrowed) is still visible.

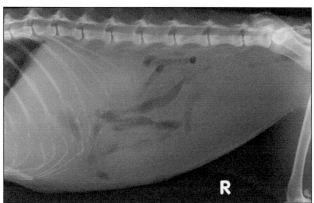

6.101 Lateral view of the abdomen of a cat with abdominal fluid. Serosal detail has been completely lost. The cat is thin with almost no fat evident within the abdomen. Despite this, the abdominal wall has a slight pendulous appearance, which indicates an abdominal effusion of significant volume.

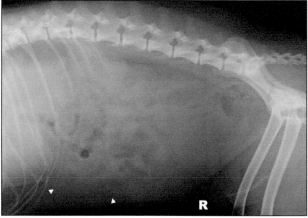

6.102 Lateral view of the abdomen of a dog with severe peritonitis. Serosal detail is blurred (arrowheads), especially ventrally where the greater omentum lies along the ventral abdominal wall. Note that the appearance is very similar to that of the patient with a small amount of free abdominal fluid in Figure 6.99. (Courtesy of the University of Bristol)

Mesenteric lymphadenopathy

Normal mesenteric lymph nodes and mild mesenteric lymphadenopathy are not radiographically apparent.

Radiological features:

- As the mesenteric lymph nodes enlarge, although they may still be too small to be individually recognizable, superimposition of a number of moderately enlarged lymph nodes may appear as a mottled, patchy increase in peritoneal opacity within the mid-abdomen.
- Large mesenteric mass lesions may be recognized as central abdominal masses of soft tissue opacity (Figure 6.103) with peripheral displacement of the small intestines.

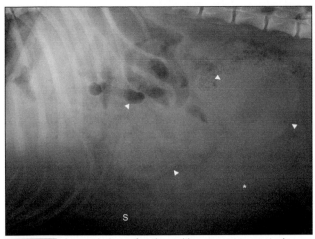

6.103 Lateral view of a dog with severe mesenteric lymphadenopathy and diffuse neoplastic infiltration of the abdomen. Some of the enlarged lymph nodes in the mid-abdomen are visible as irregularly rounded soft tissue masses (arrowheads). In the ventral abdomen, the masses are more poorly circumscribed and confluent (*) with the spleen (S) located cranioventrally. The serosal margins are blurred due to fluid or infiltrate.

- Radiologically apparent enlargement of the mesenteric lymph nodes is most likely to be due to primary multicentric neoplasia (most commonly lymphoma) or metastatic neoplasia from the intestines and/or pancreas.

Retroperitoneal effusion

Small volumes of free fluid may be difficult to detect, but sometimes result in recognizable blurring of retro-peritoneal detail.

Radiological features:

- Larger volumes can be seen as:
  - A homogeneous soft tissue opacity throughout the retroperitoneal space, obscuring the renal margins and the sublumbar muscles
  - Enlargement of the retroperitoneal space, resulting in ventral displacement of the intestines.
- Causes include:
  - Retroperitoneal haemorrhage (e.g. due to a bleeding tumour, trauma or coagulopathy) (Figure 6.104)
  - Urine (most commonly due to a traumatically ruptured or avulsed ureter).

Sublumbar lymphadenopathy

Normal sublumbar lymph nodes and mild sublumbar lymphadenopathy are not apparent radiographically.

Radiological features:

- Moderate to severe sublumbar lymphadenopathy is seen as a retroperitoneal soft tissue mass ventral to L6–L7, displacing, and possibly compressing, the descending colon and rectum ventrally.
- Radiologically apparent enlargement of the sublumbar lymph nodes is most likely to be due to primary multicentric neoplasia (most commonly lymphoma; Figure 6.105) or metastatic neoplasia from the pelvis, perineum (especially the anal glands) and possibly the hindlimbs.

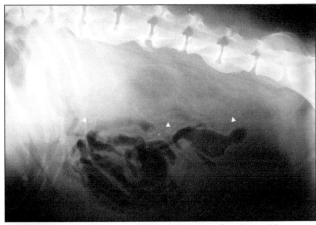

6.104 Lateral view of the abdomen of a dog with retroperitoneal haemorrhage from an adrenal gland mass. The retroperitoneal space is enlarged with ventral displacement of the descending colon. Detail within the retroperitoneal space is reduced by a streaky soft tissue opacity (arrowheads) and the left kidney is obscured. The adrenal gland mass itself cannot be distinguished from the kidneys. (Courtesy of P Mahoney)

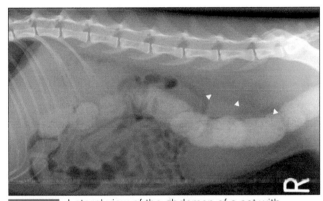

6.105 Lateral view of the abdomen of a cat with lymphoma. A large lobulated soft tissue mass (arrowheads) ventral to the caudal lumbar vertebrae is visible, consistent with marked sublumbar lymphadenopathy. The colon is displaced ventrally. (Courtesy of the University of Bristol)

Abdominal wall rupture

Radiological features:

- Disruption in the continuity of the abdominal wall.
- Displacement of the abdominal organs to lie outside the peritoneal cavity (see Figure 6.95).

References and further reading

Dennis R (1992) Barium meal techniques in dogs and cats. *In Practice* **14**, 61–82

Graham JP, Lord PF and Harrison PM (1998) Quantitative estimation of intestinal dilation as a predictor of obstruction in the dog. *Journal of Small Animal Practice* **39**, 521–524

Holt PE (2008) *Urological Disorders of the Dog and Cat: investigation, diagnosis and treatment.* Manson, London

O'Brien R and Barr F (2009) *BSAVA Manual of Canine and Feline Abdominal Surgery.* BSAVA Publications, Gloucester

O'Brien TR, Biery DN, Park RD and Bartels JE (1978) *Radiographic Diagnosis of Abdominal Disorders in the Dog and Cat: radiographic interpretation, clinical signs and pathophysiology.* WB Saunders, Philadephia

Root CR (2007) Abdominal masses. In: *Textbook of Diagnostic Radiology, 5th edn,* ed. DE Thrall, pp. 493–515. Elsevier, St Louis

Thrall DE (2013) Principles of radiographic interpretation of the abdomen. In: *Textbook of Diagnostic Radiology, 6th edn,* ed. DE Thrall, pp. 650–658. Elsevier, St Louis

Radiology of the appendicular skeleton

Gawain Hammond and Fraser McConnell

Skeletal radiology is challenging due to the complex anatomy of the skeleton and the large number of incidental findings and anatomical variants which are encountered. Degenerative changes are common within the joints, and determining the significance of lesions requires correlation with the clinical examination and history. Often it is not possible to determine the significance of lesions based on their radiological appearance alone. Bone has a limited response to injury, which means there is overlap in the radiological features of many diseases, and further tests (e.g. arthrocentesis and biopsy) are often required for a definitive diagnosis.

Key points for orthopaedic radiography

- Low kilovoltage (kV) and high milliampere second (mAs) technique.
- Small focal spot.
- Table top technique, except for proximal limbs in larger dogs.
- Keep area of interest as parallel to the cassette as possible.
- Minimize film–object distance.
- Minimize superimposed structures (e.g. retract contralateral limb).
- Use high detail screens (if available) for the distal limb.
- Obtain orthogonal views in all cases.
- Obtain separate radiographs for each joint being investigated.
- Accurate positioning and centring required for reliable interpretation.
- Label radiographs correctly.
- Use a scaler for digital radiographs (e.g. a two pence coin or other object of known size) for orthopaedic templating.
- Use radiographs of the contralateral limb for comparison to aid interpretation.

High quality radiographs are required for skeletal radiography as many significant lesions are subtle and may be missed on poor radiographs. For the joints and bones distal to the elbows and stifles, a table top technique using a detail film–screen combination and a small focal spot should be used to maximize spatial resolution. For the proximal joints and long bones in large dogs, a grid should be used, as scatter produced within the animal may be significant.

To maximize radiographic contrast, a low kV, high mAs technique should be used, and care should be taken not to overexpose the radiograph. On a properly exposed skeletal radiograph, the soft tissues and trabecular pattern of the bone should be clearly visible. In large dogs, there is marked variation in the soft tissue thickness of the proximal limbs, with significantly more muscle proximally. With conventional radiography, it may not be possible to obtain a single image that is correctly exposed for both the proximal and distal parts of the proximal limbs, and separate exposures may be required of the proximal and distal femur and humerus. When taking radiographs of the joints, the X-ray beam must be centred on the joint of interest. Due to divergence of the X-ray beam and geometric distortion, it is essential that when taking radiographs of multiple joints within one limb, separate images are obtained for each joint. Whole limb radiographs should not be taken unless screening for gross lesions (e.g. bone tumour or long bone fracture).

Orthogonal views should be obtained for all skeletal radiographic studies, as pathology is often visible on only one view (Figure 7.1). In addition, for the carpus and tarsus, lateral oblique views may be required to evaluate fully the extent of any pathology (Figure 7.2). In addition to the standard views, specific oblique views may be required to evaluate the intertubercular groove of the humerus, trochlear ridges of the tarsus and femoral trochlea. As many joint conditions are bilateral (e.g. osteochondritis dissecans (OCD), cranial cruciate disease, elbow dysplasia) it is advisable to obtain radiographs of the contralateral limb to detect occult pathology. In cases of suspected ligamentous injury, radiographs should be obtained with the joint under stress, as joint instability is often not visible on non-stressed images (Figure 7.3). Contrast radiography is rarely performed and has been largely replaced by arthroscopy, but positive contrast arthrography is occasionally helpful in the shoulder to demonstrate the location of OCD fragments and lesions affecting the biceps tendon (see Figure 7.32).

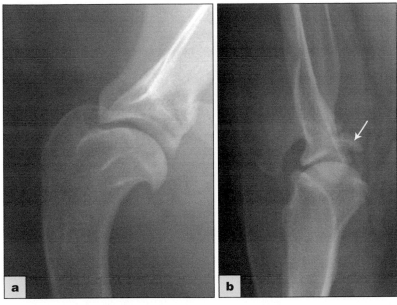

7.1 **(a)** Mediolateral and **(b)** caudocranial views of the shoulder of a 4-year-old Staffordshire Bull Terrier with acute onset lameness after falling from a height. A large articular fracture (arrowed) is visible on the caudocranial view of the shoulder, but is not visible on the mediolateral view. It is essential to obtain orthogonal views when imaging the joints to reduce the risk of missing significant pathology.

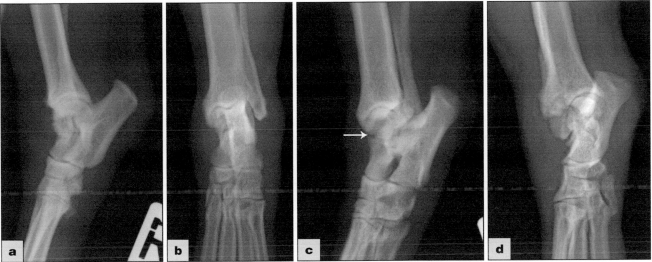

7.2 **(a)** Mediolateral, **(b)** dorsoplantar, **(c)** dorsolateral–plantaromedial oblique and **(d)** dorsomedial–plantarolateral oblique views of the tarsus of a 3-year-old White Highland West Terrier presented with lameness after being hit by a car. There is a minimally displaced articular fracture of the medial ridge of the talus (arrowed); this is best seen on the dorsolateral–plantaromedial oblique view, which skylines the dorsomedial aspect of the joint. For complex joints such as the tarsus and carpus, oblique views are required to allow full evaluation of the joint.

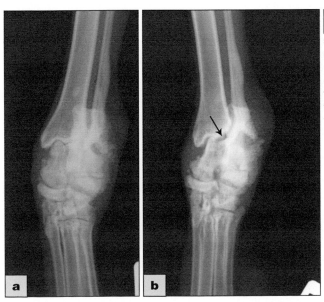

7.3 Dorsoplantar views of the tarsus of a 3-year-old Maine Coon cat presented for chronic tarsal swelling, which occurred after falling out of a window. The radiographs were obtained with the joint in **(a)** a neutral position and **(b)** a stressed position. In addition to extensive degenerative changes, there is laxity and subluxation of the tibiotarsal joint, which is only visible on the stressed view. Note the widened lateral aspect of the joint (arrowed) on the stressed view, indicating damage to the lateral collateral ligament.

Restraint and patient preparation

Since the most common indication for skeletal radiography is the investigation of lameness, general anaesthesia or heavy sedation is required as manipulation of the limbs may be painful. In cases of suspected skeletal trauma, there may be concurrent thoracic pathology, which may affect anaesthesia and should be addressed prior to radiography. Accurate positioning is required for joint radiography as rotated images may lead to lesions being missed or an erroneous diagnosis (e.g. patellar luxation). No specific patient preparation is required for skeletal radiography, but the hair coat should be dry and free from dirt, particularly for radiography of the manus or pes as dirt particles may mimic foreign bodies.

Long bones

Normal anatomy

Long bones are essentially modified cylinders, which have a hollow central diaphysis (shaft) with an epiphysis and metaphysis at either end (Figure 7.4). The external surface of the cortical bone should be smoothly marginated, but slight roughening of the cortices occurs at the insertion of muscles and tendons (e.g. between the radius and ulna at the attachments of the interosseous ligament). Normal bone is approximately 50–70% mineralized, with the compact cortical bone being denser than the spongy cancellous bone, which is less opaque and has a fine mineralized trabecular pattern. The important soft tissue component of bone cannot assessed on radiographs. Within the spongy cancellous bone, lamellae are arranged in planes according to the loading on the bone.

Bone is a dynamic organ and undergoes changes in shape and architecture according to the stresses placed on it (Wolff's law). Cortical thickness varies with the shape and loading of the bone, with thicker cortices present in areas of increased stress and loading within the diaphyseal regions. The non-articular surface of bones has an outer covering of periosteum and an inner layer of endosteum. These layers are composed of connective tissue, from which the osteoblasts involved in bone healing are generated. The marrow elements are contained within the central medullary cavity of the bone. The normal periosteum is of soft tissue opacity and is not seen as a discrete structure as it has the same opacity as the adjacent muscles. Immature bones have an open physis between the epiphysis and metaphysis, seen as a radiolucent line, which should not be confused with a fracture. The closure times for the various epiphyses are shown in Figure 7.5. The physeal plates of long bones in the dog are generally closed by 12 months of age, although those of the iliac crest may remain open for longer (or occasionally never close). In the cat, early neutering may delay growth plate closure times and it is not uncommon to see visible physes at 18 months of age. In the mature animal, the physeal scar is visible as a thin radiopaque line. Delayed closure of the growth plates, which can be associated with abnormalities of the epiphyses, may be seen with some congenital metabolic conditions, such as congenital hypothyroidism, but this is rare. The major blood supply to the long bones is via the nutrient foramina, visible as narrow radiolucent channels running through the cortex, usually within the caudal aspect of the bone in the diaphyses. Additional small arteries enter the bone at the metaphyses and cross the periosteum at the sites of muscle attachments. The smaller metaphyseal vascular channels are often not visible radiologically.

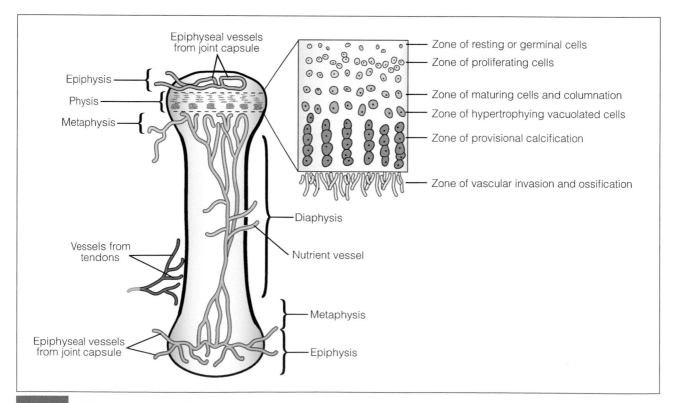

Epiphyseal vessels from joint capsule

Epiphysis

Physis

Metaphysis

Vessels from tendons

Epiphyseal vessels from joint capsule

Diaphysis

Nutrient vessel

Metaphysis

Epiphysis

Zone of resting or germinal cells
Zone of proliferating cells
Zone of maturing cells and columnation
Zone of hypertrophying vacuolated cells
Zone of provisional calcification
Zone of vascular invasion and ossification

7.4 Different regions and blood supply in an immature (top) and mature (bottom) long bone.

Growth plate/physis	Approximate age of closure
Scapula: supraglenoid tubercle	4–7 months
Proximal humerus: greater tubercle to humeral head	4 months
Proximal humeral physis	10–13 months
Distal humerus: lateral and medial parts of condyle	6 weeks
Distal humerus: medial epicondyle	6 months
Distal humerus: condyle to diaphysis	5–8 months
Proximal radius	5–11 months
Proximal ulna: olecranon	5–10 months
Proximal ulna: anconeus	3–5 months
Distal radius	6–12 months
Distal ulna	6–12 months
Accessory carpal bone	2–5 months
Proximal metacarpal i	6 months
Distal metacarpals ii–v	5–7 months
Phalanges	4–6 months
Pelvis: acetabulum	4–6 months
Pelvis: iliac crest	12–24 months
Pelvis: tuber ischii	8–10 months
Proximal femur: neck	6–11 months
Proximal femur: greater trochanter	6–10 months
Proximal femur: lesser trochanter	8–13 months
Distal femur	6–11 months
Proximal tibia: medial and lateral condyle	6 weeks
Proximal tibia: tuberosity to condyle	6–8 months
Proximal tibia: condyle to diaphysis	6–12 months
Proximal fibula	6–12 months
Distal tibia: physis	5–11 months
Distal tibia: medial malleolus	5 months
Distal fibula	5–12 months
Tuber calcis	3–8 months

7.5   Growth plate closure ages for the dog.

Indications

The indications for long bone radiography include:

- Lameness, where pain is localized to the long bones
- Assessment of abnormal limb angulation or limb deformity
- Investigation of hypercalcaemia of unknown origin
- Limb swelling.

Principles of skeletal radiology

Bone can only respond to disease in two ways: loss of bone (lysis) and production of bone (proliferation). Many diseases result in a combination of lysis and proliferation, and the radiological appearance depends on the balance between the two processes. It should also be remembered that significant bone pathology can be present with completely normal radiographs, as pathology that is predominantly within the soft tissues

of the bone (and not altering the mineral content) may not be visible radiographically.

Lysis or loss of mineralized tissue (resulting in decreased opacity of bone) can only be seen radiographically once 30–50% of the mineral content has been lost. This usually takes at least 7–10 days from the onset of changes; therefore, peracute bone injury may not result in recognizable changes. Although many diseases create a focal area of lysis (and so are easier to detect), some diseases (particularly metabolic or nutritional abnormalities) or chronic disuse of a limb (Figure 7.6) can result in a more diffuse loss of bone density, leading to diffuse osteopenia (reduction in bone opacity) (Figure 7.7). This may be more difficult to recognize and can potentially be mimicked by poor radiographic technique (e.g. overexposure).

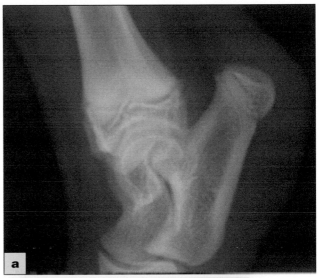

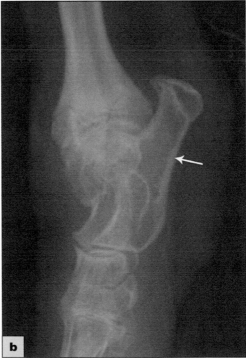

7.6   Mediolateral views of the tarsus of a Cocker Spaniel with a tibial fracture treated by casting. **(a)** On the initial examination, the bone opacity was normal. **(b)** Radiograph taken 6 weeks after casting showing severe osteopenia due to reduced weight bearing and loading of the bones. Note the thinning of the cortices (arrowed) and reduced opacity of the bone. (continues) ▶

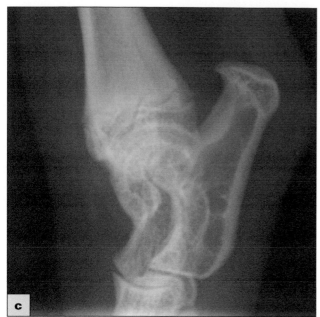

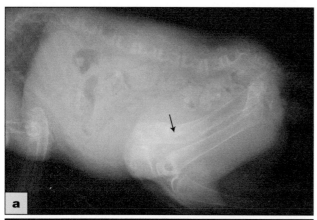

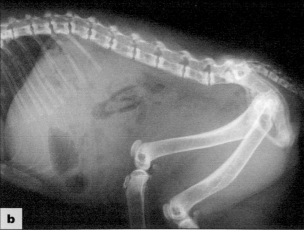

7.6 (continued) Mediolateral view of the tarsus of a Cocker Spaniel with a tibial fracture treated by casting. **(c)** Follow-up radiograph taken 5 weeks after the cast was removed showing remineralization of the bones with thicker cortices and increased opacity.

7.7 Nutritional hyperparathyroidism in a kitten. **(a)** At presentation, there was diffuse osteopenia with poor contrast between the bones and soft tissues, and the cortical thickness of the long bones was reduced. A folding (pathological) fracture (arrowed) of one of the femurs is present. Distortion and malformation of the vertebral column is associated with the reduced bone mineral content.
(b) The same kitten following 3 months of dietary correction. Bone density is now normal, although deformities resulting from the initial disease persist.

Assessment of mild alteration in bone opacity is difficult on digital radiographs which allow alteration of brightness and contrast of the image during viewing.

The appearance of increased bone opacity is referred to as sclerosis (Figure 7.8) and may be due to increased density within bone, an increase in the amount of bone within the medullary cavity, increased mineral content of bone, superimposed periosteal or endosteal new bone or superimposed bony structures (e.g. an over-riding fracture). A rare condition that can give rise to this appearance is osteopetrosis (or 'chalk bones'), which may be idiopathic. Sclerosis of subchondral bone is a useful indicator of joint pathology and often indicates pathology in the overlying cartilage.

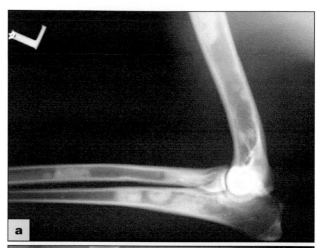

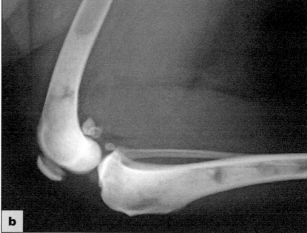

7.8 **(a)** Forelimb and **(b)** hindlimb of a dog with multifocal sclerosis within the medullary cavity. Differential diagnoses include bone infarcts associated with osteosarcoma or immune-mediated disease and osteopetrosis. Bone infarcts vary from stippled foci to large patches of dystrophic mineralization in the medullary cavity of the distal limbs. Osteopetrosis is a rare condition, resulting in polyostotic areas of marked medullary sclerosis (increased opacity) with loss of the normal trabecular pattern. Cortical thickening may be present. The changes are usually diffuse, obliterating the medullary cavity, and better recognized in the appendicular skeleton. It may be an incidental finding in older cats.

Patterns of osteolysis

Lysis of bone may occur due to a variety of mechanisms, including chronic pressure on the bone (e.g. due to a slowly expanding soft tissue mass), disruption of the blood supply to the bone (avascular necrosis), or destruction of the bone by tumour or infection. The appearance of focal osteolysis can reflect the underlying disease process, in particular whether the disease shows aggressive or benign characteristics. However, lesions can show a mixture of patterns and in such cases the lesion is best classified by the most aggressive pattern present (Figures 7.9 and 7.10).

- Geographic osteolysis is a single area of lysis with well defined margins (possibly sclerotic). It is normally found within cancellous bones and, if large, may cause distortion of the shape of the bone. This pattern is usually seen with benign diseases such as bone cysts, but also occurs with some bone tumours. The margination is important for differentiating benign from aggressive disease, with benign lesions typically having sharp, smooth, clearly defined margins.
- Moth-eaten osteolysis describes multiple, often variably sized, areas of lysis with variably defined margins (from sharply to poorly marginated). Areas may coalesce to form larger areas resembling geographic osteolysis. This pattern of lysis is indicative of more aggressive disease processes such as osteomyelitis or neoplasia (including multiple myeloma).
- Permeative osteolysis is the presence of multiple, pinpoint, poorly defined lytic areas, giving the appearance of diffuse 'erosion' of the bone (most easily seen in the cortex) (Figure 7.11). This pattern is indicative of highly aggressive disease (rapidly progressive osteomyelitis or neoplasia).

Periosteal reactions

Insult to bone results in production of new bone, usually from the periosteum and endosteum. The surface of the long bones should be carefully assessed for the presence of periosteal reactions, which may be subtle, but indicate pathology within the adjacent bone. As with osteolysis, the appearance of a periosteal reaction gives an indication of the biological behaviour of a lesion (benign or aggressive) and also the chronicity of the pathology. In general, smooth, sharply marginated periosteal reactions indicate chronicity and benign disease, whereas poorly marginated, irregular new bone indicates more active pathology. The more ill defined and irregular the periosteal reaction, the more aggressive the lesion. With very aggressive disease such as primary malignant bone tumours the new bone produced is often wispy in appearance with ill defined margination. The amount of periosteal new bone produced varies with the age of the patient and should be taken into account when interpreting periosteal reactions. Skeletally immature animals produce much more exuberant new bone than aged animals. Periosteal reactions can be divided into two broad groups (Figure 7.12):

- Continuous periosteal reactions
- Interrupted periosteal reactions.

Continuous reactions: A continuous periosteal reaction tends to suggest a slower and more benign disease process (although these reactions can be seen towards the margins of a more aggressive lesion). Smooth, sharply marginated periosteal new bone is a feature of chronic, benign lesions, e.g. a healing fracture. Continuous patterns that require a more guarded prognosis include those with a brush border or palisading block-like appearance, which are frequently seen with either more aggressive diseases or with systemic disease such as hypertrophic osteodystrophy, A further continuous pattern, the Codman's triangle (indicating new bone filling underneath an area of periosteal elevation), is commonly associated with primary bone neoplasia, although any elevation of the periosteum (e.g. associated with traumatic disease) can result in this pattern.

Interrupted reactions: These typically indicate more aggressive disease (see Figure 7.10) and frequently resemble a 'sunburst' with multiple spurs of new bone extending into the surrounding soft tissues.

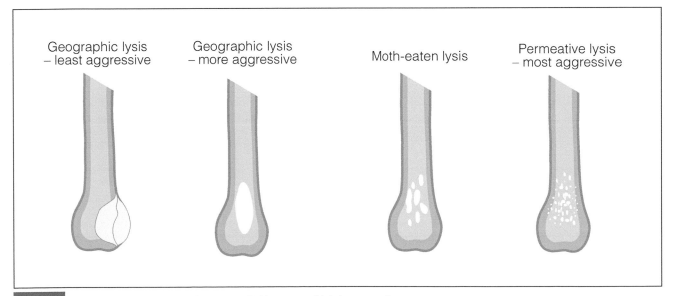

| Geographic lysis – least aggressive | Geographic lysis – more aggressive | Moth-eaten lysis | Permeative lysis – most aggressive |

7.9 Focal bone destruction from least (left) to most (right) aggressive.

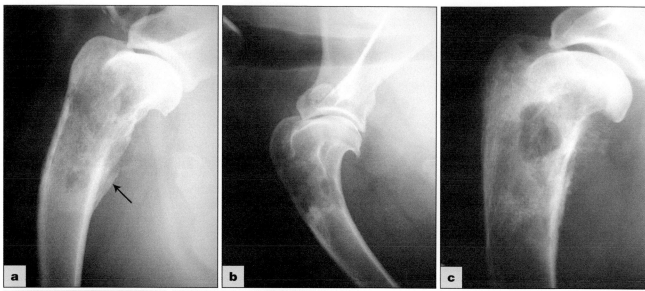

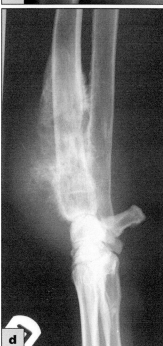

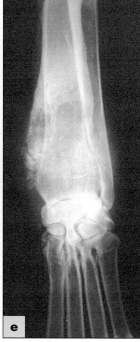

7.10 Primary osteosarcoma affecting the long bones. The radiographic features vary but are characteristic of an aggressive bone lesion and include extensive bone destruction, cortical thinning or disruption, aggressive periosteal reaction (palisading or spiculated) and poorly defined transition to normal bone. The metaphyseal location is typical for a primary bone tumour. **(a)** The lesion is characterized by moth-eaten osteolysis, a palisading periosteal reaction along the cranial cortex and a Codman's triangle at the caudal cortex (arrowed), along with some lysis of both the cranial and caudal cortices. **(b)** The lesion is predominately lytic with areas of moth-eaten and permeative lysis. **(c)** The lesion is mixed lytic–proliferative with a central mixed geographic/moth-eaten area of lysis and a caudal ill defined spiculated periosteal reaction, indicating rapid deposition of new bone. **(d–e)** Mediolateral and craniocaudal radiographs of an osteosarcoma arising in the distal radial metaphysis. The mixed lytic–proliferative lesion has moth-eaten and permeative areas of lysis, with an irregular spiculated periosteal reaction (with a Codman's triangle seen on the medial aspect of the radius) and marked soft tissue swelling around the lesion. Although in close proximity to the ulna and carpus, the lesion in the radius is monostatic (i.e. only involves the radius). This is typical of primary malignant bone tumours and helps differentiate them from soft tissue tumours and secondary bone tumours.

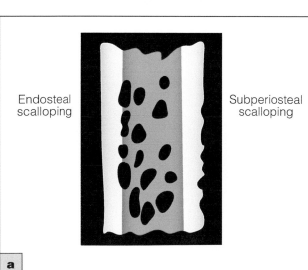

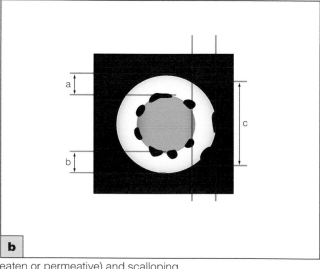

7.11 Lysis location in cortical bone destruction (e.g. moth-eaten or permeative) and scalloping.
(a) Lateral view of a long bone diaphysis. The lytic areas appear to be in the medulla but are in the superimposed cortex. **(b)** Cross-section of the bone in (a). The lytic areas are actually in the cortex but are superimposed on the medulla. It should be borne in mind that opacity is influenced by tissue thickness. Thus, distances a and b combined are about half the distance of c (radiologically seen cortex), so they appear relatively radiolucent on the lateral view.

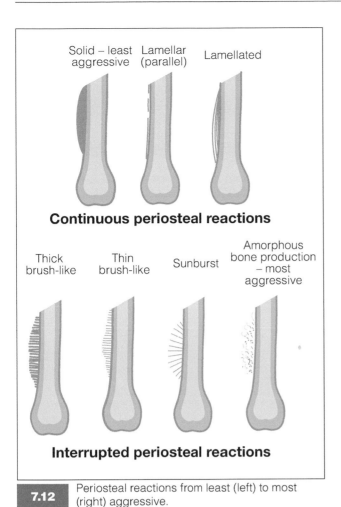

Continuous periosteal reactions

Solid – least aggressive Lamellar (parallel) Lamellated

Thick brush-like Thin brush-like Sunburst Amorphous bone production – most aggressive

Interrupted periosteal reactions

7.12 Periosteal reactions from least (left) to most (right) aggressive.

Radiological interpretation

There are a series of factors to consider when interpreting lesions affecting long bones, which can help to develop a structured differential diagnosis list (in particular, determining whether a lesion shows characteristics of benign or aggressive disease). These factors include:

- The number of bones affected:
  - Single bone (monostotic) – seen with congenital, traumatic, inflammatory and anomalous diseases and primary bone tumours
  - Multiple bones (polyostotic) – seen with metabolic disease (e.g. nutritional (see Figure 7.7) or renal secondary hyperparathyroidism), metastatic neoplasia (e.g. lymphoma, multiple myeloma, metastatic carcinoma) and diseases such as panosteitis and calcinosis circumscripta.
- Lesion distribution: diseases such as primary tumours or traumatic injuries typically result in focal changes, whereas metabolic or nutritional diseases may affect the majority of the skeleton (Figure 7.13)
- Lesion location: primary bone tumours are predominately seen in the metaphyseal regions of long bones, whereas the diaphyses are more commonly affected by trauma, metastatic neoplasia, hypertrophic osteopathy (Marie's disease) or panosteitis. Diseases affecting the physis or epiphysis include congenital diseases such as chondrodysplasia

- Presence and pattern of lysis: important in determining whether a bone lesion is aggressive or benign
- Presence and pattern of new bone formation: may allow determination of the chronicity and biological behaviour of lesions
- Zone of transition (the margin between the lesion and surrounding normal bone): if this is well defined and short, it often indicates a more benign lesion; whereas if this is long and poorly defined, more aggressive diseases should be considered. However, the zone of transition should be interpreted with caution as it is not uncommon for highly aggressive lesions to have a short zone of transition (e.g. metastatic and soft tissue tumours)
- Presence of soft tissue changes: soft tissue swelling is frequently seen with aggressive diseases, whilst chronic lesions may cause muscle atrophy and a loss of muscle mass. Traumatic disease may introduce emphysema (e.g. from an open wound) whilst more chronic disease may cause mineralization of the soft tissues
- Rate of progression: if serial radiographs are obtained, the rate of progression of the changes can be assessed. An aggressive lesion typically shows rapid changes, whilst more benign lesions show slow or no progression over time

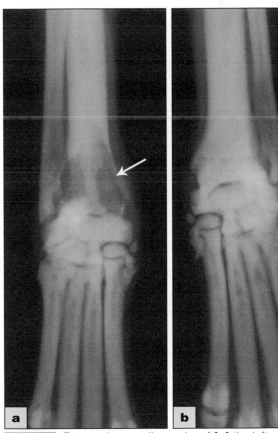

7.13 Dorsopalmar radiographs of **(a)** the left and **(b)** the right carpi of a dog with hyperostosis and a primary bone tumour (arrowed) in the distal left radius. The hyperostosis in this case was presumed to be idiopathic and has resulted in a generalized increase in opacity of all bones, with thickening of the cortices and a reduction in size of the medullary cavities. The generalized polyostotic distribution is seen with metabolic and some congenital and idiopathic diseases. In contrast, the lesion in the radius is monostotic and the distribution within the metaphysis is a predilection site for primary bone tumours.

■ History, breed and age: helpful when considering differential diagnoses as some diseases have breed and age predilections.

Mnemonic for assessing skeletal structures

A mnemonic for assessing skeletal structures, which may help radiological interpretation is:

■ A: Alignment – assess for evidence of fractures or loss of cortical integrity, alignment of the joints or evidence of malformation of the bones (e.g. chondrodysplasia, bowing due to premature closure of the growth plate)
■ B: Bone – assess the general opacity of the bone and the clarity of the corticomedullary differentiation (which may be reduced with metabolic diseases) as well as the trabecular pattern of the medullary cavity. In addition, look for evidence of focal lysis or new bone proliferation
■ C: Cartilage – assess for indirect evidence of cartilage pathology (joint effusion, subchondral sclerosis, vacuum phenomenon)
■ (D: Device – if orthopaedic implants are present, assess for evidence of loosening, failure or osteomyelitis, as well as the healing of fractures or osteotomy sites)
■ E: Envelope (or Everything Else) – assess for changes to the soft tissues (swelling or atrophy).

The key features for differentiating aggressive and benign long bone lesions are summarized in Figure 7.14.

Feature	Appearance of aggressive lesions	Appearance of benign lesions
Lysis	Typically moth-eaten or permeative patterns and likely to involve the cortical bone	Typically geographic pattern. May be some cortical thinning if there is sufficient expansion of the lesion (rare)
Periosteal new bone	Typically interrupted patterns (spiculated, sunburst) with ill defined margins to the new bone	Typically continuous patterns with well defined margins to the new bone
Lesion location	Primary bone tumours have predilection sites ('away from the elbow', 'near the knee') whilst osteomyelitis is most frequently associated with local trauma or surgical implants	No typical features, although metabolic diseases are more likely to affect multiple bones
Zone of transition (transformation from abnormal to normal bone)	Long and ill defined	Short and well defined
Soft tissue swelling around the lesion	Usually marked	Usually fairly mild
Rate of progression on serial radiographic examinations	Rapid	Slow

7.14 Features differentiating benign and aggressive bone lesions.

Röntgen signs

Size: The majority of size variation in the long bones is related to normal breed and anatomical variants. A pathological increase in the size of the bones can occur to compensate for the congenital absence or deformity of another bone in the limb, but this is rare. More common is remodelling of the bone due to altered loading, which can result in an increase in diameter (and shape) of the bone (Figure 7.15). Reduced length of the bones can be seen with congenital hypothyroidism, chondrodysplasias and premature closure of growth plates.

Shape: As with size, long bone shape alterations are most commonly related to breed variants. Most diseases that result in alterations in size also cause alterations in shape. Congenital shape abnormalities (e.g. chondrodysplasia; Figure 7.16) are usually symmetrical,

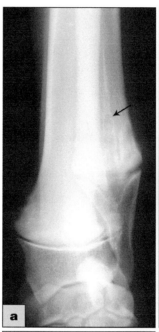
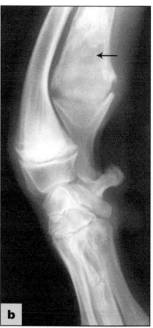
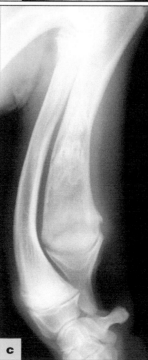

7.15

(a) Craniocaudal and (b–c) mediolateral views of the antebrachium of a dog with premature closure of the distal ulnar growth plate due to a retained cartilaginous core (arrowed). The cartilaginous core is 'candle shaped' with reduced opacity within the metaphysis and distal diaphysis. The antebrachium is bowed cranially and there is proximal displacement of the styloid process due to disturbance of the distal ulnar growth plate. Due to the increased loading, the ulna has a larger diameter than normal. This is the result of Wolffs law and illustrates the effect of altered loading on bone shape and size.

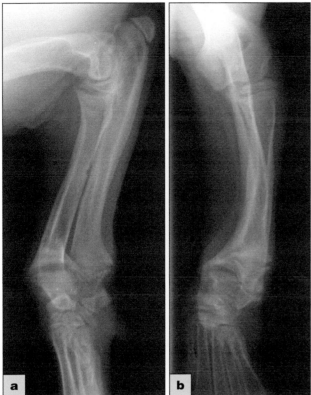

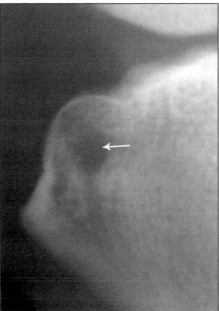

Mediolateral view of the normal tibia. Note the area of reduced opacity (arrowed) within the tibial tuberosity due to retained cartilage and thinness of the bone. This should not be mistaken for pathological lysis.

7.16 **(a)** Mediolateral and **(b)** craniocaudal radiographs of the antebrachium of a chondrodystrophic puppy. The bowing of the radius and ulna is most clearly seen on the craniocaudal view. The shape of the distal radial epiphysis is altered, as is the articulation at the radiocarpal joint. Radial and ulna lengths are approximately equal.

whereas acquired diseases (e.g. neoplasia, trauma) result in asymmetrical changes in shape. Masses arising from within the bone usually lead to focal expansion of the cortices, resulting in divergence of the cortices on orthogonal views (see Figure 7.10).

Number: Alterations in the number of bones are very rare and occur with congenital anomalies (e.g. ectrodactyly (absence of a digit) and polydactyly (additional or supernumerary digits)).

Opacity: Recognizing alterations in the opacity of bone is a key feature in radiological interpretation. Loss of bone opacity can occur due to reduced mineral content of the bone, reduced thickness of the bone or artefactual causes such as overexposure, gas within the soft tissues or loss of the overlying soft tissues. Care should be taken to account for the shape of the bone when assessing opacity. Thinner parts of the bone will be less opaque than thicker regions (e.g. the tibial tuberosity is often relatively lucent compared with the rest of the tibia, due to the triangular cross-section of the proximal tibia; Figure 7.17). The distribution of the reduced opacity, the number of bones affected and the presence of other changes (such as cortical destruction and new bone formation) should be determined.

Margination: Abnormal margination of a bone or joint is a sensitive indicator of pathology and can be subtle and easily overlooked. Margination is an important

feature in determining the chronicity of lesion and also helps to differentiate aggressive from benign pathology. Ill defined and poorly marginated lesions are usually more active or aggressive than smooth, sharply marginated lesions. It is important to distinguish between the shape of the bone lesions and their margination. It is possible to have an irregular but sharply marginated lesion and a smooth but poorly marginated lesion (Figure 7.18).

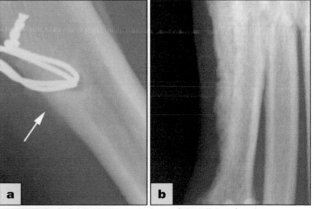

7.18 **(a)** Mediolateral view of the tibia of a dog following surgery. The periosteal new bone (arrowed) is poorly marginated with indistinct edges, which are difficult to differentiate from the soft tissues. Despite being poorly marginated, the shape of the new bone formation is smooth. **(b)** Dorsopalmar view of the metacarpus of a dog with hypertrophic osteopathy. The new bone is sharply marginated with distinct edges; however, the shape of the new bone is irregular, almost palisading.

Position, location and alignment: Abnormalities in the location of the long bones are usually due to trauma, resulting in fractures or luxation. The alignment of the joints and limb should be assessed, and it is important to differentiate abnormal alignment due to abnormalities in the shape of the bones (e.g. due to long bone fractures or secondary to premature closure of a growth plate) from abnormal joint alignment (e.g. rupture of a ligament). Stressed radiographs may be required to demonstrate ligamentous injury. In animals with varus or valgus deformities, the site of deformity can be assessed on craniocaudal views. Lines bisecting the distal and proximal parts of the limb are drawn on the radiograph. The point at which the two lines cross indicates the site of deformity (e.g. joint, physeal region, diaphysis) (Figure 7.19).

Common diseases

Fractures

Fractures are most commonly the result of trauma, although pathological fractures can be seen with underlying bone disease (e.g. tumours, osteopenia). There is a high incidence of concurrent thoracic and abdominal injuries with external trauma, especially trauma resulting in fracture of the proximal limbs. If there is any doubt as to whether there is thoracic or abdominal involvement, radiographs of these regions should be obtained (see Chapters 5 and 6). Stress fractures most commonly occur in athletic dogs and occur at specific sites due to abnormal loading of the bone. Fractures are seen as a discontinuity of the cortex with radiolucent fracture lines. With incomplete, non-displaced fractures, the fracture line may be difficult to see in the acute stages. Resorption of bone occurs at, and increases visibility of, the fracture site 3–7 days following injury, thus in some cases repeat radiographs may be required to visualize the fracture. In older animals with no history of significant trauma, the fracture site should be carefully evaluated for any evidence of new bone formation and lysis to rule out a pathological cause for the fracture. Pitfalls in fracture diagnosis may occur when radiolucent lines not associated with bone injury are superimposed over the bone (e.g. nutrient foramina, Mach lines, fascial planes; Figure 7.20). Superimposed lucencies within the soft tissues almost always occur in unusual locations for fractures, often extend beyond the bone margins and are not associated with other bony changes.

An initial assessment of the fracture should evaluate the following features:

- Location – which bone(s) is affected and which part of the bone (diaphysis, metaphysis, physis)
- Fracture configuration/classification (avulsion, simple, wedge, complex, complete, incomplete, comminuted)
- Displacement and degree of over-riding of fragments/bones – the displacement (cranial, medial) of the major distal fragment should be described relative to the proximal fragment
- Whether it is an open or closed fracture – the presence of gas or foreign bodies within the soft tissue, large soft tissue defects or extension of bone through the skin indicate an open fracture
- Age of the fracture based on sharpness of bone edges and presence of any callus
- Articular involvement
- Any evidence of underlying bone pathology
- Any growth plate involvement (in immature animals)
- Any other complicating factors.

Radiological features:

- Soft tissue swelling around the fracture site in early stages.
- Gas or foreign material may be present within the soft tissues if the fracture is open.
- Malalignment of the limb in complete fractures (may be normal with incomplete fractures).
- Discontinuity of the cortex with radiolucent lines running through the bone.

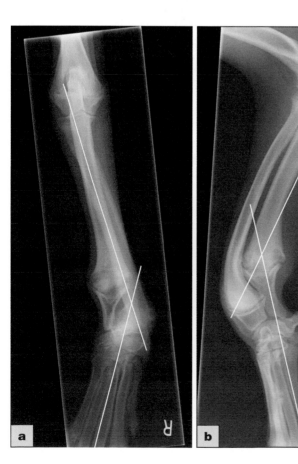

7.19 **(a)** Craniocaudal and **(b)** mediolateral views of the antebrachium of a 6-month-old Irish Wolfhound with angular limb deformity due to premature closure of the distal growth plate. With limb deformities, it can be helpful to superimpose lines on the centre of the bones proximal and distal to the deformity. The point at which the lines cross indicates the region of maximal deformity and the probable site of the primary pathology. In this case, the intersection is at the level of the distal ulnar metaphysis.

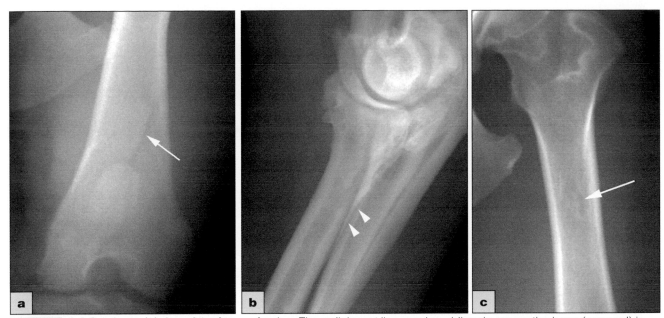

7.20 **(a)** Caudocranial view of the femur of a dog. The radiolucent line running obliquely across the bone (arrowed) is due to fat within the fascial planes between the muscle bellies. The lucency can be seen to extend beyond the margins of the bone. **(b)** Mach line/rebound artefact, resulting in an artefactual linear radiolucency (arrowheads) crossing the cranial cortex of the ulna where the edges of the radius and ulna cross. **(c)** The short linear lucency running vertically in the femur (arrowed) is the normal nutrient foramen. Nutrient foramina occur in predictable locations and are most obvious within the diaphyseal regions of the long bones.

- Fragmentation of the bone if comminuted/avulsion fracture.
- Mineralized callus formation adjacent to the fracture in subacute/chronic stages (from approximately 5–7 days).

Assessment of fracture healing: The radiographic changes of normal fracture healing are progressive and follow a series of distinct stages. Follow-up radiographs should be obtained periodically (every 2–6 weeks) post repair to monitor progression of healing and detect any complications. The frequency of repeat radiography is dependent upon the age of the patient and the expectation of any problems. There is much variation in the time for fractures to heal depending on the age of the patient, fracture configuration, type of fixation, soft tissue disruption, vascular supply, presence of infection or systemic disease. In the early stages of classical fracture healing there is haematoma

formation between the bone ends, which progressively becomes organized then resorbed. Concurrently a callus forms around the fracture site which is initially non-mineralized. The presence of haematoma and early callus appears radiologically as soft tissue swelling, which gradually resolves over 1–14 days. Also during the first 2 weeks post fracture there is resorption of bone at the fracture ends, which leads to a loss in the sharpness of the fracture margins. The maturing callus becomes mineralized from 10–12 days post fracture and in the early stages appears poorly marginated and indistinct. Significant mineralized callus formation should be visible by 3–4 weeks. Progressive callus formation and maturation around the fracture sites results in a gradual closure of the fracture line, with bridging of the fracture ends and remodelling of the cortices. This last stage is usually seen at approximately 8–12 weeks in adult animals following fracture reduction and stabilization (Figures 7.21 and 7.22).

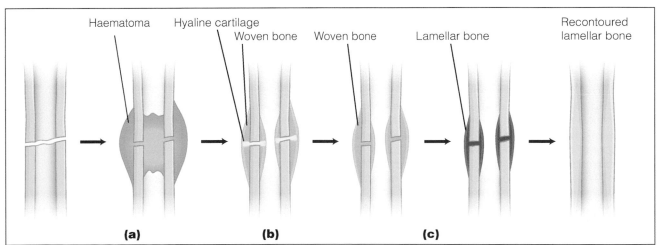

7.21 Classical fracture healing. **(a)** Haematoma at the fracture site. **(b)** Bridging callus at the fracture site mineralized peripherally but with hyaline cartilage at the level of the fracture site. **(c)** Compaction and remodelling of the mineralized callus.

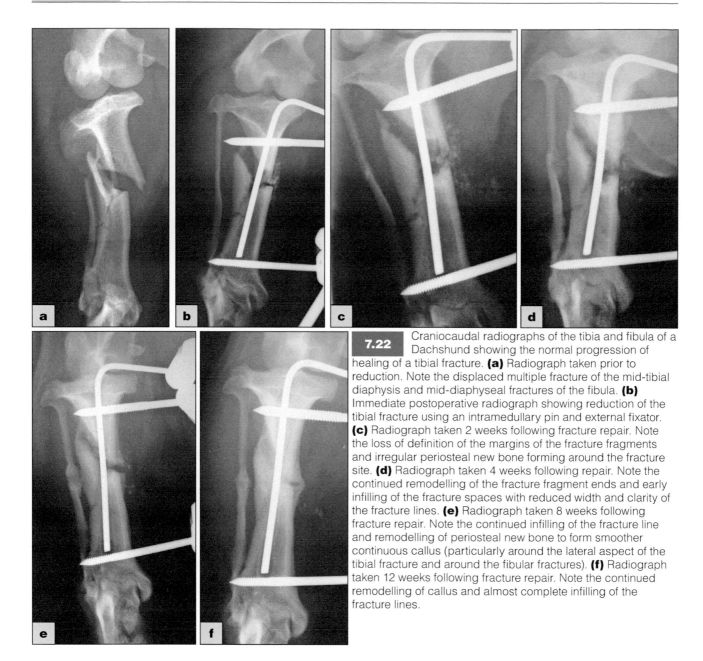

7.22 Craniocaudal radiographs of the tibia and fibula of a Dachshund showing the normal progression of healing of a tibial fracture. **(a)** Radiograph taken prior to reduction. Note the displaced multiple fracture of the mid-tibial diaphysis and mid-diaphyseal fractures of the fibula. **(b)** Immediate postoperative radiograph showing reduction of the tibial fracture using an intramedullary pin and external fixator. **(c)** Radiograph taken 2 weeks following fracture repair. Note the loss of definition of the margins of the fracture fragments and irregular periosteal new bone forming around the fracture site. **(d)** Radiograph taken 4 weeks following repair. Note the continued remodelling of the fracture fragment ends and early infilling of the fracture spaces with reduced width and clarity of the fracture lines. **(e)** Radiograph taken 8 weeks following fracture repair. Note the continued infilling of the fracture line and remodelling of periosteal new bone to form smoother continuous callus (particularly around the lateral aspect of the tibial fracture and around the fibular fractures). **(f)** Radiograph taken 12 weeks following fracture repair. Note the continued remodelling of callus and almost complete infilling of the fracture lines.

The radiological appearance of normal fracture healing is very variable and depends upon the age of the animal (more rapid healing occurs in younger animals), fracture location and configuration (slower healing in highly comminuted fractures), method of repair and stability of the fracture and presence of complicating factors (soft tissue disruption, etc.). With accurate reduction of fractures and stable fixation resulting in contact between the cortices direct bone union may occur with little or no callus formation. In addition to assessing progression of fracture healing the appearance of the implants and alignment of the bones should be evaluated. On postoperative radiographs the reduction of the fracture, alignment of the bone and position of any implants should be assessed for any problems. Loosening or infection around implants typically results in a halo of lysis around the screws or pins.

Radiological features:

- Soft tissue swelling in early stages.
- Faint mineralized callus adjacent to fracture sites from 2–3 weeks.
- Significant mineralized new bone formation from periosteum and endosteum adjacent to the fracture should be visible by 4 weeks.
- Once the fracture is bridged and is stable, progressive remodelling results in the callus becoming smaller, smoother and more sharply marginated as woven bone is converted to lamellar bone (may take months).
- Disuse osteopenia often occurs if weight-bearing is reduced and especially if the limb has been cast. The radiological changes include cortical thinning, double cortical line and reduced bone opacity with coarse trabecular pattern.
- Presence of lysis adjacent to implants indicates infection or loosening.

Abnormal fracture healing: Abnormalities of fracture healing can include malunion (Figure 7.23) and delayed or non-union (Figure 7.24). Delayed union appears the same radiologically as normal fracture healing, except that the stages occur later than normal. Malunion occurs when there is normal fracture healing but with complications due to abnormal size or shape of the bone.

In the early stages it is not possible to tell radiologically if fracture healing is simply delayed or progressing to a non-union. Non-union of fractures commonly occurs due to inadequate immobilization of the fracture ends, resulting in movement of the bones or disruption of the blood supply. Radiologically, non-union is often divided into viable (biologically active) non-unions and non-viable (biologically inactive) non-unions. Biologically viable non-unions include hypertrophic and oligotrophic types, which are characterized by the degree of callus formation. Hypertrophic non-unions suggest poor immobilization of the fracture but with adequate blood supply. With hypertrophic non-unions the fracture ends appear smooth with large amounts of sharply marginated callus formation, which may fill the medullary cavity at the fracture site. If the fracture is not stabilized a pseudoarthrosis may ultimately form, with expanded ends to the bone (elephant foot configuration). Oligotrophic non-unions have no or limited callus formation. An inadequate blood supply to the fracture site may result in a biologically inactive non-union appearing radiologically as a non-union with no or very little callus formation. A specific form is the atrophic non-union that can occur with antebrachial fractures in toy breed dogs where there is severe osteopenia and resorption of the bones, which become tapered.

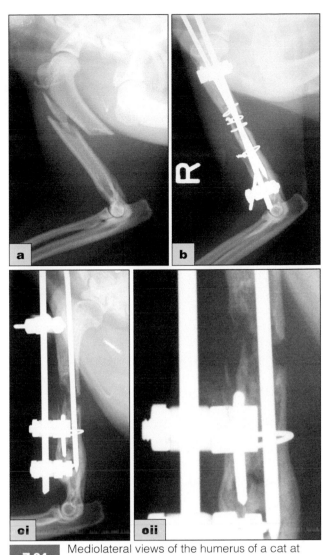

7.24 Mediolateral views of the humerus of a cat at **(a)** presentation and **(b)** at 6 weeks and **(c)** 12 weeks following reduction of a mid-diaphyseal multiple fracture. (b) At 6 weeks, there is loss of bone beneath the proximal cerclage wires, which were subsequently removed. (ci) At 12 weeks, the ends of the fracture fragments have retreated from the fracture site, indicating an atrophic non-union. (cii) Magnified view.

Growth plate injuries: Trauma to the long bones in skeletally immature animals may result in fracture of the physes. It is important to recognize when a physeal fracture is present as they may result in premature closure of the growth plate, leading to limb deformities. In cases with suspected trauma to the physes, follow-up radiographs should be obtained at 2-week intervals to rule out developing limb deformity and allow early corrective surgery. Recognizing pathology of the physes may be difficult if unfamiliar with the normal appearance and it is helpful to radiograph the contralateral limb for comparison. Some physeal injuries, especially crushing injuries (most commonly to the distal ulna physes) may not be visible on radiographs in the acute stages. Growth plate fractures are classified according to the Salter–Harris classification (Figure 7.25).

Primary bone neoplasia

The most common primary bone tumours are osteosarcoma and chondrosarcoma. There are a number of sites in the appendicular skeleton that show a

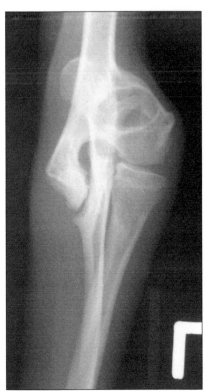

7.23 Craniocaudal view of the elbow of a dog with malunion following a lateral humeral condylar fracture. The lateral part of the humeral condyle has fused to the lateral supracondylar bone of the humerus, resulting in marked deformation of the elbow joint with proximolateral displacement of the humeroradial articulation.

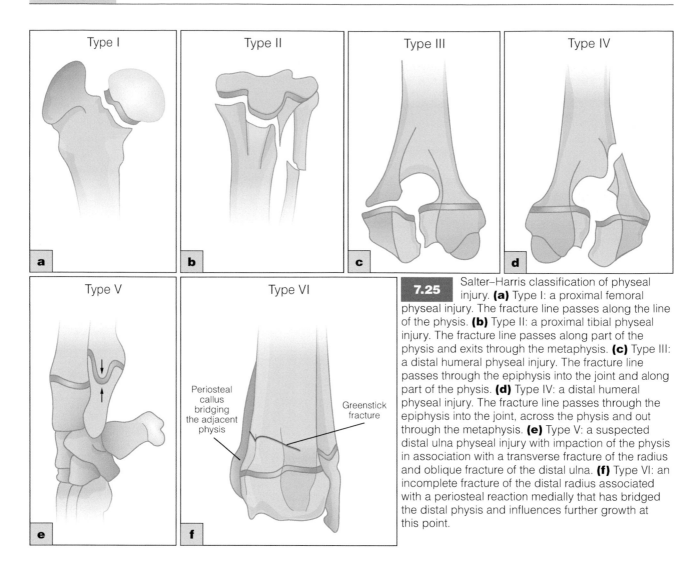

7.25 Salter–Harris classification of physeal injury. **(a)** Type I: a proximal femoral physeal injury. The fracture line passes along the line of the physis. **(b)** Type II: a proximal tibial physeal injury. The fracture line passes along part of the physis and exits through the metaphysis. **(c)** Type III: a distal humeral physeal injury. The fracture line passes through the epiphysis into the joint and along part of the physis. **(d)** Type IV: a distal humeral physeal injury. The fracture line passes through the epiphysis into the joint, across the physis and out through the metaphysis. **(e)** Type V: a suspected distal ulna physeal injury with impaction of the physis in association with a transverse fracture of the radius and oblique fracture of the distal ulna. **(f)** Type VI: an incomplete fracture of the distal radius associated with a periosteal reaction medially that has bridged the distal physis and influences further growth at this point.

predilection for the development of primary bone neoplasia. Common sites for primary bone tumours are the proximal humerus and distal radius ('away from the elbow') and the distal femur and proximal tibia ('near the knee'), although they also occur at other sites. The lesions are usually centred on the metaphysis. Tumours may show predominantly lytic, predominantly proliferative or mixed patterns of bony change. The features are typically those of an aggressive bony lesion (see Figure 7.10). Primary bone tumours in dogs show early metastatic potential, and thoracic radiographs should be obtained to screen for pulmonary metastasis. The tumour type cannot be determined by radiological assessment and a biopsy is required for a definitive diagnosis. In early cases, lesions may be subtle, but if repeat radiographs are obtained 4–6 weeks later, progression of the lesions will be seen.

Radiological features:

- Localized soft tissue swelling (may be severe).
- Aggressive bone lesion with cortical destruction.
- Variable in appearance but lysis present in all cases.
- Monostotic (affecting a single bone) with lesions arising in the region of the metaphysis.
- If in paired bones or adjacent to a joint, the lesion does not cross the joint space or involve the adjacent bone, which helps differentiate a primary bone tumour from a secondary bone tumour.
- Periosteal reaction is common and appears ill defined and poorly marginated. The periosteal reaction is interrupted, commonly with a sunburst appearance, and often extends some distance from the cortex into the adjacent soft tissue swelling. Indistinct, poorly marginated mineralization is often present within the soft tissue swelling due to tumour mineralization. Elevation of the periosteum by the tumour may result in a triangular shaped area of subperiosteal new bone known as a Codman's triangle.
- Lesions are expansile (arising from within the medullary cavity), which results in divergence of the cortices.

Bone metastases

Metastatic spread of neoplasia to long bones is most commonly seen with mammary gland or prostatic carcinomas, as well as spread from bone tumours at other sites. Radiological features are not specific to tumour type and there is usually evidence of involvement of other body areas.

Radiological features:

- Metastatic bone tumours are usually found in the mid-diaphysis adjacent to the nutrient foramen (as metastases are spread haematogenously) (Figure 7.26).

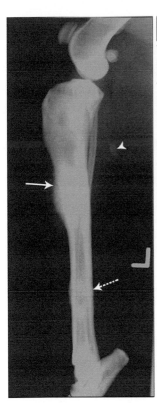

7.26 Mediolateral view of the left tibia and fibula of a dog with metastatic spread of mammary gland carcinoma to the long bones. The mid-diaphyseal tibial lesion has a dense, irregular, periosteal proliferation, resulting in increased bone opacity (solid arrow). The smaller lesion in the distal tibial diaphysis (dashed arrow) is similar and superimposed on indistinct bone lysis. A couple of small focal areas of mineralization (arrowhead) are seen caudal to the tibia: these are consistent with dystrophic soft tissue mineralization. The location of the bone lesions is not typical of a primary bone tumour. Tumours that metastasize to bone tend to be localized to the diaphysis, especially the areas around the nutrient vessels. The radiographic appearance is variable.

- May be polyostotic and arise at sites that are uncommon for primary bone tumours.
- Variable in appearance but the features are those of an aggressive bony lesion. They are most commonly lytic in appearance (especially thyroid tumours and many carcinomas), with variable (often minimal) periosteal reaction. Less common appearances are sclerotic (blastic) lesions (which may be seen with prostatic tumours or osteosarcoma metastases) or mixed (lytic and proliferative) lesions.

- Periosteal reactions are variable but when present are irregular in appearance.

Soft tissue tumours

Tumours arising from the soft tissues adjacent to bones most commonly present with a soft tissue swelling on the limb, with or without local invasion of bone. In addition to direct invasion of bone, soft tissue tumours may also potentially metastasize to bone (see above). Common soft tissue tumours of the appendicular skeleton include a variety of soft tissue sarcomas (haemangiosarcoma, fibrosarcoma, peripheral nerve tumours, rhabdomyosarcoma), squamous cell carcinomas and round cell tumours. Radiological features are not specific to tumour type and biopsy is required for histological diagnosis.

Radiological features:

- Localized soft tissue swelling.
- Focal cortical lysis, which is adjacent to a localized soft tissue swelling or mass.
- Bony lysis often results in concavity in the surface of bone, in contrast to expansion seen in primary bone tumours.
- Often polyostotic if adjacent to paired bones or joints.
- Variable in location with no predilection for metaphysis, unlike primary bone tumours.
- Often predominately lytic with little periosteal reaction.

Osteomyelitis

Osteomyelitis is most commonly associated with bacterial infection. Fungal infections may also be seen in some countries but are rare in the UK. Although osteomyelitis may arise from a haematogenous spread of infectious organisms, it is typically seen as a local lesion associated with focal trauma (or placement of surgical implants) (Figure 7.27). Systemic

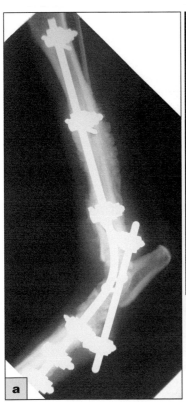

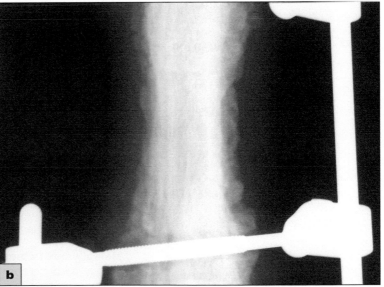

7.27 **(a)** Mediolateral and **(b)** craniocaudal (close-up) views of the tibia and fibula of a dog with osteomyelitis associated with an external fixator. There is a generalized marked palisading periosteal reaction with diffuse soft tissue swelling affecting the distal tibial diaphysis and metaphysis. Bone lysis around the external fixator pins indicates loosening and infection extending into the bone around the pins. These are features of aggressive bone disease, but the periosteal reaction is well defined and established, indicating chronic disease. The narrow transition to normal bone proximally is typical of bone infection.

osteomyelitis is rare but may be seen in immunocompromised animals (e.g. German Shepherd bitches with relative IgA deficiency).

Radiological features:

- Typically osteomyelitis is seen as a mixed lytic–proliferative lesion. When present associated with surgery, lysis occurs mainly around any surgical implants, resulting in a halo of lysis. Periosteal reactions are often palisading or irregular and florid.
- Soft tissue swelling is in most cases marked.
- With haematogenous infections, lesion may be polyostotic (see Figure 3.43).

Panosteitis

Panosteitis is most frequently seen in young male dogs (particularly German Shepherds) presenting with a history of shifting lameness. Good radiographic technique is essential to visualize these lesions as they are easily masked on overexposed or underexposed radiographs. Lesions are most easily recognized when comparing images from the contralateral limb. Panosteitis is a benign lesion with no evidence of bone lysis. Bone infarcts may look similar with focal irregular areas of increased bone opacity within the medullary cavity, but these are rare, most commonly seen in older animals, and often not associated with pain.

Radiological features:

- Most commonly appears as focal, patchy areas of increased medullary opacity – these may have the classic rounded 'thumbprint' appearance (Figures 7.28 and 7.29). Lesions can be subtle and are easily overlooked. A more diffuse increase in medullary opacity may be seen occasionally.

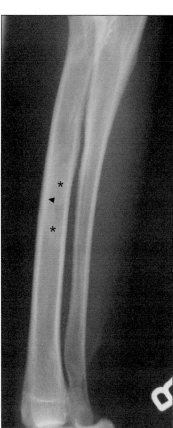

7.28 Mediolateral view of the antebrachium of a dog with panosteitis. Ill defined 'thumbprint' areas (*) of increased medullary opacity in the mid-diaphyseal area of the radius and endosteal irregularity (arrowhead) are visible. Lesions are frequently centred on the nutrient foramen and blurring of the trabeculae may be present. Areas of medullary sclerosis may coalesce. Radiographic changes may lag behind the clinical signs in the early stages and so may not be present, therefore, radiographs should be repeated in 10–14 days where the clinical suspicion remains. Radiographic changes may also remain beyond resolution of the clinical signs, with cortical thickening persisting.

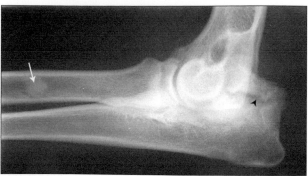

7.29 Mediolateral neutral radiograph of the elbow of a dog with an ununited anconeal process. The area of the anconeal process is altered in shape due to new bone formation, and the anconeal process is separated from the olecranon of the ulna by a radiolucent line (arrowhead). In addition, the sclerosis of the ulnar trochlear notch indicates more generalized degenerative joint disease. The radiopaque 'thumbprint' lesion (arrowed) in the medullary cavity of the radial diaphysis indicates concurrent panosteitis.

- Predilection site is mid-diaphysis, often centred in the region of the nutrient foramen.
- Usually polyostotic, affecting multiple long bones, often at different times.
- Mild smooth endosteal and periosteal bone formation.
- After lesions resolve, the medullary cavity may appear relatively lucent with reduced trabeculation.

Hypertrophic osteopathy

Hypertrophic osteopathy (Marie's disease) is most commonly seen with intrathoracic masses (particularly primary lung tumours), although it has been reported with some abdominal tumours. The exact mechanism is uncertain but is thought to be neurovascular since sectioning the vagus nerve may result in resolution of the lesions.

Radiological features:

- Polyostotic periosteal reaction affecting the distal limb bones, but sparing the joints. The periosteal reaction is most commonly a combination of an irregular continuous, and palisading pattern. More proximally, the new bone typically becomes smoother and more continuous (Figure 7.30).
- Multiple limbs are affected and there is usually associated diffuse soft tissue swelling. This does not represent metastatic spread of the tumour and if the primary cause is removed, the periosteal reaction gradually remodels and reduces over time.
- New bone formation initially starts on the abaxial surface of the bones and spares the joint spaces.

Metaphyseal osteopathy

Metaphyseal osteopathy (also known as hypertrophic osteodystrophy) is typically seen in immature dogs, usually presenting with pyrexia and lameness. It occurs most commonly in large-breed dogs (especially Great Danes, Boxers and Weimaraners) and the lameness may be severe, with affected dogs unable to stand. The main differential diagnosis is haematogenous osteomyelitis, which, in some cases, may be indistinguishable from metaphyseal osteo-

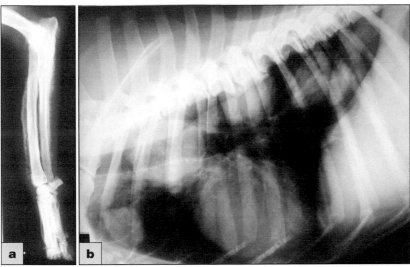

7.30 Mediolateral views of **(a)** the left antebrachium and **(b)** the left lateral thorax of a dog with hypertrophic osteopathy (Marie's disease) associated with pulmonary metastatic disease. (a) A diffuse mixed periosteal reaction surrounds the antebrachial and metacarpal bones. The appearance of the periosteal new bone is laminar cranially, with a more palisading appearance caudally. The carpal and elbow joints and adjacent metaphyses are spared. (b) Multiple variably sized pulmonary soft tissue nodules are present within the thorax. The patient's right forelimb had been amputated 5 months previously due to a proximal humeral osteosarcoma. Although usually associated with thoracic mass lesions, similar changes may also be caused by abdominal masses and, rarely, diffuse thoracic infiltrates.

pathy on radiographs. With haematogenous osteomyelitis often only one bone is involved and a collar of new bone surrounding the periosteum is not seen.

Radiological features:

- Localized soft tissue swelling surrounding the metaphyseal regions.
- The key feature is focal lysis (often crescent-shaped) in the metaphyses of multiple long bones parallel to the physis.
- Adjacent to the lysis there is usually sclerosis within the distal diaphysis.
- Generally polyostotic and affects the majority of the limbs.
- In more advanced cases, a 'collar' of new bone may surround the affected metaphyses.
- Due to damage to the physis, limb deformity may develop, even after the metaphyseal lesions have resolved (Figure 7.31).

Chondrodysplasia

This is seen in several dog breeds (e.g. Dachshund, Basset Hound) and occasionally in the Domestic Shorthaired cat. Chondrodysplasia is a disorder of endochondral ossification. It results in an abnormally bowed shape to the long bones, which can lead to altered dynamics of the associated joints and a predisposition to the development of osteoarthritis. This is most commonly seen affecting the bones of the antebrachium (see Figure 7.16).

Secondary hyperparathyroidism

This presents most commonly in skeletally immature animals, secondary to renal disease or dietary deficiency. Increased parathyroid hormone levels result in resorption of calcium from the skeleton, leading to severe osteopenia. The distribution of the osteopenia differs with the underlying cause. Renal secondary hyperparathyroidism preferentially results in demineralization within the skull, whereas nutritional causes usually affect the entire skeleton uniformly.

Radiological features:

- Cortical thinning with reduced opacity of all bones and a double cortical line may be visible. In severe

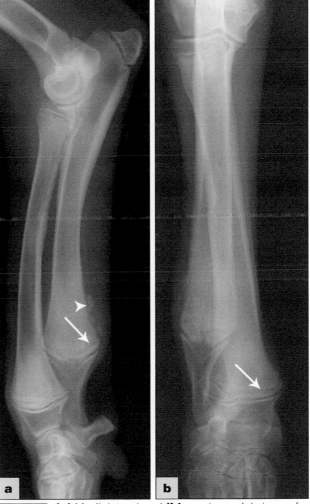

7.31 **(a)** Mediolateral and **(b)** craniocaudal views of the antebrachium of a Great Dane puppy with metaphyseal osteopathy (hypertrophic osteodystrophy). Areas or bands of radiolucency (arrowed) with mild surrounding sclerosis are present in the distal metaphyseal regions of the radius and distal metaphysis of the ulna. A collar of paraperiosteal new bone (arrowhead) is visible adjacent to the distal ulna and is seen in chronic cases of metaphyseal osteopathy. Changes in the contralateral limb and the metaphyses of the tibia and distal femur in this dog were similar. Haematogenous osteomyelitis can resemble metaphyseal osteopathy, but often only affects one limb and a collar of paraperiosteal new bone is not seen.

cases of demineralization the bones may be barely visible ('ghost-like') and difficult to distinguish from structures of soft tissue opacity (see Figure 7.7).

- In severe cases with cortical thinning, pathological (folding) fractures are common.
- There is a rapid return to normal bone opacity if the diet is corrected (if due to a nutritional cause) but deformity due to fractures may persist.
- In renal secondary hyperparathyroidism, metastatic calcification of the soft tissues (gastric mucosa, blood vessels, myocardium, kidneys) and small, irregular kidneys may be present. In renal secondary hyperparathyroidism the skull bones are often most severely affected (see Chapter 8).

Joints

Joint pathology is extremely common and frequently causes lameness, but the significance of any radiological abnormalities can often only be determined in conjunction with the history and clinical examination. Apparently incidental degenerative changes not associated with lameness are common, especially in the shoulder and metacarpophalangeal joints. The soft tissue structures of joints (cartilage, ligaments, menisci, synovium) are not visible as distinct structures and cannot be differentiated radiologically from joint fluid. Diseases associated with significant soft tissue pathology may be present with no radiological abnormalities (Figure 7.32). A normal radiograph does not mean that the joint is normal and, in many cases, additional tests are required for a definitive diagnosis or to characterize joint pathology.

Radiological interpretation

Radiographs of joints should be evaluated systemically, with specific attention paid to the soft tissues, shape and opacity of the subchondral bone, and the presence of any new bone formation at the margins of the joint or within the periarticular soft tissues. Using a bright light or altering the window and level on digital images is often necessary to visualize the soft tissues, as they are often relatively overexposed on radiographs. As many significant lesions are subtle, the use of a magnifying glass is recommended, particularly for evaluating smaller joints.

Soft tissues

Evaluation of the soft tissues of the joints is important as many diseases result in an effusion within the joint or swelling of the periarticular soft tissues. Localization of the increase in opacity to within the joint (Figure 7.33) helps differentiate effusion from other causes of periarticular soft tissue swelling such as cellulitis or ligamentous injury (Figure 7.34). The presence of joint effusion is a specific sign of joint disease, but may occur secondary to systemic disease (e.g. immune-mediated polyarthritis, bleeding disorders), as well as with primary joint disease. Joint effusion results in an increase in soft tissue opacity that is confined to the joint cavity. Effusions can only be reliably detected in the stifles, tarsi and carpi and are usually not visible in the proximal joints (shoulders and hips) and the small metacarpophalangeal and interphalangeal joints. Absence of a radiographic effusion does not exclude the presence of a small effusion and radiography is not 100 percent sensitive in demonstrating increased joint fluid. As the type of effusion within a joint cannot be determined from radiographs, arthrocentesis and analysis of joint fluid are often required for definitive diagnosis of polyarthritis or infectious arthropathies. Rarely, gas (predominately nitrogen) may be visible within the joint space (vacuum phenomenon) and in most cases indicates joint pathology. The gas accumulates when the joint is distracted, resulting in negative pressure within the joint space and causing diffusion of gas from the extracellular fluid into the joint space.

Ligamentous injury (sprain) may result in localized soft tissue swelling adjacent to the joint (see Figures 7.34 and 7.35), the location of which varies with the tendon/ligament involved. The location of soft tissue swelling due to a sprain differs from that seen with effusion. Diagnosis relies on anatomical knowledge of the insertion, origin and location of the tendons. Acute ligamentous injury may be associated with concurrent effusion due to trauma or instability of the joint, and this may make differentiation of effusion and tendon/ligament swelling impossible. In cases of severe sprain there may be instability of the joint, which occasionally may be recognized on standard radiographs as malalignment or subluxation. As joint radiographs are taken with the limb non-weight-bearing,

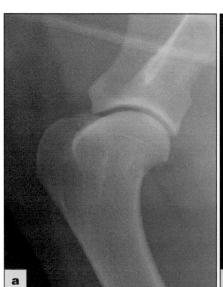 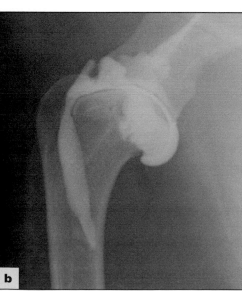

7.32 Mediolateral views of the shoulder **(a)** pre-arthrography and **(b)** post-arthrography of an 8-year-old Border Collie presented with acute onset lameness. The plain radiograph is normal but the arthrogram reveals the absence of the normal biceps muscle due to complete avulsion of the tendon. Arthrography is most commonly performed in the shoulder, where it may demonstrate cartilage flaps and osteochondral fragments secondary to OCD, in addition to allowing assessment of the biceps tendon.

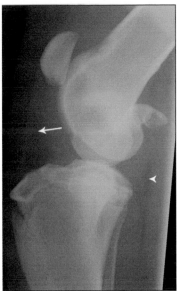

7.33 Mediolateral view of the stifle of a dog. Effusion can be seen within the stifle joint (note the reduced size of the intrapatellar fatpad (arrowed) and displacement of the fascial planes caudal to the joint (arrowhead)). The presence of effusion is a specific indicator of joint pathology. Knowledge of the extent of the normal synovial compartments is important in differentiating joint effusions from other causes of juxta-articular soft tissue swellings.

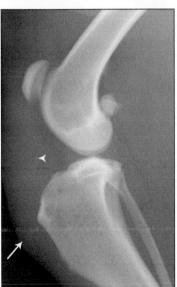

7.34 Mediolateral view of the stifle of a dog with patellar tendonitis. In this case, the soft tissue swelling is predominately extra-articular (arrowed) and extends beyond the boundaries of the stifle joint, which helps differentiate the swelling from an effusion. Small mineralized foci (arrowhead) within the swelling represent dystrophic mineralization, indicating chronicity.

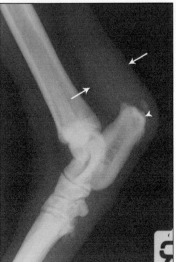

7.35 Mediolateral view of the tarsus of a Labrador Retriever with chronic Achilles tendonopathy. There is enlargement of the tendon (arrowed) just proximal to the tuber calcaneus and dystrophic mineralization within the tendon. Enthesophyte formation is present on the tuber calcaneus (arrowhead).

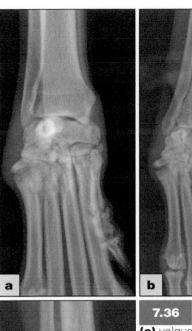
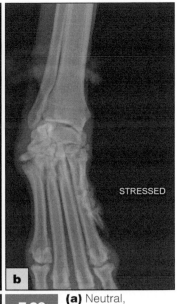

a · b · STRESSED

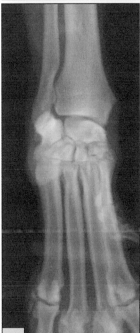

c

7.36 **(a)** Neutral, **(b)** varus and **(c)** valgus stressed dorsopalmar views of the carpus of a dog. Stressing the lateral aspect of the joint results in an abnormal varus deformity and widening of the fracture within the proximal fifth metacarpal bone, which is not visible on the neutral position.

most joint instability is not visible radiologically unless stressed views are obtained (Figure 7.36).

The interpretation of stressed radiographs can be difficult and is aided if stressed radiographs of the contralateral limb are obtained for comparison. In cases of chronic joint disease, periarticular fibrosis/

hypertrophy may result in soft tissue swelling adjacent to the joint (e.g. medial buttress in cases of cranial cruciate ligament disease) and it is often not possible to differentiate this from effusion or ligamentous injury. Soft tissue swelling that extends significantly beyond the joint (Figure 7.37) is usually the result of soft tissue pathology such as cellulitis or oedema rather than a specific radiological feature of joint disease. In cases of soft tissue tumours involving joints, a localized soft tissue swelling may be present adjacent to the joint but is associated with areas of bone lysis (Figure 7.38).

Alignment of the joint

The alignment of the joint should be assessed. Over-interpretation of apparent malalignment of joints can occur with poor radiographic positioning. For example rotation of the stifle on caudocranial views may resemble the appearance of patellar luxation. (Figure 7.39). The most common causes of abnormal joint alignment include trauma, developmental limb deformity (especially secondary to growth plate injuries) and

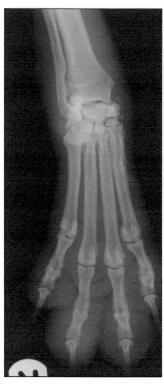

7.37 Dorsopalmar view of the carpus of a 1-year-old Boxer with cellulitis due to *Nocardia* infection. There is extensive soft tissue swelling, which extends from the digits proximally to at least the mid-antebrachium. The swelling is not confined to the joint spaces, which helps differentiate soft tissue swelling from joint effusion. The changes in the case are non-specific and could be seen with oedema.

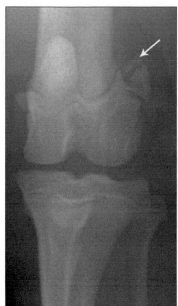

7.39 Caudocranial view of the stifle with apparent medial displacement of the patella due to poor radiographic positioning. Note the fabellae are asymmetrical relative to the medial and lateral cortices of the femur, indicating rotation of the stifle. The lateral fabella is multipartite (arrowed), which is an incidental finding of no clinical significance.

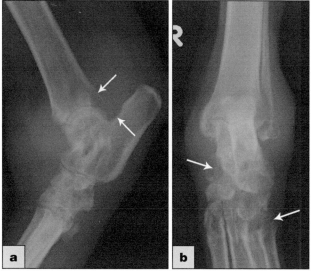

7.38 **(a)** Mediolateral and **(b)** dorsoplantar views of the tarsus showing a soft tissue tumour invading the joint. The soft tissue mass and focal areas of lysis (arrowed) affecting multiple bones are typical of soft tissue joint tumours.

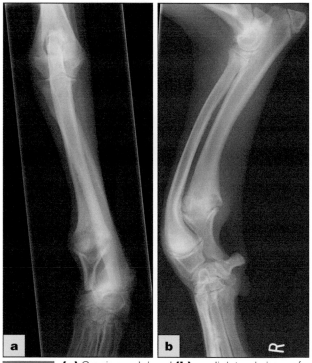

7.40 **(a)** Craniocaudal and **(b)** mediolateral views of the antebrachium of an Irish Wolfhound with an angular limb deformity due to premature closure of the distal growth plate. The cranial bowing of the antebrachium and carpal valgus are indicative of this condition. In cases of limb deformity, radiographs should include the joints proximal and distal to the deformity. Separate radiographs, centred on the joints, may be required to assess whether there is any joint incongruency.

degenerative disease. Most cases of traumatic joint injury that result in subluxation of the joint are associated with soft tissue swelling in the acute stage and signs of osteoarthritis in the chronic stages. In cases of suspected subluxation/instability, radiographs taken whilst stressing the joint will confirm the pathology. Malalignment of the joint may be secondary to long bone deformity and in cases of limb deformity radiographs of the entire limb are required (Figure 7.40).

Subchondral bone

Cartilage is not visible on radiographs unless there is pathological calcification (as occasionally seen with OCD). The subchondral bone frequently reflects the quality of the cartilage, with bone oedema, microfractures and necrosis often present in the bone. These changes in the subchondral bone often result in sclerosis and are a valuable indirect finding of cartilage and joint pathology (Figure 7.41). The thickness of the subchondral bone reflects loading of the joint, and increased thickness or abnormal sclerosis may occur secondary to abnormal loading of the joint. Osteoarthritis often results in sclerosis of the subchondral bone and geode (subchondral cyst) formation, which appear radiologically as small, often flask-shaped, subchondral lucencies.

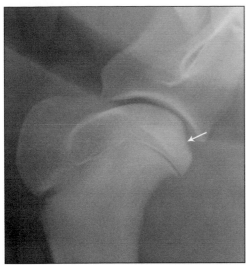

7.41 Mediolateral view of the shoulder of an Irish Setter with OCD of the humeral head. The focal flattening/defect within the subchondral bone (arrowed) is typical of OCD. OCD occurs in specific locations within joints, which helps to differentiate the disease from other causes of subchondral defects. Adjacent to the defect, there is sclerosis of the bone secondary to the cartilage pathology.

Joint space width

The joint spaces should be bilaterally symmetrical. Accurate assessment of joint space width is limited in small animals as radiographs are taken with the joint non-weight-bearing. Differences in patient positioning and centring of the X-ray beam result in variation in the apparent width of the joint space (Figure 7.42) and care should be taken when diagnosing alterations in joint space (unless the changes are severe). Comparison with radiographs of the contralateral limb is helpful (provided that positioning and centring are similar). A reduction in joint space width is seen occasionally in severe osteoarthritis (Figure 7.43) due to cartilage loss and alterations in synovial fluid viscosity. In these cases, there are additional signs of osteoarthritis.

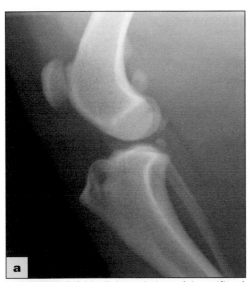

7.42 **(a)** Mediolateral view of the stifle of a dog. The apparent narrowing of the joint space on (b) the caudocranial view is artefactual due to the alignment of the X-ray beam relative to the joint space. The steep angle of the tibial plateau means that the X-ray beam is not parallel with the joint space. Radiological assessment of joint space width is often unreliable. (continues) ▶

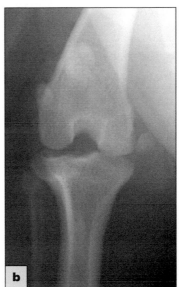

7.42 (continued) **(b)** Caudocranial view of the stifle of a dog. The apparent narrowing of the joint space is artefactual due to the alignment of the X-ray beam relative to the joint space. The steep angle of the tibial plateau means that the X-ray beam is not parallel with the joint space. Radiological assessment of joint space width is often unreliable.

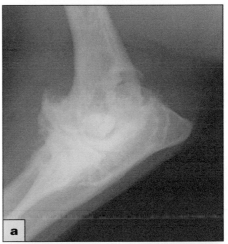

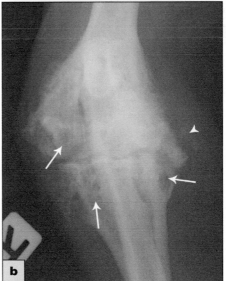

7.43 **(a)** Mediolateral and **(b)** caudocranial views of the elbow of a Labrador Retriever with severe chronic osteoarthritis. Marked new bone formation is seen surrounding the joint. The subchondral bone is irregular and collapse of the joint space is visible on the craniocaudal view. The small irregular regions of mineralization within the periarticular soft tissues (arrowhead) represent dystrophic mineralization. Due to the large amount of irregular new bone superimposed on the elbow, there are areas of relative lucency (arrowed) which can be misinterpreted as lysis. With severe osteoarthritis, the primary cause is often not visible.

Apparent narrowing of joint spaces may also be seen with joint fractures (Figure 7.44). Widening of the joint space (Figure 7.45) may occur with large joint effusions, joint tumours, diseases that cause destruction of the subchondral bone and subluxation/damage to the supporting ligaments and joint capsule.

Congruency of the joint

Most joints (other than the stifle) should be relatively congruent, with the contour of the subchondral bone on either side of the joint space matching. This is most apparent in the elbows, hips and hocks where

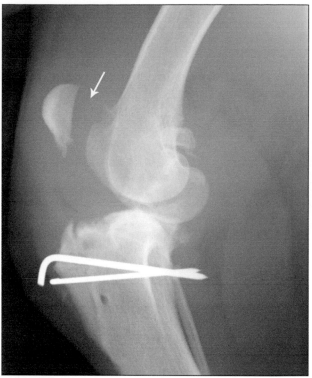

7.45 Mediolateral view of the stifle of a dog with septic arthritis. Note the widening of the femoropatellar joint space (arrowed) with cranial displacement of the patella. Joint widening is an uncommon feature of large effusions and can also be seen with intra-articular soft tissue masses.

the joint surfaces are in close apposition. There is a degree of physiological incongruency in the elbows and shoulders, which allows for deformation of the bone and the spread of load when weight bearing. Pathological incongruency may occur with fractures, developmental disease (Figure 7.46), neoplasia and erosive arthropathies (e.g. sepsis, rheumatoid arthritis). The consequences of incongruency are alterations in joint loading, which are seen radiologically as sclerosis and potentially remodelling of the subchondral bone. Pathological incongruency often results in osteoarthritis.

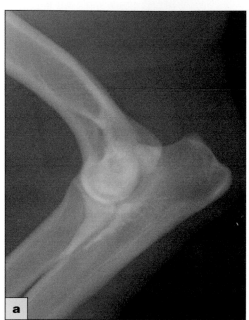

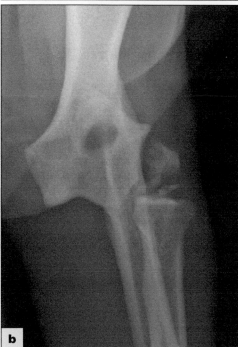

7.44 **(a)** Mediolateral and **(b)** craniocaudal views of the elbow of a dog with traumatic luxation. On the mediolateral view, the normal humeroradial joint space is not clearly visible and the humeral condyle and radial head are superimposed. On the craniocaudal view, the radius and ulna are displaced laterally relative to the humerus, indicating complete luxation of the elbow. The small triangular bony fragment lateral to the humeral epicondyle is likely to involve the collateral ligament.

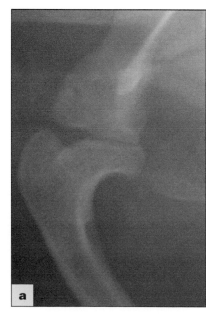

7.46

(a) Mediolateral view of the shoulder of a 16-month-old Yorkshire Terrier with unilateral (presumed congenital) shoulder dysplasia. The joint is incongruent with an abnormal shallow glenoid cavity. Abnormal joint loading in immature animals may lead to severe incongruency. (continues) ▶

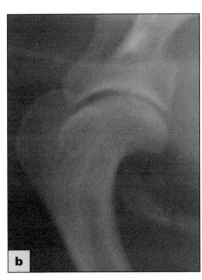

7.46

(continued)
(b) Mediolateral view of the normal contralateral shoulder for comparison.

Presence of osteophyte or enthesophyte formation

Osteophytes represent new bone formation; they occur at the margins of a synovial joint (Figure 7.47) and are a radiological feature of osteoarthritis. Osteophytes are usually irregular in shape and have specific predilection sites within each joint. Osteophytes need to be differentiated, if possible, from enthesophytes, which represent new bone formation at the origin of insertion of a ligament or tendon (see Figure 7.35). Osteophytes and

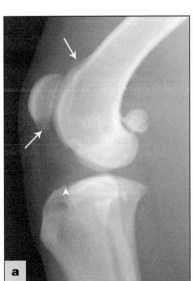

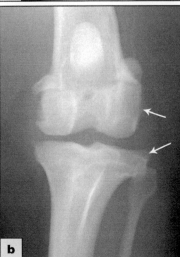

7.47

(a) Mediolateral and **(b)** caudocranial views of the stifle of a dog with osteoarthritis. Note the small osteophytes (arrowed) on the poles of the patella, trochlear ridges and at the margin of the femorotibial joint. In addition to the osteophytes, there is a large joint effusion and focal sclerosis and new bone formation on the tibial plateau (arrowhead) at the site of insertion of the cranial cruciate ligament.

enthesophytes have a similar radiological appearance but differ in their location within the joint. Enthesophytes are a feature of ligament/tendon injury, which may require different treatment and have a different prognosis to osteoarthritis.

Number of joints affected and symmetry of changes

Assessment of the number of joints affected and the symmetry of any lesions provides information that may help with the differential diagnoses. Trauma, septic arthritis and joint neoplasia usually only affect one joint, polyarthritis (by definition) affects multiple joints, and many developmental diseases (such as hip dysplasia, elbow dysplasia and OCD) affect pairs of joints with pathology often appearing relatively symmetrical. In older animals, osteoarthritis affecting multiple joints is common and should not be mistaken for immune-mediated polyarthritis (the absence of degenerative changes is an important feature of immune-mediated polyarthritis).

Signs of aggressive joint disease

Aggressive joint diseases include infectious arthritis, neoplasia and erosive arthritis. They result in lysis and destruction of the subchondral bone. Aggressive joint disease is usually associated with soft tissue swelling or joint effusion. Lysis of the bone usually occurs on both sides of a joint space (Figure 7.48), which helps differentiate it from focal subchondral cyst formation that occurs as a feature of osteoarthritis (most commonly within the tibial plateau at the insertion of the cranial cruciate ligament). Normal variation in bone thickness affects the radiological opacity of bone. Thicker areas of bone appear more opaque and can create the illusion of lysis in normal bone. Areas of thin

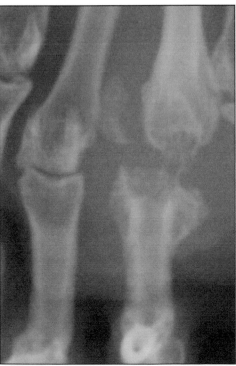

7.48 Dorsopalmar view of the manus of a 1-year-old cat with lameness and swelling of the digit. There is extensive destruction of the sesamoid bones and bones on either side of the joint. The changes are non-specific but highly aggressive and could represent neoplasia, infection or erosive monoarthritis.

bone, such as the tibial tuberosity, appear relatively lucent compared with the adjacent bone and this should not be mistaken for pathological lysis (see Figure 7.17). Extensive, large, irregular osteophytes superimposed over normal bone can also result in the appearance of areas of relative lucency in the normal bone, which are less opaque than the osteophytes.

Presence of articular and juxta-articular mineralization

Mineralization and mineralized bodies are commonly seen within, or adjacent to, the joints. There are numerous potential causes and many are incidental findings or normal anatomical variants which are of no clinical significance. The shape, margination and location should be evaluated. There are several sesamoid bones (Figure 7.49) which can potentially be mistaken for pathology. For example, the sesamoid bone within the supinator muscle (Figure 7.50) could

be mistaken for a fragmented medial coronoid process in the elbow, but this sesamoid bone occurs laterally not medially. Sesamoid bones are smoothly marginated and have a regular oval to triangular shape and, if sufficiently large, have a trabecular pattern. Sesamoids occur at predictable locations, which helps differentiate them from pathological mineralized bodies. Fragmentation or multipartite sesamoid bones are common and are usually of no clinical significance (Figure 7.51).

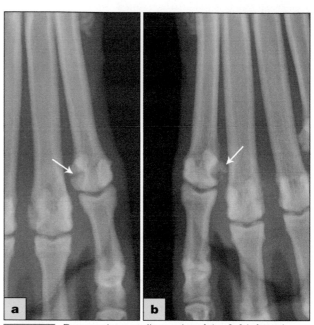

Joint	Sesamoid bone
Shoulder	Clavicle (medial end of tendinous insertion of brachiocephalic muscle)
Elbow	Tendon of origin of supinator muscle
Carpus	Tendon of abductor pollicis longus muscle
Hip	None
Stifle	Patella (tendon of insertion of quadriceps femoris muscle) Fabellae (lateral and medial origin of gastrocnemius muscle) Popliteal sesamoid (tendon of popliteus muscle)
Tarsus	Lateral plantar tarsometatarsal bone Intra-articular tarsometatarsal bone
Metacarpo/ metatarsophalangeal	Paired palmar/plantar sesamoid bones (tendons of insertion of the interosseous muscles) Single dorsal sesamoid (in the extensor tendons)

7.49   Sesamoid bones around joints of the appendicular skeleton of dogs and cats.

7.51   Dorsopalmar radiographs of the **(a)** left and **(b)** right manus of an Airedale Terrier with non-localizable lameness. The second palmar sesamoid bones are fragmented (arrowed) in both manus with the changes in the left appearing smooth and the sesamoid bone divided symmetrically into two parts. The fragmentation in the right manus is irregular with several small fragments. Multipartite sesamoid bones are common, often involve the second or seventh palmar sesamoid bones and are usually of no clinical significance. In this case, gamma scintigraphy showed increased radiopharmaceutical uptake in the sesamoid bone of the right manus. Surgical removal of the sesamoid bone resulted in resolution of the lameness. The second right sesamoid bone was presumed to be fractured, rather than a congenital anomaly. Radiological differentiation of a multipartite from a fractured sesamoid bone is difficult and may not be possible.

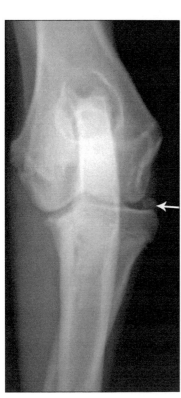

7.50
Craniocaudal view of the elbow of a normal dog. The rounded ossified body (arrowed) superimposed on the lateral aspect of the radial head is a sesamoid bone within the origin of the supinator muscle. This is a normal anatomical variant and should not be mistaken for a fragmented coronoid process.

Most pathological mineralization within the soft tissues of a joint is the result of dystrophic mineralization due to tissue damage and therefore usually indicates chronic soft tissue pathology. Dystrophic calcification is often irregularly but sharply marginated. Potentially, any soft tissue can undergo dystrophic calcification, but in dogs it is most commonly seen within the supraspinatus tendon adjacent to the shoulder superimposed on the greater tubercle (Figure 7.52), within the origin of the flexor muscles adjacent to the medial epicondyle of the elbow and adjacent to the hips within the gluteal muscles (Figure 7.53). Intra-articular mineralized bodies are less commonly seen in dogs and are usually significant. They may occur if OCD flaps mineralize, if there are intra-articular fractures and with dystrophic mineralization of intra-articular soft tissues. In cats, joint-associated mineralization is commonly present

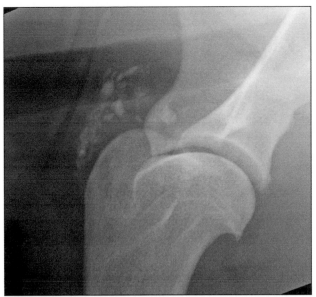

7.52 Mediolateral view of the shoulder of a dog with supraspinatus mineralization and osteoarthritis. Mineralization of the soft tissues within and adjacent to the joints is common and often of no clinical significance. Supraspinatus mineralization is common and seen as irregular areas of mineralization overlying/adjacent to the greater tubercle of the humerus. The location of the osteophytes on the caudal aspect of the humeral head and glenoid is typical of shoulder osteoarthritis.

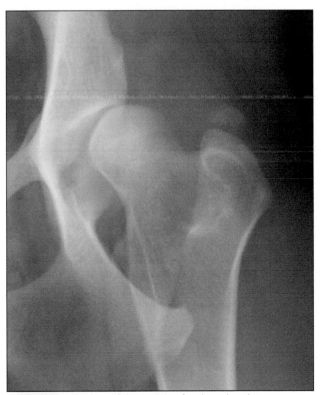

7.53 VD view of the pelvis of a dog showing dystrophic mineralization within the gluteal muscles adjacent to the left greater trochanter. This is usually an incidental finding. Note also the presence of hip dysplasia.

with osteoarthritis when there is often extensive calcification present within the periarticular soft tissues (e.g. synovial osteochromatosis) (Figure 7.54). Meniscal mineralization is not uncommon in cats (Figure 7.55) and is associated with cartilage pathology.

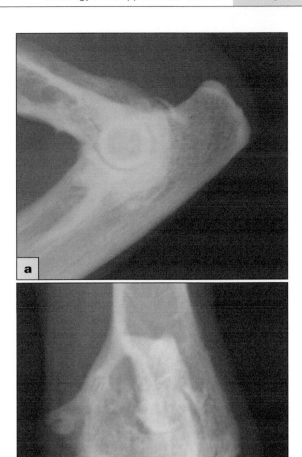

7.54 **(a)** Mediolateral and **(b)** craniocaudal views of the elbow of a cat with osteoarthritis. The extensive mineralization within the juxta-articular soft tissues is commonly seen in feline joints with osteoarthritis. In severe cases, cartilaginous nodules may form in the synovium and mineralize (synovial osteochondromatosis).

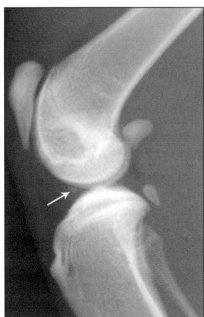

7.55 Mediolateral view of the stifle of a cat with mineralization within the medial meniscus (arrowed). This has been associated with significant cartilage pathology, but can also be seen as an apparently incidental finding.

Anatomical variants and pathology unlikely to be associated with clinical signs

- Distomedial displacement of the medial fabella in terriers (Figure 7.56).
- Multipartite sesamoid bones (fabellae and palmar sesamoid bones; see Figures 7.39 and 7.51).
- Secondary ossification centre of the caudal glenoid (Figure 7.57).

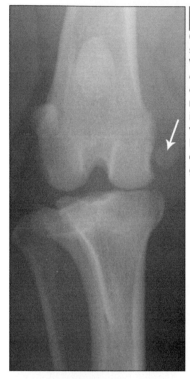

7.56
Caudocranial view of the stifle of a West Highland White Terrier. The distomedial displacement of the medial fabella (arrowed) is a normal anatomical variant and should not be mistaken for avulsion of the head of the gastrocnemius muscle.

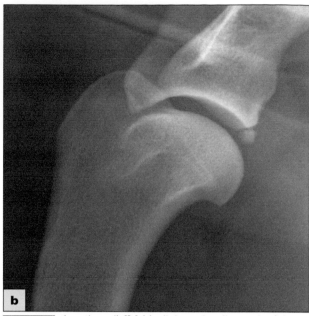

7.57 (continued) **(b)** Mediolateral radiograph of the shoulder of a mature dog. The small triangular bony fragment on the caudal aspect of the glenoid represents a separate centre of ossification. In immature animals, the fragment may unite fully with the remainder of the glenoid. In young dogs, the greater tubercle may have irregular margins, which is a normal finding and should not be mistaken for bone lysis. Fragments at the caudal aspect of the glenoid are common and usually incidental findings.

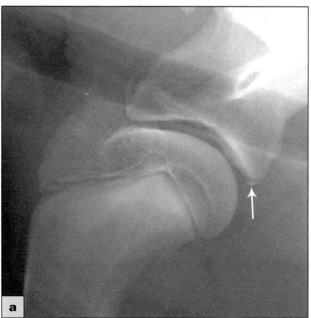

7.57 **(a)** Mediolateral radiograph of the shoulder of a 6-month-old dog. The small triangular bony fragment (arrowed) on the caudal aspect of the glenoid represents a separate centre of ossification. In immature animals, the fragment may unite fully with the remainder of the glenoid. Note also the irregular margins to the greater tubercle in this case, which is a normal finding in young dogs and should not be mistaken for bone lysis. Fragments at the caudal aspect of the glenoid are common and usually incidental findings. (continues) ▶

- Mineralization within gluteal muscles adjacent to the greater trochanter (see Figure 7.53).
- Supraspinatus mineralization (see Figure 7.52).

Common diseases

There is overlap between the radiological features of different joint diseases with abnormalities often non-specific and many arthritides (e.g. developmental, traumatic, septic or, uncommonly, immune-mediated diseases) ultimately result in osteoarthritis. Differential diagnoses should be based upon history, signalment, clinical examination and the results of other diagnostic tests, in addition to radiological abnormalities. The clinician should try to differentiate aggressive joint disease (due to neoplasia, sepsis or erosive arthritides) from non-aggressive disease (osteoarthritis, non-erosive arthritides).

Osteoarthritis

Osteoarthritis is extremely common and there is an increasing prevalence with age. Affected animals typically present with lameness and stiffness, especially after rest. This may result in reluctance to exercise, reduced grooming or behavioural changes (particularly in cats). Osteoarthritis is the most common disease affecting the joints and in dogs is almost always secondary to an underlying pathology (e.g. instability, incongruency). The primary cause may not be visible on radiographs, especially in severe cases, but an attempt should be made identify the underlying pathology, as this should be treated if possible. In cats, a primary cause is often not found. Irrespective of the underlying cause, the radiological appearance of osteoarthritis is similar in all synovial joints.

Radiological features:

- Joint effusion – this occurs early in the development of osteoarthritis (see Figure 7.33).
- Periarticular soft tissue swelling due to synovitis/fibrosis, which is often indistinguishable from effusion.
- Development of osteophyte formation. Osteophytes are small, irregular areas of new bone formation which arise from the margins of the joint (see Figure 7.47). Each joint has predilection sites for osteophyte formation. The rate at which osteophytosis develops varies from 3–4 weeks in cranial cruciate disease to months for hip or elbow dysplasia. The severity of osteophytosis also varies between individual animals and breeds.
- In the later stages, there is often sclerosis and irregularity of the subchondral bone (Figure 7.58).
- Less commonly seen signs are enlargement of the joint surfaces and collapse of the joint space.
- In feline osteoarthritis, mineralization of the soft tissues in and around the joint are common and may be extensive (see Figure 7.54).

Polyarthritis

Polyarthritis is divided radiologically into two groups: non-erosive and erosive. In dogs, the most common type is non-erosive polyarthritis, which is typically immune-mediated. Involvement of other organs may occur and imaging of the thorax and abdomen may be indicated to screen for underlying causes of polyarthritis. Erosive polyarthritis is rare in dogs. Polyarthritis is relatively rare in cats with the most common form being periosteal proliferative polyarthritis. Most animals with polyarthritis have systemic signs (commonly pyrexia) in addition to the stiffness/lameness due to the joint pathology.

Non-erosive polyarthritis: The radiological features of non-erosive polyarthritis include the presence of joint effusion and soft tissue swelling in multiple joints. Joint effusions are easiest to recognize on radiographs within the stifle joints, followed by the hocks, carpi and elbows. By definition, there is no lysis nor subchondral bone changes associated with non-erosive polyarthritis.

Radiological features:

- Multiple joints are affected and there is usually a symmetrical distribution (Figure 7.59).

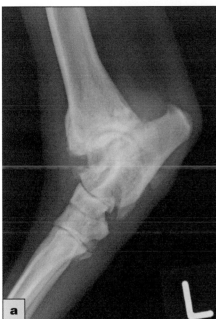

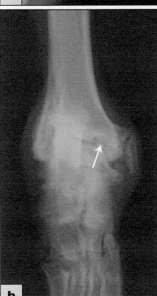

| **7.58** | **(a)** Mediolateral and |

(b) dorsoplantar views of the tarsus of a Labrador Retriever with severe chronic osteoarthritis secondary to OCD of the medial ridge of the talus. The typical features of osteoarthritis can be seen, along with joint effusion and osteophyte formation. In this case, the primary pathology (OCD) is also visible with flattening of the medial ridge of the talus (arrowed). The subchondral bone is sclerotic and irregular due to the chronicity and severity of the cartilage pathology.

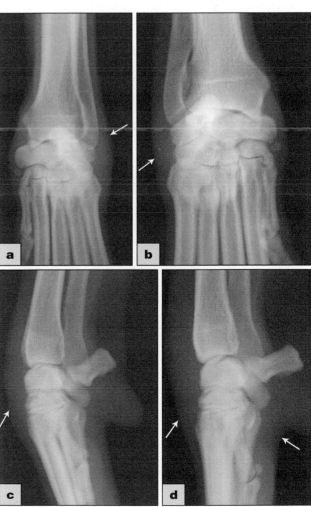

| **7.59** | **(a–b)** Dorsopalmar and **(c–d)** mediolateral views of both carpi in a dog with non-erosive |

immune-mediated polyarthritis. There is swelling of the soft tissues (arrowed) confined to the limits of the joint and no signs of bone pathology. Radiographs of both tarsi also showed the presence of effusion.

- Joint effusion and soft tissue swelling are confined to the margins of the joints.
- Osteophytes are usually absent.
- Subchondral bone is normal in appearance.

Erosive polyarthritis: As with non-erosive polyarthritis, effusion is present in multiple joints. In addition, there are small focal areas of lysis within the subchondral bone. The subchondral lysis is often subtle and most commonly seen in the hocks and carpi. In severe cases, destruction of the soft tissues results in laxity of the joints, leading to subluxation and collapse of the joint spaces.

Radiological features:

- Multiple joints are affected and there is usually a symmetrical distribution.
- Joint effusion and soft tissue swelling are confined to the margins of the joints.
- Focal lucencies are present within the subchondral bone of multiple joint surfaces, most commonly in the tarsi and carpi (Figure 7.60).
- Subluxation of joints in chronic or severe cases (Figure 7.61).

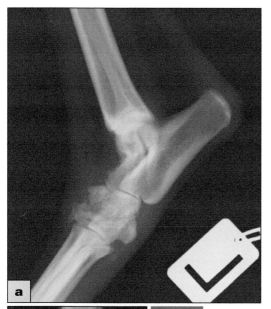

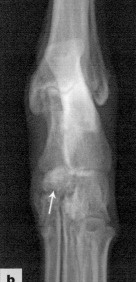

7.60

(a) Mediolateral and **(b)** dorsoplantar views of the tarsus of a dog with erosive polyarthritis. Note the subchondral lysis (arrowed) involving multiple tarsal bones and resulting in an irregular subchondral surface and loss of definition to the intertarsal joints.

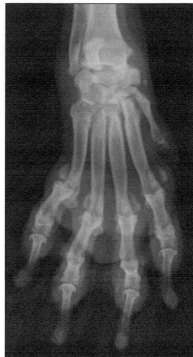

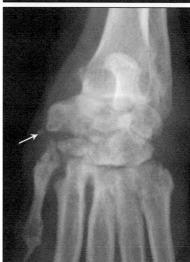

7.61

Dorsopalmar views of the carpus of a dog with erosive polyarthritis. In severe cases of erosive arthritis, there may be subluxation of the joints. In this patient, all the metacarpophalangeal joints are luxated. Note also the carpal effusion and lysis of the carpal bones (arrowed).

Periosteal proliferative/chronic progressive polyarthritis: This is a rare condition, most commonly seen in young male cats. Radiologically, it resembles erosive canine polyarthritis with erosions variably present and enthesophyte formation at the insertion of the ligaments/tendons adjacent to the affected joints.

Septic arthritis

In cats and dogs, septic arthritis occurs most commonly as a sequel to surgery or, less frequently, secondary to penetrating trauma or haematogenous spread (rare). Affected joints are often swollen and painful and may feel hot; arthrocentesis is required to reach a diagnosis. In acute cases, there is initially an effusion and in some cases more diffuse soft tissue swelling surrounding the joints. In chronic cases, infection results in destruction of the subchondral bone with irregular lysis affecting both sides of the joint. If secondary to surgery, there is often lysis surrounding the surgical implants. The radiological changes are non-specific, and in chronic cases radiological changes associated with osteoarthritis are superimposed on the pathology due to joint infection.

Radiological features:

- Single joints are affected most commonly, particularly the stifles, elbows, carpi and tarsi (Figure 7.62).
- Joint effusion.
- Soft tissue swelling adjacent to the joint, which may be extensive.
- In chronic cases there is subchondral lysis (Figure 7.63).
- Disuse osteopenia occurs in chronic cases.
- If there is a haematogeneous aetiology (e.g. bacterial endocarditis), septic arthritis may affect multiple joints, in which case radiological changes resemble immune-mediated erosive polyarthritis.
- If secondary to surgery, there is often lysis surrounding the surgical implants (Figure 7.64).

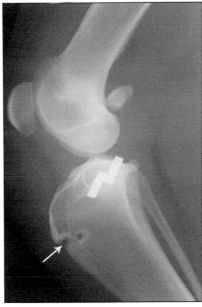

7.64 Mediolateral view of the stifle of a dog with septic arthritis following surgery for cranial cruciate ligament disease. In the acute stages septic arthritis is indistinguishable from any other cause of joint effusion. In cases secondary to surgery, lysis is usually centred around the implants. Note the lysis around the suture tract (arrowed) within the tibial tuberosity in this case.

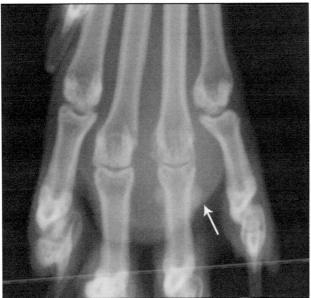

7.62 Dorsopalmar view of the carpus of a cat with septic arthritis involving the fourth metacarpophalangeal joint (this is the same cat as in Figure 7.40, but 4 weeks earlier). Note the subtle lysis of the subchondral bone and the indistinct, poorly marginated periosteal new bone (arrowed) at the margins of the joint as well as the marked soft tissue swelling.

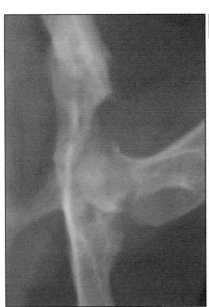

7.63 VD view of the pelvis of a dog with septic arthritis involving the hip joint. In chronic cases, destruction of the bones either side of the joint is common. In this case, the infection was presumed to be haematogenous in origin.

Neoplasia

A wide variety of soft tissue tumours may invade the joints, but synovial cell sarcoma is most common. Joint neoplasia is rare but is seen most commonly in larger breed dogs and usually involves the proximal joints, particularly the stifle and elbow. The radiological features are non-specific and a biopsy is required to determine the histological type. Soft tissue swelling occurs adjacent to the joint and may extend into the joint, where is can resemble a joint effusion. Focal areas of lysis affecting multiple bones indicate aggressive joint disease, and the presence of a soft tissue swelling/mass (see Figure 7.38) in an older animal is suggestive of joint neoplasia.

Radiological features:

- Soft tissue mass/swelling adjacent to the joint. The soft tissue changes are often larger and more extensive than those seen with joint effusion.
- Focal areas of lysis on the bones adjacent to the joint (easily overlooked).
- The presence of lysis on both sides of the joint helps to differentiate joint/soft tissue tumours from primary bone tumours, which are monostotic.
- Usually predominantly lytic; significant new bone formation is uncommon.

Fractures

Most joint fractures occur secondary to external trauma (e.g. a road traffic accident) and detecting an intra-articular component of a fracture is important for surgical planning and treatment. Fractures lines are only visible if the X-ray beam is parallel with the fracture line, and oblique views may be required to visualize the full extent of the joint trauma. Radiology often underestimates the complexity and number of fractures, particularly in the carpus and tarsus where computed tomography (CT) is considerably more accurate in assessing the fracture configuration. In skeletally immature animals, the bone is relatively weaker than the ligaments/tendons and avulsion fractures may occur, with small fractures arising at the origin or insertion of the ligaments/tendons (Figure 7.65).

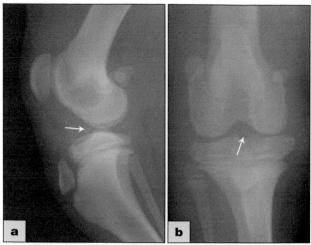

7.65 **(a)** Mediolateral and **(b)** caudocranial views of the stifle of a 4-month-old Labrador Retriever with a cranial cruciate ligament avulsion fracture. Note the small avulsed mineralized fragments (arrowed) at the location of the insertion of the cranial cruciate ligament. Avulsion fractures are most commonly seen in immature animals due to the relative weakness of the bone compared with the tendon/ligament. In mature animals, rupture of the tendon/ligament is more commonly seen.

In older animals, the tendon/ligament is relatively weaker than the bone and avulsion fractures are rare. Fractures occurring secondary to other joint diseases (e.g. incomplete ossification of the humeral condyles) or due to chronic repetitive trauma/stress (central tarsal bone fractures in racing Greyhounds) may show signs of pre-existing joint disease such as new bone formation or sclerosis. Fractures in athletic animals (especially Greyhounds) often occur in specific bones and configurations due to repetitive stress on the bone.

Radiological features:

- Soft tissue swelling adjacent to the joint, which may be extensive. There may be gas and foreign material within the soft tissues in cases of external trauma or significant soft tissue loss in cases of shearing injury.
- Radiolucent fracture lines within the bones of the joint or extending into the subchondral bone from the long bone.
- A step or defect in the subchondral bone/joint surface.
- Displacement of bones.
- In avulsion fractures, there are small fragments of bone adjacent to the origin or insertion of a ligament/tendon and corresponding defects in the parent bone. Avulsed fragments are usually displaced due to the pull of the tendon/ligament.

The forelimb

Scapula, shoulder joint and humerus

Standard radiographic views: scapula

- Mediolateral view:
  - The animal should be placed in lateral recumbency with the side of interest closest to the cassette (dependent) and the upper forelimb retracted as far as possible

- The X-ray beam is centred over the midpoint of the scapular spine (identified by palpating the lower scapula) and collimated to include the dorsal aspect of the scapula (dorsal aspect of the skin), the shoulder joint (identified by palpating the acromion of the scapula) and the cranial and caudal borders of the scapula.
- Caudocranial view:
  - The animal should be placed in dorsal recumbency and slightly rotated to the side of interest, so that the scapula is perpendicular to the table top
  - The leg should be extended as far cranially as possible
  - The X-ray beam is centred on the midpoint of the scapula (identified by palpating the scapular spine) and collimated to include the shoulder, the dorsal border of the scapula and the lateral skin surface.

Standard radiographic views: shoulder joint

- Mediolateral view:
  - The animal should be placed in lateral recumbency with the side of interest dependent, the upper limb retracted as far as possible and the limb of interest protracted as far as possible (Figure 7.66)
  - The X-ray beam is centred over the acromion process at the distal end of the scapular spine, which can be palpated as a prominence at the distal end of the scapula. Collimation should include the distal third of the scapula and the proximal third of the humerus. A grid should be used if the area of interest is >8 cm thick.
- Caudocranial view:
  - The animal is placed in dorsal recumbency (using a trough if necessary) with the leg of interest extended as far as possible (Figure 7.67)
  - The X-ray beam is centred medial to the acromion process and collimated to include the distal third of the scapula and the proximal third of the humerus.

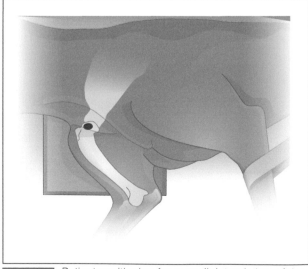

7.66 Patient positioning for a mediolateral view of the shoulder.

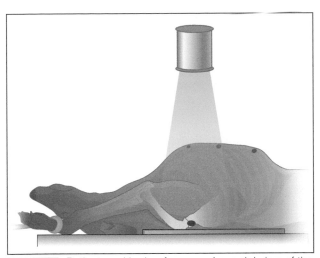

7.67 Patient positioning for a caudocranial view of the shoulder.

Special views:

- Cranioproximal–craniodistal (skyline) view of the intertubercular groove:
  - The animal is placed in sternal recumbency with the leg of interest positioned with both the elbow and shoulder flexed
  - Sandbags should be placed lateral to the limb to prevent adduction
  - The cassette rests on the cranial surface of the antebrachium and should be pushed into the crook of the elbow. Foam wedges are used to stabilize the cassette
  - The head and neck are flexed away from the shoulder being imaged and the head supported with a foam block
  - The X-ray beam is centred over the greater tubercle of the shoulder (identified by palpation) and collimated to include just the shoulder joint.

Standard radiographic views: humerus

- Mediolateral view:
  - The animal is placed in lateral recumbency with the side of interest dependent, the limb of interest protracted and the upper limb retracted as far as possible
  - The X-ray beam is centred on the midpoint of the humerus and collimated to include the shoulder and elbow joints.
- Caudocranial view:
  - The animal is placed in dorsal recumbency with the leg of interest extended as far as possible
  - The X-ray beam is centred on the mid-humerus and collimated to include the shoulder and elbow joints.

Contrast studies

Shoulder arthrography (see Chapter 4) can be used to demonstrate osteochondrosis affecting the caudal humeral head and diseases of the bicipital tendon sheath. A small volume (1–4 ml) of diluted contrast medium (100 mg/ml) is injected into the shoulder joint under aseptic conditions and a mediolateral radiograph taken within 5 minutes. Contrast medium fills

the joint and bicipital tendon sheath, and these should have smooth and well defined margins. Contrast medium can demonstrate a loose cartilage flap, joint mice and irregularities of the tendon sheath.

Radiological interpretation

- Scapula – bone integrity, any alterations in continuity of the scapular spine and the definition of the borders and shape of the scapular neck and glenoid cavity are evaluated. Scapula pathology is uncommon but easily overlooked due to superimposition by the thorax and contralateral scapula. Fractures and neoplasia of the scapula occur uncommonly, and other pathologies within the proximal scapula are extremely rare.
- Shoulder joint – an assessment should be made of the joint space (should be an even width) and integrity of the subchondral bone (particularly the humeral head). Evidence of degenerative changes (especially osteophytosis of the caudal humeral head) should also be sought (see Figure 7.52).
- Proximal humerus – the shape (humeral head, greater tubercle) and normal appearance (cortex, medullary cavity with normal trabecular pattern) of the proximal humerus are evaluated.
- The soft tissues around the shoulder are difficult to assess on a radiograph and the presence of any shoulder joint effusion is rarely visible radiologically.

Common diseases: scapula

Separate centre of ossification of the glenoid: In skeletally immature animals, there is a separate centre of ossification of the supraglenoid tubercle (Figure 7.68). This fuses to the rest of the glenoid by 4–7 months and should not be confused with an avulsion fracture. A separate centre of ossification may also be present on the caudal rim of the glenoid (see Figure 7.57) and may fail to fuse with the remainder of the glenoid. This is usually an incidental finding.

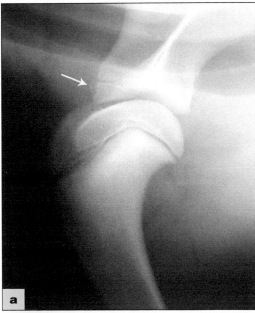

a

7.68 **(a)** Mediolateral view of the shoulder of a dog with osteochondrosis at 4 months of age. Note the separate centre of ossification of the supraglenoid tubercle (arrowed). (continues) ▶

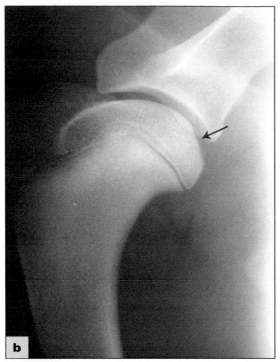

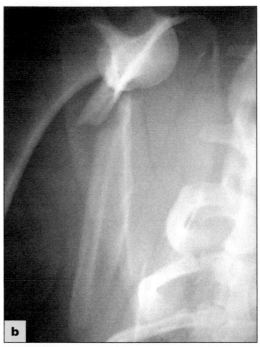

7.68 (continued) **(b)** Mediolateral view of the shoulder of a dog with osteochondrosis at 7 months of age. Progressive development of an osteochondral lesion has resulted in flattening of the caudal humeral head. Close inspection reveals a faint mineralized line (arrowed) parallel to the defect in the humeral head, which is consistent with a mineralized cartilage flap. Note that the physis of the supraglenoid tubercle has closed in the time between the two radiographs.

Fractures: Fractures of the body of the scapula are most easily seen as discontinuity and angulation of the scapular spine on lateral radiographs (Figure 7.69a). Caudocranial and/or craniocaudal radiographs (Figure 7.69b) should also be obtained to demonstrate displacement of part of the scapula. Fractures of the glenoid (including avulsion of the supraglenoid tubercle) are most easily seen on a lateral radiograph (Figure 7.70).

7.69 (continued) **(b)** Craniocaudal (with shoulder flexed) view of the scapula of dog showing a fracture of the body of the scapula. An interruption in the line of the scapular spine is seen on both radiographs. Note that the altered shape of the scapula is due to the caudal rotation of the proximal fragment.

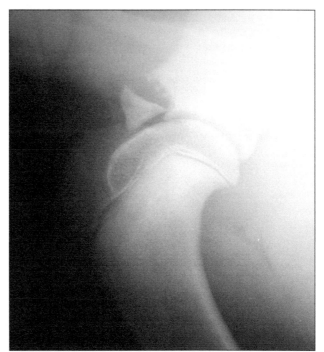

7.70 Mediolateral view of the shoulder of a skeletally immature dog. An avulsion fracture of the supraglenoid tubercle is visible with distal displacement of the tubercle due to the draw of the biceps brachii muscle. Note the marked displacement of the supraglenoid tubercle compared with the normal location seen with an open physis (as seen in Figure 7.69a). Further fragments are present within the fracture bed. Avulsion injuries through the physes of accessory ossification centres are not uncommon in puppies following trauma, particularly falls from a height. At other sites, such as the insertion of the cranial cruciate ligament, avulsion of a fragment of bone rather than rupture of the ligament may occur.

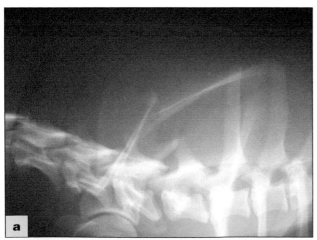

7.69 **(a)** Mediolateral view of the scapula of dog showing a fracture of the body of the scapula. An interruption in the line of the scapular spine is seen on both radiographs. Note that the altered shape of the scapula is due to the caudal rotation of the proximal fragment. (continues) ▶

Neoplasia: Chondrosarcoma is the most common tumour of the scapula and is usually seen as a poorly defined mass showing some mineralization and disrupting or distorting the normal scapular architecture (Figure 7.71).

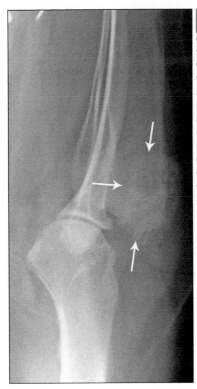

7.71

Caudocranial view of the scapula of a dog with a primary bone tumour of the scapular spine. Note the bone lysis and expansile nature of the lesion (arowed). It is not possible to differentiate chondrosarcoma from osteosarcoma reliably on radiographs. Scapular lesions are easily overlooked on lateral views due to superimposition of the thorax.

Common diseases: shoulder joint

Osteochondritis dissecans: OCD of the shoulder is most commonly seen in young male large-breed dogs. Occasionally, in very young animals, the lesion may not be particularly obvious and repeating radiographs at a later date can be useful (see Figure 7.68). Osteochondrosis is frequently bilateral, so, if identified, the contralateral shoulder should also be imaged. Rarely, an osteochondral lesion of the glenoid cavity of the scapula may be seen.

Radiological features:

- Abnormal shape of the caudal part of the humeral head on the mediolateral view, with localized flattening of the subchondral bone and, occasionally, a saucer-shaped defect in the subchondral bone (see Figure 7.41). The subchondral defect may not be visible on standard mediolateral views and mediolateral views with the limb pronated and supinated may be required to skyline the defect.
- Subchondral bone defect/flattening, which is usually accompanied by surrounding sclerosis.
- Occasionally, a calcified cartilage flap or mineralized body is seen in the caudal joint space (joint mouse). Shoulder arthrography may be helpful to demonstrate the contrast medium beneath the defective articular cartilage.
- Rarely, calcified osteochondral fragments migrate to within the biceps tendon sheath.
- Gas arising within the joint space due to vacuum phenomenon can outline the cartilage surface.

- Signs of secondary osteoarthritis are usually present in older animals.

Osteoarthritis: Osteoarthritis of the shoulder is best visualized on a mediolateral view and usually appears radiologically as osteophytosis of the caudal humeral head. In many older dogs this may be seen as a clinically insignificant finding with no visible primary pathology.

Osteophyte formation is also commonly seen on the caudal aspect of the glenoid (see Figure 7.53) and within the intertubercular groove. New bone formation within the intertubercular groove is best seen on the cranioproximal–craniodistal (skyline) view, when small irregular spurs of bone are visible projecting into the groove. On the mediolateral view, focal irregular sclerosis may be seen superimposed over the intertubercular groove. The presence of new bone formation within the intertubercular groove may also be seen with bicipital tenosynovitis.

Radiological features:

- Irregular spurs of periarticular new bone present on the caudal aspect of the humeral head.
- New bone formation commonly present on the caudal aspect of the glenoid.
- Small separate mineralized bodies adjacent to the caudal rim of the glenoid are not uncommon and may represent concurrent separate centres of ossification, fragmentation of the glenoid or dystrophic mineralization.
- New bone within the intertubercular groove results in focal, often patchy sclerosis in this region.

Luxation: Shoulder luxation is most commonly the consequence of trauma, and orthogonal views are required to confirm the degree and direction of the luxation. On a mediolateral view, there may be the impression of either a reduced joint space or the humeral head overlying the glenoid (Figure 7.72). Luxation may be accompanied by fractures, particularly avulsion fractures of the supraglenoid tubercle of

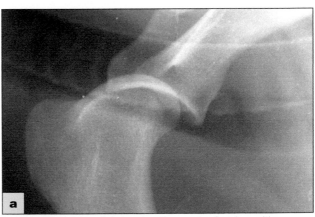

a

7.72 **(a)** Mediolateral radiograph of a dog with craniolateral luxation of the shoulder. Superimposition of the humeral head and glenoid cavity results in a curvilinear sclerotic band. The normal conformation of the humeral head and glenoid indicate that this is an acquired luxation (compare with Figure 7.46a). This is easily overlooked on radiographs not centred on the shoulder, and, in cases of trauma where thoracic radiographs are obtained, this sign can draw attention to the shoulder injury. (continues) ▶

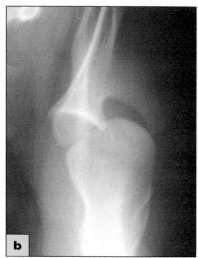

7.72 (continued) **(b)** Caudocranial radiograph of a dog with craniolateral luxation of the shoulder. Superimposition of the humeral head and glenoid cavity results in a curvilinear sclerotic band. The normal conformation of the humeral head and glenoid indicate that this is an acquired luxation (compare with Figure 7.46a). This is easily overlooked on radiographs not centred on the shoulder, and, in cases of trauma where thoracic radiographs are obtained, this sign can draw attention to the shoulder injury.

the scapula (Figure 7.73). Rarely congenital shoulder luxation may be associated with an underdeveloped and shallow glenoid cavity (shoulder dysplasia); this is most commonly seen in toy breeds (see Figure 7.46).

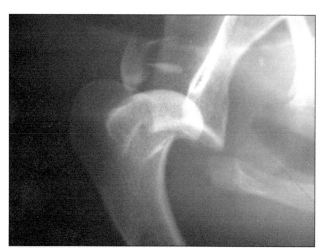

7.73 Mediolateral view of a dog with a fracture–luxation of the shoulder. The humeral head is displaced cranially with marked superimposition over the glenoid. The triangular bone fragment cranial to the neck of the scapula is consistent with displacement of the fractured supraglenoid tuberosity. (Courtesy of M Sullivan)

Mineralized bodies outside the shoulder: Mineralization within or adjacent to the shoulder is common and in many cases is of no clinical significance or represents anatomical variants. Cats have residual clavicles seen as curvilinear mineralized structures immediately cranial to, or overlying, the shoulder joint. Dogs may have very fine mineralization of the clavicular remnant, seen as fine linear mineralization craniomedial to the shoulder joint on a caudocranial view (this may also be seen on dorsoventral (DV)

radiographs of the thorax) on digital radiographs. In larger dogs, a calcifying tendinopathy is not uncommon. This most commonly affects the supraspinatus tendon and is recognized on radiographs as mineralized or ossified opacities adjacent to or superimposed on the greater tubercle of the humerus (Figure 7.74). The significance of this finding is uncertain but is usually of no clinical significance. Infraspinatus tendon/bursal mineralization is most

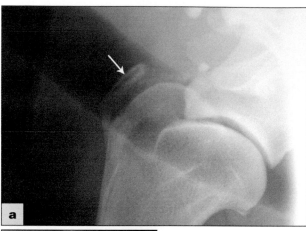

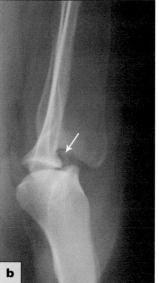

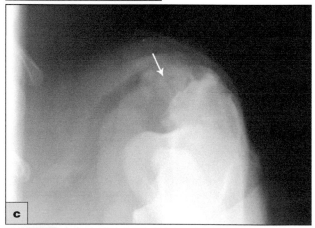

7.74 **(a)** Mediolateral, **(b)** caudocranial and **(c)** skyline bicipital groove views of the shoulder of a dog with periarticular mineralizations (arrowed) in the supraspinatus tendon. Note that the new bone at the craniolateral aspect of the glenoid extends on to the greater tubercle of the humerus. The clinical significance of these findings is unknown.

commonly seen in Labrador retrievers and is commonly associated with lameness. Mineralization within the infraspinatus occurs lateral to the shoulder, adjacent to the distal aspect of the greater tubercle.

Bicipital tenosynovitis: This is typically seen in middle-aged, medium- and large-breed dogs. The radiographic findings can be subtle and are often non-specific, and include sclerosis and new bone formation around the bicipital groove, which may be visible on skyline views. In addition, there may be remodelling of the supraglenoid tubercle associated with the origin of the bicipital tendon due to focal enthesopathy. Arthrography may show irregular filling of the tendon sheath with loss of the normal well defined margins to the contrast medium column. In severe cases there may be dystrophic mineralization of the biceps tendon, which can be difficult to differentiate from supraspinatus tendon mineralization. The location of the mineralization on the cranioproximal–craniodistal view may be helpful in determining which structures the mineralization is located in. In cases of biceps mineralization the pathology is centred within the groove, whereas with supraspinatus mineralization the changes are typically more cranially located adjacent to the greater tubercle. Arthrography is useful in determining location of the mineralization within or adjacent to the intertubercular groove relative to the biceps tendon.

Common diseases: humerus

Primary bone tumours: These are most commonly seen in older, large-breed dogs and usually involve the proximal metaphysis (see Figure 7.10). The radiographic signs are consistent with an aggressive bony lesion (moth-eaten or permeative lysis, cortical lysis, irregular interrupted periosteal proliferation and a long/poorly defined zone of transition) (see above).

Fractures: Humeral fractures most commonly involve the distal third of the diaphysis, although traumatic fractures of the proximal humerus can occur, typically at the level of the deltoid tuberosity.

Elbow

Standard radiographic views

- Mediolateral view:
  - The animal is placed in lateral recumbency with the leg of interest dependent and the upper leg retracted (Figure 7.75)
  - The X-ray beam is centred on the medial epicondyle and collimated to include one-third of the long bone on either side
  - For the neutral view, the joint should be at about 90–100 degrees
  - For the flexed view, the joint should flexed maximally. Foam wedges and sandbags are used to maintain the leg position
  - For an extended view, the joint should be extended fully.
- Craniocaudal view:
  - The animal is placed in sternal recumbency with the leg of interest extended (Figure 7.76)
  - The olecranon should be aligned with the humerus ensuring there is no rotation of the joint
  - Foam wedges are placed beneath the contralateral axilla to tilt the animal towards the side of interest
  - The head and neck are flexed away from the side of interest, with the head supported on a foam block
  - The X-ray beam is centred on the elbow joint (by palpating the medial epicondyle) and collimated to include the medial and lateral skin edges and one-third of the long bones on either side of the joint.

Special views:

- Cranio 15 degrees lateral–caudomedial oblique (Cr15°L-CdMO) view:
  - The animal is positioned as for a craniocaudal view and the limb is then pronated by approximately 15 degrees
  - This view is used to improve visibility of medial coronoid process and medial humeral condyle pathology

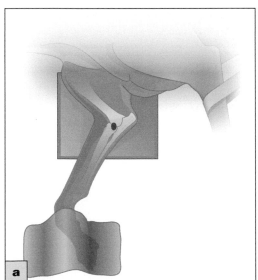
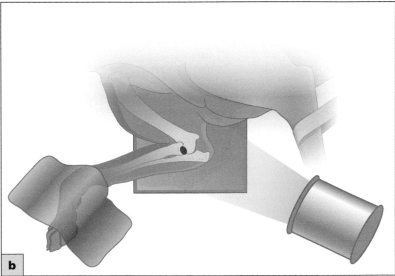

7.75 Patient positioning for **(a)** neutral and **(b)** flexed mediolateral views of the elbow.

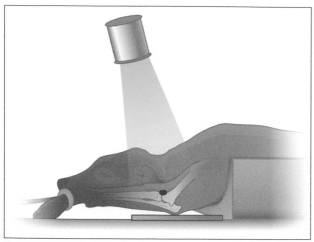

7.76 Patient positioning for a craniocaudal view of the elbow.

- Cranio 15 degrees medial–caudolateral oblique (Cr15°M-CdLO) view:
  - The animal is positioned as for a craniocaudal view and then the elbow supinated by approximately 15 degrees
  - This view is used to improve visualization of incomplete ossification of the humeral condyle (IOHC) fissures within the humeral condyle

Radiological interpretation

The components of the elbow joint are the proximal radius and ulna (including the olecranon, anconeal process, trochlear notch and coronoid process) and the distal humerus (including the condyle, medial and lateral epicondyles and supratrochlear foramen (dog) and supracondyloid foramen (cat)). Full assessment of these structures requires craniocaudal, mediolateral flexed and mediolateral neutral radiographs. As many diseases occur bilaterally, radiography of the contralateral limb should be considered. Elbow effusion is difficult to detect on radiographs and is rarely seen unless it is very severe.

The key features to assess include:

- Joint spaces (particularly on the craniocaudal view) – any gross incongruency between the radial head and coronoid process should be noted
- Anconeal process of the ulna (on the mediolateral flexed view) – any new bone formation on the craniodorsal aspect should be noted
- Medial and lateral epicondyles of the humerus (on the craniocaudal view) – inspect for any new bone on or adjacent to the epicondyles
- Humeral condyle – evaluate for the presence of subchondral sclerosis and any defects within the bone (most commonly medially)
- The shape of the medial coronoid process (on the mediolateral and craniocaudal views) – should be triangular and sharply marginated
- The shape of the radial head (on the mediolateral view) – any osteophyte formation on the cranioproximal aspect
- Shape and opacity of the trochlear notch of the ulna (on the mediolateral view) – sclerosis of the subtrochlear region is a feature of osteoarthritis. Humeroulnar incongruency may result in an abnormal ellipsoid trochlea

- The supinator sesamoid bones (on the lateral aspect of the joint) adjacent to the radial head should not be mistaken for a fragmented coronoid process
- Presence of mineralization within periarticular soft tissues.

Common diseases

Dysplasia: Elbow dysplasia is a common developmental condition in larger dogs, particularly in retriever breeds, with a complex genetic component involved. There are three primary lesions associated with elbow dysplasia, which typically lead to the development of osteoarthritis. All lesions can (and frequently do) occur bilaterally and so both elbows should be imaged if dysplasia is suspected.

Medial coronoid process disease: This has a spectrum of severity, ranging from mild changes in bone density to full fragmentation (fragmented coronoid process). Mild changes can be extremely difficult to detect on radiographs and even fragments can be challenging to identify due to superimposition of the adjacent bones. Radiographs have low sensitivity and poor specificity for the primary lesions. Features to recognize include altered shape (size, margins) of the medial coronoid process on mediolateral and craniocaudal radiographs and separate mineralized bodies in the region of the medial coronoid. In many cases, the presence of medial coronoid disease is suspected on the basis of secondary osteoarthritic changes (see Figures 7.43 and 7.77).

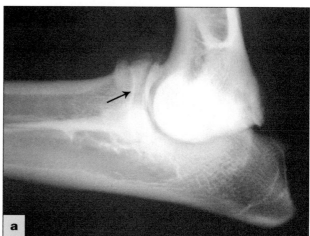

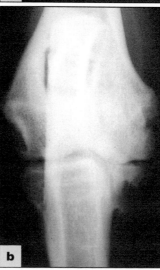

7.77 **(a)** Neutral mediolateral and **(b)** craniocaudal radiographs of the elbow of a dog with a fragmented medial coronoid process and secondary degenerative joint disease. The fragment from the medial coronoid is a triangular mineralized area superimposed on the radial head (arrowed) on the mediolateral view, and medial to the radial head on the craniocaudal view. New bone formation is present on the radial head and medial and lateral humeral epicondyles. (continues) ▶

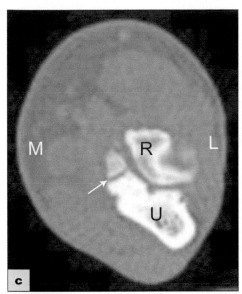

7.77 (continued) **(c)** CT image of the elbow of a dog with a fragmented medial coronoid process and secondary degenerative joint disease showing a line crossing the base of the medial coronoid process (arrowed). New bone formation is present on the radial head and medial and lateral humeral epicondyles. L = lateral; M = medial; R = radial head; U = body of the ulna.

Osteochondritis dissecans: In the elbow, OCD commonly affects the medial part of the humeral condyle and is seen most clearly on the craniocaudal view. It appears as a focal, saucer-shaped subchondral bone defect in the articular surface (Figure 7.78). In contrast to OCD in other joints, it is rare to identify mineralized fragments associated with OCD in the elbow. The major differential diagnosis for this appearance is an erosive 'kissing' lesion resulting from a fragmented coronoid process causing lysis of the humeral articular surface. There may be an area of sclerosis within the subchondral bone adjacent to the defect.

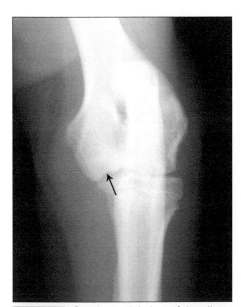

7.78 Craniocaudal view of the elbow of a dog with OCD. The defect in the articular surface of the medial part of the humeral condyle (arrowed) is surrounded by some sclerosis of the adjacent bone. (Courtesy of M Sullivan)

Ununited anconeal process: This primary dysplasia lesion is more commonly seen in German Shepherd Dogs, setters and Bassett Hounds. The aetiology is uncertain and there may be some implication of short ulna (or long radius) syndrome creating pressure on the ossification centre of the anconeus. Trauma has also been proposed as a possible cause. The anconeus should fuse to the olecranon at about 4–5 months of age, so an ununited anconeal process (UAP) should not be diagnosed in dogs younger than approximately 6 months of age. The condition is most easily diagnosed on a flexed mediolateral view. A radiolucent line separates the anconeal process from the olecranon (see Figure 7.27). There is frequently marked remodelling of the anconeal process due to secondary degenerative changes.

Elbow dysplasia scoring

In the UK, there is a scheme run by the Kennel Club and British Veterinary Association (BVA) that grades the changes associated with elbow dysplasia with a view to identifying individuals that are suitable for breeding purposes. The scheme works in a similar manner to the Hip Scoring Scheme (see below) with radiographs being submitted for grading by an expert panel.

Radiographs to be submitted

Neutral (approximately 110 degree angle between the humerus and radius) and flexed (joint at 45 degrees) mediolateral radiographs of each elbow should be submitted (submissions can be either conventional films or digital images). Radiographs should be labelled with the animal's Kennel Club number, microchip number, date the image was obtained and an appropriate L/R marker.

Grading scheme

The grading scheme is based on the International Elbow Working Group system:

- Grade 0 – Normal elbow with no osteoarthritis or primary lesion
- Grade 1 – Mild osteoarthritis with no osteophytes >2 mm
- Grade 2 – Moderate osteoarthritis with osteophyes between 2 and 5 mm
- Grade 3 – Severe osteoarthritis with osteophytes >5 mm.

In addition, the BVA scheme adjusts the grading according to the presence of a primary lesion (OCD, UAP or fragmented coronoid process):

- Grade 2 – Primary lesion present with no osteoarthritis
- Grade 3 – Primary lesion present with any osteoarthritis.

The overall grade for the animal is that of the higher elbow, and it is recommended only to breed from animals with an overall grade of 0 or 1. Further information and detailed procedure notes can be obtained from the BVA.

Osteoarthritis: Elbow osteoarthritis commonly occurs secondary to diseases such as elbow dysplasia and trauma. Mild primary degenerative changes may be seen as clinically silent changes in older animals. Osteophytosis around the elbow is most commonly seen on the cranial radial head, anconeal process and medial humeral epicondyles. Less commonly, there may be osteophytes on the lateral aspect of the joint. Early signs of osteoarthritis in the elbow include sclerosis of the region adjacent to the trochlear notch of the ulna and osteophyte formation on the dorsodistal aspect of the anconeal process. The early changes are subtle and easily overlooked. Care must be taken when interpreting mild new bone formation on the dorsal anconeus as a small fusiform-shaped protuberance of bone is normal in larger dogs. Soft tissue swelling and/or effusion associated with elbow pathology is uncommonly seen radiologically. The extent of the osteoarthritic changes is used in the grading of changes associated with elbow dysplasia (see above).

Incongruency: This may be seen in dogs predisposed to elbow dysplasia, and the altered joint dynamics are thought to increase the pressure on the anconeal or medial processes, predisposing them to fragmentation. Incongruency may result from a shallow ulnar trochlear notch (Figure 7.79), long radius (which creates increased pressure on the anconeal process) or long ulna, which results in an increased radiohumeral joint space and increased pressure on the medial coronoid process. Radiology is insensitive for demonstrating incongruency in the elbow and changes must be severe to be reliably assessed. A degree of physiological incongruency in the elbow is normal.

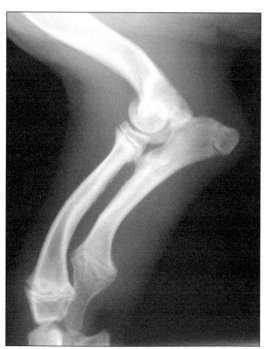

7.79 Mediolateral view of the elbow and antebrachium of a dog with severe ulnar chondrodystrophy (elbow incongruity). The trochlear notch of the ulna is abnormally shallow, leading to a widened humeroulnar joint space. The distal ends of both the radius and ulna are bowed cranially. Incongruency of the elbow has to be relatively severe to be reliably detected radiologically.

Incomplete ossification of the humeral condyles: The growth plate between the medial and lateral halves of the humeral condyle usually fuses at about 6 weeks of age. In spaniel breeds (particularly Springer Spaniels) there is a predisposition to failure of ossification of this growth plate. This failure of ossification may be partial or complete and can cause chronic intermittent lameness as well as predispose the joint to condylar fractures (see below). Diagnosis of incomplete ossification of the humeral condyles (IOHC) on radiographs is difficult. In some cases, it may be possible to visualize the fissure on either a craniocaudal (Figure 7.80) or a cranio 15 degrees medial–caudolateral oblique (Cr15°M-CdLO) view. Care should be taken not to mistake the Mach lines resulting from the superimposition of the olecranon on the distal humerus on these views with genuine fissure lines. CT is the preferred method for diagnosing IOHC (Figure 7.81). IOHC is frequently bilateral and both elbows should be imaged. Concurrent medial coronoid pathology is commonly seen in association with IOHC.

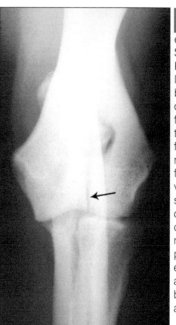

7.80 Craniocaudal view of the elbow of an English Springer Spaniel with IOHC. A fine radiolucent line (arrowed) extending between the two halves of the humeral condyle, from the articular surface to the supratrochlear foramen, can be seen. In many IOHC cases, the fissure cannot be visualized due to superimposition by the olecranon. In some cases, focal periosteal new bone may be present on the humeral epicondyles due to abnormal stresses on the bone (and may precede a condylar fracture).

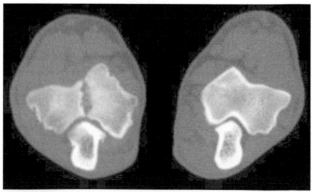

7.81 CT images of the elbows of an English Springer Spaniel with unilateral IOHC. The elbow of the left has a fissure line between the two halves of the humeral condyle.

Radiological features:

- Vertically orientated radiolucent fissure within centre of the humeral condyle on craniocaudal views.
- Sclerosis of the humeral condyle adjacent to the fissure.
- Smooth periosteal new bone formation may be present on the lateral epicondyle.

Fractures: The most common type of fracture affecting the elbow involves the humeral condyles. A lateral condylar fracture, resulting from a force transferred from the paw along the radius to the lateral condyle, is most often seen with fracture lines through the humeral condyle (involving the articular surface) and lateral supracondylar bone. 'Y'-shaped fractures involving both sides of the humeral condyle are also frequently encountered (Figure 7.82). IOHC

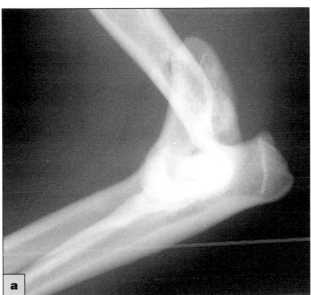

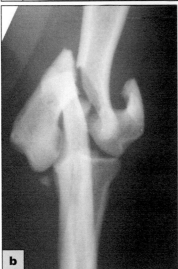

7.82 **(a)** Mediolateral and **(b)** craniocaudal views of the elbow of a dog with a 'Y'-shaped fracture of the distal humerus. On the craniocaudal view, a fracture extends into the elbow joint, resulting in separation and displacement of both halves of the humeral condyle. A small triangular bony fragment distal to the medial part of the humeral condyle indicates a fracture of the medial coronoid process. On the mediolateral view, the distal humerus is fractured and the normal elbow joint cannot be visualized.

predisposes spaniel breeds to condylar fractures, which can often occur following relatively minor trauma. In spaniels with condylar fractures, the contralateral elbow should be screened for the presence of IOHC.

Mineralized bodies: Mineralized structures may be seen around the elbow joint. Sesamoid bones associated with the supinator muscle are commonly seen in dogs (and some cats) as smooth, rounded, osseous shadows craniolateral to the radial head (see Figure 7.50). Other mineralized structures that may be seen include enthesophytes extending from the humeral epicondyles. These are most commonly associated with the medial epicondyle in the origins of the flexor muscles. Severe elbow osteoarthritis can also result in extensive mineralization in the periarticular region, especially in cats (see Figure 7.54).

Luxation: Luxation or subluxation may be congenital or traumatic. Congenital (sub)luxation is commonly seen in small dogs as a result of a deformity of the elbow and antebrachium or due to severe elbow incongruity (particularly a shallow ulnar trochlear notch). The most common variant is lateral luxation of the radial head caused by an overlong radius (or short ulna). Traumatic luxation can be seen following road traffic accidents or where the limb gets caught in a fence. With traumatic luxation, the mediolateral view may appear normal and the craniocaudal view is required to confirm displacement of the joint structures (see Figure 7.44). Luxation of the radial head is seen with Monteggia fractures: the proximal ulna is fractured and seen in conjunction with cranial luxation of the radial head and displacement of the distal part of the ulna.

Antebrachium

Standard radiographic views

- Mediolateral view:
    - The animal is placed in lateral recumbency with the leg of interest dependent and the upper limb retracted
    - The X-ray beam is centred on the mid-antebrachium and collimated to include the elbow and carpus.
- Craniocaudal view:
    - The animal is placed in sternal recumbency with the leg of interest extended
    - The olecranon should be in line with the humerus ensuring that there is no rotation. Foam wedges can be placed underneath the contralateral axilla to tilt the animal towards the side of interest
    - The head and neck are flexed laterally away from the side of interest, with the head supported on a foam block
    - The X-ray beam is centred on the mid-antebrachium and collimated to include the elbow and carpus.

Radiological interpretation

The approach to interpretation of radiographs of the antebrachium follows the general assessment of the long bones. The overall bone opacity and relative appearances of the cortex and medulla should be assessed, along with scrutiny for evidence of periosteal or endosteal changes and evidence of soft tissue disease. The elbow and carpal joints should be included on the radiograph and assessed. Care should be taken not to over-interpret irregular mineralization between the radial and ulnar diaphyses in the interosseous space; this is a normal radiological finding. It is not uncommon to see small spurs of new bone on the medial aspect of the distal radial physis/epiphysis at the origin of the short medial collateral ligament. Whilst representing pathology, this is usually an incidental finding.

The key features to assess include:

- Shape and integrity of the radius and ulna
- Presence of any new bone formation or bone lysis
- Evidence of increased medullary opacity of the radius or ulna
- Metaphyseal areas (immature animals)
- Distal radial metaphysis (older animals) – common site for neoplasia.

The radius and ulna may be affected by many of the diseases that affect the long bones in general, such as metaphyseal osteopathy, hypertrophic osteodystrophy, primary bone tumours (most commonly within the distal radial metaphysis) and fractures. There are also some conditions that are more specific to the antebrachium.

Common diseases

Fractures: The antebrachium is a common site for fractures, which can occur in a wide range of configurations and commonly involve both bones.

Primary bone tumours: The distal antebrachium is a common site for osteosarcoma, which can arise from either the radius or ulna. Despite the close proximity of the bones, primary bone tumours (see above) are usually monostotic.

Panosteitis: The radius and ulna are commonly involved in panosteitis (see above).

Premature closure of the distal ulnar growth plate: The conical distal ulnar physis can show early closure following compression fractures (Salter–Harris type V fracture): the shape of the physis renders the growth plate relatively more susceptible to damge than other physes. As a result, where this occurs before the animal has reached skeletal maturity, ulnar growth ceases whilst radial growth continues, leading to a bowed shape to the radius (usually in a cranial direction) and a malformation of the antebrachium (Figure 7.83). The caudal cortex of the radius is thickened (due to stress remodelling) and there may be separation of the ulnar styloid process from the ulnar carpal bone. Treatment usually involves corrective osteotomy of the ulna. In extreme cases, the deformation may extend proximally, leading to elbow subluxation.

Retained cartilaginous core: This is most commonly seen in the distal ulnar metaphysis of giant-breed dogs. A region of the physeal cartilage fails to ossify, leading to an area of lucency (often with a 'candle flame' shape) in the distal ulna (see Figure 7.15).

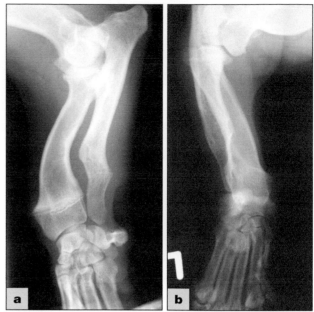

7.83 **(a)** Mediolateral and **(b)** craniocaudal views of the antebrachium of a dog with premature closure of the distal ulnar physis. On the mediolateral view, the distal ulnar physis can no longer be recognized. There is marked cranial bowing of the radius and incongruity of the humeroulnar joint. On the craniocaudal view, the paw is deviated laterally (carpal valgus) below the carpal joint.

Whilst this has been suggested as a predisposing cause of premature closure of the distal ulnar growth plate (see above), it is also frequently seen with an absence of associated clinical signs.

Carpus

The carpus is a compound joint comprising eight carpal bones and sesamoid bones plus the distal antebrachium and proximal metacarpal bones. The carpal bones are arranged into proximal and distal rows with the majority of motion occurring within the radiocarpal joint. Numerous ligaments are associated with the carpus but are not visible radiologically as discrete structures. The complex nature of the carpal joint can make interpretation difficult due to superimposition of the small carpal bones, and comparison with the contralateral limb is often extremely useful. Stressed views can also be useful to demonstrate or confirm the site of any instability. Features to be considered include the subchondral bone surfaces of the carpal bones (which should be smooth and of even thickness and show no evidence of erosion), evidence of alteration of the carpal joint spaces and evidence of osteophytosis of the carpal joints. The relative positions of the carpal bones and relationship to the antebrachial and metacarpal bones should also be considered. Soft tissue swelling around the joint should also be considered, although this is likely to be more easily assessed on clinical examination.

Standard radiographic views

- Mediolateral view:
  - The animal is placed in lateral recumbency with the leg of interest dependent, the upper limb retracted and the carpus in a neutral position (Figure 7.84)

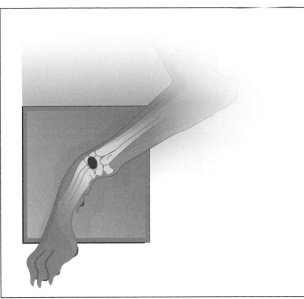

7.84 Patient positioning for a mediolateral view of the carpus.

- The X-ray beam is centred on the carpus and collimated to include the distal third of the antebrachium and digits.
- Dorsopalmar view:
  - The animal is placed in sternal recumbency with the leg of interest extended (Figure 7.85)
  - The olecranon should be in line with the humerus to ensure that there is no rotation. Placing sandbags lateral to the elbow may be helpful to prevent adduction of the limb
  - Foam wedges can be placed underneath the contralateral axilla to tip the animal across to the side of interest

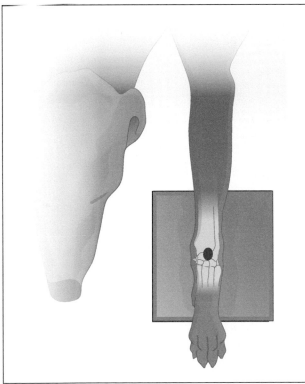

7.85 Patient positioning for a dorsopalmar view of the carpus.

- The X-ray beam is centred on the carpus and collimated to include the digits and the distal third of the antebrachium.

Special views: If insufficiency of the carpal ligaments is suspected, stressed radiographs should be obtained to evaluate for joint laxity (Figure 7.86). Depending on the aspect of the joint that is suspected to be affected, tension (using rope ties and sandbags) can be applied in the contralateral direction to widen the joint spaces on the affected side. A foam wedge and sandbag can be used to maintain the joint position when stress is applied. The flexed mediolateral view separates the dorsal surface of the carpal bones and is useful to identify small chip fractures or mineralization associated with the dorsal aspect of the joint.

- Flexed mediolateral view:
  - The animal is placed in lateral recumbency with the leg of interest dependent, the upper limb retracted and the carpus flexed. The flexed position can be maintained with the use of sandbags or tape (Figure 7.87)
  - The X-ray beam is centred on the carpus and collimated to include the distal third of the antebrachium and digits.

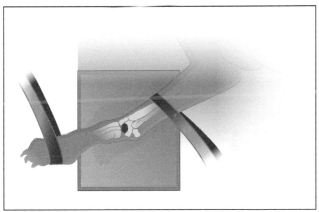

7.86 Patient positioning for a stressed extended view of the carpus.

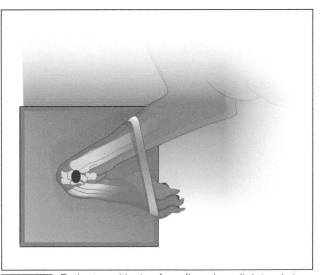

7.87 Patient positioning for a flexed mediolateral view of the carpus.

Radiological interpretation

As in all joint radiology, the soft tissues should be assessed for any joint effusion and periarticular soft tissue swelling. In extension, the joint spaces are narrow with the articular surfaces in close apposition (congruent) but they should be clearly defined on the dorsopalmar view. Osteoarthritis of the radiocarpal joint commonly results in new bone formation on the dorsal margins of the distal radius, radial carpal bone and metacarpal bones. New bone formation is also frequently seen on the base of the accessory carpal bone. Small spurs of smooth new bone are often present on the medial aspect of the distal radius at the origin of the short radial collateral ligament and are often incidental findings.

Key features to assess include:

- Congruency of joints
- Subchondral bone for sclerosis and irregularity
- Periarticular new bone formation
- Number and location of the carpal bones
- Margins of the carpal bones
- Margins of the antebrachiocarpal and carpometacarpal joint spaces
- Evidence of soft tissue swelling
- Evidence of laxity (stressed radiographs required).

Common diseases

Luxation: There are several possible causes of carpal (sub)luxation:

- Carpal hyperextension injury – associated with jumping from a height. Although plain radiographs may appear normal, stressed radiographs (with the carpus stressed into extension) show hyperextension, which may arise from any of the joints associated with the carpus
- Collateral ligament damage – plain radiographs are likely to appear normal, but radiographs with the carpus stressed medially or laterally show widening of the joint spaces on the affected side of the joint (Figure 7.88)
- Antebrachiocarpal subluxation – may be seen with angular limb deformities, leading to altered dynamics at the joint. The articulation of the radius and radial carpal bone is often altered, with the radial carpal bone displaced in a palmar direction relative to the distal end of the radius.

Fractures:

Accessory carpal bone fractures: Fractures of the accessory carpal bone are often associated with avulsion of the ligaments attached to the bone, and are particularly seen in Greyhounds and other athletic breeds. These fractures are most clearly seen on mediolateral radiographs.

Radial carpal bone fractures: These may be seen in the absence of obvious trauma and are postulated to be associated with a closure defect of the radial carpal bone (which develops from two centres of ossification). These fractures are most clearly seen on dorsopalmar radiographs.

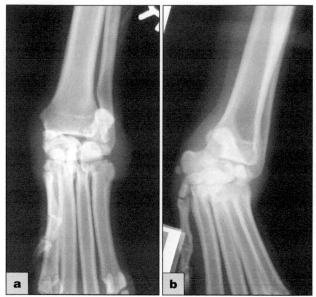

7.88 **(a)** Neutral dorsopalmar and **(b)** stressed dorsopalmar views of the carpus of a dog with rupture of the medial carpal collateral ligaments. (a) A degree of soft tissue swelling around the carpal joint is consistent with joint effusion. (b) The antebrachium and digits are pulled laterally, placing stress on the medial aspect of the carpal joint, resulting in medial subluxation of the radiocarpal joint. The radial carpal bone is displaced medially due to the loss of support from the medial collateral ligament.

Osteoarthritis: Osteophytosis and enthesophytosis may be seen around the carpal joint, particularly the medial aspect of the antebrachiocarpal and carpometacarpal joints (Figure 7.89). Whilst mild osteoarthritis may be seen as an incidental finding in older animals, the degree of new bone formation does not correlate with the degree of lameness attributed to the degenerative change.

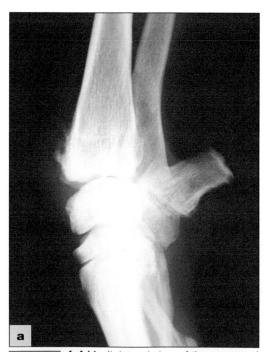

7.89 **(a)** Mediolateral view of the carpus of a dog with carpal osteoarthritis. Osteophytes are present on the distal radius and dorsal and medial aspects of the carpal bones. A mild joint effusion is visible as a mild degree of soft tissue swelling around the joint. (continues) ▶

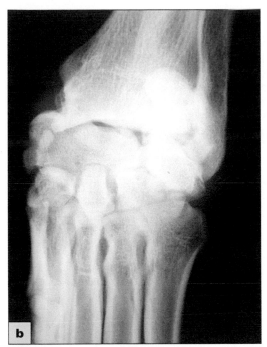

7.89 (continued) **(b)** Dorsopalmar view of the carpus of a dog with carpal osteoarthritis. Osteophytes are present on the distal radius and dorsal and medial aspects of the carpal bones. A mild joint effusion is visible as a mild degree of soft tissue swelling around the joint.

Polyarthropathies involving the carpus: The carpal joints are frequently involved in polyarthritic diseases. Whilst diseases such as immune-mediated polyarthritis are likely to result only in joint effusion (Figure 7.90), rheumatoid and other erosive arthropathies cause bilateral erosive lesions in the carpal bones and are associated with significant joint effusion.

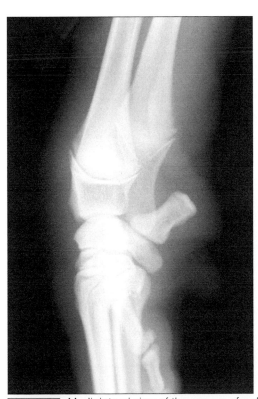

7.90 Mediolateral view of the carpus of a dog with carpal joint effusion. Soft tissue swelling is present dorsal to the carpal bones and is confined to the limits of the carpal joint.

Septic arthritis: Septic arthritis may affect the carpus. It is seen radiologically as an erosive disease causing lysis of the subchondral bone of the carpal bones and is usually accompanied by a marked joint effusion (Figure 7.91). Septic arthritis is usually seen in only one joint, whereas erosive polyarthropathies (such as rheumatoid arthritis) more commonly affect multiple joints.

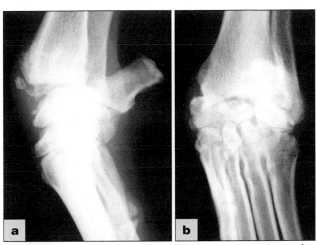

7.91 **(a)** Mediolateral and **(b)** dorsopalmar views of the carpus of a dog with septic arthritis. There is marked joint effusion with irregular lytic erosions of the subchondral bone of the distal radius and proximal row of carpal bones. Mineralized fragments are present in the dorsal aspect of the antebrachiocarpal joint, which may represent dystrophic mineralization or fragmentation of the bone. In cases of septic arthritis, where there is pre-existing osteoarthritis, it is often difficult to detect the signs of bone lysis, which occur in the later stages of sepsis.

Manus

Standard radiographic views

- Mediolateral view:
  - The animal is placed in lateral recumbency with the leg of interest dependent, the upper limb retracted and the carpus in a neutral position
  - The X-ray beam is centred on the distal metacarpals and collimated to include the carpal joint and digits
  - This view results in significant superimposition of the digits, and splaying the digits may be of benefit (see below).
- Dorsopalmar view:
  - The animal is placed in sternal recumbency with the leg of interest extended
  - The olecranon should be in line with the humerus to ensure that there is no rotation. Foam wedges can be placed underneath the contralateral axilla to tip the animal across to the side of interest
  - The X-ray beam is centred on the distal metacarpals and collimated to include the digits and the carpal joint.

Special views: If close inspection of the digits is required (e.g. for the investigation of foreign material) then using porous tape to splay the digits on a mediolateral view (Figure 7.92) or placing cotton wool

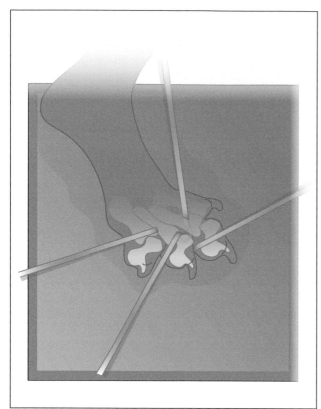

7.92 Patient positioning for a mediolateral view of the foot. Note the separation of the toes.

between the digits to separate them on a dorsopalmar view may increase the visibility of the soft tissues around the digits. Due to superimposition of the digital structures (particularly on the mediolateral view), splayed views with the digits separated can be used to allow complete visualization of the digital anatomy. In addition, due to the normal flexed position of the digits, it can be very difficult to visualize all of the interphalangeal joints (particularly the distal joints), although these can usually be seen reasonably clearly on a mediolateral radiograph. Care should be taken to clean the paw (including the interdigital spaces) to remove dirt and other material, which could be mistaken for foreign bodies on a radiograph.

Radiological interpretation

Considerations when assessing a paw radiograph include evaluating the metacarpal and phalangeal bones for evidence of dislocation or fracture. The metacarpophalangeal and interphalangeal joints should be assessed for evidence of degenerative changes, dislocation or more aggressive erosive disorders. The soft tissues (particularly around the distal phalanges) should be assessed for swelling and scrutinized (using a bright light) for evidence of foreign material. Finally, the palmar sesamoid bones should be checked for both number and position.

Key features to assess include:

- Number and relationship between the metacarpal and phalangeal bones
- Joint spaces
- Evidence of traumatic injury
- Evidence of soft tissue swelling
- Evidence of foreign material.

Common diseases

Traumatic injury: Metacarpal and phalangeal fractures, and interphalangeal luxations are fairly commonly seen in association with road traffic accidents or other trauma (Figure 7.93). Multiple bones (or joints) may be involved. The degree of displacement is variable and intact bones may act as an integral splint, minimizing the displacement of the fractures. In some cases, stressed views may be useful to demonstrate subluxations or fractures.

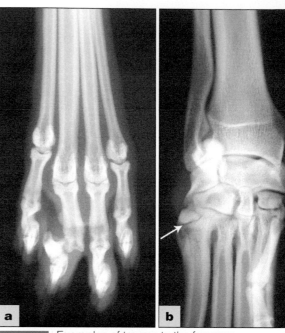

7.93 Examples of trauma to the forepaw.
(a) Dorsopalmar view of the digits with medial and proximal luxation of the second and third phalanges of the third digit. **(b)** Dorsopalmar view of the carpus with a minimally displaced fracture (arrowed) of the lateral aspect of the proximal end of the fifth metacarpal.

Osteoarthritis: Degenerative changes on the metacarpophalangeal and interphalangeal joints are common findings in older animals and may be incidental (Figure 7.94). Radiographic changes frequently include deposition of new bone around the joint margins (osteophytosis).

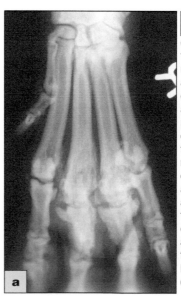

7.94

(a) Dorsopalmar view of the forepaw of a dog with marked digital osteoarthritis. There is extensive new bone seen around the proximal interphalangeal joints, most obviously in the third and fourth digits, which represents enthesopathy of the collateral ligaments and osteophyte formation. Although dramatic, these changes are commonly seen as apparently incidental findings (especially in large-breed dogs). (continues) ▶

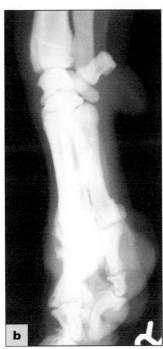

7.94 (continued) **(b)** Mediolateral view of the forepaw of a dog with marked digital osteoarthritis. There is extensive new bone seen around the proximal interphalangeal joints, most obviously in the third and fourth digits, which represents enthesopathy of the collateral ligaments and osteophyte formation. Although dramatic, these changes are commonly seen as apparently incidental findings (especially in large-breed dogs).

Foreign bodies: Depending on the nature of the foreign body, it may be seen on a radiograph of the paw. Glass is slightly more radiopaque than soft tissue and may be seen as a well defined opacity within the soft tissues (which usually also show some swelling) (Figure 7.95). Plant foreign bodies (such as grass seeds) tend to have the same opacity as the soft tissues and can be very difficult to detect on a

radiograph. If there is some abscessation of the soft tissues, then small bubbles of gas may be seen on close examination of the film. If the foreign body is recent, then some radiolucency associated with the entry tract may also be seen.

Soft tissue masses: Soft tissue swellings of the paw are usually appreciated on clinical examination. When evaluating a radiograph, it is vital to assess for evidence of lysis of the phalangeal (and/or metacarpal) bones. Some soft tissue tumours (particularly melanoma) have a predilection for the digit and may show aggressive characteristics. In cats, a digital soft tissue mass can be seen with distant metastases from a pulmonary carcinoma ('lung–digit syndrome') and it is important that in any case where neoplasia is suspected that thoracic radiographs are obtained to evaluate for further neoplastic disease (Figure 7.96). Most tumours involving the digits arise from P3 and often result in focal lysis of the ungual process. It is not possible from radiographs to differentiate soft tissue tumours involving the digits from osteomyelitis and a biopsy should be performed. Most soft tissue masses are localized to one digit; the presence of diffuse swelling involving the whole foot is suggestive of oedema or cellulitis.

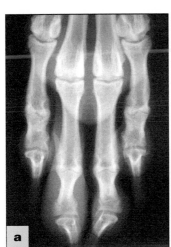

7.95 **(a)** Dorso-palmar and **(b)** splayed mediolateral views of the digits of a dog with glass foreign bodies. There is soft tissue swelling around the distal phalanx of the third digit and, on the mediolateral view, two small well defined radiopacities (arrowed) are seen in the region of the digital pad (small glass fragments). The linear opacities seen on the mediolateral view are due to the tape used to splay the digits.

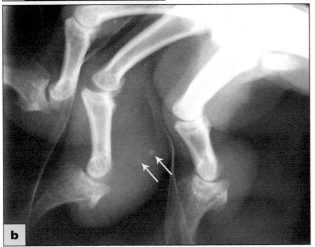

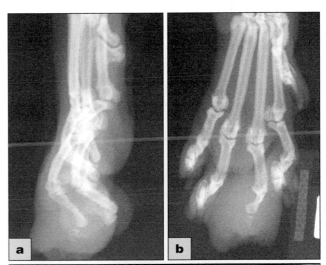

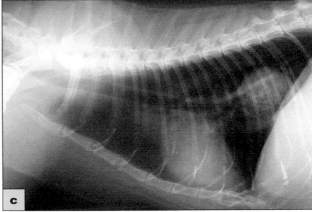

7.96 **(a)** Mediolateral and **(b)** dorsopalmar views of the manus and **(c)** lateral view of the thorax of a cat with a pulmonary carcinoma and metastasis to the digit. There is marked soft tissue swelling around the distal end of the third digit with almost complete lysis of the distal phalanx. The changes are consistent with an aggressive soft tissue tumour destroying the bone. The rounded mottled pulmonary nodule present in the lungs in the caudal thorax is consistent with a primary lung tumour.

The hindlimb

Hip and pelvis

For routine radiographic examination of the hip joints an extended ventrodorsal (VD) and a lateral view should be obtained. Sedation or general anaesthesia is required for hip radiography. If there is severe pain on extension of the hips or a high index of suspicion of hip/pelvic trauma, a flexed (frog-legged) VD view is often less painful and easier to obtain, and is usually sufficient to demonstrate significant pathology. Some pathology affecting the femoral neck and head (especially physeal fractures in young animals) are most easily seen on the flexed (frog-legged) view. On the lateral view the hip joints are superimposed and better separation can be seen on lateral oblique radiographs. A specific view to visualize the dorsal acetabular rim has been described but is rarely used as it is of limited value for most hip diseases.

Standard radiographic views

- VD view:
  - A table top technique for cats and small dogs, with a detail film–screen combination, should be used. For larger dogs, a grid (ideally a moving grid) should be used
  - The animal is placed in dorsal recumbency with both pelvic limbs fully extended to the same degree using ties or a sandbag over the hocks (Figure 7.97). In dogs that have limited extension of the femurs due to hip pathology, the hocks should be supported using a foam block

- It is essential to ensure that the entire body is straight to prevent axial rotation/tilting of the pelvis. Placing the thorax in a positioning trough to reduce axial rotation should be considered
  - The stifles should be internally rotated so that the patellae are centrally located over the trochleae. This requires tape or ties to be wrapped around the stifles whilst internally rotating the hindlimbs
  - The femora should be parallel and placing a foam block between the tarsi helps keep the femora parallel and reduce external rotation of the stifles
  - The greater trochanters should be palpated to ensure that the hips are at the same level and height above the table. Both stifles should be level
  - The X-ray beam is centred on the greater trochanters (which can be easily palpated in most animals) and collimated laterally to the skin edges, cranially to the iliac crests and caudally to the mid-femur.
- Flexed (frog-legged) VD view:
  - This view is often preferred in sedated animals, particularly those that may resent extension of the hindlimbs due to hip pain. Assessment of any subluxation of the hips is less reliable than on the standard VD view, but some conditions (such as femoral head and neck fractures) are better visualized on the frog-legged view
  - In cases where the standard VD view is normal but there is clinically significant hip pain (especially in trauma cases) both extended and frog-legged VD views should be obtained
  - The animal is positioned as for the extended VD view but with the pelvic limbs in a neutral flexed position (Figure 7.98)
  - Foam wedges can be placed under the stifles/proximal limbs to prevent axial rotation of the pelvis
  - The X-ray beam is centred and collimated as for the standard VD view.
- Lateral view:
  - The animal is placed in lateral recumbency with the legs in a neutral position (Figure 7.99)

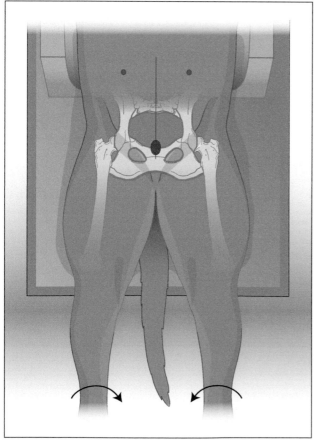

7.97 Patient positioning for a VD view of the hip and pelvis.

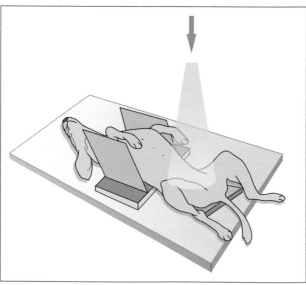

7.98 Patient positioning for a flexed (frog-legged) VD view of the hip and pelvis.

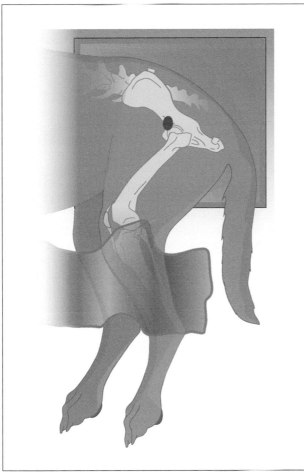

7.99 Patient positioning for a lateral view of the hip and pelvis.

- A foam wedge should be placed under the sternum to ensure that it is level with the thoracic spine
- To prevent axial rotation of the pelvis, padding should be placed between the stifles/femora. The femora should be parallel, which can be ensured by positioning the iliac wings at the same level and perpendicular to the cassette
- For larger animals, a grid with a Bucky should be used
- The X-ray beam is centred on the hip joints using the greater trochanter as a landmark
- On the lateral view the hip joints are superimposed. A lateral oblique view is required to allow the hip joints to be visualized without superimposition. Angling the X-ray tube head cranially by approximately 20 degrees separates the hip joints on the image.

Radiological approach

The following should be assessed when reviewing hip and pelvic radiographs:

- The size and shape of the obturator foramina, iliac wings and sacroiliac joints to determine whether there is axial rotation of the pelvis due to poor positioning. Differences between the left and right sides indicate tilting of the pelvis, which should be noted as this affects interpretation of the hip joints (tilting may artefactually give the appearance of subluxation of the hip joint). If there is axial rotation

of the pelvis, the side that is closest to the table (i.e. the side towards which the pelvis is tilted) will have the smaller obturator foramen and larger iliac wing (Figure 7.100)

- The size, symmetry and opacity of the pelvis and thigh muscles. Reduced volume of gluteal and thigh muscles may help localize the side of lameness (Figure 7.101) as muscle atrophy is common with chronic lameness and peripheral

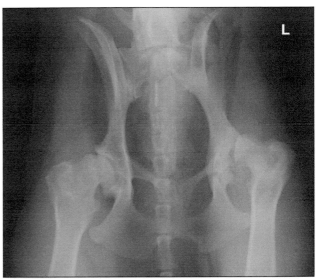

7.100 VD view of the pelvis with axial rotation to the left. Note the asymmetry of the iliac wings and obturator foramina. The pelvis is rotated towards the side with the smaller obturator foramen and larger iliac wing, in this case on the left (i.e. the left side of the patient is closest to the cassette). The dog has severe hip dysplasia and osteoarthritis with extensive osteophyte formation, irregular sclerosis of the subchondral bone and marked remodelling of the joints.

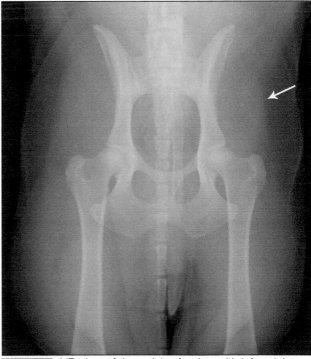

7.101 VD view of the pelvis of a dog with left pelvic limb lameness showing muscle atrophy. Note the reduced size of the left gluteal (arrowed) and thigh muscles compared with the right side.

nerve disease. Dystrophic mineralization within the gluteal and psoas muscles is occasionally seen and is usually an incidental finding of no clinical significance (see Figure 7.53)

■ Congruency of the hip joints and the presence of any subluxation. The hip joints are ball and socket joints and the femoral heads and acetabulae should be congruent with similar curvature to the femoral heads and cranial acetabulum. Subluxation of the femoral head results in widening of the joint space and lateral displacement of the femoral head relative to the acetabulum

■ The presence of any new bone formation on the femoral heads, necks and acetabulae (Figure 7.102)

■ The presence of any lysis within the femur or pelvis. Care should be taken not to mistake superimposition of faeces or gas within the large intestine or anal sacs for pathology, as they can mimic lytic lesions in the ischia or sacrum (Figure 7.102). Fascial planes between the muscle bellies of the thigh and nutrient foramina in the femurs may be mistaken for fissure fractures

■ Due to superimposition by overlying muscles, effusion within the hip joints is not visible radiologically.

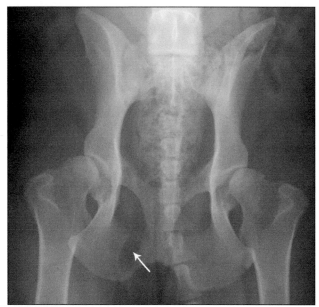

7.102 VD view of the pelvis of a dog with hip dysplasia and gas within the right anal sac (arrowed). The ovoidal-shaped lucency caused by the gas is superimposed over the right ischium and should not be mistaken for an area of lysis. There is moderately severe osteoarthritis with irregular osteophytes around the femoral heads and necks, and subluxation of both hips.

Key features to assess include:

■ Positioning of the pelvis
■ Soft tissues for any atrophy, swelling or mineralization
■ Joint congruency
■ Periarticular new bone.

Common diseases

Pathology involving the non-articular parts of the pelvis is rare (other than fractures and neoplasia). In contrast, lesions involving the hip joints are extremely common but can be clinically silent.

Hip dysplasia: Hip dysplasia is an inherited developmental disease resulting in laxity of the hip joint and secondary osteoarthritis. The disease is multifactorial with environmental and genetic factors involved in the development of the disease. Dysplasia is the most common condition affecting the hip in dogs, occurring in almost all breeds but with clinical signs most apparent in large and giant breeds. In chondrodystrophic breeds, subluxation of the hip joints can be considered almost normal but is usually asymptomatic. The age of onset of clinical signs is bimodal, with young dogs (<1 year old) having clinical signs due to joint laxity and microfractures of the acetabular rim and older animals presenting with signs of osteoarthritis. Hip dysplasia occurs less commonly in cats with Maine Coon, Persian, Devon Rex and Himalayan breeds predisposed. Clinical signs include a bunny-hopping gait, reluctance to exercise, pelvic limb lameness and difficulty rising. Clinical signs may overlap with lumbosacral disease as both hip dysplasia and degenerative changes affecting the lumbosacral junction are common in older animals.

An accurate diagnosis requires careful clinical examination as imaging changes are often unhelpful in differentiating the cause of the lameness. The primary pathology of hip dysplasia is laxity of the hip joint, and passive laxity may be assessed using dynamic distraction radiography (PennHIP Scheme). Assessment of joint laxity on an extended VD view is problematical as extending the pelvic limbs may result in the erroneous appearance of good joint congruency. There is poor correlation between the severity of radiological changes and clinical signs with hip dysplasia. Determination of the significance of the radiological changes needs to be made in conjunction with the history and clinical examination.

Radiological features: Radiological abnormalities are divided into two groups: changes due to joint laxity and changes due to secondary osteoarthritis. Careful radiographic positioning is important and tilting of the pelvis must be avoided to allow accurate assessment of subluxation.

■ Laxity of the joint results in subluxation of the hip joints and as the femoral head moves laterally there is medial divergence of the cranial joint space (Figure 7.103).

■ Subluxation also results in a reduced Norberg angle (Figure 7.104), which is an objective measure of the degree of subluxation and depth of the acetabulum. The Norberg angle is measured using a device called an ischiometer (or if this is not available, a protractor). The centre of each of the femoral heads is determined using the ischiometer and marked. A baseline is then drawn between the centres of the femoral heads. For each hip, a line is drawn from the centre of the femoral head to the craniolateral aspect of the acetabulum. Using the ischiometer (or protractor), the angle between the baseline and the line to the craniolateral acetabulum is measured. If the acetabulum is shallow or the femoral head is subluxated, there is a reduction in the Norberg angle. There are breed variations in the Norberg angle, with a mean angle of 105 degrees in normal

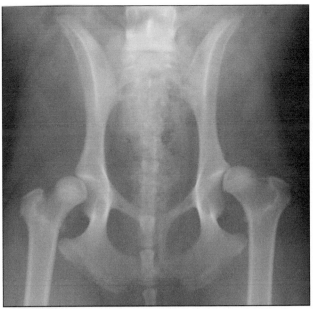

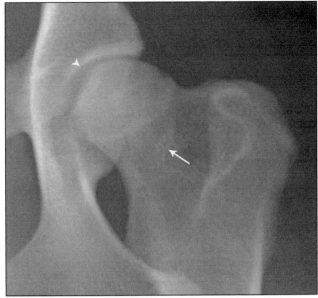

7.103 Severe hip dysplasia in a 6-month-old Tibetan Terrier. There is marked subluxation of both femoral heads and shallow acetabulae. Due to the lateral displacement of the femoral heads, there is reduced coverage of the femoral heads by the dorsal acetabulae.

7.105 VD view of the pelvis of a dog with mild hip dysplasia and osteoarthritis. The subtle curvilinear osteophyte (arrowed) on the femoral neck is an early sign of hip osteoarthritis. The hip dysplasia is associated with only mild subluxation, resulting in medial divergence of the joint space cranially (arrowhead).

- Predilection sites for osteophyte formation are around the femoral head and neck and adjacent to the cranial acetabulum.
- Remodelling of the femoral head and neck often results in a mushroom-shaped femoral head (Figure 7.106).
- The subchondral bone of the femoral head may appear irregular and sclerotic in severe cases (see Figure 7.100).

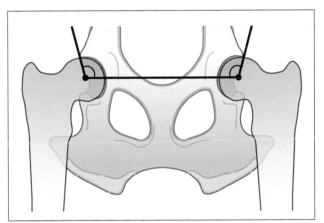

7.104 Norberg angle measurement. On the extended VD view of the hip, it is the angle between a line connecting the femoral head centres and a line from the centre of the femoral head to the craniodorsal acetabular rim.

dogs. A Norberg angle <105 degrees is considered abnormal. In cats, a Norberg angle >93 degrees is considered normal.

- The percentage of the femoral head covered by the dorsal acetabulum is reduced by lateral displacement of the femoral head (see Figure 7.103). In normal dogs, the centre of the femoral head should lie medial to the dorsal acetabular rim, with >50% coverage of the femoral head considered normal.

In more chronic cases, there is remodelling of the femoral head and acetabulum with secondary osteoarthritis. The radiological changes associated with osteoarthritis of the coxofemoral joint are as for other joints, but neither joint effusion nor soft tissue swelling is visible on radiographs.

- The earliest sign of osteoarthritis is the presence of a small curvilinear osteophyte on the femoral neck ('Morgan's line') (Figure 7.105).

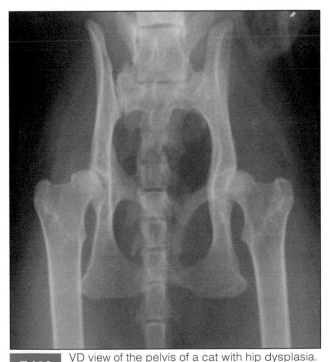

7.106 VD view of the pelvis of a cat with hip dysplasia. There is subluxation of both hips and shallow acetabulae. In cats with osteoarthritis of the hips, osteophyte formation is often most severe on the craniodorsal acetabulum, with relative sparing of the femoral neck compared with dogs. Mushroom-shaped femoral heads can be seen in asymptomatic/normal cats.

Hip dysplasia scoring

Several radiological-based scoring systems are used to try and reduce the incidence of hip dysplasia. The majority of schemes (including the BVA/ Kennel Club Scheme in the UK) use the extended VD view and grade or score the radiological features of joint laxity and osteoarthritis. The diagnosis of mild laxity is most reliable on stress radiographs. The PennHIP Scheme uses dynamic radiographs with the hips in a compressed position and then distracted, using a patented distractor to measure primary joint laxity. The difference in position of the centre of the femoral head when compressed and distracted is measured and given as a ratio (the distraction index) to the radius of the femoral head. The greater the degree of laxity, the larger the distraction index. A good correlation exists between the distraction index and the development of osteoarthritis. The PennHIP Scheme involves the use of a special distractor and is not widely used in Europe because of the lack of trained personnel and radiation safety issues.

BVA/Kennel Club Scheme

The BVA/Kennel Club Scheme has been used since 1983 to score hips, and a large number of dogs have been screened and the results published. Submission of radiographs prior to breeding is advisable to try and reduce the prevalence of hip dysplasia. Dogs that have radiographs submitted for scoring must have permanent identification (usually a microchip) and for pedigree dogs, the Kennel Club number must be permanently marked on the image. Dogs need to be a minimum of 12 months old for their hips to be scored. Films or digital images submitted to the Scheme are assessed by two experienced scrutineers and a consensus decision is reached on the score. Scoring uses a 9-point grading scheme that measures the Norberg angle, degree of subluxation, appearance of the cranial acetabular edge, dorsal acetabular edge, cranial acetabular rim, acetabular fossa and caudal acetabular edge, femoral head remodelling and the presence of femoral head and neck exostoses.

Each feature is given a numerical score and each hip is scored separately, giving a maximum score of 106 for both hips. The larger the score, the greater the degree of subluxation and secondary osteoarthritis. A total score of 0–4 indicates perfect or near perfect hips and a score of <10 indicates borderline changes which are unlikely to worsen with age. A score of >20 indicates hips with moderate to marked dysplasia with the presence of osteoarthritis. Statistics of the scores are published for each breed and it is recommended that breeding only takes place from dogs whose worst hip score is below the breed median score, taking into account the scores of related animals (if available).

Hip luxation: Hip luxation occurs most commonly following extrinsic trauma (e.g. road traffic accidents) but may rarely occur spontaneously due to severe hip dysplasia. Hip luxation occurs in animals >1 year old when the proximal femoral physes have closed. Luxation may occur in a craniodorsal, caudodorsal or ventral direction, but craniodorsal luxations are most common (approximately 90%). Orthogonal radiographs should be obtained prior to reduction to determine the direction of the luxation (Figure 7.107) and enable detection of avulsion fractures of the teres ligament and the presence of any pre-existing pathology which may affect reduction. Radiographs should also be taken after reduction of the luxation to ensure that the hip is in its normal location.

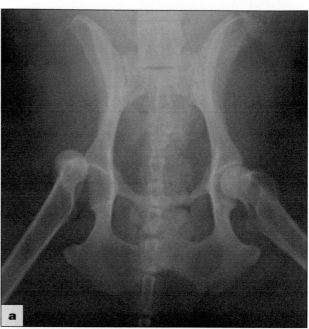

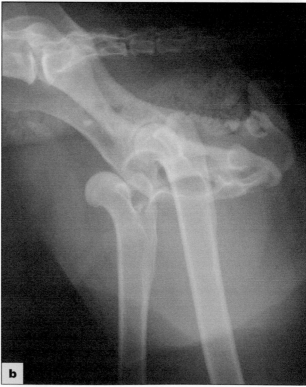

7.107 **(a)** VD and **(b)** lateral views of the pelvis of a dog with cranioventral hip luxation. On the VD view it is not possible to determine whether the luxation is dorsal or ventral. In cases of traumatic hip luxation, a careful evaluation should be made for an avulsion fracture on the femoral head or evidence of pre-existing hip dysplasia, which may alter treatment options and prognosis.

Fractures: Pelvic fractures are common but it may be radiologically difficult to determine the fracture configuration. Studies have shown that radiographs underestimate the number of pelvic fractures present. Faeces within the colon overlying the sacrum on a VD view can make detection of sacral fractures and sacroiliac subluxations difficult. Radiological interpretation of pelvic fractures is aimed at determining whether there is articular involvement, whether the fracture is stable and whether there is any gross displacement that may lead to stenosis of the pelvic canal (Figure 7.108). Trauma to the urethra and bladder is common with pelvic fractures and, if there is doubt as to the integrity of the lower urinary tract, a positive contrast retrograde urethrocystogram should be performed (see Chapters 4 and 6).

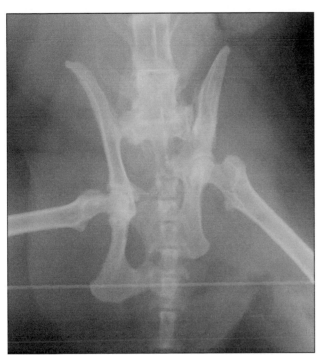

7.108   VD view of the pelvis of a cat with a left sacral fracture, a right sacroiliac subluxation and fractures of the pubis and left ischium. The pelvis can be thought of as a rigid box and there are usually multiple fractures. Radiography often underestimates the number of pelvic fractures.

Aseptic necrosis of the femoral head and neck (Legg–Calvé–Perthes disease): This is an uncommon disease of immature or young adult toy breeds, most commonly terriers. The aetiology of the condition is unknown, but in at least one breed a genetic component with high heritability has been shown. The primary pathology is ischaemic necrosis of the femoral head and neck, but the cause of the ischaemia is unknown. Affected dogs present with progressive pelvic limb lameness and hip pain. The disease may be unilateral or bilateral, but most cases are unilateral and the disease may result in pathological fractures of the femoral necks. In larger dog breeds, the main radiological differential diagnosis is spontaneous Salter–Harris type I fracture of the femoral neck (Figure 7.109) and if the blood supply to the femoral capitus is disrupted then aseptic necrosis of the femoral head may occur. A flexed (frog-legged) VD view may be helpful to visualize lesions and determine the presence of any femoral neck fractures.

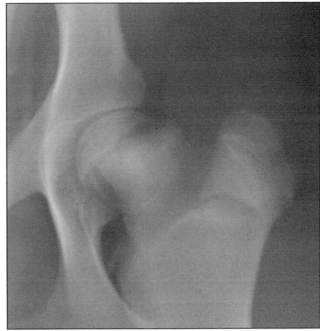

7.109   VD view of the pelvis of a young dog with a Salter–Harris type I fracture of the femoral head. This type of fracture may occur spontaneously with no history of external trauma and may be bilateral. If there is damage to the blood supply, there may be avascular necrosis of the femoral head.

Radiological features:

- In the early stages, there is widening of the joint space and subtle irregularity and often reduced opacity of the subchondral bone of the femoral head (Figure 7.110).
- Irregular areas of focal lucency within the femoral neck, which may progress to collapse of the femoral head.
- Necrosis of the femoral head, leading to incongruency of the joint.

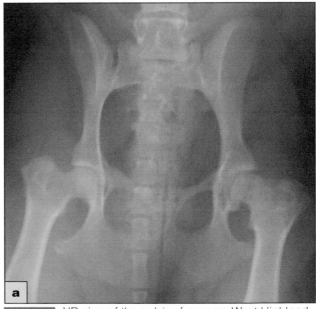

7.110   VD view of the pelvis of a young West Highland White Terrier. **(a)** There is lysis and reduced opacity of the left femoral head and neck and widening of the joint space on the initial examination, but the right hip is normal in opacity. (continues) ▶

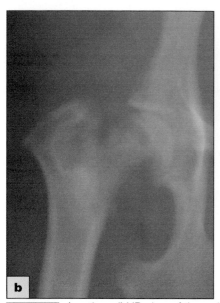

7.110 (continued) VD view of the pelvis of a young West Highland White Terrier. **(b)** Radiograph taken 2 months following the initial examination. Note the presence of lysis on the right femoral neck, which has an 'apple core' appearance.

- The femoral neck commonly becomes thickened and sclerotic.
- In severe cases, pathological fracture of the femoral neck may occur.
- Secondary osteoarthritis is a feature of more chronic cases.

Slipped capital epiphysis/epiphysiolysis: This is an idiopathic condition that occurs occasionally in cats and larger breed dogs and is associated with separation of the proximal femoral epiphysis despite minimal/ no history of trauma. It also occurs in young animals with open physes. The physeal separation is often most easily visualized on the flexed (frog-legged) VD view.

Radiological features:

- In the acute stage, widening of the proximal femoral physes and displacement of the epiphysis, resulting in an abnormal contour to the femoral neck with a step between the femoral neck and head (see Figure 7.109).
- In chronic cases, reduced opacity of the femoral head with adjacent sclerosis of the femoral neck.

Neoplasia: The pelvic bones are commonly involved with multiple myeloma, which also often involves the spine (see Chapter 9) (Figure 7.111). Multiple myeloma most commonly occurs in dogs, which may have bio-chemical (hypergammaglobulinaemia) and/or haem-atological abnormalities. Radiological features of multiple myeloma include punched out areas of lysis involving multiple bones. Areas of lysis are often irregular in shape and entirely lytic, with no new bone formation. In dogs, care must be taken not to misinterpret gas within the anal sacs overlying the ischium on VD pelvic radiographs as pathology, as it can resemble a lytic lesion. Primary bone tumours (osteosarcoma, chondrosarcoma) also occasionally involve the pelvic bone and proximal femur and resemble bone tumours elsewhere in the limbs.

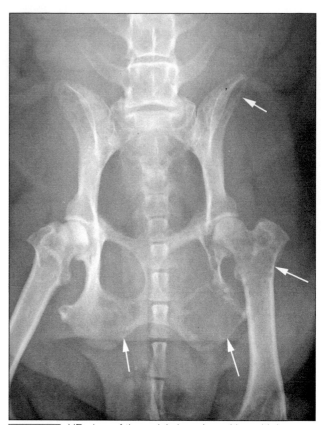

7.111 VD view of the pelvis in a dog with multiple myeloma. There are multiple punched out areas of lysis within multiple bones of the pelvis and femur (arrowed).

Femur

Standard radiographic views

- Mediolateral view:
  - The animal is placed in lateral recumbency with the side of interest dependent, the limb of interest in a neutral position and the upper limb adducted as far as possible
  - In male dogs, the prepuce may need to be retracted dorsally using a bandage around the caudal abdomen to prevent it from overlying the distal femur
  - The X-ray beam is centred on the midpoint of the femur and collimated to include the hip and stifle joints
  - Due to the large variation in tissue depth between the proximal and distal femur in large dogs, two separate radiographs may need to be taken if conventional film is being used.
- Craniocaudal view:
  - The animal is positioned as for a VD view of the pelvis
  - The X-ray beam is centred on the mid-diaphysis of the femur under investigation and collimated to include the hip and stifle.

Common diseases

Congenital abnormalities of the femur, leading to abnormal alignment, usually present with stifle or hip problems due to the abnormal conformation. The femur is a common site of trauma or neoplasia, which are easily recognizable. The approach to the interpretation of radiographs of the femur is the same as for other long bones. On the caudal aspect of the distal femur, the supracondylar tuberosities project from the cortex and should not be mistaken for enthesopathy/new bone formation.

Primary bone tumours: The distal femur is a predilection site for primary bone tumours, which typically arise in the metaphyseal region. Their appearance is as bone tumours in other long bones (see Figure 7.10).

Fractures: Femoral fractures are one of the most common long bone fractures and occur in a wide variety of configurations. Complications during fracture healing occur more frequently in the femur than in other long bones.

Panosteitis: The femur is often involved in cases of panosteitis (see above).

Stifle

Standard radiographic views
A standard radiographic examination comprises a mediolateral view with the stifle in a neutral position and a caudocranial view. Lateral oblique views are occasionally helpful for visualizing OCD lesions within the femoral condyles. A cranioproximal–craniodistal oblique (CrPr-CrDiO) (skyline) view of the femoral trochlea can be used to assess the depth of the trochlea and to visualize some patellar lesions, but is rarely required.

- Mediolateral view:
  - A table top technique with a detail film–screen combination should be used
  - The patient is placed in lateral recumbency with the leg of interest dependent and the upper limb retracted (Figure 7.112)
  - The stifle should be in a neutral position and overflexion should be avoided
  - In male dogs, the prepuce should not overlie the stifle

- To prevent axial rotation of the stifle, a small foam wedge/pad can be placed under the hock. It may also be helpful to place a thin pad under the hip in larger dogs
  - The X-ray beam is centred just distal to the femoral condyles and caudal to the patellar ligament, and collimated to include the distal third of the femur and the proximal third of the tibia.
- Caudocranial view:
  - This view results in less magnification compared with the craniocaudal view. The main problems are axial rotation of the stifle due to tilting of the thorax/abdomen and failure to internally rotate the stifle
  - A table top technique should be used
  - The animal is placed in a prone position and sandbags placed beside the thorax to prevent tilting
  - The affected stifle should be extended and internally rotated, and then placed on the cassette. A sandbag should be placed over the hock
  - The contralateral leg should be elevated with the limb flexed and placed on a foam pad/block
  - The X-ray beam is centred in the midline just distal to the femoral condyles and collimated to include the distal third of the femur and proximal third of the tibia.
- Craniocaudal view:
  - This view may be difficult to perform in animals with restricted extension of the hips and results in greater magnification than the caudocranial view (Figure 7.113)
  - The animal is placed in dorsal recumbency in a positioning trough with the hindlimb under investigation fully extended
  - The limb should be straight (tilting the thorax slightly away from the side under investigation may help)

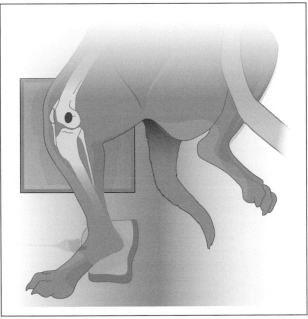

7.112 Patient positioning for a mediolateral view of the stifle.

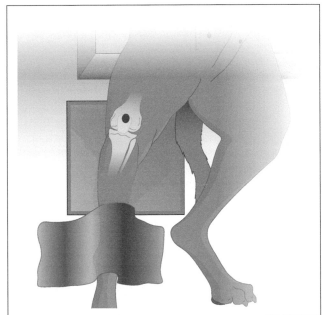

7.113 Patient positioning for a craniocaudal view of the stifle.

- The affected stifle is positioned over the cassette
- A sandbag can be placed over the hock and, if necessary, over the thigh
- The X-ray beam is centred in the midline just distal to the femoral condyles and collimated to include the distal third of the femur and the proximal third of the tibia.

Special views: The craniodistal–cranioproximal oblique (CrDi-CrPrO) (skyline) view of the patella (Figure 7.114) can be used to assess the depth of the femoral trochlea and patella. This rarely adds useful information to that obtained from the clinical examination and standard radiographic views.

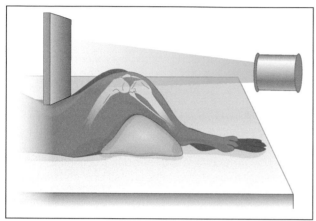

7.114 Patient positioning for a craniodistal–cranioproximal oblique (CrDi-CrPrO) (skyline) view of the patella.

Radiological interpretation

As for all joints, radiographs of the stifle should be assessed for the presence and location of any swelling and the presence of mineralization/gas within the soft tissues. It is important to evaluate the size and shape of the infrapatellar fatpad on the mediolateral view. The infrapatellar fatpad should contact the patellar tendon cranially and the femoral condyle caudally. Many conditions affecting the stifle cause effusion, which results in a reduced size of the fatpad (see Figure 7.33). The fatpad is displaced cranially with a soft tissue opacity between the surface of the femur and the caudal margin of the fatpad. If only a mild stifle effusion is present, the fatpad typically has a streaky appearance due to the superimposition of fluid. In normal dogs, a small soft tissue opacity is present caudal to the fatpad and represents the cruciate ligaments and menisci. Osteophyte formation is most commonly seen on the poles of the patella, trochlear ridges, fabellae and margins of the femoro-tibial joint.

Key features to assess include:

- Presence of any stifle effusion
- Margination, shape and opacity of the subchondral bone
- Presence of osteophyte formation
- Position of the popliteal sesamoid bone and fabellae
- Alignment of the patella.

There are a number of incidental findings and anatomical variants that should not be mistaken for genuine pathology. In cats and small dogs, the medial fabella may be absent. In some small terrier breeds (e.g. West Highland White Terriers) the medial fabella is often located distomedial to the lateral fabella (see Figure 7.56) and should not be mistaken for avulsion of the gastrocnemius muscle. The proximal part of the tibial tuberosity is thin and appears as a focal area of relative radiolucency, which should not be mistaken for a localized area of bone lysis. On the caudodistal aspect of the femur, at the origin of the gastrocnemius muscles, there is a ridge of bone that is highlighted if there is slight rotation of the femur on the lateral view and should not be mistaken for new bone formation.

Common diseases

Cranial cruciate disease: This is the most common cause of pelvic limb lameness and in almost all cases results in radiographic changes. The radiographic changes primarily reflect secondary osteoarthritis, and cranial displacement of the tibia is rarely seen (since the radiographs are taken in a non-weight-bearing position). The underlying aetiology is multi-factorial and may be secondary to trauma, limb conformation and degenerative changes. Mediolateral and caudocranial views should be obtained of both stifles, as cranial cruciate disease is commonly bilateral. If a tibial osteotomy is planned, then additional mediolateral radiographs of the entire crus are required to allow measurement of the tibial angle.

Predisposing factors: Several anatomical factors have been reported to predispose to the development of cranial cruciate ligament disease. These may be seen radiologically as:

- A steep caudal slope to the tibial plateau due to premature closure of the caudal part of the proximal tibial physis. This is reported mainly in terrier breeds
- A narrow intercondylar notch has been associated with cranial cruciate ligament disease.

Radiological features: The radiographic changes due to osteoarthritis include:

- Reduced size of the infrapatellar fatpad
- Osteophyte formation on the poles of the patella, trochlear ridges, fabellae and margins of the femorotibial joint
- Specific changes include:
  - Distal displacement of the popliteal sesamoid bone (Figure 7.115)
  - Localized subchondral cyst formation and sclerosis in the tibial plateau in the region of the intercondylar eminences
  - Cranial displacement of the tibia relative to the femoral condyles (uncommonly seen, but occasionally present with total rupture of the cranial cruciate ligament)
  - Small focal areas of dystrophic mineralization within the joint in the region of the cruciate ligaments
  - In traumatic cases (usually young adult dogs), an avulsion fracture within the intercondylar eminence or tibial plateau at the level of the insertion or origin of the cruciate ligaments may be seen (see Figure 7.65).

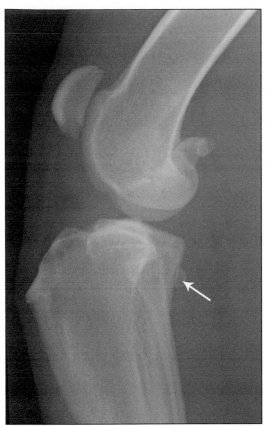

7.115 Mediolateral view of a dog with cranial cruciate ligament disease. Note the distal displacement of the popliteal sesamoid bone (arrowed), which is suggestive of the disease. Other changes seen with cranial cruciate ligament disease are non-specific and largely relate to secondary osteoarthritis.

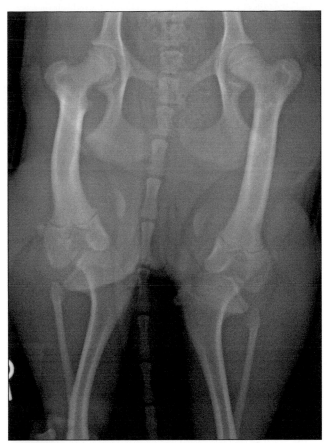

7.116 VD view of the pelvis and pelvic limbs of a dog with severe medial patellar luxation. The patellae are visible lying medial to the stifle joints and there is deformity of the femoral and tibial bones. The tibial tuberosities are rotated medially.

Medial patellar luxation: This is a common condition, particularly in terriers and small breeds. Animals present with skipping lameness. There are four grades of severity, with grades 1 and 2 usually having no radiographic abnormalities. There is usually concurrent deformity of the femur and tibia, which results in malalignment of the quadriceps apparatus. To assess long bone deformity, the entire pelvic limb should be imaged.

Radiological features:

- Medial displacement of the patella relative to the femoral trochlea. The apparent position of the patella on the caudocranial view varies with the degree of internal rotation and, unless the stifle is straight, accurate assessment of the patella is difficult.
- Medial displacement of tibial tuberosity relative to femoral trochlea.
- Medial bowing of the distal femur and lateral bowing of the proximal crus ('bow-legged' conformation) (Figure 7.116).
- Hypoplasia of the medial femoral condyle.
- The mediolateral view is usually normal, unless grade 4 disease is present, in which case the patella appears caudally positioned overlying the femoral condyles.
- There is usually minimal/no joint effusion.
- A craniodistal–cranioproximal oblique (CrDi-CrPrO) (skyline) view may show shallow trochlea.

Lateral patellar luxation: This is less common than medial patellar luxation and occurs primarily in large- and giant-breed dogs. It is usually associated with genu valgum deformity of the femur and tibia, which results in a 'knock-kneed' conformation (Figure 7.117). Radiographs are required to assess for abnormal conformation and should include the femur.

Trauma: Severe external trauma may result in ligamentous and soft tissue injuries, in addition to fractures and osseous injury. Instability of the stifle is normally easily detected on clinical examination, but instability and subluxation may not be visible on standard radiographic views.

Osteochondritis dissecans: This is an uncommon condition and primarily occurs in large-breed dogs. Affected animals often present as young adults. A lateral oblique view may be helpful in visualizing flattening of the femoral condyle. OCD lesions occur most commonly on the medial aspect of the lateral femoral condyle, usually on the distal or caudal surface. Lesions are less commonly seen on the medial condyle (lateral aspect). Defects are often more easily visualized on the mediolateral view. Visualization of condyle flattening on the caudocranial view is only possible if the X-ray beam is tangential to the lesion. The normal focal depression of the extensor fossa within the lateral condyle at the origin of the long digital extensor tendon should not be mistaken for an OCD lesion.

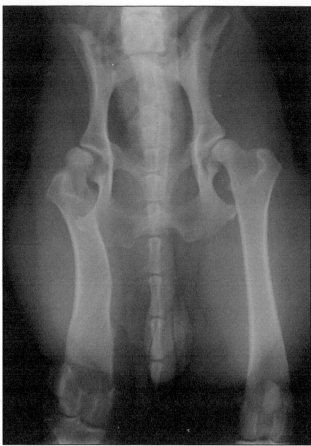

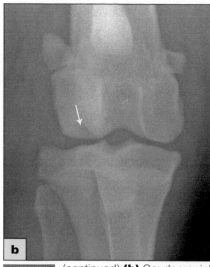

7.118 (continued) **(b)** Caudocranial view of the stifle of an Akita with OCD of the stifle. The predilection site for OCD in the stifle is the medial aspect of the lateral femoral condyle. The typical saucer-shaped defect (arrowed) is often easiest to see on slightly oblique mediolateral views. A mineralized fragment is present within the recess of the joint cavity proximal to the patella. On the caudocranial view, the normal extensor fossa should not be mistaken for an OCD lesion. In this case, the flattening of the lateral condyle is visible.

- In some cases, a mineralized cartilage flap may be present and fragments can be seen adjacent to the flattened condyle or within the joint space following migration (Figure 7.118).

Avulsion of the long digital extensor tendon: This is a rare condition, primarily see in immature large- and giant-breed dogs.

Radiological features:

- Defect in the extensor fossa of the lateral femoral condyle.
- Localized new bone formation on the lateral femoral condyle centred on the extensor fossa.
- Localized mineralization/fragments within the soft tissues immediately distal to the extensor fossa (Figure 7.119).

7.117 VD view of the pelvis and pelvic limbs of a Bullmastiff with lateral patellar luxation. There is genu valgum deformity with medial bowing of the limb and the patella can be seen lying lateral to the stifle. Note the abnormal conformation of the hip joint, which can also be associated with patellar luxation.

Radiological features:

- Signs of stifle effusion in most cases, with reduced size of the infrapatellar fatpad.
- Localized flattening of the caudodistal part of the lateral femoral condyle with focal lucency in the subchondral bone (Figure 7.118).
- Localized sclerosis of the condyle adjacent to the defect.

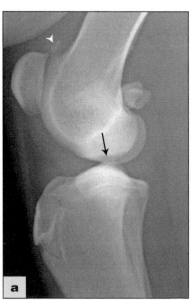

7.118 **(a)** Mediolateral view of the stifle of an Akita with OCD of the stifle. The predilection site for OCD in the stifle is the medial aspect of the lateral femoral condyle. The typical saucer-shaped defect (arrowed) is often easiest to see on slightly oblique mediolateral views. A mineralized fragment (arrowhead) is present within the recess of the joint cavity proximal to the patella. (continues) ▶

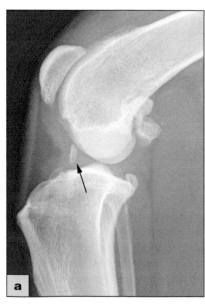

7.119 **(a)** Mediolateral view of the stifle of a dog with avulsion of the long digital extensor tendon. The avulsed bony fragment (arrowed) is usually seen immediately distal to the extensor fossa and there may be a defect visible within the lateral femoral condyle at the origin of the tendon. (continues) ▶

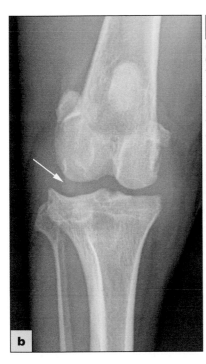

7.119

(continued)
(b) Caudocranial view of the stifle of a dog with avulsion of the long digital extensor tendon. The avulsed bony fragment (arrowed) is usually seen immediately distal to the extensor fossa and there may be a defect visible within the lateral femoral condyle at the origin of the tendon.

7.120 Mediolateral views of **(a)** the right and **(b)** the left stifle of a dog showing tibial tuberosity avulsions in both limbs. Avulsion fractures occur predominately in young animals and may occur spontaneously with no history of external trauma. The proximal displacement of the tibial tuberosity is the consequence of pull from the quadriceps muscle.

Crus

Standard radiographic views

- Mediolateral view:
  - The animal is placed in lateral recumbency with the leg of interest dependent and the upper limb retracted
  - The X-ray beam is centred on the mid-crus and collimated to include the stifle and tarsal joints.
- Craniocaudal/caudocranial view:
  - The animal is placed in dorsal recumbency, ensuring that the crus is straight (as for the dorsoplantar view of the tarsus; see below)
  - The X-ray beam is centred on the mid-crus and collimated to include the stifle and tarsus.

Radiological interpretation
The approach to interpretation of radiographs of the crus follows the same principles as for the other long bones. The radiological abnormalities seen mirror those of the other long bones.

Common diseases

Fractures: The crus is a common site for fractures, which can occur in a wide range of configurations and commonly involve both the tibia and fibula.

Avulsion of the tibial tuberosity: This occurs in young animals when the tibial tuberosity physis is open. It may occur with a history of minimal trauma and is occasionally bilateral. The pull from the quadriceps muscle results in widening of the physis and, if there is complete avulsion, the tibial tuberosity and patella may be abnormally proximally located (Figure 7.120).

Primary bone tumours: The proximal tibia is a common site for osteosarcoma, which despite the close proximity does not extend to involve the fibula (see above).

Tarsus
The tarsus is a complex joint involving seven tarsal bones, four major joints (talocrural/tibiotarsal joint, proximal intertarsal joint, centrodistal joint and tarsometatarsal joint) and multiple intertarsal joints between the individual tarsal bones. The only joint with significant motion is the talocrural joint, which is a hinge joint exhibiting predominately flexion and extension. Limited motion occurs between the intertarsal and tarsometatarsal joints due to the numerous intertarsal ligaments. There is little soft tissue covering the tarsus and radiologically the soft tissues largely conform to the bone surface.

Standard radiographic views
A standard radiographic examination should include mediolateral and dorsoplantar views. In cases of tarsal fractures, and if lesions are not clearly seen on standard views, lateral oblique views should be obtained. Stressed radiography is useful in cases of suspected instability or ligamentous injury. Evaluation of the lateral ridge of the talus may be difficult due to superimposition of the calcaneus.

- Mediolateral view:
  - A table top technique with a detail film–screen combination should be used
  - The patient is placed in lateral recumbency with the leg of interest dependent and the upper limb retracted (Figure 7.121)
  - The tarsus should be in a neutral position (overflexion and overextension should be avoided). To prevent axial rotation of the tarsus, placing a sandbag over the proximal part of the limb should be considered
  - The X-ray beam is centred just distal to the medial and lateral malleoli on the tibiotarsal joint, and collimated to include the distal third of the tibia and the distal metatarsal bones.
- Plantarodorsal/dorsoplantar view:
  - Either a plantarodorsal or dorsoplantar view can be obtained, but if there is restricted extension

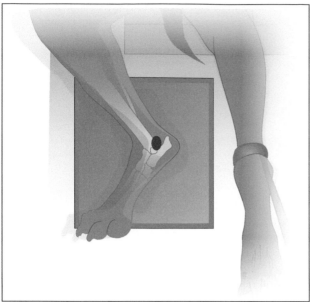

7.121 Patient positioning for a mediolateral view of the tarsus.

of the limb (e.g. due to hip disease) it is easier to extend the tarsus for a plantarodorsal view. The main problems are axial rotation of the tarsus due to tilting of the thorax/abdomen and failure to rotate the stifle internally

- A table top technique should be used
- For a plantarodorsal view, the animal should be placed in a prone position. For a dorsoplantar view, the animal should be placed in dorsal recumbency with a sandbag placed over the stifle/proximal limb to extend the limb (Figure 7.122)

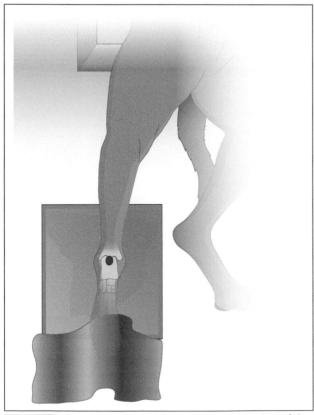

7.122 Patient positioning for a dorsoplantar view of the tarsus.

- Excessive tilting can be prevented by placing sandbags beside the thorax
- For a plantarodorsal view it can be helpful to adduct and elevate the contralateral limb, which is flexed and placed on a foam pad/block. This counters the tendency of the affected limb to rotate externally
- The affected tarsus should be extended with care taken not to rotate the limb
- The affected tarsus should be positioned on the cassette
- The X-ray beam is centred in the midline, just distal to the malleoli, and collimated to include the distal third of the tibia and the distal metatarsal bones.

Special views:

- Flexed dorsoplantar view:
  - This view is used to skyline the trochlear ridges of the talus and tibiotarsal joint without superimposition of the calcaneous
  - A table top technique should be used
  - The animal is placed in dorsal recumbency in a positioning trough to prevent tilting of the thorax and abdomen
  - The joint under investigation should be elevated and placed on a block so that both the stifle and tarsus are flexed approximately 90 degrees (Figure 7.123)
  - The cassette is placed on top of the block and under the caudal aspect of the distal tibia and tarsus
  - The tibiotarsal joint should be flexed approximately 90 degrees by placing a sandbag or pad adjacent to the plantar surface of the metatarsal bones
  - The X-ray beam is centred on the tibiotarsal joint and collimated to include the distal third of the tibia.

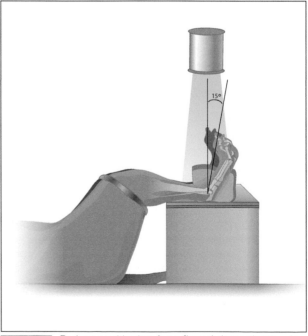

7.123 Patient positioning for a flexed dorsoplantar view of the tarsus.

- Plantaromedial–dorsolateral oblique (PIM-DLO) and plantarolateral–dorsomedial oblique (PIL-DMO) views:
  - Many tarsal fractures and some OCD lesions may not be clearly visible on standard views. Oblique views should be obtained in cases of suspected tarsal trauma or lameness where the cause is not apparent on standard radiographic views
  - The animal should be positioned as for a standard plantarodorsal/dorsoplantar view, but for a plantaromedial–dorsolateral or dorsomedial–plantarolateral oblique view the thorax and abdomen should be rotated towards the side being investigated. For the opposite oblique view, the limb and body should be rotated away from the side being investigated
  - The tarsus should be rotated approximately 45 degrees
  - The X-ray beam is centred in the midline, just distal to the malleoli and collimated to include the distal third of the tibia and the distal metatarsal bones.

Radiological assessment

The many small bones of the tarsus make interpretation of radiographs challenging, particularly in small dogs and cats. As with all joints, the soft tissues should be assessed for the presence of joint effusion (Figure 7.124), periarticular soft tissue swelling and swelling in the region of the Achilles tendon. The soft tissues of the tarsus are in close apposition with the bones, making soft tissue swelling or effusion easily seen. The talocrural joint space is a narrow joint space with articular surfaces in close apposition. The talocrural joint space should be uniform in width and is best assessed on the dorsoplantar view. On the mediolateral view, the talar ridges should form a smooth even curve. The intertarsal and tarsometatarsal joint spaces are only clearly visualized if the X-ray beam is parallel with the joint space. Poor visualization of the dorsal aspect of the distal intertarsal joint space is often normal due to the poor alignment of the X-ray beam and the joint space. Osteoarthritis of the tibiotarsal joint commonly results in new bone formation on the margins of the distal tibia, especially on the plantar aspect, on the malleoli, talus and calcaneus adjacent to the malleoli. New bone formation on the plantar aspect of the tarsus or on the tuber calcanei usually indicates chronic ligamentous injury. Smooth, bridging new bone on the dorsal aspect of the centrodistal joint is often seen as an apparently incidental finding in dogs but can be associated with lameness (see below).

Key features to assess include:

- Congruency and width of the joint spaces
- Presence and location of any soft tissue swelling
- Subchondral bone for sclerosis or irregularity
- Periarticular new bone formation.

Common diseases

Osteochondritis dissecans: This is commonly seen in medium and large-breed dogs, with Labrador Retrievers and Rottweilers predisposed. OCD lesions most commonly affect the medial ridge of the talus, but can be seen on the lateral ridge. Lateral ridge lesions may be difficult to visualize due to superimposition of the calcaneus.

Radiological features:

- Joint effusion and soft tissue swelling associated with the tibiotarsal joint is present in almost all cases. This is often easiest to see on the plantarodorsal view.
- Flattening of the talar ridge, which results in focal widening of the tibiotarsal joint space.
- Sclerosis of the talar ridge adjacent to the area of flattening (Figure 7.125).
- If the cartilage flap is mineralized, small intra-articular mineralized bodies may be seen adjacent to the area of flattening or the defect in the talar ridge.
- Secondary osteoarthritis may be present.
- Fragmentation of the medial malleolus/small areas of calcification within the soft tissues distal the medial malleolus may represent a manifestation of OCD or dystrophic calcification.

Plantar ligament degeneration/rupture: Degeneration of the plantar ligament occurs most commonly in Rough Collies and Shetland Sheepdogs. As the changes are often bilateral, the contralateral hock should be imaged. Degeneration of the plantar ligaments results in hyperextension of the proximal intertarsal joint. There is often concurrent degeneration/rupture of the palmar carpal ligaments. Stressed radiographs may be required to demonstrate hyperextension and subluxation/luxation of the

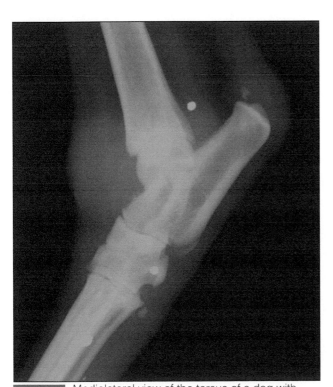

7.124 Mediolateral view of the tarsus of a dog with severe tibiotarsal joint effusion. Note that the swelling is confined to the margins of the tibiotarsal space. There is also concurrent swelling of the Achilles tendon and gunshot pellets within the tarsus.

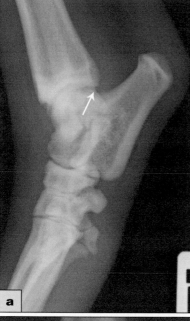

7.125

(a) Mediolateral and **(b)** dorsoplantar views of the tarsus of a Labrador Retriever with OCD. There is a moderately severe joint effusion, which is present in most cases of tarsal OCD. Due to the defect in the medial ridge of the talus, there is widening of the medial aspect (arrowhead) of the tibiotarsal joint space. The mediolateral view shows flattening of the talus proximally (arrowed), but this is easily overlooked due to superimposition.

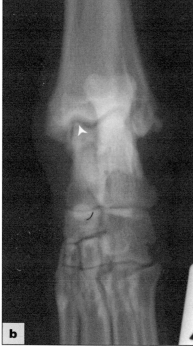

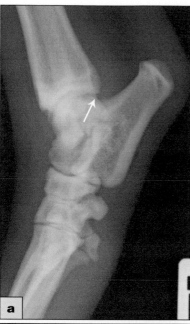

7.126 Mediolateral view of the tarsus of a dog with chronic plantar ligament degeneration and rupture. There is hyperextension of the proximal intertarsal joint and swelling of the soft tissues on the plantar surface of the tarsus. Extensive new bone formation on the plantar surface of the joint is common.

- Enthesophyte formation on the dorsal aspect of the talocentral and centrodistal joints is often present.
- Subluxation of the proximal intertarsal joints.

Fractures: A large number of fracture configurations occur within the hock. The majority of tarsal fractures are the result of external trauma, except in working dogs where fractures may occur during exercise. In racing Greyhounds, the hock (almost invariably the right hock) is the most common location for fractures. Radiological evaluation of the extent of hock fractures can be difficult due to the complex anatomy and lateral oblique views should be obtained (Figure 7.127). Fractures of the malleoli are common and often associated with damage to the collateral ligaments, which may be seen on stressed radiographs. Fragmentation of the malleoli (most commonly the medial malleolus) may occur in association with tarsal OCD and can be difficult radiologically to differentiate from small avulsion fractures.

Calcanean (Achilles) tendon injuries: The majority of Achilles tendon injuries are chronic and occur in medium and large-breed dogs (especially Dobermanns and Labrador Retrievers). Acute injuries may also occur, often following penetrating injury.

Radiological features:

- Soft tissue swelling proximal to the tuber calcanei, with the swelling centred on the Achilles tendon.
- In chronic cases, there are usually small irregular areas of calcification within the soft tissue swelling proximal to the tuber calcanei (see Figure 7.35).

hock. Traumatic rupture of the plantar ligaments may occur in any breed and, as it is an acute injury, radiographic changes show no signs of chronicity (new bone formation, dystrophic mineralization). Subluxation of the tarsometatarsal joint is less commonly seen than proximal intertarsal joint subluxation and is usually traumatic in origin.

Radiological features:

- Soft tissue swelling along the plantar aspect of the hock.
- Dystrophic mineralization within the soft tissues plantar to the tarsus (chronic cases) (Figure 7.126).
- Periosteal new bone formation on the plantarodistal aspect of the calcaneus, the plantar process of the central tarsal bone, the plantar aspect of the fourth tarsal bone and the plantaroproximal aspect of the metatarsal bones.

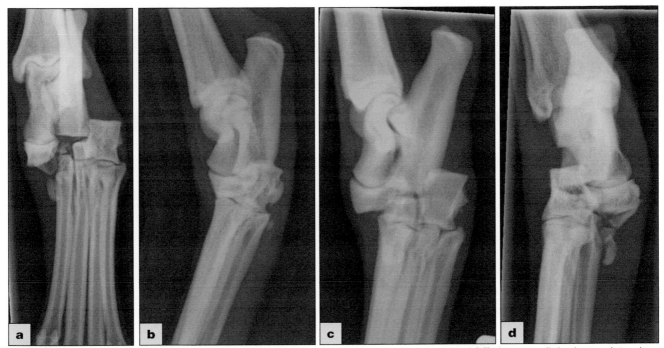

7.127 **(a)** Mediolateral, **(b)** dorsoplantar, **(c)** dorsolateral–plantaromedial oblique and **(d)** dorsomedial–plantarolateral oblique views of the tarsus of a dog with multiple tarsal fractures. Due to the complex anatomy of the tarsus, radiography underestimates the severity and degree of comminution of tarsal fractures. In this case, there is subluxation of the centrodistal joint and calcaneoquartal joint and comminuted fractures of the central tarsal bone.

- Avulsion of the insertion of the tendon from the calcaneus often results in a focal defect within the cortex of the tuber calcanei.
- In chronic cases, sclerosis and localized enthesophyte formation is present on the proximal aspect of the tuber calcanei.

Centrodistal joint lameness: Lameness associated with the centrodistal joint is seen as a cause of lameness, typically in athletic dogs (e.g. Greyhounds and Border Collies). Clinical examination shows pain when stressing the medial axis of the tarsus. The radiological changes seen with centrodistal lameness are also seen in asymptomatic dogs and careful clinical examination is required to determine the significance of the radiological changes. Lesions are often bilateral and both hocks should be radiographed.

Radiological features:

- Focal new bone formation on dorsal aspect of the centrodistal joint visible on the mediolateral views.
- Enthesopathy of the central plantar ligament on the distal calcaneous.
- Sclerosis of the central and 1st to 3rd tarsal bones.

Pes

The radiographic technique and radiological interpretation of the pes are the same as for the manus (see above).

References and further reading

Adams WM (2000) Radiographic diagnosis of hip dysplasia in the young dog. *Veterinary Clinics of North America: Small Animal Practice.* **30**(2), 267–280
Barr FJ and Kirberger RM (2006) *BSAVA Manual of Canine and Feline Musculoskeletal Imaging.* BSAVA Publications, Gloucester
Dennis R (2012) Interpretation and use of BVA/KC hip scores in dogs. *In Practice* **34**, 178–194
Douglas SW, Herrtage ME and Williamson HD (1987) Canine Radiography: Skeletal System. In: *Principles of Veterinary Radiography, 4th edn.* pp. 141–176. Bailliere Tindall, Eastbourne
Guilliard MJ (2005) Centrodistal joint lameness in dogs. *Journal of Small Animal Practice* **46**(4), 199–202
Mahoney PN and Lamb CR (1996) Articular, periarticular and juxta-articular calcified bodies in the dog and cat: a radiographic review. *Veterinary Radiology and Ultrasound* **37**, 3–19
Marchevsky AM and Read RA (1999) Bacterial septic arthritis in 19 dogs. *Australian Veterinary Journal* **77**(4), 233–237
Thrall DE and Robertson ID (2011) The Thoracic Limb and The Pelvic Limb. In: *Atlas of Normal Radiographic Anatomy and Anatomic Variants in the Dog and Cat.* Elsevier Saunders, St Louis

Radiology of the head

Andrew Holloway and Avi Avner

There is little doubt that the cross-sectional imaging modalities of computed tomography (CT), magnetic resonance imaging (MRI) and diagnostic endoscopy are superior to radiography for the assessment of diseases involving the head. The limitations of radiography for imaging the head are that, whilst it is sensitive for detecting some diseases, it is insensitive for detecting others, and when disease is detected the extent of the changes may be underestimated. Despite this, radiography remains a primary diagnostic technique as it is widely available and inexpensive. In addition, it also allows the head to be surveyed before deciding if, and which, more expensive further investigations should be undertaken.

The skull is a complex bony structure enclosing the brain and the communicating air-containing structures of the nose, nasopharynx, oropharynx and auditory bullae. Surrounding soft tissue structures are limited to the masticatory muscles, salivary glands and supporting muscles of the neck. Therefore, although the skull has high inherent radiographic contrast and can be imaged using an X-ray tube with limited output, the principal challenge is posed by the superimposition and geometric complexity of the bones of the skull. However, as the skull is a symmetrical structure and disease frequently has a unilateral presentation, radiological assessment is aided by comparison with the unaffected side.

Interpretation of skull radiographs is assisted by achieving consistency in all aspects of radiographic technique. Accurate positioning of the animal with correct centring and collimation is essential, especially for dorsoventral (DV), ventrodorsal (VD) and rostrocaudal views, which allow the left and right sides to be compared. Even slight asymmetry in positioning may mimic disease or obscure pathology.

Indications

The clinical signs and localization of abnormalities determine how the radiographic study is performed, as specific oblique views are required for different parts of the skull (see below). General indications for survey radiography of the head include:

- Swelling of the head
- Pain associated with the head
- Airway obstruction
- Dysphagia
- Exophthalmos
- Nasal disease
- Aural disease.

Restraint and patient preparation

To avoid frustration and errors, and to ensure a consistent technique, general anaesthesia is preferred for studies of the head. Heavy sedation, or conscious radiographs in unstable animals, may be sufficient to obtain limited studies. Not all structures can be assessed on a single view and certain structures are better evaluated on specific views. Radiographic studies of the head, therefore, usually require at least two views.

A high-definition conventional film–screen combination (e.g. as used for mammography) or digital radiography should be used. Dental non-screen film is helpful for radiography of the teeth and, occasionally, the nasal cavity and mandibles in cats and small dogs. A grid is not necessary, except perhaps when imaging the skull of giant-breed dogs such as the St Bernard or mastiff breeds. Positioning devices such as radiolucent foam wedges or plastic gags for open-mouth views are essential. Any tape or ties used for positioning or fixing the endotracheal tube should be radiolucent. Radiopaque monitoring devices and the endotracheal tube may have to be temporarily removed to avoid obscuring important structures.

Standard radiographic views

The lateral and DV views described below are general views and usually performed in all cases. These views are supplemented and modified to assess specific anatomical structures, depending on the clinical signs. Additional views are described in detail in the relevant anatomical sections.

Laterolateral view: skull

- For a laterolateral view, the animal is positioned in lateral recumbency with the nose supported by a radiolucent foam wedge to achieve a mid-sagittal plane that is parallel to the cassette (Figure 8.1). In some animals, a foam wedge placed under the cranial neck is useful to prevent the nose from tilting upwards. Axial rotation should be avoided and the hard palate should be perpendicular to the table. The mandibles can be kept partially open to reduce superimposition of the dental structures and to better assess the air-filled oropharynx and structures over the base of the skull.

- Centring and collimation depends on the area of interest, which may be the whole skull or a more defined area such as the frontal sinuses. For the whole skull, the beam is centred midway between the orbit and the ear.
- On a correctly positioned lateral view, the bullae (and wings of the atlas) are superimposed on the contralateral structure.

superimposed. Thus, even significant unilateral disease of the nasal cavity and bony margins may be overlooked.

Dorsoventral and ventrodorsal views

- A DV or VD view can be performed. It is more difficult to position the head for a VD view. The DV view is often preferred as the skull is more stable and less likely to rotate axially when resting on the mandibles compared with the dorsum of the skull.
- For a DV view, the animal is positioned in sternal recumbency with the head extended and hard palate horizontal to the table (Figure 8.2). The cassette is placed on the table top underneath the

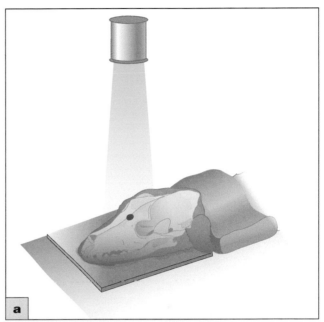

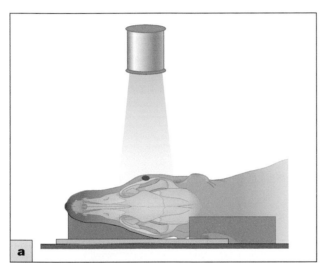

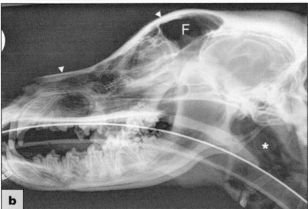

8.1 **(a)** Patient positioning for a lateral view. The nose is elevated to keep the sagittal plane parallel to the cassette. Centring depends on the region of interest, but is usually between the orbit and external ear canal. **(b)** The dorsal margins of the nasal and frontal bones (arrowheads) and the air-filled nasopharynx (*) and frontal sinus (F) are well visualized.

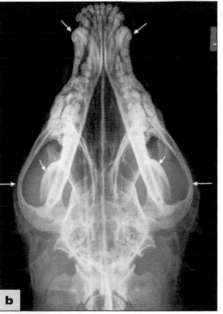

8.2 **(a)** Patient positioning for a DV view. For deep-chested dogs, the cassette can be elevated and supported on a block. Centring depends on the region of interest, but for survey radiographs it is usually between the eyes. For the bullae, the beam is centred on the horizontal ear canal. **(b)** On a well positioned radiograph, the maxillary canines, coronoid processes of the mandible and the zygomatic arches should all be symmetrical (arrowed).

The laterolateral view is used to evaluate the dorsal nasal cavity and frontal sinuses, the margin of the nasal and frontal bones, and the dorsal margin of the calvarium. This view can also be used to assess the cribriform plate. It is the view best suited to examine the nasopharynx, the retropharyngeal area and hyoid apparatus. The limitation of the laterolateral view is that bilateral structures are mandibles. In deep-chested dogs, it may be necessary to elevate the head and cassette on a level pad or box to ensure that the hard palate remains perpendicular to the cassette. The film–focal distance should be adjusted accordingly. Adhesive tape placed across the bridge of the nose or a sandbag placed across the neck may be used to achieve stable positioning.

■ For a VD view, the animal is positioned in dorsal recumbency in a trough with a foam pad beneath the neck and the forelimbs extended caudally (Figure 8.3). The head is extended so that the hard palate is horizontal to the table. The cassette is placed on the table underneath the head. It may be necessary to use foam wedges to avoid axial rotation.

■ Centring depends on the clinical signs, but for survey radiographs the beam is centred between the eyes. For middle ear disease, collimated views centred on the bullae should be obtained.

■ The endotracheal tube may need to be removed prior to exposure to prevent midline structures from being obscured.

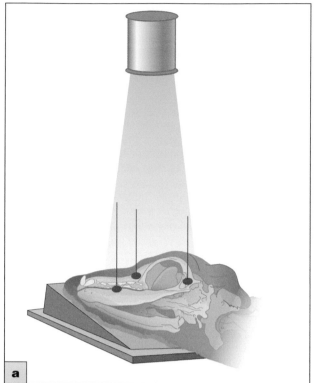

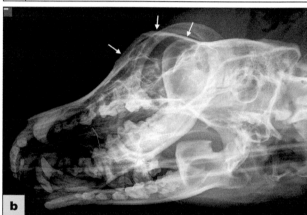

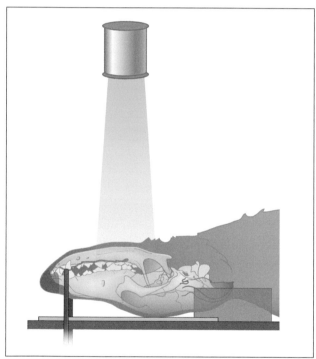

8.3   Patient positioning for a VD view. The hard palate must be parallel to the cassette. Supporting the neck and taping the muzzle help stabilize the skull.

DV and VD views are used to assess the lateral and caudal aspects of the skull, the external ear canal and middle ear, and the temporomandibular joints. VD/DV views are limited by superimposition of the mandibles on the lateral part of the nasal cavities and frontal sinuses. Thus, these views restrict assessment to the medial aspect of the nasal chambers, the caudal vomer, medial frontal sinuses and the cribriform plate. This view should not be used as a substitute for intraoral views of the nose.

Lateral oblique view

Lateral oblique views (Figure 8.4) are used to assess the bullae, the maxillary and mandibular premolars,

8.4   **(a)** Patient positioning for a lateral oblique view of the skull. Lateral oblique views are used to assess the frontal sinuses, the bullae and the maxillary and mandibular dental arcades. The skull is rotated axially toward the DV or VD position (approximately 30 degrees) in order to place the region of interest closest to the film. Rotation toward the DV position (shown) is used to evaluate the frontal sinuses and mandibular dentition, whilst rotation toward the VD position is used to assess the tympanic bullae and maxillary dentition. To examine the dental arcades, the jaw is opened. **(b)** The lateral region of the frontal sinus is projected dorsally (arrowed) and skylined using a lateral oblique view.

and the frontal sinuses. Patient positioning for imaging each of these structures is described later in the text. All involve axial rotation of the skull around the sagittal plane. The degree of rotation is dictated by the area under investigation. The jaws are open when assessing the dental arcades. Where structures are not adequately visualized, exposures must be repeated after adjusting the degree of obliquity. The degree of obliquity can be dictated to some extent by skull conformation. Wider skulls require less rotation to separate structures located laterally, whereas narrow skulls require greater rotation.

Rostrocaudal view: sinuses and calvarium

- For a closed-mouth rostrocaudal view, the animal is positioned in dorsal recumbency in a trough with the forelimbs extended caudally (Figure 8.5). The head is flexed so that the nose is vertical. The cassette is placed beneath the back of the head. The hard palate should be perpendicular to the cassette.

- The profile of the frontal sinuses is projected dorsal to the nasal chambers by centring the vertical X-ray beam on the hard palate/nose. If the nose is rotated too far dorsally, or if the beam is centred too far ventrally, then the nasal chambers are projected over the frontal sinuses. The degree of flexion depends on skull conformation and area of interest. A greater degree of flexion is required to visualize the cranium. In animals with a brachycephalic conformation, or dome-shaped calvarium, the sinuses are attenuated or absent, which limits the usefulness of this view.

- Positioning can be technically difficult and the use of positioning aids (e.g. foam pads, sandbags) and tape is inevitably necessary.

- Care should be taken to prevent the endotracheal tube kinking and obstructing air flow.

The rostrocaudal view is used to evaluate the frontal sinuses. It can also be used to examine the calvarium, particularly the zygomatic arches, to assess for displacement of fracture fragments in cases of trauma and for temporomandibular joint disease associated with lateral displacement of the coronoid process, resulting in 'open-mouth' jaw locking.

Intraoral views

Dorsoventral view

- For a DV intraoral view, the animal is placed in sternal recumbency with the head extended and hard palate parallel to the table top (Figure 8.6). In deep-chested dogs, it may be helpful to raise the head on a block or pad.

- For conventional radiography, a flexible cassette comprising a protective plastic envelope containing an intensifying screen, the film and rigid backing is used. For computed radiography systems, the detector plate can be removed from a conventional cassette and placed in the protective envelope, although care must be taken not to damage the detector phosphor. After exposure, the detector plate is replaced in the conventional cassette, and identified and processed by the digitizer as normal.

- The flexible cassette is placed in the mouth, corner first, as far caudally as possible. The beam is centred on the midline midway between the nasal planum and the orbits. To avoid damage to the envelope–screen and to relax the masticatory muscles, allowing the envelope to be positioned sufficiently caudally, the procedure must be performed under general anaesthesia. Pressure damage to the screen and envelope should then be avoided.

- In most mesaticephalic and dolichocephalic dogs, well positioned intraoral films visualize the entire nasal cavity including the cribriform plate. As any rotation of the head results in asymmetry, the flexible cassette should be supported with foam pads to ensure that it is parallel to the hard palate and the table. In smaller dogs and cats, the endotracheal tube frequently causes rotation of the head. This can be minimized by securing the endotracheal tube to the mandible, supporting the flexible cassette and the anaesthetic circuit. In brachycephalic dogs it may be difficult to push the envelope sufficiently caudally and the study is limited to evaluation of the rostral nasal chambers and the premaxilla.

As there is no superimposition of extraneous structures, the DV intraoral view is preferred for assessing

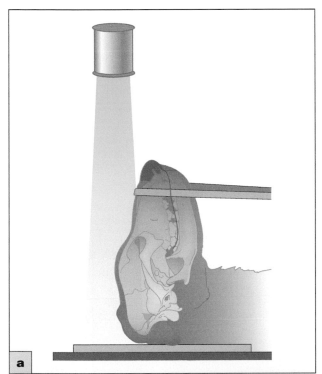

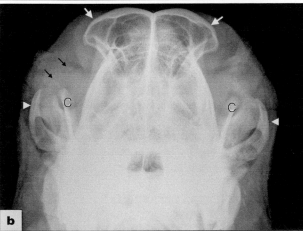

8.5 **(a)** Patient positioning for a rostrocaudal view of the frontal sinuses and calvarium. On this view, the frontal sinuses are projected above the nose and remainder of the calvarium. **(b)** The zygomatic arches (arrowheads), frontal sinuses (white arrows) and coronoid processes (C) of the mandible can be assessed. The orbital ligament is occasionally recognized as a dense opaque structure, extending between the zygomatic arch and frontal bone (black arrows).

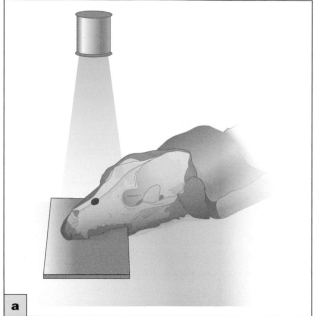

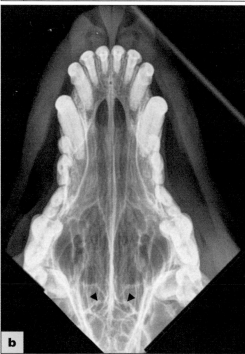

8.6 **(a)** Patient positioning for a DV intraoral view of the nasal chambers. The flexible cassette must be placed in the mouth as far caudally as possible. **(b)** Dental and nasal structures should be symmetrical and the cribriform plate (arrowheads) included on the film.

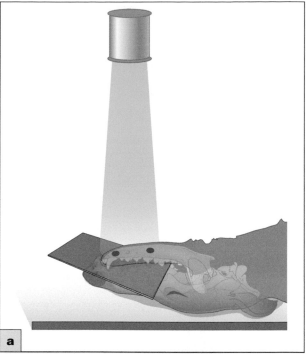

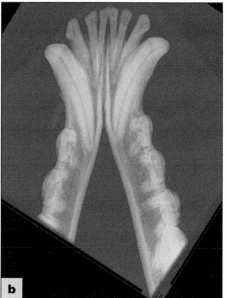

8.7 **(a)** Patient positioning for a VD intraoral view of the mandible. The plate is advanced as far caudally as possible whilst avoiding rotation. **(b)** The mandibular rami and arcades should be symmetrical.

and comparing the nasal cavities and paranasal sinuses. The maxilla and premaxilla, and in some animals the cribriform plate, can also be assessed.

Ventrodorsal view: mandible

- For the VD intraoral view, the animal is placed in dorsal recumbency with the head extended (Figure 8.7). A flexible cassette is placed corner first within the mouth as far caudally as possible. Both the mandible and the cassette should be parallel to the table. To support the head and cassette, a foam wedge is placed caudally beneath the neck; this also helps to prevent axial rotation and the nose from tipping up.

- The beam is centred midway between the mandibular symphysis and the angle of the jaw to assess the mandible. To assess the mandibular incisors and canines, the beam is centred on the symphysis. The beam can be angled to obtain a minimally distorted view of these teeth (see bisecting angle technique).

The VD intraoral view can be used to assess the mandibular symphysis, the incisor and canine teeth, the rostral mandibular rami and provide a limited assessment of the dental arcades.

Lesion-oriented oblique views

Oblique views are used to evaluate the surface and margins of swellings or changes otherwise projected *en face* or superimposed by other structures on conventional views. Lesion-oriented oblique views highlight swellings on the surface of the skull bones. The swelling is placed as close to the cassette as possible, to avoid magnification, and the beam or skull angled to produce the largest, true, undistorted shadow of the swelling. Exposure factors may have to be adjusted (usually reduced) to avoid overexposure.

Contrast studies

Contrast studies of the skull are only occasionally performed (see Chapter 4). MRI and CT have widely replaced the need for such studies because they are cross-sectional techniques, which overcome the limitations of superimposition that occur with two-dimensional (2D) radiographic images, and provide excellent contrast resolution of the skull tissues. Nonetheless, contrast procedures may still prove valuable as long as case selection is appropriate, the expectations of the study are carefully considered and the study is correctly performed. Dacryocystography, sialography and sinography (occasionally) are the most commonly performed procedures using positive contrast media. These studies are used primarily to demonstrate the integrity of the ducts and communication with abnormal structures. CT using the same radiographic techniques would be the method of choice if available.

Radiological interpretation

A systematic evaluation of the skull is required. As for other structures, the soft tissues should be evaluated first but are often easily overlooked. On DV, intraoral and rostrocaudal views, the two sides are projected as mirror images of each another, and the left and right sides should be compared. It is useful to examine the radiograph from right to left. Bony structures should be assessed for changes in shape and integrity, and air-filled structures compared to determine whether there has been any increase in soft tissue opacity.

The radiographic interpretation should focus on determining whether:

- All structures remain symmetrical. This applies to the bones of the skull in particular, but the symmetry of the soft tissue air-filled structures must not be overlooked
- The air in the nasal chambers, paranasal sinuses, nasopharynx and bullae has been displaced or replaced by soft tissue or osseous changes
- Bone and dental structures are intact
- Masses palpated or visualized involve bone
- Extraneous (foreign) material is present.

Normal anatomy

The normal anatomy of the skull is complex and varies markedly with breed and species (Figure 8.8). The conformation of the skull can be divided into three morphological groups:

- Dolichocephalic: nasal area (facial length) is longer than the cranium (cranial length) (Figure 8.9a). Breed examples include Greyhounds, Rough Collies and Whippets

- Mesaticephalic: nasal area is equal in length with the cranium (Figure 8.9b). Breed examples include Labrador Retrievers, spaniels and most crossbreeds
- Brachycephalic: nasal area is shorter than the cranium and the facial part of the skull is broad (Figure 8.9c). Breed examples include Cavalier King Charles Spaniels, Boxers, Bulldogs, Pekingese and Pugs. This conformation represents a form of chondrodysplasia, which results in shortening and widening of the skull. It is associated with many differences in skull anatomy compared with dolichocephalic and mesaticephalic dogs. For example, the frontal sinuses are small or absent, the nares are narrowed, the turbinates are crowded and distorted, the soft palate is thickened and elongated, and dental and laryngeal abnormalities as well as tracheal hypoplasia may be present. Some, but not all, of these changes may be associated with disease. In brachycephalic airway syndrome, many of the changes mentioned above result in increased airway resistance, leading to obstructive airway disease. The challenge to the clinician when evaluating radiographs from brachycephalic breeds, is to distinguish 'normal' brachycephalic anatomical traits from those associated with disease in individual animals. When general anaesthesia is planned for radiographic studies in brachycephalic breeds, consideration should be given to any potential complications that may arise, in particular during recovery from the anaesthetic.

Anatomically, the head can be divided into six main divisions:

- Nasal cavity and paranasal sinuses
- Cranial cavity and calvarium
- Masticatory structures (maxillofacial and dentition)
- Temporomandibular joint
- Auditory structures
- Oropharynx, nasopharynx and larynx (the oesophagus is covered in Chapter 5).

Nasal cavity and paranasal sinuses

- The nose forms part of the facial skull and is one of the areas most affected by the variation in skull morphology in the dog and to a lesser extent in the cat. The nasal cavity (Figure 8.10) extends from the external nares rostrally to the cribriform plate and nasopharynx caudally. It is divided into two halves by the nasal septum and is lined by scrolled conchae (turbinates). The air in the nasal chamber allows the turbinates and nasal conchae to be identified.
- The turbinates have a fine, alternating pattern of mineralization and air. The turbinate detail is best recognized in long-nosed dogs. There are two major types of turbinates present in the nasal cavity: the nasal turbinate and the ethmoidal turbinates. The nasal turbinates consist of the dorsal and ventral conchae, which arise from the medial maxilla. Rostrally, these conchae fill the nasal vestibule. The dorsal conchae are small. The

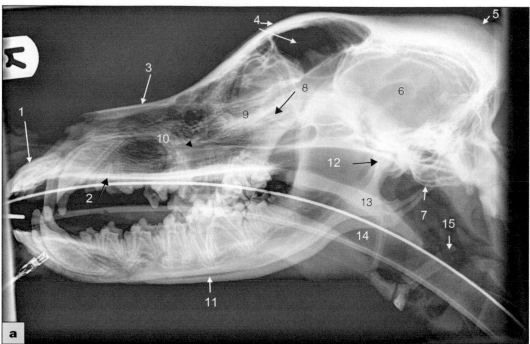

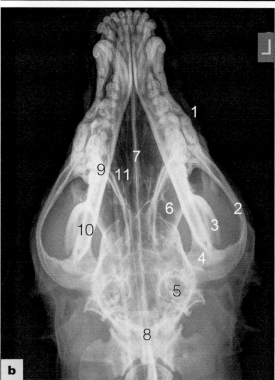

8.8 Normal skull anatomy of the dog. **(a)** Lateral view.
1 = incisive bone; 2 = hard palate (maxilla); 3 = nasal bone;
4 = frontal bone and sinuses; 5 = external occipital protuberance
(calvarium); 6 = cranial vault; 7 = tympanic bullae; 8 = cribriform plate;
9 = ethmoturbinates; 10 = nasal (or maxillary) turbinates; 11 = body of
the mandible; 12 = temporomandibular joint; 13 = soft palate;
14 = oropharynx; 15 = pharynx and hyoid bone. **(b)** VD view.
1 = maxillary teeth; 2 = zygomatic arch; 3 = coronoid process of the
mandible; 4 = condyloid process of the mandible; 5 = tympanic bulla;
6 = frontal sinus; 7 = vomer; 8 = external occipital protuberance;
9 = body of the mandible; 10 = ramus of the mandible; 11 = nasal cavity
(obscured rostrally by mandible).

larger ventral conchae (or maxilloturbinates)
extend caudodorsally to fill the middle section of
the nasal chamber. The ethmoturbinates, which
arise from (and extend rostral to) the cribriform
plate, fill the caudal nasal cavity. There is a subtle
difference in the appearance from rostral to
caudal. The rostral nasal conchae have a fine,
linear, parallel appearance. The maxilloturbinates
in the middle third have a 'bubbly' or irregular
honeycomb appearance. The caudal
ethmoturbinates also have a linear, parallel
arrangement, but are thicker and more dense than
the rostral conchae. The basic turbinate anatomy
of the cat is similar to that of the dog, except that
in the cat the ethmoidal turbinates are larger and

the nasal turbinates are correspondingly smaller.
The turbinates are best seen on a DV intraoral view
in dogs and a lateral view in cats. The cribriform
plate, which is an extension of the ethmoid bone,
is a sieve-like division between the nasal cavity
and the cranial vault. It is seen in the caudal nasal
cavity as an opaque C or V shape on DV or VD
views. Destruction of any portion of the cribriform
plate suggests invasion into the cranial vault and
warrants cross-sectional imaging to determine the
true extent of any change.

■ The vomer is a grooved bone that extends the
length of the nasal cavity, dividing it into a left and
right nasal chamber. It only extends one-third of
the height of the nasal chamber. The cartilaginous

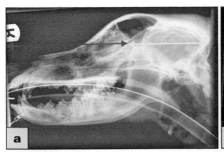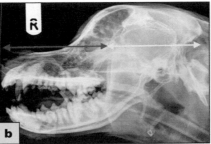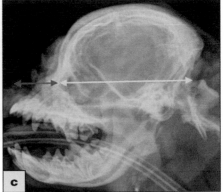

8.9 Lateral radiographs showing **(a)** dolichocephalic, **(b)** mesaticephalic and **(c)** brachycephalic skull conformation in the dog. Note that the facial length (red arrows) is markedly reduced in brachycephalic breeds compared with the length of the calvarium (yellow arrows).

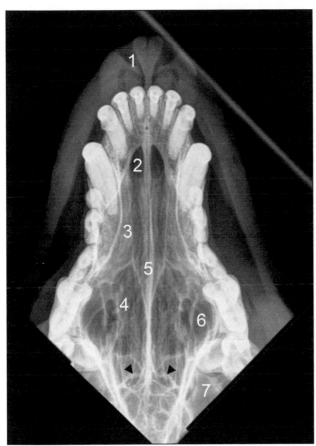

8.10 DV view showing the anatomy of the nose. The arrowheads denote the cribriform plate.
1 = nares; 2 = palatine fissure; 3 = maxilloturbinates;
4 = ethmoturbinates; 5 = vomer; 6 = maxillary recess;
7 = frontal sinus (medial recess).

They communicate with the nasal chambers via the frontonasal opening, which is not visible on radiographs.

■ On the DV view, the caudal aspect of the rami of the mandible is superimposed on, and obscures, the large lateral recesses of the frontal sinuses, so that only the medial aspect of the sinuses can be assessed. On the lateral view, the superimposed frontal sinuses are oval to triangular and should be air-filled on adequately exposed radiographs; any soft tissue opacity is abnormal. If the lateral view is axially rotated, the margin of the more dorsally projected sinus may mimic expansion or swelling of the bone. The two frontal sinuses are separated by an internal bony septum. This is best recognized on rostrocaudal skyline views. Partial internal separation is visible on skyline and lateral views.

■ The maxillary recesses can be identified on DV intraoral views in the dog. They lie medial to the caudal roots of the third premolar and the fourth premolar. They are not true sinuses, but air-filled expansions of the medial wall of the maxillary bone that communicate with the nasal chambers dorsally. This communication cannot be seen on radiographs but can be appreciated on cross-sectional images. The medial wall of the recess is a thin curved bony plate. The recess can fill with secretions or neoplastic tissue and the destruction of the bony margin is an important indicator of neoplasia. Cats do not have a maxillary recess.

■ The sphenoidal sinuses are large and air-filled in the cat and can be seen on lateral views dorsal to the nasopharynx. In the dog, they are filled with endoturbinates and cannot be visualized.

Cranial cavity and calvarium

■ The bony cranium is formed of 14 bones (four paired and six single) joined together by sutures (Figure 8.11).

■ The fontanelles are areas where two or more sutures join. Fontanelles and suture lines may remain open throughout life in some dogs with dome-shaped heads. They should not be mistaken for fractures on radiographs.

■ The calvarium is the roof of the cranium (excluding the facial and basal parts) and comprises flat bones (Figure 8.12). Some breeds tend to have a thick calvarium (e.g. English Bull Terrier, Bullmastiff, West Highland White Terrier).

septum is not seen on radiographs. The term composite vomer/septum is often used to refer to the combined entity. Displacement or erosion of the septum can only be inferred when a soft tissue mass is present, displacing the midline structure.

■ The paranasal sinuses in the dog comprise the frontal sinus and maxillary recess. These air-filled structures communicate with the nasal cavity. They are all paired structures. Each frontal bone is a diamond-shaped expansion, immediately rostral to the cranium, which contains the air-filled frontal sinuses. These are the largest of the paranasal sinuses in the dog and cat. They may be small or absent in brachycephalic breeds.

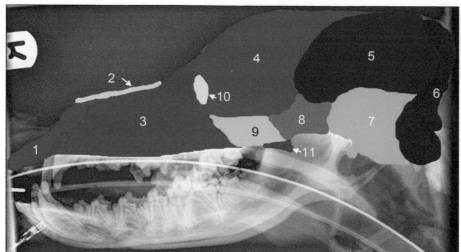

8.11   Bones of the skull.
1 = incisive; 2 = nasal;
3 = maxilla; 4 = frontal; 5 = parietal;
6 = occipital; 7 = temporal;
8 = sphenoid; 9 = palatine;
10 = lacrimal; 11 = pterygoid.

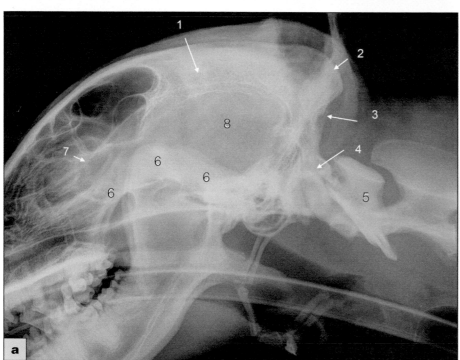

8.12   Normal anatomy of the calvarium. **(a)** Lateral view.
1 = parietal bone; 2 = external occipital
protuberance; 3 = occipital bone (basal); 4 = occipital condyle;
5 = atlas; 6 = zygomatic arch; 7 = cribriform plate; 8 = cranial
vault. **(b)** DV view. 1 = mandibular fossa; 2 = zygomatic arch;
3 = maxilla; 4 = vomer; 5 = frontal sinus; 6 = body of the
mandible; 7 = coronoid process of the mandible; 8 = condyloid
process of the mandible; 9 = tympanic bulla; 10 = occipital
condyle; 11 = mastoid process; 12 = paracondylar process.

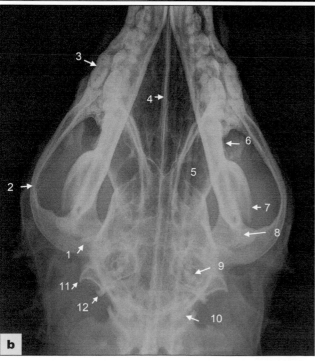

- The internal margin of the normal cranium has a slightly varying bone opacity, resulting in a 'copper beaten' appearance, due to the difference in thickness as it conforms to the underlying sulci and gyri of the brain. Some brachycephalic and toy breeds tend to have a dome-shaped cranium with thin constituent bones and a featureless internal margin. These dogs may have enlarged lateral ventricles of the brain (subclinical hydrocephalus).
- The basicranium forms the floor of the cranium, including the sphenoid and pterygoid bones, the dense petrous temporal bones, the mandibular fossa for articulation with the mandibles and the middle ear.
- The cranium is divided into a cranial and caudal fossa. On radiographs, this division is partially defined by the tentorium cerebelli osseum (a thin curvilinear plate of cortical bone, extending rostrally from the dorsal aspect of the occipital bone). The tentorium is indistinct on radiographs in many dogs, but is more obvious in the cat. The cranium of the cat is comparatively larger (compared with the rest of the skull) than that of the dog.
- The sagittal crest forms the dorsal margin of the calvarium and extends caudally to form the external occipital protuberance. It is very thick and prominent in some breeds of dog and less distinct in the cat. The occipital condyles are rounded protuberances of the caudal basicranium which articulate with the atlas (C1). They may be small and poorly defined in some brachycephalic and toy breeds or those with dome-shaped heads.
- The cribriform plate demarcates the boundary between the cranial and nasal cavities. It is a paired structure of thin, dense cortical bone. It appears as a bilobed U or V shape on DV views and a flattened C shape on lateral views.
- Ventrally, the petrous temporal bone forms the mandibular fossa (the dorsal aspect of the temporomandibular joint). The mandibular fossa is a semilunar depression in the petrous temporal bone, within which the condyloid process of the mandible articulates. The fossa is oriented perpendicular to the long axis of the skull, although in some breeds the fossa has a more oblique or even curved orientation (e.g. Cavalier King Charles Spaniels), with the medial aspect of the fossa advanced more rostrally than the lateral aspect. The retroarticular process of the mandibular fossa prevents caudal displacement of the condyloid process of the mandible. The cartilaginous meniscus of the temporomandibular joint is radiolucent.
- The bony orbit is formed medially by the caudal maxilla, lacrimal bone and rostroventral cranium, dorsolaterally by the lateral aspect of the frontal sinus, and laterally and rostrally by the zygomatic arch. The orbit is incomplete laterally. On rostrocaudal views of the skull, the orbital ligament may be identified as a dense soft tissue opacity, extending from the zygomatic arch to the frontal bone. It should not be mistaken for a foreign body.

Masticatory structures

Dentition:

- Deciduous or primary teeth are present at birth and erupt between 3 and 6 weeks of age (Figure 8.13). Permanent teeth erupt between 2 and 7 months and a 'full mouth' should be present by 7 months of age.

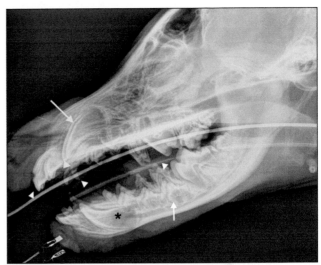

8.13 Lateral view of the skull of a dentally immature dog. Both deciduous (arrowheads) and (unerupted) permanent (arrowed) teeth are visible. The permanent teeth lie beneath the deciduous teeth. In the permanent tooth, the pulp cavity is wide (*) and the dentine walls are thin. Once the tooth apices of the erupted permanent teeth have formed, the animal is considered dentally mature.

- All teeth consist of a crown and single or multiple roots.
- The crown is covered by a layer of enamel, which is the most radiopaque tissue in the body. The bulk of the tooth consists of dentine, which is less radiopaque than enamel. The root is covered by a layer of cementum, which has a similar radiopacity to dentine, so is indistinguishable from it on radiographs.
- Lying within the centre of a tooth is the radiolucent soft tissue of the pulp, which runs from the pulp chamber in the crown along each root canal to the root apex, through which the neurovascular bundles enter. In the immature animal, the pulp cavity of the tooth root is wide, the dentine is thin and the apical foramen is open. When the apical foramen closes, the animal is considered to be dentally mature. The widened pulp cavity then narrows as secondary dentine is laid down.
- The tooth is supported in the alveolar bone by the periodontal ligament (Figure 8.14), which is of soft tissue opacity and lucent compared with the adjacent alveolar bone. The lamina dura is the dense line of compact bone surrounding the root and periodontal ligament. The alveolar bone should extend to the crown–root junction at the interdental spaces as well as the furcation (area between the roots).
- The mandibular dental arcade is narrower than the maxillary arcade, resulting in a shearing action, especially caudally, against the lingual surfaces of the maxillary dental arcade.

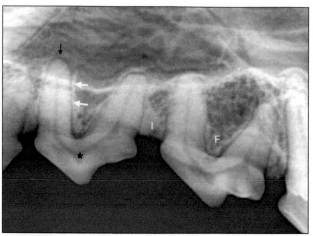

8.14 Lateral oblique view of the normal second and third maxillary premolar teeth using an extraoral parallel technique. Each tooth has two roots surrounded by the thin, dense cortical bone of the lamina dura (white arrows). The lamina dura is separated from the tooth root by the radiolucent periodontal ligament. The apex of the tooth root is closed (black arrow). The pulp cavity (*) is narrowed in the mature dog. F = furcation; I = interdental space.

Normal dental formulae

The normal dental formulae for the dog and cat are:

Deciduous teeth (immature)
Dog: 2 x [I3/3 C1/1 PM3/3] = 28
Cat: 2 x [I3/3 C1/1 PM3/2] = 26

Permanent teeth (mature)
Dog: 2 x [I3/3 C1/1 PM4/4 M2/3] = 42
Cat: 2 x [I3/3 C1/1 PM3/2 M1/1] = 30
Where: I = incisor; C = canine; PM = premolar; M = molar.

The second and third maxillary premolars have two roots, the fourth premolar and first molar have three roots, and the second molar has one root. All mandibular premolars and molars have two roots.

Modified Triadan system

The modified Triadan system is used by veterinary dentists to identify the teeth. Using this system, the maxillary and mandibular arcades are divided into quadrants and numbered in a clockwise fashion (as viewed from the front of the animal) starting with the right maxilla (1), left maxilla (2), left mandible (3) and right mandible (4).
Using this system, the teeth in the right maxillary arcade are numbered as follows:

Incisors: 101–103
Canine: 104
Premolars: 105–108
Molar: 109–110

Mandible:

■ The mandibles are paired flattened bones joined rostrally by a cartilaginous symphysis (Figure 8.15). They consist of horizontal bodies which diverge caudally, vertically oriented rami, and condyloid processes which articulate with the mandibular fossa at the base of the skull. The coronoid process forms the dorsal margin of the vertical ramus and the angular process is the triangular bony protuberance seen along the caudoventral aspect of the ramus. The coronoid process should lie medial to the zygomatic arch.

■ The mandible is slightly narrower than the maxilla. The degree of divergence of the mandible varies with skull conformation and between breeds. It is greater in breeds with a broad facial morphology and in brachycephalic breeds. The angle created by the bodies of the mandible is smaller in dogs and cats with a longer, narrower facial conformation and is greater in those animals with shorter or brachycephalic features. Radiological assessment of the mandibles is improved by using open-mouth views.

■ The mandibular symphysis is a connective tissue or fibrocartilaginous joint. The cortical bone margins may develop a somewhat ragged appearance in older animals. The symphysis accommodates rotational movements and slight widening of the mandibles during the shearing and crushing actions of mastication.

■ The mental foramina are lucent areas in the rostral mandible, which are partially superimposed on the distal roots of the canines. The inferior alveolar nerve, supplying the rostral mandible and teeth, exits via the foramen. The mental foramina are best seen on a lateral view and should not be mistaken for lytic lesions.

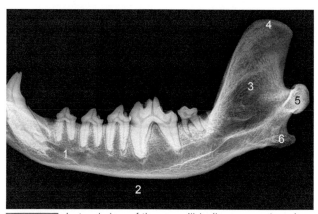

8.15 Lateral view of the mandible (bone specimen). 1 = mental foramen; 2 = mandibular body; 3 = mandibular ramus; 4 = coronoid process; 5 = condyloid process; 6 = angular process.

Premaxilla:

■ The premaxilla or incisive bone is the rostral part of the maxilla which contains the upper incisors and canines (Figure 8.16).

■ The alveolar bone has a foamy appearance due to coarse trabeculation.

■ The soft tissues of the nasal planum are projected rostral to the premaxilla and the nares are visible as symmetrical air-filled channels, which should be patent, on radiographs. They can be occluded with nasal discharge, especially in animals with destructive rhinitis.

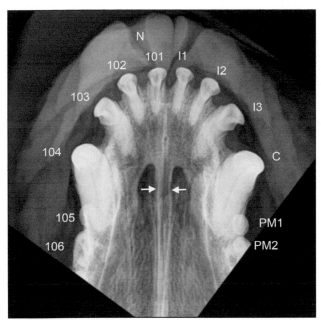

8.16 DV view of the premaxilla. The trabeculation of the premaxilla has a coarse and foamy appearance. The lateral margins of the rostral vomer bone (arrowed) and paired palatine fissures can be seen. The modified Triadan numbering system is shown for the right premaxilla and maxilla, and conventional numbering is shown for the left premaxilla and maxilla. N = nares.

Maxilla:

■ The maxilla is the largest of the facial bones. It forms the upper dental arcade, the floor and lateral walls of the nasal cavity, and caudally it forms the ventromedial wall of the bony orbit.

Palate:

■ The hard palate is a dense plate-like bony opacity, extending from the premaxilla rostrally to the soft palate caudally. The soft palate reaches the epiglottis caudally.
■ The palatine fissures are paired symmetrical linear–oval openings in the rostral hard palate. They should not be mistaken for bone lysis.

Temporomandibular joint

The temporomandibular joint of the dog and cat is a transversely elongated condylar synovial joint formed between the mandibular condyle and the mandibular fossa of the temporal bone at the base of the zygomatic process (Figure 8.17). The retroarticular process is a caudoventral extension of the mandibular fossa, which cups and prevents caudal luxation of the mandibular condyle. The temporomandibular joint acts mainly as a hinge joint, allowing opening and closing of the mouth. The flattened meniscus is not visible on radiographs. It is attached to the skull medially and to the mandibular condyloid process laterally. This limits lateral movement of the condyle when the carnassial teeth are aligned during the shearing movements of mastication. The appearance of the temporomandibular joint space varies slightly between different breeds of dog, but as a general rule it should appear as a sharply demarcated, curved, radiolucent

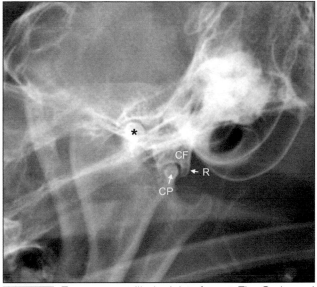

8.17 Temporomandibular joint of a cat. The C-shaped mandibular fossa (CF) and the condyloid process (CP) form the temporomandibular joint. The retroarticular process (R) prevents caudal displacement of the condyloid process. The opposite temporomandibular joint is projected dorsally (*).

band of constant width between the convex mandibular condyle and concave mandibular fossa on the sagittal oblique or 'nose-up' view (see below). In young dogs (up to 6 months of age), the joint space appears wider. It is slightly less curved and poorly marginated. This is a normal feature caused by the incompletely ossified cartilage and should not be confused with temporomandibular joint dysplasia.

Auditory system

■ The external ear canals are air-filled tubular structures. The horizontal canal appears as a lucent ring superimposed on the bulla. The external auditory meatus creates the impression of compartmentalization of the bulla, but true compartmentalization is only present in the cat (not the dog). The ear canals, usually the distal (horizontal) canal, may become mineralized with age, although this is more commonly due to otitis externa.
■ The tympanic bulla (Figure 8.18) is the largest part of the middle ear and is separated from the external ear by the tympanic membrane. The tympanic membrane cannot be recognized on radiographs. The tympanic bullae also communicate with the oropharynx via the Eustachian tubes.
■ The bullae lie ventral to the dense petrous temporal bone. The bullae should be filled with air but this is not always easy to appreciate on all views. Superimposition of the tongue on the bulla on open-mouth rostrocaudal views may mimic increased opacity within the bulla.
■ The bony wall is thin ventrally, expanding slightly where it merges with the basicranium dorsally. The bullae in some dogs appear small, hypoplastic and thick-walled (e.g. Bulldogs, Cavalier King Charles Spaniels). It is difficult to project hypoplastic bullae separately, beneath the skull, to

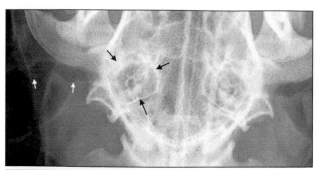

8.18 DV view of the skull showing the normal anatomy of the tympanic bulla. The external ear canals are filled with air (white arrows). The bony bullae (black arrows) are superimposed on the dense petrous temporal bone.

obtain diagnostic radiographs. This finding, which may be associated with secretory otitis, is frequently recognized on MRI and is usually of no clinical significance.

Pharynx and larynx

- The normal radiographic appearance of the larynx and pharynx are shown in Figure 8.19.
- The posterior nares (choanae) are the air-filled communication between the nasal chambers and the nasopharynx. Their location is defined by the junction of the hard and soft palates. The posterior nares are narrower than the nasopharynx.
- The nasopharynx lies dorsal to the soft palate and extends to the larynx. The dorsocaudal compartment of the nasopharynx lies dorsal to the palatine arches and surrounds the opening of the oesophagus. The caudal boundary of the nasopharynx is defined on radiographs by the hyoid apparatus and larynx. The intrapharyngeal ostium (the air space cranial to the larynx) is created where the oropharynx and nasopharynx cross.
- The four laryngeal cartilages (epiglottis, arytenoids (paired), cricoid and thyroid) are of soft tissue opacity, and in the younger animal only those margins bordered by air or fat within the fascial planes can be recognized. The epiglottis should be routinely recognized as it is surrounded by the air in the pharynx. It extends rostrally as a soft tissue curvilinear band, with the tip reaching dorsal to the caudal aspect of the soft palate. The position of the epiglottis relative to the soft palate varies with function, but usually lies just dorsal to the soft palate. Laryngeal gas often outlines the cuneiform and corniculate processes of the arytenoid cartilage and rostral cornu of the thyroid cartilage dorsally. This is more easily recognized in large-breed or giant-breed dogs.
- The position of the larynx relative to the cervical spine is influenced by the degree of flexion of the head. The base of the epiglottis usually falls between the occipital condyles and the body of C2. However, in chondrodystrophic breeds, the larynx is frequently more caudally positioned (often below the body of C3).
- The laryngeal cartilages mineralize with age in many dogs. The diameter of the trachea along its length is similar to that of the larynx.

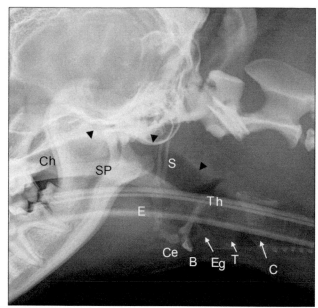

8.19 Lateral view of the pharynx and larynx. The dorsal margin of the nasopharynx is denoted by arrowheads. B = basihyoid; C = cricoid cartilage; Ce = ceratohyoid; Ch = choane; E = epihyoid; Eg = epiglottis; S = stylohyoid; SP = soft palate; T = thyroid cartilage; Th = thyrohyoid.

- The hyoid apparatus lies superimposed on the base of the tongue. It is a roughly U-shaped, slightly caudally rotated structure. All hyoid bones are paired except for the basihyoid. All hyoid bones are mineralized except for the tympanohyoid (the most dorsally located hyoid bone) which is cartilaginous. The basihyoid bone should not be mistaken for a foreign body. Evaluating the hyoid apparatus is important to help assess laryngeal position.
- None of the salivary glands are visible on radiographs. Changes in the salivary glands are only recognized when there is mineralization of salivary secretions (sialoliths) or enlargement of the glands.
- The oesophagus cannot be recognized on radiographs unless it contains air or opaque material. A small amount of gas is occasionally present within the cranial oesophagus, outlining the caudal margin of the cricopharyngeus muscle (cranial oesophageal sphincter). The normal cricopharyngeus muscle should not be mistaken for an oesophageal foreign body or retropharyngeal mass. Persistent and large amounts of cervical oesophageal air are abnormal findings that warrant investigation.

Breed and species variations

Brachycephalic breeds: The shape of the head is determined primarily by the shape of the facial region of the skull (Figure 8.20). The differences between brachycephalic animals and other breeds with longer facial features include:

- Reduced broadened facial component to the skull
- The nasal chambers are reduced in size
- The vomer may have a sigmoid appearance on DV intraoral radiographs

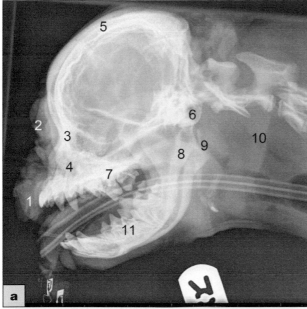

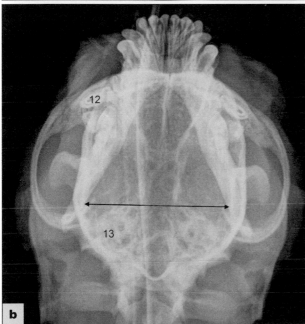

8.20 Brachycephalic skull. **(a)** Lateral view. 1 = nasal planum; 2 = facial folds; 3 = frontal sinuses markedly attenuated or absent; 4 = nasal chambers – attenuated; 5 = dome-shaped calvarium; 6 = hypoplastic tympanic bullae; 7 = short maxilla (and hard palate); 8 = thickened soft palate; 9 = narrowed nasopharynx; 10 = thickened retropharyngeal soft tissues; 11 = crowded mandibular dentition. **(b)** DV view. The wide mandible is denoted by the arrow. 12 = crowded maxillary dentition; 13 = bullae.

- The frontal sinuses are attenuated or absent
- The occipital protuberances may be small
- The calvarium in toy breeds and breeds with dome-shaped heads may be thin-walled
- Teeth may be crowded or missing – variations in dentition are more common with brachycephalic breeds
- The maxilla is often shorter than the mandible, resulting in a jaw that is prognathic (undershot lower jaw or mandibular prognathism). In comparison, dogs with a longer nose tend to have a relative mandibular brachygnathism or receding mandible

- The nasopharynx is narrowed and the soft palate elongated and thickened
- Eversion of the laryngeal saccules may obliterate the air space within the larynx. The epiglottis may be trapped by the vocal folds
- The orbits are directed more rostrally.

It should be noted that the term brachycephalic refers only to the head or facial part of the skull and not to the body conformation. Some breeds that have a chondrodysplastic appendicular skeleton (e.g. Dachshunds) do not have facial chondrodysplasia; they have a mesaticephalic skull.

Cats: There is more uniformity in the appearance of the skull in the cat (Figure 8.21), although extreme variations still occur (e.g. Persian, Chinchilla). Some oriental breeds may have quite elongated facial features. Structures are small and excellent quality radiographs are essential.

- The calvarium has a more rounded appearance than that of the dog.
- The nasal bone is more curved.
- The sagittal crest is less prominent.
- The tentorium cerebelli osseum is conspicuous on the lateral view.
- The cranium is large and facial length is reduced in relation to the cranium.
- The bullae are large and divided into two components by a bony shelf.
- The orbits are large and face more rostrally. The zygomatic arches extend more laterally and have large postorbital processes. The lateral extension of the zygomatic arches may confound attempts to image the last maxillary molar, especially with intraoral techniques.
- The nasal turbinates are extremely fine and poorly visible on the lateral view.
- The ethmoturbinates present prominently on the lateral view ('seashell' appearance).
- Dentition is reduced. The premolars are reduced in size, resulting in lengthening of the post-canine space. The molars do not have any grinding action.

Röntgen signs

Size

- The assessment of size and shape are closely associated in the skull.
- Masses involving the calvarium, basicranium and caudal maxilla tend to be significant in size and the course of the disease is usually advanced before they are recognized on radiographs. Large masses can result in only minor swelling, subtle facial asymmetry or secondary signs such as difficulty opening the jaw. Mass lesions of the calvarium are covered by a large amount of muscle in most dogs and are usually extensive before they are recognized by palpation.
- Similarly, orbital masses may be sizable before they are detected, or may be overlooked unless substantial destructive changes of the orbital wall are present. In comparison, masses of the premaxilla and rostral mandible are detected earlier.

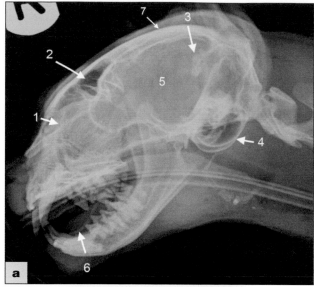

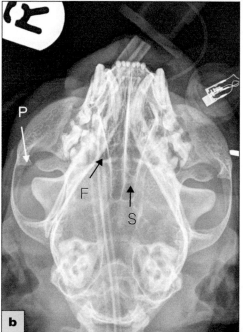

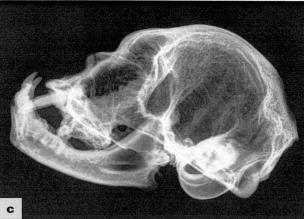

■ Expansile change in the shape of the skull (Figure 8.22) can be present with both non-neoplastic disease (e.g. lacrimal cysts, congenital or developmental tumours) and malignant disease (e.g. neoplasia of the middle ear). Differentiating benign from aggressive disease depends on assessment of the integrity of the expansile structure. With expansion of the frontal sinus due to fungal infection, the cortical bone, although reactive, normally remains intact. In neoplastic disease, the bone is often breached. Thinning of the cortical bone without destruction suggests benign behaviour, whereas disruption of the cortices and displacement of the bone elements suggests an aggressive process.

■ Cystic lesions are most commonly present in the maxilla, mandible and lacrimal bones. They deform and remodel the skull and facial bones.

■ Thickening of the bones (Figure 8.23) without a distinct mass lesion being present can be associated with periosteal thickening as in craniomandibular osteopathy (CMO), cortical

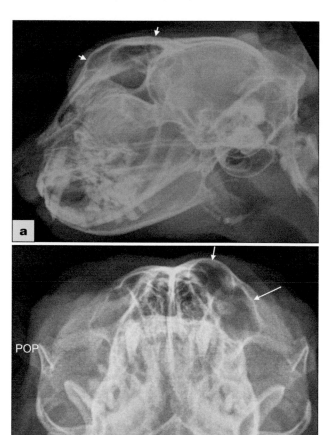

8.21 Normal skull anatomy of the cat. **(a)** Lateral view. The nasal bone is curved and the tympanic bullae are large and project ventrally. 1 = ethmoturbinates; 2 = frontal sinuses; 3 = tentorium cerebelli ossium; 4 = tympanic bullae; 5 = calvarium; 6 = mandible with widened interdental space; 7 = sagittal crest less prominent. **(b)** DV view. F = frontal sinus; P = postorbital process; S = sphenoidal sinus. **(c)** Brachycephalic skull. Note the reduced facial length and extreme mandibular prognathism.

8.22 Röntgen sign: size. **(a)** Lateral oblique and **(b)** rostrocaudal views of the skull of a cat with facial swelling. (a) There is dome-shaped enlargement of the frontal bones (arrowed). The sinus still appears air-filled but the frontal sinuses are better skylined on the rostrocaudal view. (b) The swelling is a focal expansion of the lateral recess of the left frontal sinus (arrowed). The cortices of the frontal sinus are intact and the sinus is air-filled. These changes are typical of a benign process. POP = postorbital process. (Courtesy of A Dupuy, Mandeville Veterinary Hospital)

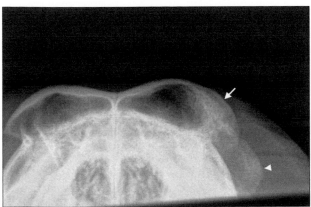

8.23 Röntgen sign: size. Rostrocaudal view of the skull of a dog with swelling around the left orbit. The frontal sinuses are skylined and the zygomatic process of the left frontal bone (arrowed) is thickened and sclerotic. Further thick crescentic organized new bone extends ventrally along the dorsal orbit and parietal bones (arrowhead). The changes are non-destructive, chronic and relatively organized, consistent with a low-grade (bacterial) osteitis.

thickening as in calvarial hyperostosis, or metabolic bone disease or inflammatory disease (osteitis or osteomyelitis). The thickening is best recognized when projected in profile, which requires specific views or lesion-oriented oblique views.

- Reduction in the size of skull structures is difficult to assess.
  - Narrowing of the airways is probably the feature that is most important to assess, although the role of radiography is quite limited. Nonetheless, the posterior nares and nasopharynx should be assessed for narrowing due to congenital disease or soft palate thickening of mass lesions, including polyps extending into the nasopharynx.
  - Thinning of the bones may be present due to expansile lesions, destructive or erosive processes and in developmental or congenital diseases (calvarium).
  - Reduction in the size of the nasal chambers or paranasal sinuses due to congenital or developmental lesions, or displaced (depression) fractures following trauma.

Shape

- Large alterations in the skull contour can usually be assessed using conventional radiographic views.
- Skyline views are required to identify subtle changes. Depression fractures (Figure 8.24) are difficult to appreciate and assess by palpation and radiographic views must be tailored to demonstrate changes.
- Comparison of the left and right sides is necessary to detect subtle changes (e.g. cribriform plate destruction and intracranial extension of nasal neoplasia).
- Shape and margination are closely associated.
- Some changes in shape are normal (e.g. sigmoid shape to the vomer in cats and brachycephalic breeds) and must be distinguished from displacement due to pathology.

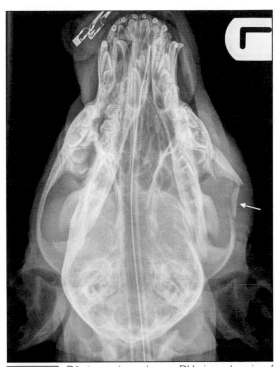

8.24 Röntgen sign: shape. DV view showing fracture of the left zygomatic arch (arrowed). Displacement and altered contour are easily overlooked if the lateral view is relied upon alone.

Number

- Most important in assessment of the dentition (Figure 8.25).
- Where dental structures are absent on clinical examination, radiographs are indicated to determine whether dentigerous or eruption cysts are present.

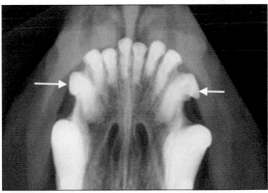

8.25 Röntgen sign: number. All skull bones and teeth should be paired and symmetrical. Occasionally, additional structures, usually (supernumerary) teeth, as in this dog with an extra pair of incisors, (arrowed) are recognized. However, the absence of one of a paired structure is usually a more important finding, indicating destruction or displacement of the structure.

Opacity

- As there is high contrast within air-filled structures and between bone and soft tissue, changes in opacity are invaluable when assessing the skull (Figure 8.26).
- The displacement of air by a soft tissue opacity confirms the presence of disease, but is not specific for an underlying cause.

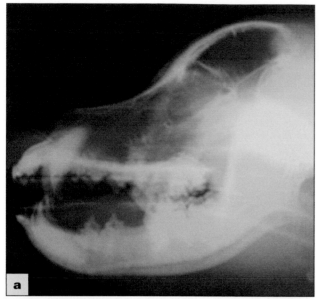

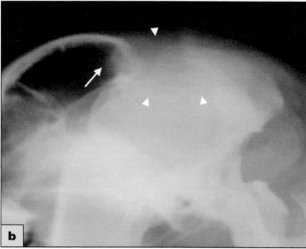

8.26 Röntgen sign: opacity. **(a)** The gas opacity of the caudal part of the frontal sinus has been replaced by a subtle, rounded soft tissue opacity bulging into the sinus. **(b)** Centring the beam on the lesion demonstrates an extensive destructive calvarial mass (arrowheads) breaking into the frontal sinus (arrowed).

- For structures such as the nasal turbinates, blurring of fine detail but preservation of the underlying turbinate pattern suggests the accumulation of secretions, congestion or haemorrhage.
- Reduced opacity is seen with bone or turbinate lysis. Recognition of turbinate lysis in the presence of a large volume of nasal secretion is difficult.
- Markedly opaque structures usually indicate an osteoblastic process. Osteosarcoma of the facial bones is often predominantly lytic, whereas osteosarcoma of the calvarium is predominantly osteoproductive.
- Lytic areas of the skull can be difficult to assess where bones are thin, superimposed on structures normally filled with air or projected *en face*.
- Dystrophic mineralization or mineralization with neoplastic lesions is uncommon in the nasal chambers but may be present in some neoplasms arising from the calvarium (e.g. multilobular tumour of bone, also termed multilobular osteochondrosarcoma).

Margination

- Inflammatory diseases and neoplasia can result in bony proliferation. The change simply indicates a reactive process. Neoplastic bone proliferation is generally indistinguishable from the reactive process, with the exception of lesions such as multilobular tumour of bone (multilobular osteochondrosarcoma) where the fine stippled appearance is characteristic.
- Sharp margination usually implies a less aggressive process (e.g. periapical abscessation) or a locally invasive process (e.g. tumours arising from the periodontal ligament).
- Smooth margination without bone disruption implies a benign process. Expansile, thin-walled structures also imply slowly progressive, non-aggressive or minimally aggressive lesions.
- Assessment of margination is particularly important in the evaluation of dental disease. Loss of the thin cortical bone of the alveolus is a sign of significant dental disease.
- Ragged margins are present with more aggressive disease, especially neoplastic and inflammatory diseases. Periosteal reactions may change or obscure the margin of the bone in a limited number of diseases such as CMO or calvarial hyperostosis. Aggressive spiculated periosteal reactions are less common in the skull, but are seen with squamous cell carcinomas involving the mandible.
- Within the nose, blurring of the turbinates (Figure 8.27) is a non-specific sign indicating congestion, swelling, the accumulation of secretions, haemorrhage, inflammation or early neoplastic disease. Despite this, recognizing the location of this change can help focus other investigations (e.g. rhinoscopy) to a particular area.

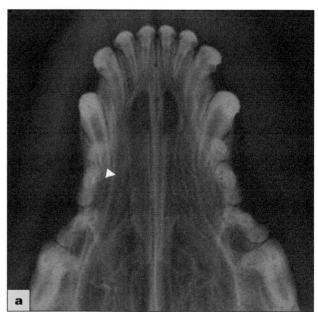

8.27 Röntgen sign: margination. DV intraoral nasal radiographs of two dogs presented with sneezing and epistaxis. **(a)** The rostral nasal turbinates on the right (arrowhead) are blurred and indistinct due to inflammation and the accumulation of fluid as a result of a nasal foreign body (grass seed). (continues) ▶

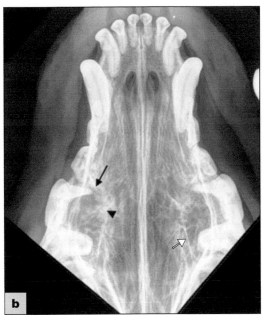

8.27 (continued) Röntgen sign: margination. DV intraoral nasal radiographs of two dogs presented with sneezing and epistaxis. **(b)** The thin line of cortical bone demarcating the right maxillary recess is indistinct (arrowhead). Compared with the normal air-filled left maxillary recess (white arrow), the right maxillary recess is of increased soft tissue opacity. The ethmoturbinates medial to the right maxillary recess are blurred. In addition, a poorly circumscribed area of lysis surrounds the mesial root of the fourth maxillary premolar (black arrow). The changes are subtle, but by assessing the margins the presence of bone destruction can be confirmed, although the extent cannot be determined from the radiograph. On MRI, a maxillary mass that had eroded into the right nasal chamber was visible.

Position and location

- Displacement of normal structures, most commonly due to neoplasia (Figure 8.28) but also as a result of trauma (fractures) and congenital

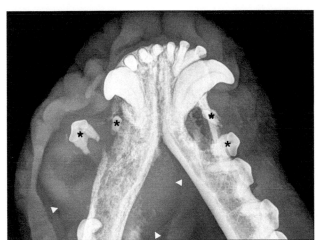

8.28 Röntgen sign: location. VD intraoral radiograph of a dog with an aggressive soft tissue mass (squamous cell carcinoma) invading the rostral mandible (arrowheads). Multiple mandibular premolars (*) on both the left and right have been displaced by the mass. Note the extensive lysis of both hemimandibles and the irregular, somewhat spiculated periosteal reaction on the medial aspect of the right hemimandible. Involvement of both hemimandibles is more typical of a soft tissue tumour invading bone; it is unusual for a mass arising from one hemimandible to involve the contralateral hemimandible.

malformations, is a useful indicator of disease. Displacement of the teeth is the most common example of this effect.

- The position of the larynx and hyoid apparatus is an indicator for retropharyngeal disease (masses, cysts or abscessation).

Function

Assessment of function in the skull is limited to fluoroscopic studies of swallowing disorders.

Nasal cavity and frontal sinuses

Common indications

- Persistent nasal discharge.
- Epistaxis.
- Sneezing.
- Facial swelling.
- Trauma.
- Exophthalmus.
- Epiphora.

Radiographic views

- Lateral view (see Figure 8.1).
- DV intraoral view of the nose (see Figure 8.6).
- Open-mouth ventro 20 degrees rostral–caudodorsal oblique (V20°R-CdDO) view.
- Caudo 30 degrees ventral–rostrodorsal oblique (Cd30°V-RDO) view.
- Rostrocaudal view of the frontal sinuses (see Figure 8.5).
- Caudorostral view of the frontal sinuses (horizontal beam).

Open-mouth ventrodorsal oblique views

- An alternative to the DV intraoral view of the nasal chambers is the open-mouth V20°R-DCdO view (Figure 8.29). This view can be used when a flexible cassette is not available or when it is not possible to include most of the caudal nasal cavities and the cribriform plate on the image (e.g. in brachycephalic breeds).
- For the VD oblique view, the animal is positioned in dorsal recumbency in a trough and the forelimbs are extended caudally. The head is extended so that the hard palate is horizontal to the table and the mouth is held open using a tie, gag or positioning frame.
- The cassette is placed beneath the head and the X-ray tube head is angled caudally so that the beam is centred on the mid-nasal cavity. The angle of the tube head/beam (approximately 20 degrees) should be approximately parallel to the mandible. If the beam is centred or angled too far caudally, or the mouth is not opened sufficiently, the rostral mandible will be superimposed on the caudal nasal chambers. The tongue should be secured so that it is not superimposed on the nasal chambers. The endotracheal tube can be removed for the exposure or secured to the mandible.

The open-mouth V20°R-DCdO view allows the caudal nasal chambers and maxilla to be evaluated. However, it should be noted that there is some

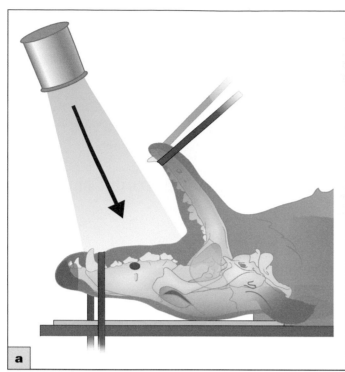

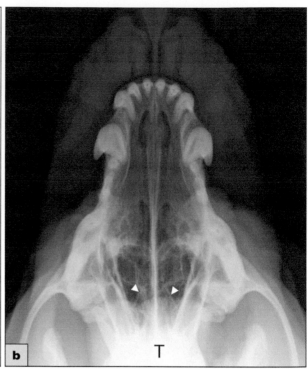

8.29 Open-mouth V20°R-DCdO view. **(a)** Patient positioning. The X-ray beam should be parallel to the long axis of the mandible. The most common error is that the jaw is not opened sufficiently. **(b)** This view is used to assess the caudal aspect of the nasal chambers, maxilla and the cribriform plate (arrowheads). The tongue (T) and endotracheal tube must be secured so that they are not superimposed on the nasal chambers.

geometric distortion as the beam is not parallel to the cassette. In the cat, it may not be possible to include all premolars and molars when using an intraoral technique. The open-mouth VD oblique view allows the caudal maxilla to be fully visualized.

An alternative in brachycephalic dogs is the ventro 30 degrees caudal–dorsorostral oblique (V30°Cd-DRO view (Figure 8.30). Positioning is the same as for the

VD view. The X-ray tube head is positioned caudal to the skull and the beam is angled rostrally, centred at the widest part of the jaw. Angulation is similar to the V20°R-DCdO view. The wider angle made by the mandibles results in less superimposition and allows the caudal nasal chambers and cribriform plate to be assessed.

Caudorostral view: frontal sinuses

- An alternative to the rostrocaudal view of the frontal sinuses (see Figure 8.5) is a skyline view of the frontal sinuses using a horizontal beam (Figure 8.31).
- With the animal in sternal recumbency and the head elevated on a pad, the cassette is placed vertically immediately rostral to the nose.
- The horizontal beam is directed rostrally toward the cassette and centred on the dorsal aspect of the frontal sinuses.
- This view has the advantages that it can demonstrate fluid levels in affected sinuses and it is easier to position and obtain symmetrical images of the frontal sinuses more consistently. There may be slightly greater magnification than with a rostrocaudal view. As a horizontal beam is being used, appropriate radiation safety requirements must be observed (see Chapter 2).

8.30 V30°Cd-DRO view. The wide angle of the caudal mandible allows the caudal aspect of the nasal chambers (*), the cribriform plate (arrowed) and lateral recesses of the frontal sinuses (F) to be assessed. The temporomandibular joints are also well demonstrated.

The caudorostral view is used to assess the frontal sinuses. Other diagnostic procedures such as rhinoscopy and biopsy should follow radiography. In young animals with nasal discharge, and where it may be necessary to exclude unusual conditions such as ciliary dyskinesia, radiographs of the thorax should be obtained.

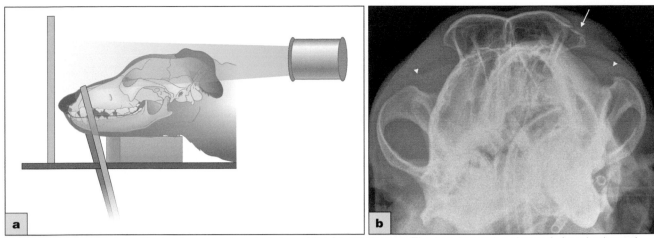

8.31 **(a)** Patient positioning for a caudorostral view of the frontal sinuses. The head must be elevated. As a horizontal beam is used, fluid levels may be recognized. **(b)** Depression fracture (arrowed) of the lateral recess of the frontal sinus. Note the region in which the orbital ligament may be recognized (arrowheads).

Specific approach to interpretation

The entire sinonasal region must be imaged (see Figure 8.26). The signs of nasopharyngeal disease or frontal sinus disease may be indistinguishable from disease involving the nasal cavities alone. Normal radiographs do not rule out nasal disease. In the sinonasal area, interpretation is focused on whether:

- Disease is unilateral or bilateral
- Distribution is focal, multifocal or diffuse
- The turbinates and vomer are intact
- The turbinate destruction is replaced by a mass lesion
- Erosion or extension into the maxilla or nasal bone is present
- There is evidence of extension into the cranium
- Frontal sinus and/or nasopharyngeal involvement is present
- Foreign material can be identified.

Common diseases

Neoplasia

Nasal tumours: Nasal neoplasia is recognized most frequently in older (>8 years old) medium to large mesaticephalic and dolichocephalic dogs (Figure 8.32abc). With the exception of the Boxer, nasal tumours are uncommon in brachycephalic breeds. Nasal tumours are typically slow-growing and, in most cases, disease is advanced at the time of diagnosis. Clinical signs are usually related to nasal discharge, epistaxis or facial deformity. Occasionally, dogs present with neurological disease alone due to extension of the tumour through the cribriform plate and into the cranial vault. Although the biological behaviour of nasal neoplasia is principally associated with local invasion, and distant metastasis is uncommon, thoracic radiographs are usually obtained. This is primarily to assess for concurrent disease prior to radiotherapy as most dogs are old at the time of diagnosis. The most common nasal tumours arise from secretory tissue (adenocarcinoma and undifferentiated carcinoma) or squamous tissue (squamous cell carcinoma). Mesenchymal or connective tissue tumours are less commonly reported and include chondrosarcoma, fibrosarcoma and undifferentiated sarcoma/osteosarcoma. Nasal lymphoma is uncommon in the dog but may present with involvement of both nasal chambers. The most common nasal tumours in the cat are lymphoma and carcinoma. Most tumours arise in the middle and caudal thirds of the nasal chamber.

Radiological features:

- Nasal tumours are locally aggressive and lead to turbinate destruction with replacement by a soft tissue mass.
- Nasal neoplasms arise unilaterally, although, in advanced cases, bilateral involvement of the nasal chambers may occur.
- Erosion or destruction of the vomer may be present. In animals presented at an early stage of the disease, no changes (or only thinning of one side of the vomer) may be present. A normal appearance of the vomer does not rule out neoplasia.
- Involvement of the cartilaginous septum cannot be determined, although displacement of the septum towards the unaffected nasal chamber, a mass lesion within both nasal chambers and destruction of the vomer usually suggest septal involvement.
- The frontal sinuses may be opacified due to extension of the tumour into the frontal sinus or obstruction of the nasofrontal opening by the subsequent accumulation of mucus and debris in the frontal sinuses.
- Destruction of bone may be present with extensive or aggressive tumours involving the nasal and maxillary boundaries, with extension into the soft tissues and facial deformity, or extension through the cribriform plate into the calvarium.
- The maxillary recess may be filled with soft tissue opacity, as a result of tumour extension into the recess. Destruction of the thin medial wall of the recess may be present.
- Extensive involvement of the maxilla may result in extension of the tumour into the orbit, displacing the globe or obstructing the nasolacrimal duct.

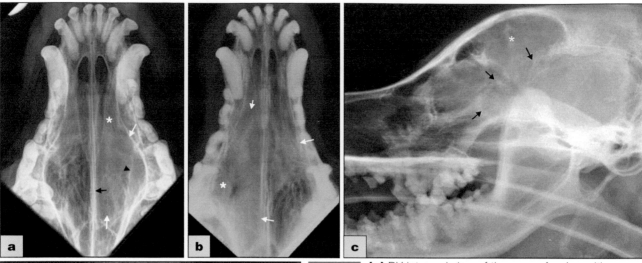

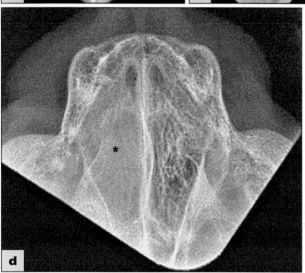

8.32 **(a)** DV intraoral view of the nose of a dog with epistaxis due to a nasal carcinoma. A poorly defined soft tissue mass (white arrows) fills the mid and caudal left nasal chamber. Turbinates are not recognized within this area. Bone destruction of the maxilla is not present. The vomer is thinned caudally (black arrow). The maxillary recess is filled with a soft tissue opacity, but the thin bony medial wall is still intact (arrowhead). Note that the rostral turbinates (*) are blurred, probably due to the accumulation of secretions, but still intact. **(b)** In this dog, the mass (arrowed) fills most of the right nasal chamber, including the maxillary recess (*), but also extends across the midline to fill the middle region of the left nasal chamber. **(c)** In this dog, there is extension into the calvarium. There is lysis of the bony margin of the rostral calvarium and cribriform plate (arrowed). The frontal sinus (*) is filled with a mass or fluid. **(d)** Nasal lymphoma in a cat. The right nasal chamber is completely filled with a homogeneous soft tissue mass (*). The turbinates are not recognized. The bony margins are intact.

- Tumours arising from the mid-portion of the nasal chamber (most common location) may obstruct the posterior nares, leading to the accumulation of secretions throughout the obstructed nasal chamber and within the frontal sinuses. In these cases, the integrity of the remaining intact maxilloturbinates and ethmoturbinates cannot be distinguished from the mass. Therefore, it must be recognized that radiological assessment of the extent of any mass lesion is limited. If the mass extends beyond the posterior nares, a soft tissue mass may be recognized in the rostral nasopharynx.
- Nasal mass lesions are usually of uniform soft tissue opacity. Occasionally, unstructured mineralization within a nasal mass is present (typically mesenchymal tumours) which is indicative of neoplasia.

The combination of turbinate destruction, increased soft tissue opacity in the nasal passages, and destruction of the vomer and/or facial bones should raise the index of suspicion for nasal neoplasia. The diagnosis of advanced disease by radiography may not be challenging, but the extent of the changes should be assessed by CT and MRI to establish which treatment options are possible. The diagnosis of less advanced disease poses a greater diagnostic challenge. However, recognition of unilateral loss of turbinate detail without associated focal lucency of the nasal chamber, the impression of increased soft tissue opacity (even if a discrete mass is not recognized) and thinning or an asymmetrical appearance of the vomer is suggestive of a neoplastic lesion. In the cat, lymphoma may present on radiographs as a soft tissue mass involving both nasal chambers. Although a turbinate pattern may not be recognized, destruction is not necessarily present and the turbinates may be recognized as intact on post-treatment radiographs.

Benign masses are unusual in both the dog and cat but include nasal polyps (cats) and nasal cysts. Radiographic diagnosis is characterized by normal studies or a focal soft tissue mass without evidence of turbinate destruction. Frontal sinus obstruction is less common.

Frontal sinus tumours: Primary frontal bone neoplasia (Figure 8.33) is not uncommon. The usual aetiology is squamous cell carcinoma.

Radiological features:

- Opacification of one or both frontal sinuses.
- With more extensive disease, there may be a mixture of soft tissue opacification and frontal bone destruction.
- Destruction and expansion of the frontal bone, and extension into the soft tissues or calvarium.

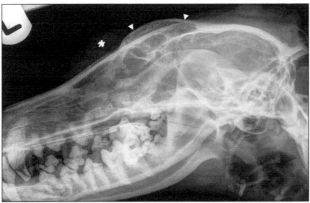

8.33 Frontal sinus tumour in a dog. The soft tissue mass filling the frontal sinus has expanded and thinned the frontal bone (arrowheads). The mass extends rostrally within the soft tissues (*) dorsal to the frontal sinus and into the caudal nasal chambers.

Canine rhinitis

Destructive or fungal rhinitis: Destructive rhinitis in the dog (Figure 8.34) is usually caused by fungal infection, although turbinate destruction is occasionally associated with foreign body inhalation and lymphoplasmacytic rhinitis. The two most common causes of nasal fungal disease in the dog are *Aspergillus fumigatus* and *Penicillium* species. *Aspergillus fumigatus* is the most common isolate. Fungal infections that cause destructive rhinitis are considered opportunistic diseases. Young to middle-aged dolichocephalic and mesaticephalic breeds are most commonly affected. Destructive rhinitis should not be excluded in brachycephalic breeds (e.g. Boxers), although the restricted nasal chambers make diagnosis challenging. The infection tends to arise in the rostral to middle sections of the nasal chambers. Infection usually arises unilaterally, but extension to involve both sides of the nose is not uncommon. Although radiography is a useful diagnostic technique for fungal rhinitis, a definitive diagnosis is usually made using rhinoscopy, biopsy and visualization, and culture of the plaques. Radiography is used as a survey technique to try and exclude other differential diagnoses such as neoplasia and to guide rhinoscopy.

Radiological features:

- Typically a multifocal destructive pattern: changes may be unilateral or bilateral.
- Destructive pattern appears as ill defined radiolucent areas due to turbinate lysis.
- Changes usually arise in the rostral nasal chamber. In areas bordering lysis, the turbinate pattern is blurred due to the accumulation of secretions, fungal plaques and early turbinate destruction.

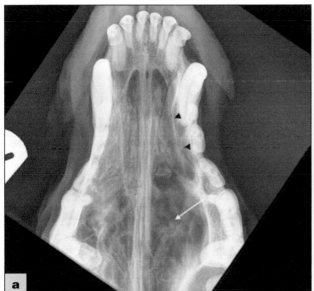

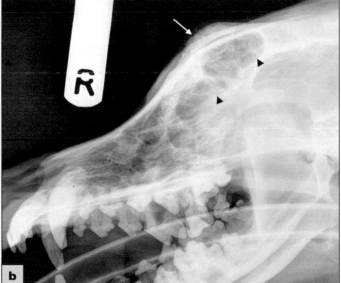

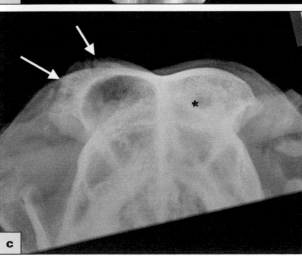

8.34 **(a)** DV intraoral, **(b)** lateral and **(c)** rostrocaudal (skyline) views of the nasal chambers of a dog with destructive rhinitis due to nasal aspergillosis. (a) There is unilateral destruction of turbinates in the rostral (black arrowheads) and caudal (arrowed) left nasal chamber. The left nasal chamber is reduced in opacity (more air; fewer turbinates) compared with the right side. The amorphous soft tissue opacity in the caudal nasal chamber and superimposed on the maxillary recess represents accumulated discharge and debris. The degree of involvement of the right nasal chamber cannot be established based on radiographs alone. (b) At least one of the frontal sinuses is filled with material of soft tissue opacity (black arrowheads). The dorsal aspect of at least one of the frontal bones is thickened with a prominent lamellar periosteal reaction recognized in profile (arrowed). (c) On the skyline view, both frontal sinuses are recognized to be affected. The left sinus is almost completely opacified (*) and the right sinus is partially affected but with a marked reaction and thickening of the frontal bone (arrowed) due to fungal osteomyelitis.

- Larger patches of increased radiopacity are more common in the caudal nasal chambers, but there is no discrete soft tissue mass.
- Punctate lucencies may be present in the surrounding nasal and maxillary bones due to local extension.
- Vomer and/or septum involvement is not common. Where destruction of the vomer is present, the interruption is multifocal or piecemeal.
- Extension of the infection into the frontal sinuses may be associated with opacification of the frontal sinuses due to the retention of secretions and the accumulation of discharge. The overlying frontal bone may be thickened and mottled due to osteomyelitis.

It is not possible to differentiate neoplasia from destructive rhinitis using radiography alone in all cases. Predominantly unilateral changes, turbinate destruction, replacement by soft tissue mass, mineralization of the soft tissue mass, displacement of midline structures, bone destruction or facial distortion and frontal sinus obstruction are all more likely with neoplasia, but this is not absolute. Destructive rhinitis, by comparison, is more likely to be associated with multiple or multifocal lesions, lucent foci, and absence of a discrete mass lesion or bony wall destruction. Frontal sinus involvement is less common or not recognized on the radiograph.

Foreign body rhinitis: Intranasal foreign bodies (Figure 8.35), although seen most frequently in younger active dogs, can be present in animals of all ages and breeds. Radiography can be useful to localize radiopaque foreign bodies and to screen for changes. Only

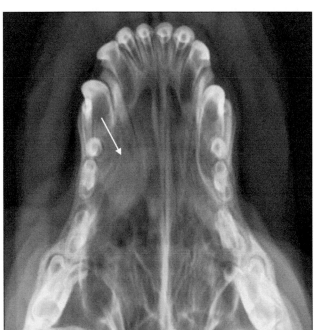

8.35 DV intraoral view of the nasal chambers of a dog presented with sneezing and discharge from the right naris. There is a focal area of soft tissue opacity (arrowed) in the right rostral nasal chamber, medial to the right maxillary canine, obscuring the turbinates. Gross destruction cannot be recognized. The rostral location, focal changes, young age and unilateral location are suggestive of an inhaled foreign body. A grass seed was retrieved at rhinoscopy.

foreign bodies with a high atomic number, metal, mineral or teeth can be identified. Radiolucent foreign bodies (most common) such as plant awns cannot be recognized on radiographs. Radiographic changes, where present, are associated with surrounding inflammation or mucopurulent secretion.

Radiological features:

- The diagnosis is suggested by the presence of focal areas of increased soft tissue opacity.
- The absence of radiographic change does not rule out disease. Rhinoscopy is the technique of choice to evaluate suspicious areas.
- Follow-up radiographs should demonstrate resolution of the area of focal, increased radiopacity in the nasal cavity following removal of the foreign body.
- Destruction may be more extensive in rare cases of foreign body complicated by destructive (fungal) rhinitis.

Lymphoplasmacytic rhinitis: Lymphoplasmacytic rhinitis is an inflammatory chronic rhinitis of unknown aetiology. The condition is characterized by a serous, mucopurulent or haemorrhagic bilateral nasal discharge. Turbinate destruction may be a feature of the radiological changes. However, these changes are typically less severe compared with the bony destruction associated with fungal infection. Radiological assessment is used to exclude other mass lesions or extensive destruction. The diagnosis is confirmed by rhinoscopy, histopathology and the elimination of other differential diagnoses.

Radiological features:

- Changes are usually subtle, diffuse and non-specific.
- Mild to moderate diffuse increase in soft tissue opacity and blurring of the rostral nasal turbinates due to the accumulation of a large amount of nasal discharge.
- Mild symmetrical or asymmetrical turbinate destruction is relatively common, particularly in the rostral half of the nasal cavity.

Other causes of rhinitis: In the dog, rhinitis may also be associated with allergic, infectious, hyperplastic and parasitic (nasal mite) disease or occur secondary to dental disease. Radiographic changes are usually subtle and bilaterally symmetrical (except in cases with nasal foreign bodies). It may be helpful to perform radiography both before and after flushing to remove the nasal discharge. Rhinitis in the dog, particularly chronic rhinitis, is not normally associated with turbinate destruction unless complicated by fungal infection.

Radiological features:

- Bilateral changes.
- Increased soft tissue opacity and blurring of the nasal turbinates, which may be slightly thickened.
- Opacification of the frontal sinuses due to trapped secretions in severe cases.

Feline rhinitis

Acute rhinitis: Acute rhinitis in the cat is usually associated with infectious disease (primarily feline respiratory diseases, although atypical infectious agents such as *Bordetella bronchiseptica* may be recognized occasionally). Diagnosis is usually based on the history and clinical findings and radiography is rarely necessary.

Chronic rhinitis: Chronic unilateral or bilateral, mucopurulent or haemorrhagic discharge in the cat (Figure 8.36) can be caused by neoplasia (lymphoma, adenocarcinoma) or fungal infection (cryptococcosis, aspergillosis) or can occur secondary to viral or bacterial infection, nasal foreign body, nasopharyngeal stenosis or dental-related diseases.

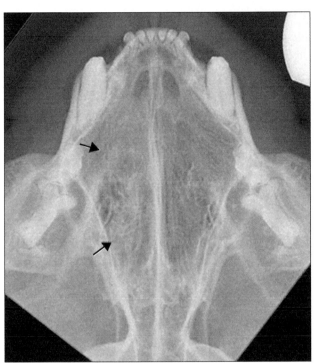

8.36 DV intraoral view of the nose of a cat with chronic rhinitis. The right nasal turbinates are indistinct due to irregular foci of soft tissue opacity (arrowed). The areas are not confluent. The deviation and variable thickness of the vomer is not uncommon in the cat.

Clinical signs may result from a destructive process within the nasal cavity initiated by the infectious agent (e.g. feline herpesvirus-1). Bacterial rhinitis is more common in the cat than the dog due to the association with viral infection. Chronic rhinitis is generally characterized by a hyperaemic mucosa, a large amount of mucoid to purulent discharge and increased space between the irregular looking turbinates. Regardless of the underlying cause, pathological changes to the turbinate can result in chronic osteitis, necrosis and destruction. The nasal discharge may become caseous and inspissated, and necrotic turbinates may never be resorbed. Necrotic turbinates can form sequestra; however, recognition of this change on radiographs is almost impossible. These pathological changes result in a mixed appearance of the nasal cavity on radiography.

Radiological features:

- Changes are mixed, representing a variable degree of turbinate lysis and increased fluid radiopacity within the nasal cavity.
- Changes are frequently bilateral.
- The frontal sinuses are often affected and subsequently become filled with fluid opacity.

Foreign body rhinitis: Nasal foreign bodies are less common in the cat, although entrapment of grass blades in the posterior nares or nasopharynx can result in signs of rhinitis. Radiography may demonstrate the accumulation of discharge within the nasopharynx, but flexible rhinoscopy is required to reach a diagnosis. Rarely, unusual foreign bodies such as airgun pellets or tooth fragments (due to inhalation or displacement into the nasal cavity during prophylactic dentistry) are recognized on survey radiography.

Trauma
The only soft tissues protecting the nasal bone are the skin and subcutis.

Radiological features:

- Nasal bone fractures may be depressed and comminuted.
- Subcutaneous emphysema is usually present.
- Increased intranasal soft tissue opacity and blurring of the turbinates due to haemorrhage.
- Traumatized turbinates may be devitalized and sequestra may develop.
- Malunion can lead to acquired nasal disease and occasionally airway obstruction.

Cranium and calvarium
Common indications

- Swellings and facial asymmetry.
- Trauma.
- To rule out radiopaque foreign body.
- Exophthalmos.
- Head pain.
- Epiphora.

Radiographic views

- DV view.
- Lateral view.
- Lesion-oriented oblique view.
- Rostrocaudal (skyline) view of the frontal sinuses and calvarium. Collimation should be widened to include the zygomatic arches.

Specific approach to interpretation
Radiography of the calvarium and cranium is limited by the superimposition of structures (it is a biplanar rather than a cross-sectional technique) and low contrast, especially of the soft tissues. However, a radiographic study should allow:

- Assessment of aggressive versus non-aggressive features where bone changes can be recognized
- Localization of bone changes where recognized

- Rapid localization of metal foreign bodies (especially projectiles)
- Survey assessment for skull fractures and the location of gas (if any) within the tissues.

Common diseases

Hydrocephalus

Congenital hydrocephalus is recognized as an extreme dome-shaped appearance to the cranium. This may be relatively easy to recognize in breeds that should have a mesaticephalic or dolichocephalic conformation, but is more difficult to recognize in toy breeds. Clinical signs are usually evident within the first year of life, although the late onset of signs is occasionally recognized. The appearance may not be associated with clinical signs, although whether this represents subclinical disease is not known.

Radiological features:

- The calvarium is enlarged and the bones are thinned (Figure 8.37).
- Calvarial markings are absent or difficult to recognize. The internal aspect of the calvarium has a smooth appearance.
- The bregmatic fontanelle may remain open and can be recognized as a smoothly marginated defect dorsally at the junction of the frontal, parietal and occipital bones.
- Open sutures are usually easier to recognize on a DV view.

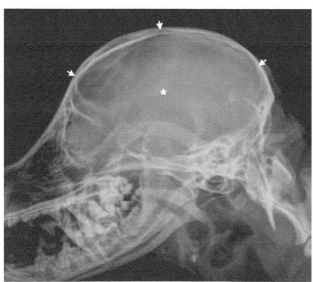

8.37 Lateral view of the skull of a young dog with hydrocephalus. The cranium is enlarged, rounded and dome-shaped with thinning of the calvarial bones (arrowed). Note that the calvarium has a smooth internal appearance (*) and lacks the normal groove-like markings.

Occipital dysplasia

Occipital dysplasia is defined as an abnormally large foramen magnum due to incomplete ossification of the ventromedial supraoccipital bone during gestation. Occipital dysplasia has been reported in toy and brachycephalic breeds such as the Cavalier King Charles Spaniel, Yorkshire Terrier, Maltese, Chihuahua and Beagle. It has infrequently been associated with

the presence of clinical signs. The disease may be associated with a congenital abnormality of the caudal occipital bone, resulting in overcrowding of the caudal fossa and compression at the level of the cervicomedullary junction (caudal occipital malformation or Chiari-like malformation), leading to anomalies of cerebrospinal fluid (CSF) flow dynamics. Crowding of the caudal fossa and syringomyelia of the spinal cord is diagnosed using MRI. The relationship between occipital dysplasia and caudal occipital malformation and the clinical signs associated with caudal fossa crowding remains unclear. The condition may be associated with atlantoaxial malformation and instability, deformities of the atlas and hydrocephalus.

Radiological features:

- The foramen magnum is best visualized on an open-mouth rostrocaudal view; however, considering the association with the conditions detailed above, conventional lateral, VD and carefully flexed lateral views centred on the atlas and axis should be obtained first.
- The open-mouth rostrocaudal view is contraindicated if there is any evidence of atlantoaxial instability and due consideration should be given to performing MRI or CT studies in any animal with clinical signs localized to caudal fossa crowding or the cranial cervical spine.
- The radiographic appearance of occipital dysplasia is dorsal extension and enlargement of the foramen magnum, resulting in a keyhole shape. The appearance of this enlargement varies greatly.
- C1 (atlas) and the occipital condyles may be abnormal in shape. The atlas may be shortened with a tightly curved dorsal arch, which appears to overlap the base of the occipital bone. The occipital condyles may be hypoplastic.

Trauma

Fractures of the calvarium are often associated with blunt trauma due to road traffic accidents, but bite wounds and penetrating foreign bodies can also occur. Most dogs have a relatively thick calvarium and bulky masticatory muscles, which protect the head; therefore, fractures tend to occur in the less well protected regions of the skull, frontal sinuses and teeth, and these areas should not be overlooked.

Radiological features:

- Radiological changes may be limited to soft tissue swelling/haematoma and, if accompanied by open wounds, subcutaneous emphysema.
- Fractures with minimal displacement may appear as curvilinear radiolucent defects. In the immature animal, normal suture lines should not be mistaken for skull fractures. Fractures displaced inwards are known as depressed fractures.
- Depressed fractures of the frontal sinus (Figure 8.38) are associated with extensive subcutaneous emphysema. Open fractures may be complicated by infection and displaced fragments can form sequestra. Depressed fractures of the calvarium are usually associated with significant, life-threatening trauma to the brain parenchyma.

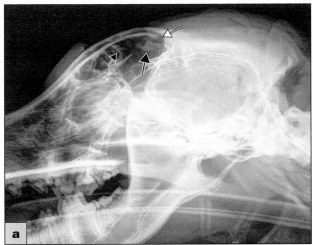

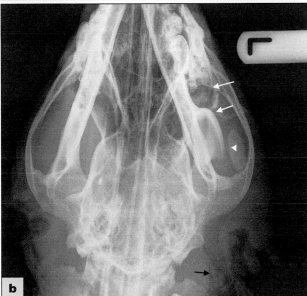

8.38 **(a)** Lateral and **(b)** DV views of the skull of a dog following vehicular trauma. Fracture of the frontal sinus is present. (a) A cortical defect is present in one of the frontal bones adjacent to the calvarium (white arrow). Multiple depressed fracture fragments (black arrows) are superimposed on the sinus. (b) On the DV view, the lateral aspect of the frontal sinus is partially obscured by the coronoid process of the mandible. Although the defect in the lateral wall can be recognized (white arrows) the full extent is not appreciated. A displaced bone fragment is seen end-on (arrowhead). Subcutaneous emphysema is present (black arrow). Skyline radiographs of the frontal sinus would be useful in this animal.

- For a fracture to be recognized, the fracture line needs to be tangential to the X-ray beam (Figure 8.39). Overlapping fracture fragments are recognized as a focal increase in bone opacity, resulting in a sclerotic appearance.
- Recent fractures are sharply marginated. Features that allow non-displaced fractures of the calvarium to be distinguished from suture lines include fracture lines tapering or widening at one end, and fracture lines radiating asymmetrically from areas of the skull remote from the fontanelles (the bregmatic fontanelle is usually the only fontanelle recognized in the dog) (Figure 8.40).
- Fractures of the skull may be multiple or comminuted and the search for fractures in cases with known trauma should not be suspended when one fracture is found.

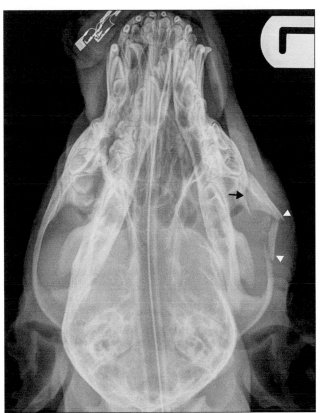

8.39 DV view of the skull of a 4-month-old dog following trauma. A comminuted fracture of the left zygomatic arch is present. The fragments (arrowheads) are displaced. The temporal process of the arch is also displaced at the suture with the maxilla (arrowed). Failure to recognize displaced zygomatic bone fractures can lead to difficulties in mastication, which are delayed in onset. This is due to callus interfering with movement of the coronoid process, development of false anklyosis or degenerative joint disease of the temporomandibular joint.

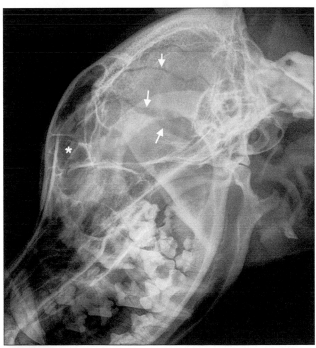

8.40 Lateral view of the skull of a dog that had been kicked by a horse. Several lucent lines (arrowed) radiate from dorsal to ventral from an area of the calvarium just caudal to the frontal sinuses. Note that the fracture lines widen ventrally. The frontal sinus (*) is partly filled with a soft tissue opacity (haemorrhage).

- Lesion-oriented oblique views of the affected area should be taken in order to skyline the displaced fragments.
- As the nasal bone is not covered with much soft tissue, depression fractures can be associated with sequestra, facial deformity or sinusitis.

The clinical signs and radiological findings associated with trauma may be delayed. In fact, knowledge of a traumatic event may not be available as part of the history. Therefore, previous trauma, historical or recent, should be considered when evaluating bony swellings, deformities or lysis involving the skull. Examples of the delayed, unrecognized or unmanaged consequences of trauma include:

- Trauma to the calvarium may cause a subperiosteal haematoma (Figure 8.41), which initially appears as a localized soft tissue swelling associated with the dorsal or dorsolateral aspect of the cranium. Normally the lesion gradually disappears over time. However, in some instances these lesions become partially calcified or ossified and could be mistaken for a bone tumour. Haematomas are usually well marginated without underlying lysis. The pattern of mineralization is usually smooth and homogeneous. A known history of trauma, the absence of bone destruction or lysis, and a narrow zone of transition to normal bone may be helpful features to differentiate a calcified haematoma from a bone tumour
- Facial deformity, bone sequestration and sinusitis
- Frontal sinus mucocoele. On radiographs these appear as focal, expansile, bony swellings in the frontal sinus region with a central soft tissue opacity. The lesion arises due to obstruction of the frontonasal opening. The retention of secretions leads to enlargement of the sinus

- Degenerative changes or ankylosis of the temporomandibular joint
- Malunion of displaced fragments (Figures 8.42 and 8.43). Malunion of zygomatic arch fractures or unmineralized callus may interfere with the coronoid process of the mandible and prevent the jaw from closing.

Radiography of the cranium also allows the bony portions of the orbit to be evaluated in cases of trauma (e.g. zygomatic arch fracture resulting in exophthalmos) and assists in detecting radiopaque foreign bodies (such as projectiles). Wooden or plastic foreign bodies are usually of soft tissue opacity. If any air surrounds or is incorporated within the foreign body, then geometric shapes may be recognized.

Neurological disease

Radiography of the skull is rarely useful in cases of neurological disease, except for investigating suspected nasal disease extending into the calvarium, mineralized meningioma in the cat (occasionally) and bony masses of the calvarium causing facial deformity or extending into the cranial vault.

- Meningiomas can present with focal thickening of the adjacent calvarium (hyperostosis) or as a circumscribed sclerotic mass arising from the inner aspect the calvarium.
- Hyperostosis is only recognized when the X-ray beam is tangential to the thickened area. As the calvarium is curved or dome-shaped, it can be challenging to demonstrate hyperostosis and recognizing the change may be fortuitous.
- Mass lesions extending into the cranial vault may arise from the bone itself or from the adjacent structures.
- Lesion-oriented oblique views may need to be obtained.

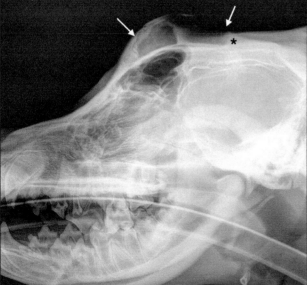

8.41 Lateral view of the skull of a dog with a swelling on the head. An expansile, thin-walled swelling (arrowed) arising from the dorsocaudal aspect of the frontal bone is visible. The transition to normal bone at the periphery is short and smooth new bone, consistent with a Codman's triangle, is present at the margin, indicating elevated periosteum (*). Internally there is ill defined mineralization. Considering the history of known trauma, the appearance is consistent with a subperiosteal haematoma.

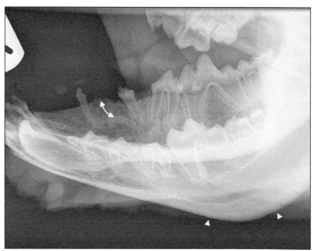

8.42 Open-mouth lateral oblique view of the mandible of a 6-month-old dog presented with difficulties opening its mouth. A fracture of the body of the right mandible had been repaired with an external fixator at 3 months of age. The fracture has healed but there is abnormal angulation of the bodies of both hemimandibles (arrowheads). Note the dental abnormalities: absent teeth, crown fractures, retained root (double-headed arrow) and malalignment of the fourth mandibular premolar as a result of the trauma.

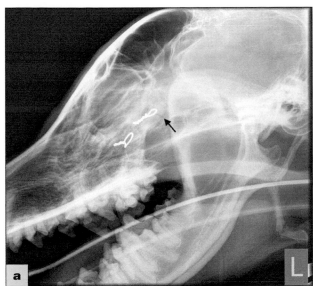

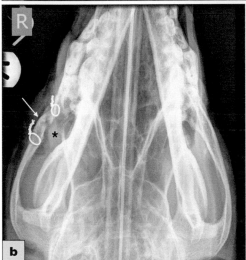

8.43 **(a)** Lateral and **(b)** DV views of the skull of a dog with a chronic non-healing fracture of the right zygomatic arch. Gas is present in the soft tissues (sinus tract). An attempt has been made to stabilize the fracture using cerclage wire; however, the central fragment of the comminuted zygomatic fracture has not healed. (a) Assessment on the lateral view is limited to recognizing the fracture line (arrowed) and the irregular margin of the rostral aspect of the zygomatic bone. (b) On the DV view, the fragment (arrowed) is seen to be displaced medially. The fragment is probably non-viable (sequestrum). The discomfort and inability to open the mouth was due to the fibrous callus along the medial zygomatic arch (*), which restricted movement of the coronoid process. The fibrous callus cannot be recognized on radiography but was visible on MRI.

Neoplasia

- The most common primary malignant bone tumours are osteosarcoma, chondrosarcoma and osteochondrosarcoma (also known as multilobular tumour of bone). Multilobular tumour of bone arises on the skull, mainly in the calvarium, maxilla and mandible. It is slow-growing and locally invasive, often recurring after excision and may spread elsewhere. The mass is often large at the time of diagnosis.
- Mass lesions of the basicranium occur but are often only recognized when advanced. Most involve intracranial extension of masses arising from the

nose, maxilla, tympanic bullae or oral cavity/salivary glands. Signs may only be evident when there is discomfort associated with opening the mouth, nasal discharge or neurological disease.

Radiological features:

- Osteosarcoma of the calvarium tends to be osteoproductive with amorphous or unstructured periosteal new bone, leading to deformity of the contour of the cranium and destruction of the underlying bone.
- As with many lesions of the calvarium, unless the periosteal reaction is skylined or the areas of greatest cortical loss are projected perpendicular to the X-ray beam, significant masses can be overlooked.
- Large masses arising in the temporal fossa region may be obscured by the bulk of the temporal muscles.
- Osteochondrosarcoma (multilobular tumour of bone; Figure 8.44) is characterized by variable osteolysis of the underlying cortical bone, granular or stippled mineralization throughout the mass (which can vary from indistinct to dense) and extension or expansion within the cranium. Intracranial extension can be difficult to appreciate unless the mass is densely mineralized or the cortical defect is tangential to the beam.
- Masses of the basicranium tend to cause extensive destruction. The extent of the bone destruction can often be underestimated due to superimposition of adjacent structures. Radiographs should be scrutinized for signs of destruction of the temporomandibular joint, tympanic bullae and maxilla. Displacement of teeth is frequently seen with maxillary masses.

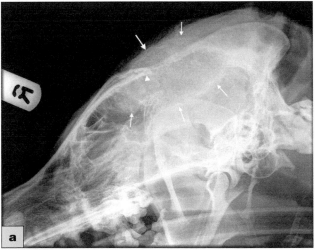

8.44 Lateral views of the skulls of two dogs with osteochondrosarcoma. **(a)** The large mass is egg-shaped and contains fine mineralization (arrowed). It has expanded, creating a large cortical defect extending rostrally into the caudal frontal sinuses, ventrally into the calvarium, dorsally into the soft tissues and caudally into the parietal and occipital bones. There is no periosteal reaction: the bone at the margins is rarefied (arrowhead), consistent with the slow growth of the mass. The dog presented with neurological signs and the mass was not palpable. (continues) ▶

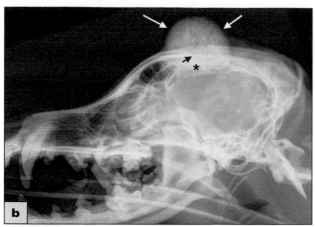

8.44 (continued) Lateral views of the skulls of two dogs with osteochondrosarcoma. **(b)** The mass is rounded with a typical granular, densely mineralized appearance (white arrows). The destruction of the calvarium is indistinct (black arrows) and the mass extends into the calvarium (*).

- Osteoma is the most common benign bone tumour (Figure 8.45). It is seen as a sclerotic, discrete, dome-shaped to cauliflower-like bony mass without associated bone lysis. Feline skull osteomas have a characteristic radiographic pattern, appearing as well circumscribed, very radiopaque masses on the periosteal surface of otherwise unaffected bone.
- Osteochondroma (multiple cartilaginous exostoses) in the cat often involve the calvarium. They appear as well mineralized juxtacortical masses. A linear lucent band representing the cartilaginous scar may remain.

Renal secondary hyperparathyroidism

Renal secondary hyperparathyroidism ('rubber jaw') is a metabolic osteopenic bone disease that occurs secondary to chronic renal failure. It is most commonly seen in young dogs with congenital renal dysplasia. Chronic renal failure results in increased levels of parathyroid hormone in order to maintain calcium homeostasis. The elevated parathyroid hormone concentration increases osteoclastic bone resorption.

As lamellar bone is resorbed, it is replaced by fibrous tissue and poorly organized woven bone, which lacks the strength of normal osseous tissue. The most marked changes associated with renal secondary hyperparathyroidism occur in the skull, although changes in the long bones may also occur. The changes are more dramatic in younger animals due to increased bone turnover. Although hyperparathyroidism may also be attributed to dietary calcium deficiency (nutritional secondary hyperparathyroidism), a feature of low calcium, all-meat diets or unbalanced diets, the changes seen with nutritional secondary hyperparathyroidism are usually limited to the appendicular skeleton.

Radiological features:

- Radiographs show reduced opacity of the skull bones (osteopenia or demineralization) resulting in a lacy trabecular pattern (Figure 8.46).
- The cortices are thinned and, in those bones with a medulla, the distinction between the cortex and medulla is lost.
- Soft tissue structures are unusually prominent relative to the bone (e.g. the soft palate and tongue may become prominent compared with the teeth and surrounding bones).
- Bones, especially the mandibles, are abnormally soft and flexible ('rubber jaw') and prone to pathological fractures. Pathological fractures may appear as folding structures with only one cortex involved or as incomplete fractures with mild sclerosis of overlapping cortices.
- The nasal turbinates may be blurred. Fibrous dysplasia of the nasal turbinates leads to thickening of the turbinate mucosa, retention of secretions and may lead to breathing difficulties.
- Loss of the lamina dura results in an ill defined halo around the teeth. This is best appreciated on DV views of the maxilla and VD views of the mandible as 'floating' teeth embedded in soft tissue.
- Abdominal radiographs may reveal small, irregular kidneys and calcification of some soft tissues (gastric rugal folds, blood vessels, kidneys).

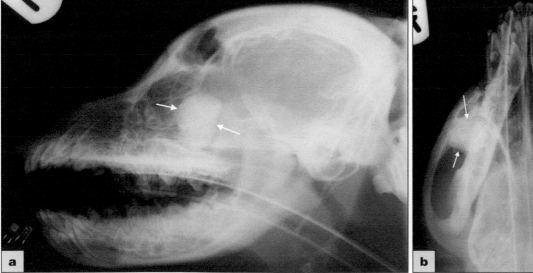
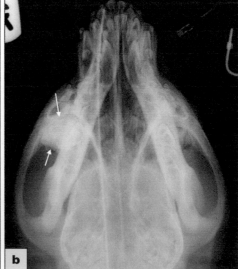

8.45 **(a)** Lateral and **(b)** VD views of the skull of a young dog with an osteoma. Note the smoothly marginated oval mass (arrowed) arising from the caudal aspect of the temporal process of the right zygoma. The mineralized mass is dense and homogeneous in appearance.

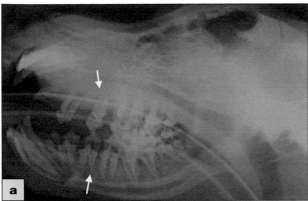

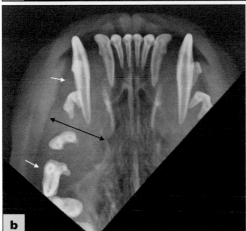

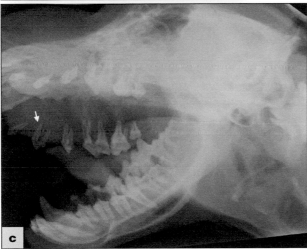

8.46 Renal secondary hyperparathyroidism. **(a)** Lateral, **(b)** DV intraoral and **(c)** open-mouth lateral oblique radiographs of the skull. There is severe demineralization of the skull, resulting in loss of the alveolar bone surrounding the teeth and poor contrast between the bone and soft tissue. The teeth appear to 'float' within the soft tissues (white arrows). The changes are consistent with fibrous osteodystrophy. The demineralized bone is replaced by thickened fibrous tissue (black arrow) and within the nasal chambers this restricts the turbinates and airflow. The changes are more dramatic in young animals as a result of the more rapid turnover of bone.

Mucopolysaccharidosis

Mucopolysaccharidosis (MPS) is a rare lysosomal disease. The most common and severe form is MPS IV. In this disease, facial dysmorphism is characterized by a short, broad face and an abnormal nasal turbinate pattern. Spinal and skeletal changes predominate, resulting in paraparesis.

Orbital disease

The orbit is formed from structures of facial origin (maxilla, lacrimal bone and zygomatic bone) as well as the ventral aspects of the cranium.

- Soft tissue causes of exophthalmos and difficulty or pain when opening the jaw (e.g. orbital cellulitis or abscessation, sialoadenitis or mass lesions of the orbit) are difficult to detect on radiography. Even where facial deformity is palpated clinically, the extent of the lesion is often underestimated. Radiographs are primarily used to assess for changes associated with the orbital wall and to establish the extent of these changes (Figure 8.47a).

- Frontal sinus or caudal nasal masses can extend into the orbit. This extension can only be identified if destruction of the orbital wall is seen. For this purpose, the open-mouth VD oblique view provides the best assessment of the caudal nasal chambers, maxilla and frontal sinuses.

- Lacrimal cysts may be developmental or acquired due to obstruction. Distortion of the maxilla is produced by an expansile, well marginated lucent cyst in the caudodorsal maxilla/lacrimal bone. Marked dilatation of the duct may cause expansion of the lateral maxilla or extend into the nasal cavity. The cysts may be demonstrated using contrast radiography (Figure 8.47b). Lacrimal cysts that communicate with the lacrimal duct become filled with contrast medium following dacryocystorhinography (see Chapter 4). Non-communicating cysts are demonstrated by injecting contrast medium directly into the cyst.

- The lacrimal duct may be obstructed by intraluminal foreign bodies or exudate. Extraluminal obstruction may occur due to masses, fractures or dental disease.

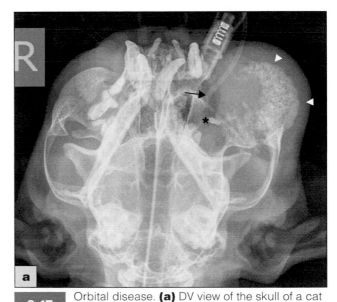

8.47 Orbital disease. **(a)** DV view of the skull of a cat with exophthalmos of the left eye and facial swelling. Clinical assessment often underestimates the extent of facial swelling as in this cat, which has a mass that has replaced most of the rostral left zygoma and maxilla. The mass is of mixed opacity with a large rounded densely mineralized area (arrowheads) arising from the lateral zygomatic arch. An extensive soft tissue component (arrowed) extends into and replaces the left maxilla and frontal sinus. Multiple teeth are absent and the first molar (*) is surrounded by the mass. (continues) ▶

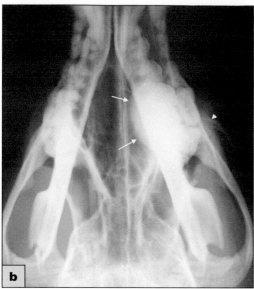

8.47 (continued) Orbital disease. **(b)** Lacrimal cyst in a dog with facial swelling and epiphora. A large contrast-filled cavity (arrowed) is superimposed on the dorsocaudal nasal chamber and lacrimal bone region. Dacryocystography (arrowhead) has been performed to demonstrate the communication between the lacrimal duct and the cyst.

- Contrast studies (e.g. dacryocystography) are required to demonstrate the location and cause of the obstruction.

Mandible, maxilla and dentition

Common indications

- Oral swellings or masses.
- Facial deformity.
- Trauma.
- Dental disease.
- Inability to close the mouth.
- Oral pain, malodorous breath, reluctance to eat and loose teeth.
- Swellings of the maxilla and mandible or gingiva.
- Malocclusion.
- Head trauma.

Equipment

Dental radiography can be performed using a conventional X-ray tube or a dedicated dental radiographic unit. The disadvantage of conventional X-ray tubes is that they are not usually in the room where dentistry is performed, which is inconvenient as radiographs may be required before, during or after the dental procedure. Furthermore, dental radiographic units can be swivelled into any position or angle required. The collimation and film–focal distance of dental radiographic units are usually fixed and the range of exposures required is limited.

Radiographic views

Radiographs can be obtained using either extraoral or intraoral techniques.

- Extraoral techniques:
  - Open-mouth ventro 20 degrees rostral-dorsocaudal oblique (V20°R-DCdO) view to evaluate the caudal maxilla (see Figure 8.29)
  - Lateral oblique view of the mandibular and maxillary dental arcades.
- Intraoral techniques:
  - Parallel technique
  - Bisecting angle technique.

To obtain radiographs using an extraoral technique, the film is placed outside the mouth. Either conventional screen cassettes or non-screen dental film can be used for these exposures. To obtain radiographs using an intraoral technique, the film is placed within the mouth. Either a conventional film–screen combination in a flexible cassette or non-screen dental film can be used for these exposures. Non-screen dental film allows the fine detail required for assessment of dental anatomy to be obtained. When used with a dedicated dental radiographic unit, the film–focal distance is determined by the size of the collimator (usually 10–20 cm). Non-screen film is usually processed using conventional chemical processing, although digital units are becoming increasingly used. Conventional processing is performed using a dedicated table top mini-darkroom or chamber.

In order to obtain an accurate representation of the teeth, radiographs should ideally be obtained with the long axis of the tooth parallel to the film. However, due to the conformation of the maxilla and mandible in the dog and cat, this is not possible for all teeth.

- Parallel technique – this technique is used to obtain radiographs with the long axis of the tooth parallel to the film. A parallel technique with intraoral film can only be used to radiograph the mandibular premolars and molars, excluding the first premolar (the film is placed medial to the body of the mandible). Near parallel radiographs of the mandibular and maxillary premolars can be obtained using an extraoral technique. However, there is always a degree of geometric distortion (foreshortening or elongation) and superimposition of the roots of teeth with multiple roots using these techniques.
- Bisecting angle technique – this technique is based on the principle of geometric projection and is an alternative to the parallel technique. The X-ray beam is centred on the imaginary line that bisects the angle formed by the X-ray film and long axis of the tooth. This results in minimal geometric distortion and a more accurate anatomical representation of the tooth. The bisecting angle technique with intraoral film is used to radiograph the maxillary and mandibular incisors and canines and the maxillary premolars.

For the purposes of this chapter, the description of radiographic techniques is limited to radiography using conventional film–screen combinations. For a detailed description of dental radiographic techniques, the reader is referred to the *BSAVA Manual of Canine and Feline Dentistry*.

Extraoral techniques

The lateral oblique view of the dental arcades (near parallel technique) is illustrated in Figure 8.48. The animal is placed in lateral recumbency with the head extended. The mouth is opened as wide as possible using a radiolucent gag. The arcade being examined is positioned closest to the film.

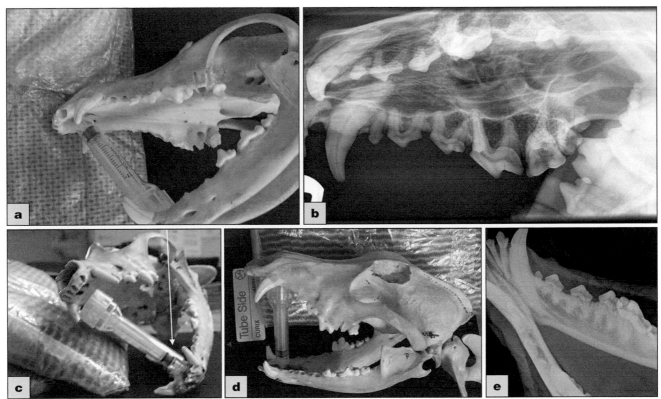

8.48 Patient positioning for lateral oblique views of the maxillary and mandibular dental arcades. **(a)** The mouth is opened and the head rotated in a VD direction. **(b)** The roots of the maxillary premolars are almost parallel to the cassette using this extraoral technique. Caudally the roots of the molars are not parallel to the film and are geometrically distorted and superimposed. **(c–d)** For the mandibular teeth, the head is rotated in a DV direction and supported. The arrow denotes the X-ray beam. **(e)** The angle formed rostrally by the converging bodies of the mandible is narrow and it is more difficult to avoid superimposition of the opposite mandible. The roots of the first three premolars are near parallel and there is greater geometric distortion of the fourth premolar and first molar.

■ For the maxillary arcade, the endotracheal tube and monitoring devices are secured to the mandible away from the region of interest. The head is rotated axially towards a VD position (usually by 20–40 degrees) so that the roots of the maxillary teeth are parallel to the cassette. The long axis of the maxilla must also be parallel to the film. A foam pad placed beneath the body of the mandible helps to achieve this position. The X-ray beam is centred on the gingival margin at the level of the fourth premolar.

■ For the mandibular premolars, the endotracheal tube is secured to the maxilla. The head is rotated towards a DV position by supporting the nose with a foam wedge. The long axis of the mandibular teeth and mandible should be positioned parallel to the cassette. The X-ray beam is centred on the fourth premolar. Due to the narrow angle of the mandible rostrally, it may not be possible to obtain an image of the first premolar without superimposition of the contralateral rostral mandible. A degree of geometric distortion of the molars is inevitable.

Intraoral techniques

■ The intraoral technique for imaging the maxillary and mandibular incisors and canines (bisecting angle technique) is similar to that described for intraoral radiography of the nasal chambers (see Figure 8.6) and mandible (see Figure 8.7), except the X-ray beam is centred on the rostral maxilla and mandible, respectively (Figure 8.49).

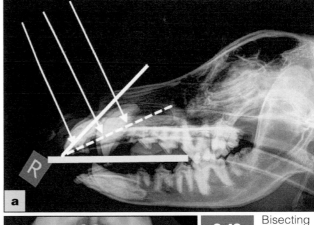

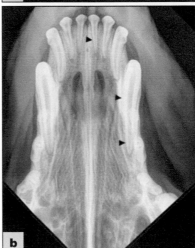

8.49 Bisecting angle technique to image the incisors and canines. **(a)** The X-ray beam is centred on an imaginary line bisecting the angle between the cassette and the long axis of the tooth. **(b)** Using this technique, the incisor and canine roots are not geometrically distorted and the entire length of the root (arrowheads) can be assessed.

- To avoid elongation or foreshortening of the teeth, the beam is angled by approximately 20 degrees in a rostrocaudal direction. Thus, the angle of the beam is perpendicular to the approximate line bisecting the angle formed by the long axis of the teeth and the cassette.

Specific approach to interpretation

Radiographic studies are performed to determine whether:

- Oral mass lesions extend to involve bone (for surgical planning)
- The origin of mass lesions can be established (e.g. gingival or periodontal ligament origin)
- Mass lesions can be distinguished from inflammatory disease (abscessation)
- Dentition changes are present that may influence treatment planning (i.e. fractured roots, fused roots and eruption abnormalities).

Common diseases

Craniomandibular osteopathy

Craniomandibular osteopathy is a self-limiting proliferative disease of the bones of the head that affects young immature dogs and mostly small breeds (West Highland White Terrier, Cairn Terrier and Scottish Terrier), although it is sporadically seen in large breeds (Labrador Retriever, Dobermann, German Shepherd Dog and Boxer). The aetiology is uncertain but in West Highland White Terriers the disease is inherited as an autosomal recessive trait. The bony lesions tend to regress at skeletal maturity. A similar condition, termed idiopathic calvarial hyperostosis, has been described in young Bullmastiffs and hyperostosis is also anecdotally suggested to occur in other giant-breed dogs.

Radiological features:

- Symmetrical deposition of florid, lamellar periosteal new bone along the ventral margin of the mandibles and tympanic bullae (Figure 8.50). Occasionally there may be involvement of the temporomandibular joint and calvarium (frontal and temporal bones).
- Affected bones become thickened and sclerotic but there is no evidence of cortical destruction. The medullary cavity may be obliterated.
- Radiographic changes may persist for a considerable time beyond the resolution of clinical signs.

With calvarial hyperostosis there is marked thickening and sclerosis of the calvarium, including the frontal, parietal and occipital bones (Figure 8.51). The changes are asymmetrical. Although usually self-limiting, the thickening can be so severe that it extends intracranially and has been associated with neurological signs.

Fractures and trauma

Maxillary and mandibular fractures are usually caused by road traffic accidents or falls from a height, and may be accompanied by concurrent injuries to the thorax or long bones. Traumatic fractures may be multiple, comminuted or complicated (open fractures)

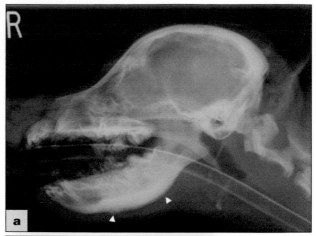

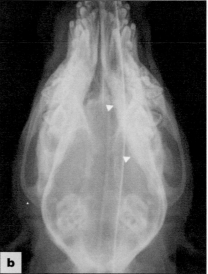

8.50 **(a)** Lateral and **(b)** DV views of the skull of a skeletally immature dog with swelling of the mandibles due to craniomandibular osteopathy. (a) Florid new bone extends along the ventral aspect of the bodies of the mandible (arrowheads). There is no cortical destruction. (b) On the DV view, although the condition is bilateral, the changes are thicker and more proliferative on the left side (arrowheads).

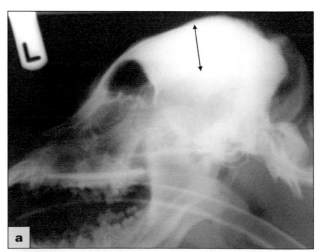

8.51 Lateral radiographs of the skulls of two dogs with calvarial hyperostosis. There is marked thickening and sclerosis of the calvarium. **(a)** The frontal, parietal and occipital bones are involved (arrowed). The changes are severe with probable encroachment upon the dorsal cranial fossa. Note that the mandibles and bullae are not affected. (continues) ▶

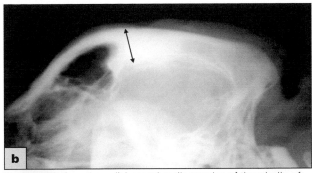

8.51 (continued) Lateral radiographs of the skulls of two dogs with calvarial hyperostosis. There is marked thickening and sclerosis of the calvarium. **(b)** The changes are more localized to the frontal bone (arrowed).

and CT studies may be required for accurate evaluation. Mandibular fractures occasionally occur as a result of bone loss associated with severe periodontitis or invasive soft tissue neoplasia.

- The teeth are frequently damaged by traumatic injuries. They may be partly or completely avulsed or the crown or roots may be fractured.
- Fractures of the mandibular body and ramus are more common in the dog.
- Mandibular symphysis fractures are more common in the cat as they are usually associated with facial impact following a fall from a height.
- Maxillary fractures are often minimally displaced and easily overlooked.
- Condylar fractures are uncommon.

Radiological features:

- With pathological fractures, the bone adjacent to the fracture may appear to lack a normal alveolar pattern with areas of lucency, and the associated cortex may be thinned and scalloped. Fracture lines may be indistinct rather than sharply marginated as seen with fractures of healthy bone. Periodontal disease, periosteal reaction or soft tissue swelling, suggestive of a mass, may be present. Pathological fractures associated with dental disease most often occur in the caudal mandible at the level of the molars.
- Midline maxillary fractures of the hard palate are usually recognized as a tapering lucent line extending from rostral to caudal (Figure 8.52). Therefore, these fractures are minimally displaced and easily overlooked. In addition, they are frequently associated with nasal discharge and blurring of the turbinates. Splitting of the hard palate is usually seen in animals that have fallen from a height (particularly cats).
- Fractures of the coronoid and condyloid processes can be difficult to identify (Figure 8.53). It is important to identify whether there is dental involvement or fractures of the teeth. These fractures may be associated with dislocation of one or both temporomandibular joints.
- In the cat, fractures of the mandibular symphysis (Figure 8.54) can be associated with swelling of the rostral mandible (due to squamous cell carcinoma or osteomyelitis due to end-stage resorptive lesions of the teeth). They appear as separation of the symphysis with minimal displacement.

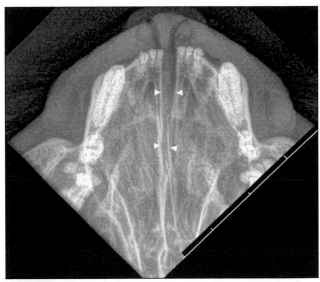

8.52 Fracture of the maxilla. There is a sagittal split (arrowheads) with mild displacement in the hard palate, which extends to the level of the third premolar.

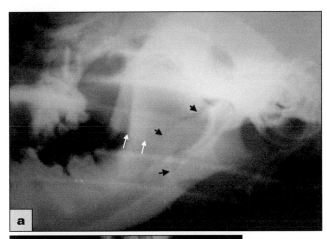

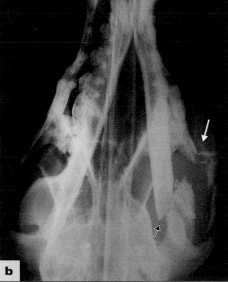

8.53 Comminuted fracture of the left mandible. **(a)** On the lateral view, a complete fracture at the junction between the body and ramus of the mandible (white arrows) is visible. An undulating fracture line between the ramus and coronoid process is also present (black arrows). **(b)** On the VD view, a concurrent comminuted fracture of the zygomatic arch (white arrow) is also seen. The mandibular fracture (black arrow) is extra-articular as the temporomandibular joint is not involved. (Courtesy of Cambridge Veterinary School)

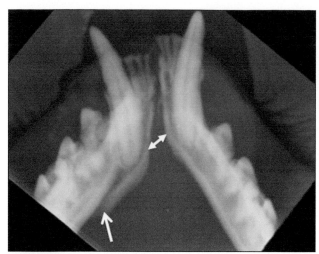

8.54 Symphysis separation in a cat. The symphysis is widened (double-headed arrow) and the right hemimandible is displaced caudally relative to the left. Note the fracture of the right mandible (arrowed) between the canine and third premolar.

With traumatic fracture, the teeth should be scrutinized carefully for small hairline cracks and fissures. Non-displaced tooth root fractures may not be seen on the initial examination and only become evident on follow-up radiographs. If the pulp cavity is exposed, infection may extend into the root of the tooth, eventually causing apical abscesses and osteomyelitis. Therefore, periodic radiographic evaluation of these teeth for evidence of infection may be necessary.

Neoplasia

Oral tumours are common in the dog and cat. Many mandibular and maxillary tumours are associated with masses arising from the surrounding soft tissues, and radiography is used to assess for extension into the underlying bone or structures. Common tumours include squamous cell carcinoma (rostral mandibular swelling in the cat) and masses arising from the periodontal elements (epulides) or gingiva (melanoma, squamous cell carcinoma, sarcoma). Primary bone tumours, especially of the mandible, are uncommon but include osteosarcoma, fibrosarcoma, undifferentiated sarcoma and (rarely) osteochondrosarcoma (multilobular tumour of bone). Benign masses of the maxilla and mandible are rare.

Radiological features:

■ The radiological features of neoplasia are illustrated in Figures 8.55 to 8.60.
■ Tumours may extend into or from the bone, resulting predominantly in a destructive pattern. The presence or extent of bone lysis is often underestimated. Periosteal new bone is often limited.
■ Tumours can be associated with displacement or loss of teeth.
■ A mixed osteolytic/osteoproductive pattern needs to be differentiated from the extensive changes associated with osteomyelitis. This distinction can be difficult.
■ Tumours arising from the caudal maxillae can be difficult to differentiate from periapical abscessation. The diagnosis may be impossible to reach without cross-sectional imaging studies or biopsy. Reliance on a radiograph may lead to misdiagnosis.

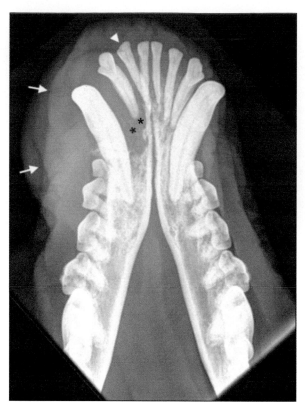

8.55 VD intraoral view of a dog with a squamous cell carcinoma of the rostral mandible. There is a soft tissue swelling (arrowed). The invasive mass is primarily destructive with loss of bone around the right incisors (*). Despite the extent of destruction there is limited displacement of the incisors (arrowhead).

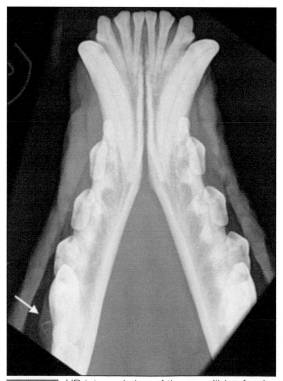

8.56 VD intraoral view of the mandible of a dog with an ossifying epulis. Note the soft tissue swelling (arrowed) lying along the gingival margin adjacent to the right first molar. Faint linear mineralization is superimposed on the swelling. The appearance is consistent with that of a tumour of periodontal ligament origin (epulis). There is no evidence of bone destruction. The mass is small and easily overlooked and would be obscured on VD views where the mandible is superimposed on the maxilla.

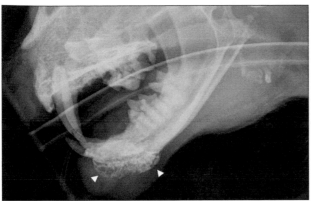

8.57 Lateral view of the skull of a cat with a fibroma of the rostral mandible. There is a dense, well defined but irregular bony mass (arrowheads) arising from the rostral mandibular cortex. The pattern is predominantly productive rather than destructive.

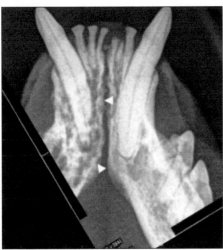

8.58 VD intraoral view of a cat with a soft tissue swelling along the rostral right hemimandible due to a plasmacytoma. An extensive irregular osteolytic pattern surrounds the root of the right mandibular canine There is slight expansion of the bone. The cortex is thinned and ragged (arrowheads) but the symphysis is intact. Differential diagnoses for the destructive pattern include neoplasia (especially squamous cell carcinoma) and severe focal osteomyelitis. However, the appearance suggests a process arising from within, rather than a soft tissue mass invading into, the mandible. Lack of specificity of the radiographic changes emphasizes the importance of obtaining a histopathological diagnosis by biopsy.

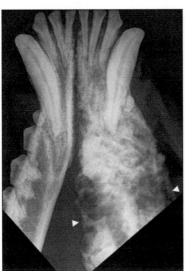

8.59 VD intraoral view of a dog with an osteo-sarcoma of the mandi-ble. An extensive mass of mixed appearance is visible. The cortices of the mandible have been destroyed and there is florid disorganized amorphous new bone. The expansion of the hemimandible (arrow-heads), destruction and amorphous new bone are consistent with a primary tumour arising from bone.

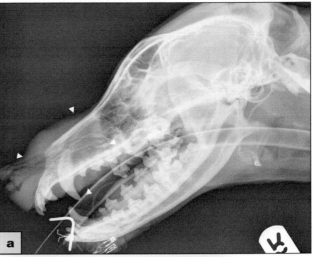

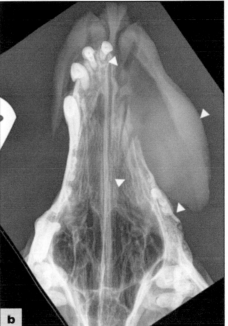

8.60 **(a)** Lateral and **(b)** DV intraoral views of the maxilla of a dog with a soft tissue sarcoma. (a) Extensive soft tissue swelling (arrowheads) is visible on the lateral view. (b) The extent of the bone destruction involving the left premaxilla and maxilla (arrowheads) is only appreciated on the DV intraoral view. As with many maxillary masses, there is little or no periosteal reaction.

Dental diseases

Radiography is most often performed in cases in which there is an external facial swelling or a draining sinus and the affected tooth is not visible on oral examination. Radiography can also be performed rapidly as part of the dental procedure using dental film and a dental X-ray unit. Pre-extraction radio-graphs should be taken to ensure that the procedure is properly planned and that no developmental abnor-malities or resorptive lesions and/or ankylosis are pre-sent. Post-extraction radiographs should be taken to ensure that all root fragments have been removed and that no iatrogenic damage has been caused.

Radiological assessment of the teeth should include:

- Tooth number
- Tooth contour, integrity and density of the dentine

- Level of the bone around the teeth, both at the furcation and interdental levels
- Size of the pulp chamber and periodontal space
- Number of roots
- Bone density around the teeth and the integrity of the lamina dura
- Evaluation for mass lesions.

Periodontitis and periodontal abscesses

Periodontitis is the most common dental disease in the dog and cat. Small dogs are most often affected. In the cat, periodontal disease is often associated with resorptive lesions at the junction between the crown and root, leading to crown fractures and retention of the roots (Figure 8.61).

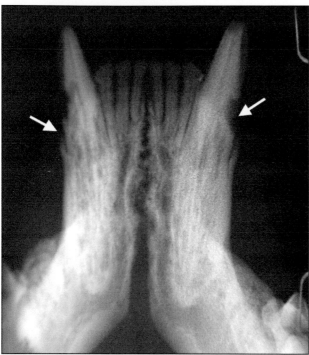

8.61 Radiograph of the rostral mandible of a cat obtained using the bisecting angle technique. Both canines have extensive enamel and dentine defects (arrowed) of the crown and crown–root junction. These changes are advanced (early resorptive lesions are difficult to recognize on radiographs). The irregularity of the mandibular symphysis is normal for an aged cat. (Courtesy of L Milella, The Veterinary Dental Practice)

A periodontal abscess may be formed secondary to periodontitis, a neoplastic process or haematogenous infection. Fracture of a tooth root and/or adjacent bony structures can lead to infection entering via the pulp cavity and formation of an apical tooth root abscess. The maxillary carnassial teeth are most commonly affected by periapical abscessation. Destruction of the tooth root may be present. The root canal may be widened if pulp necrosis is present. A consequence of previous traumatic extraction can be the presence of sequestra. These are non-vital fragments of bone. They appear sclerotic and may be surrounded by an area of lucency, representing necrotic or purulent material. Occasionally, periapical abscessation progresses to a more extensive chronic osteomyelitis with periosteal new bone and cortical destruction. This is often difficult to differentiate from soft tissue tumours invading the bone and if there is

extensive destruction or the radiological changes are not typical of periapical abscessation, then biopsy should be performed.

Radiological features:

- Resorption and loss of bone at the interdental spaces and the furcation. Bone loss can be horizontal (in the DV plane) or vertical (parallel to the roots of the teeth).
- In the cat, resorptive lesions at the crown–root junction may lead to tooth fracture and retention of the roots. Lesions may only involve the dentine or extend into the pulp cavity.
- With advanced disease, a periapical lucency (halo of lysis) around the affected root may be present. The tooth root may become irregular. Enlargement of the pulp cavity represents pulp/tooth root necrosis. At this stage, the radiological changes represent periapical abscessation (Figures 8.62 to 8.64). Periapical abscesses may occur discretely around a single tooth root or involve multiple roots. The lamina dura is not recognized.
- Facial or mandibular swelling may be present. This is usually associated with the fourth maxillary premolar, resulting in a swelling ventral to the eye. Root fragments not removed during extraction may act as sequestra with abscesses developing around them. If a mandibular tooth is affected, the ventral cortex may be thinned, eventually leading to a pathological fracture of the mandible.
- Sclerosing osteitis is a dense area of (reactive) bone formation, which may form around the root of a tooth due to pulp necrosis. This represents

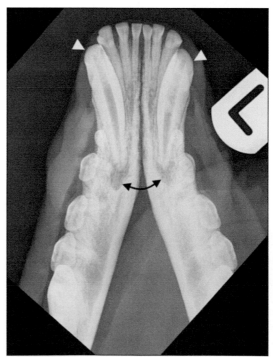

8.62 VD intraoral view of the rostral mandible of a dog with periapical abscessation of both maxillary canines. Focal lysis surrounding the apices of both incisors is visible (double-headed arrow). Note that crown fractures (arrowheads) exposing the pulp canal are present on both the left and the right and that the pulp canal is widened. These changes are consistent with bilateral periapical abscessation and pulpitis.

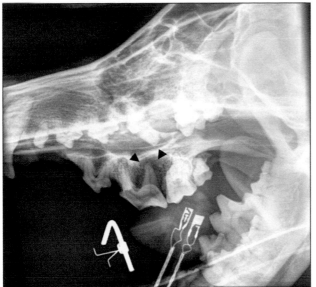

8.63 Lateral oblique view of the maxilla of a dog with a facial swelling due to a periapical abscess. The lamina dura surrounding the caudal root of the fourth premolar is indistinct (arrowheads). The trabecular bone is reduced in density and has a coarse appearance. These changes are consistent with an early periapical abscess.

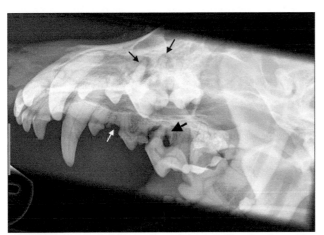

8.64 Lateral oblique view of the maxilla of a dog with periapical abscesses of both fourth premolars. Note the extensive bone loss due to periapical abscessation surrounding the rostral roots of the right (large black arrow) and rostral and caudal roots of the left (small black arrows) maxillary fourth premolars. Other radiological changes include horizontal bone loss between the first and third premolars and retention of the rostral root of the second premolar (white arrow).

low-grade stimulation, resulting in reactive bone formation. It appears as an irregularly shaped, largely uniform area of dense bone around the affected root.

- Severe periodontal disease or extensive periapical abscessation can lead to osteomyelitis, pathological fractures and formation of an oronasal fistula (Figure 8.65).
- Displacement of teeth is not usually a feature of periodontal disease and should raise suspicion for a mass lesion. Soft tissue swelling is also unusual with periodontal disease associated with periapical abscessation, with the exception of that associated with the fourth maxillary premolar.

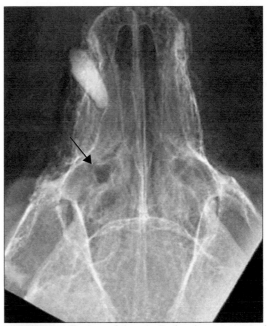

8.65 VD view of the skull of a dog presented with nasal discharge and reverse sneezing due to an oronasal fistula. A focal area of lysis (arrowed) is superimposed on the right nasal chamber and hard palate (maxilla) medial to the maxillary recess. The adjacent turbinates are blurred due to the accumulated secretions or inflammation and there is also focal turbinate destruction. All teeth apart from the right maxillary canine are absent. The diagnosis can be confirmed by visual inspection and probing the defect.

Congenital and developmental anomalies

Congenital and developmental anomalies are usually associated with abnormalities in the number, orientation and eruption of teeth. Radiography is performed to evaluate swellings, persistent deciduous teeth or permanent teeth that have not erupted, and absent or additional teeth. Dentigerous cysts are developmental anomalies or defects associated with the abnormal eruption of a tooth. These cysts are of odontogenic origin, occur infrequently and usually develop spontaneously; however, they can be acquired following iatrogenic trauma during the extraction of a deciduous tooth. These cysts are associated with the crown of an unerupted or only partially erupted tooth and are recognized as focal swellings of the gingiva. In addition, they can be associated with pathological fractures of the underlying bone and are usually extracted.

Radiological features:

- Supernumerary teeth, fusion of teeth, malpositioned teeth and impacted teeth.
- Developmental problems associated with teeth include those related to impacted or delayed eruption. Ankylosis (fusion of the root within the alveolus) is one cause of abnormal eruption. The cause may be traumatic and in the immature animal may delay eruption of the permanent teeth. The radiological feature is that the tooth root appears not to be surrounded by a lucent periodontal space. The affected tooth may be shorter in length than the adjacent teeth.
- Detection of missing permanent teeth.

- Dentigerous cysts (Figure 8.66) appear as lucent, thin-walled cyst lesions containing an unerupted tooth. The unerupted tooth is abnormally oriented. The roots of adjacent teeth can be located within the cyst. They do not normally displace other teeth. Differentiating dentigerous cysts from other cystic developmental lesions is not possible on radiographs. Differential diagnoses include periodontal cysts, eruption cysts, maxillary cysts and nasal cysts.
- Radicular cysts appear as cystic structures associated with the root of an erupted tooth.
- Pulpal stones (Figure 8.67) appear as small mineralized bodies within the pulp cavity.

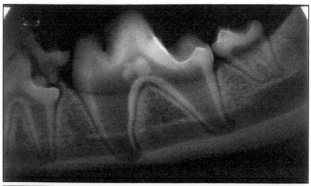

8.67 Intraoral radiograph of the mandibular molars. The pulp cavity of the first molar contains several small mineral opacities. These concretions represent pulpal stones and are an incidental finding. They are only relevant if endodontics is to be performed. (Courtesy of L Milella, The Veterinary Dental Practice)

Dental tumours

Tumours of periodontal ligament origin: These are the most common dental tumours and tend to occur in older dogs. Tumours of periodontal ligament origin or epulides originate from the periodontal stroma and are recognized along the gingival margins. Epulides are separated into three types based on histological origin:

- Fibromatous or fibrous epulides
- Ossifying epulides
- Acanthomatous epulides (canine acanthomatous ameloblastoma).

Fibromatous and ossifying epulides are pedunculated, non-ulcerating, non-invasive masses. They arise mainly around the canines in dogs and the carnassial teeth in brachycephalic breeds. They are rare in cats. Acanthomatous epulides (acanthomatous ameloblastoma or peripheral ameloblastoma) arise from the vestigial layers of the dental laminae of the mandible, typically in the incisor region. Although benign, they have characteristics of malignancy including local invasiveness and bone destruction. They do not mineralize or metastasize.

Radiological features:

- Fibromatous and ossifying epulides (Figure 8.68) contain a varying amount of bone as well as osteoid, dentinoid and cementum-like substances. The appearance of an epulis depends on the degree of mineralization and may be limited to wispy or tufted bone extending from the gingival margin or, when denser, as single or multiple bony islands with a trabecular pattern. They are usually well defined. Teeth may be displaced but there is usually no osteolysis.
- Acanthomatous epulides (Figure 8.69) do not produce dental hard products. They are usually lytic and expansile in appearance and grow slowly. A gingival soft tissue mass with infiltration and destruction of the adjacent alveolar bone may be present.

Tumours of developmental or odontogenic origin: Odontomas are of odontogenic origin and resemble the embryonic pattern of tooth development. The

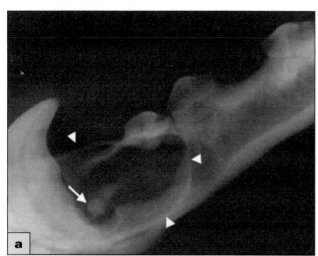

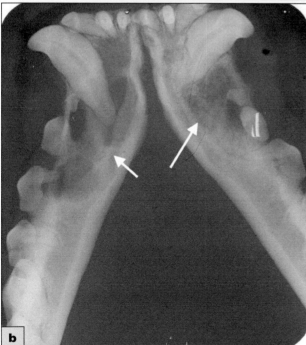

8.66 **(a)** Lateral rostral oblique and **(b)** VD views of the mandibles of two dogs with dentigerous cysts. (a) A well defined lucent cystic area (arrowheads), consistent with a dentigerous cyst, is present in the rostral mandible at the level where a tooth was absent on visual inspection. The unerupted first premolar is oriented horizontally (arrowed) and the cyst also surrounds the roots of the second premolar. (b) In this dog, the cysts are bilateral (arrowed) and surround multiple roots. (Courtesy of L Milella, The Veterinary Dental Practice)

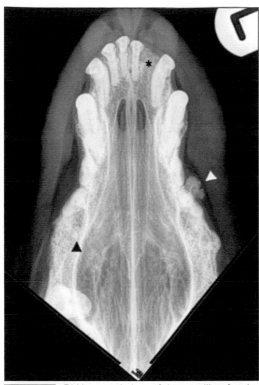

8.68 DV intraoral view of the maxilla of a dog with an ossifying epulis. A cauliflower-like ossified mass is visible adjacent to the rostral aspect of the third premolar (white arrowhead). There is no evidence of bone destruction. Other findings include the absence of the second left maxillary premolar (*) and the left and right fourth maxillary premolars, with the palatal root of the right fourth premolar being retained (black arrowhead).

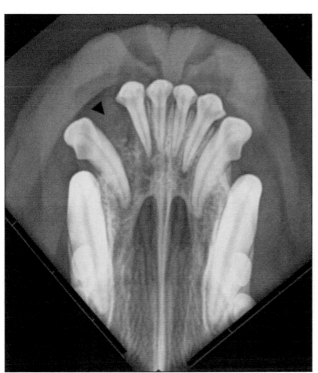

8.69 Canine acanthomatous ameloblastoma (acanthomatous epulis) demonstrating infiltration of the bone. DV intraoral view of the premaxilla. The second right maxillary incisor is missing. A poorly defined soft tissue swelling is present between the third and first incisors. The poorly marginated lysis (arrowhead) of the alveolar bone is consistent with infiltrative growth of the tumour.

mass may comprise enamel, dentine, cementum and sometimes small teeth. Odontomas may form on or near the crown or roots of a normal tooth and may resemble displaced or extra teeth.

Radiological features:

- Usually expansile masses with smooth borders and lysis of adjacent bone due to pressure atrophy.
- Internal focal mineralized opacities due to dental elements. If they contain advanced dental elements these masses are referred to as compound odontomas (Figure 8.70).
- Adjacent teeth can be displaced.

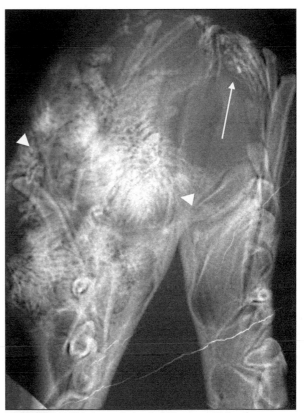

8.70 VD intraoral view of the mandible of a young dog with compound odontomas of the rostral left and right hemimandibles. The expansile masses contain multiple advanced dental components (enamel, dentine and cementum), indicating that it is of odontogenic origin. The changes are more dramatic on the right side (arrowheads). There is marked displacement of the deciduous and permanent dentition (arrowed). The swelling may only become apparent later in life. (Courtesy of L Milella, The Veterinary Dental Practice)

Temporomandibular joint

Common indications

- Difficulty in opening or closing the jaw.
- Pain/reluctance to open or close the mouth.
- Salivation, drooling and inability or reluctance to masticate.
- Facial swelling centred on the caudal jaw, orbit and zygoma.
- Head trauma.
- Bite asymmetry and malocclusion of teeth.

Radiographic views

- Lateral view (see Figure 8.1).
- DV view (see Figure 8.6)
- Caudo 30 degrees ventral–rostrodorsal oblique (Cd30°V-RDO) view.
- Open-mouth and closed-mouth sagittal oblique views.
- Open-mouth and closed-mouth rostrocaudal views.

Sagittal oblique views

- With the animal in lateral recumbency and the side of interest (temporomandibular joint) closest to the table, the nose is tilted up from a true lateral position. With the right side of the head closest to the cassette, this result in a left 20 degrees rostral–right caudal oblique (Le20°R-RtCdO) view of the right temporomandibular joint or, with the left side of the head closest to the cassette, a right 20 degrees rostral–left caudal oblique (Rt20°R-LeCdO) view of the left temporomandibular joint (Figure 8.71). The nose is elevated using a foam wedge.
- The X-ray beam is centred on the temporomandibular joint by palpating the articulation.
- The mouth is usually open.
- Brachycephalic dogs may require greater elevation of the nose (30 degrees) from a true lateral position in order for the dependent joint to be parallel to the X-ray beam. The goal is to align the condyloid process of the mandible perpendicular to the cassette, so that the joint space is visualized without superimposition. For a complete investigation of dogs with temporomandibular joint dysplasia (shallow mandibular fossa) both open- and closed-mouth sagittal oblique views may be required.

Sagittal oblique views are used to separate and assess the temporomandibular joints.

Specific approach to interpretation

Radiographic assessment is focused on:

- Identifying whether the temporomandibular joints are involved primarily or secondary to adjacent disease (bulla/muscle disease) or conformational abnormalities (zygomatic arch changes)
- Confirming whether changes are unilateral or bilateral (i.e. are the joints symmetrical in appearance)
- Ruling out degenerative changes on the temporomandibular joint and zygomatic arch
- Establishing whether the disease is congenital or acquired
- Determining whether traumatic intra-articular changes are present
- Confirming whether the changes are aggressive or non-aggressive and ruling out bone destruction.

Common diseases

Luxation and subluxation

Temporomandibular joint luxation occurs as a consequence of dysplasia, malformation (Figure 8.72) or trauma. The mandibular condyle is usually luxated rostrodorsally, leading to dental malocclusion. Fractures of the retroarticular process and mandibular condyle may allow caudal luxation of the mandibular condyle. Subluxation can be caused by dysplastic, degenerative, traumatic and idiopathic conditions, and is difficult to detect on radiography. Both open- and closed-mouth views should be obtained.

Radiological features:

- Rostral subluxation of the mandibular condyle.
- Increased width of the temporomandibular joint space. This is best detected on VD radiographs.

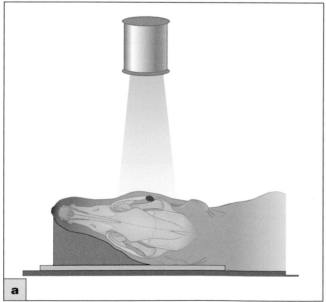 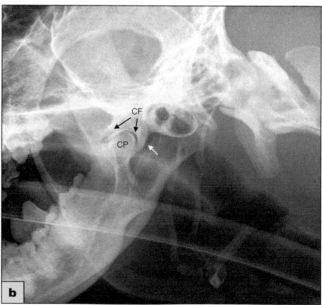

8.71 **(a)** Patient positioning for a sagittal oblique view of the temporomandibular joint. The joint being assessed is positioned closest to the plate, the nose is elevated in the sagittal plane using a foam wedge, and the X-ray beam is centred on the base of the skull at the level of the dependent temporomandibular joint. For evaluation of the left temporomandibular joint, this results in a right 20 degrees rostral–left caudal oblique (Rt20°R-LeCdO) view. **(b)** Elevation of the nose separates the temporomandibular joints and the lower joint is rotated cranially. The joint space (black arrows) is parallel to the beam. The white arrow denotes the retroarticular process. CF = mandibular fossa; CP = condyloid process.

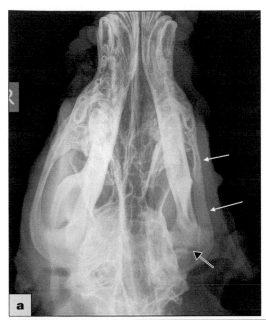

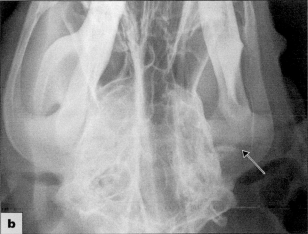

8.72 (a) DV and (b) magnified DV views of an immature dog with a malformation of the zygomatic arch. Note that the asymmetry of the mandibles is a consequence of the restriction caused by the malformation of the zygomatic arch (white arrows) and not the slight axial rotation as a result of positioning. The left temporomandibular joint is widened (black arrows).

Dysplasia

Temporomandibular joint dysplasia is a rare congenital or developmental condition affecting Basset Hounds, Dachshunds, Irish Setters, American Cocker Spaniels, Cavalier King Charles Spaniels, Pekingese, Boxers, Golden Retrievers, Labrador Retrievers and Bernese Mountain Dogs. Malformation results in laxity of the temporomandibular joint. This may lead to luxation or subluxation of the joint, with or without lateral dislocation (open-mouth jaw locking) of the coronoid process lateral to the zygoma.

Radiological features:

- Flattening of both the condyloid process of the mandible and the mandibular fossa.
- The joint space is irregularly widened.
- Changes are bilateral.
- The retroarticular process is hypoplastic and misshapen.

- The temporomandibular joints may be angled more obliquely (rostromedial orientation).
- Periarticular degenerative changes can develop.
- Periosteal bone proliferation may be seen on the zygomatic arch or coronoid process secondary to chronic irritation.

Fractures

Intra-articular fractures of the temporomandibular joint are relatively uncommon, whilst extra-articular fractures at the base of the mandibular condyle (Figure 8.73), ramus of the mandible and the zygomatic arch are more commonly recognized. Fractures of the mandibular fossa and retroarticular process are often comminuted and found in association with a fractured zygomatic arch. Fractures may be unilateral or bilateral.

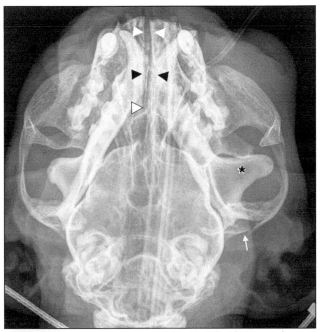

8.73 DV view of the skull of a cat following an unknown trauma. Multiple fractures are present. There is a minimally displaced midline fracture of the hard palate (white arrowheads), separation of the mandibular symphysis (black arrowheads) and a fracture of the lateral aspect of the temporomandibular joint with rostral displacement of the mandibular condyle (arrowed). Consequently, the coronoid process (*) has rotated outwards.

Radiological features:

- On sagittal oblique views, luxation results in overlapping of the condyloid process and mandibular fossa.
- A sclerotic band is visible where these bones are superimposed.
- Increased width of the temporomandibular joint space.
- The condyloid process is usually displaced rostrally. If the retroarticular process is fractured, luxation may be in a caudal direction.

Ankylosis

Ankylosis refers to restricted or complete immobility and consolidation of the temporomandibular joint. It is usually a consequence of untreated intra-articular (true ankylosis) or extra-articular (false ankylosis) trauma.

True ankylosis is more common in the cat than in the dog. False ankylosis and progressive restriction of jaw movement may occur following untreated zygomatic and mandibular fractures or due to mandibular or zygomatic masses, extensive new bone formation in chronic otitis media, aural and retro-orbital abscesses and extensive new bone formation associated with craniomandibular osteopathy in the dog.

Radiological features:

- True ankylosis – loss of the regular temporomandibular joint space and mandibular condyle contour and associated irregular bone formation. In the cat, periarticular new bone is seen as the main radiological feature.
- False ankylosis – may be possible to identify the underlying cause by inspecting the remainder of the mandible, the bullae and the zygoma (see Figure 8.76). Periarticular new bone may be the predominant feature, but the joint space and condyle may be recognized as normal on individual views.

Degenerative joint disease and infection

Osteoarthritis of the temporomandibular joint can be a sequel to trauma, dysplasia or contralateral mandibulectomy. Infection of the temporomandibular joint is rare, usually due to extension of osteomyelitis from the ipsilateral tympanic bulla, or a local penetrating bite.

Radiological features:

- With degenerative temporomandibular joint disease, osteoproductive changes alone are present. Changes are usually bilateral.
- With infection, the appearance may not differ significantly from that seen with degenerative joint disease, although occasionally bone lysis may be present. Unilateral changes and associated soft tissue swellings should raise the index of suspicion for infection.

Neoplasia

Primary neoplasia of the temporomandibular joint is rare in the dog and cat. The most common tumours in the dog are osteosarcoma and osteochondrosarcoma (multilobular tumour of bone). The extension of mass lesions of the skull base to involve the mandibular fossa is more common.

Radiological features:

- Identifying tumours involving the temporomandibular joint is challenging due to the superimposition of multiple structures on both views. The most reliable radiographic signs include:
  - Asymmetrical appearance to the temporomandibular joint, especially on the VD view
  - Rostral displacement of the temporomandibular joint on the affected side
  - Osteolysis of the mandibular fossa and zygoma or condyloid process
  - Axial rotation of the coronoid process on well positioned VD or DV views.

- Osteochondrosarcomas (multilobular tumour of bone) appear as well defined, rounded, osseous masses with coarse, granular mineralization arising from the mandible. Underlying bone destruction may be impossible to recognize in the laterally flattened mandible. These neoplasms more commonly arise from the zygomatic arch or other flat bones of the skull.
- Osteosarcomas and other aggressive bone tumours are characterized by extensive lysis of the affected bone, a marked irregular periosteal reaction and poor margination. These lesions do not usually extend across the joint space to involve adjacent bones.
- Tumours arising from the maxilla, bullae or base of the skull may be locally invasive and extend to secondarily involve the temporomandibular joint.
- Skull osteomas in cats have a characteristic radiographic pattern, appearing as well circumscribed, very radiopaque masses on the periosteal surface of otherwise unaffected bone.

Ears and bullae

Although clinical disease associated with the middle ear is most often unilateral, the radiographic signs are frequently bilateral.

Common indications

- To complement otoscopy when assessing the extent of stenosis in the external ear canal.
- Para-aural swelling.
- Middle ear disease and head tilt.

Radiographic views

- DV view (see Figure 8.2).
- Lateral oblique views (e.g. left 30 degrees ventral–right dorsal oblique (Le30°V-RtDO) view and right 30 degrees ventral–left dorsal oblique (Rt°30V-LeDO) view).
- Open-mouth rostrocaudal view.
- Rostro 10 degrees ventral–caudodorsal oblique (R10°V-CdDO) view (cat).

Lateral oblique view: bullae

- The animal is placed in lateral recumbency with the head extended and the side of interest closest to the table. The skull is then rotated about its long axis towards a VD direction. Axial rotation is achieved by placing a wedge beneath the ventral aspect of the mandible. As the head tapers towards the nose, the head is placed slightly across the wedge to keep the nose parallel to the cassette. Dogs with floppy ears should have the ears taped back.
- To image the bullae, the degree of rotation required from a true lateral position is 20–30 degrees. For the right bulla, a left 20 degrees ventral–right dorsal oblique (Le20°V-RtDO) view should be obtained and for the left bulla, a right 20 degrees ventral–left dorsal oblique (Rt20°V-LeDO) view should be obtained.
- The X-ray beam should be centred on the lower

bulla. The positional marker is placed below the dependent bulla to avoid confusion with labelling.

- The dependent bulla is projected ventrally beneath the skull base and the upper bulla is superimposed on the skull base and poorly visualized (Figure 8.74).

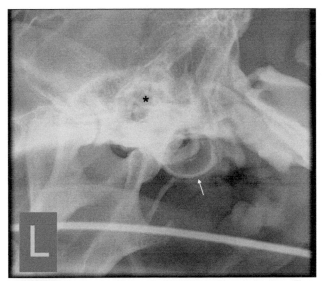

8.74 Lateral oblique view of the tympanic bullae. The dependent bulla is projected ventral to the skull base and is filled with air (arrowed). The upper bulla (*) is superimposed on the skull base.

Lateral oblique views are used to separate the tympanic bullae.

Open-mouth rostrocaudal view: bullae

- The animal is positioned in dorsal recumbency in a trough and the forelimbs are extended caudally. The head is flexed and the mouth is held wide open with the hard palate rotated to form an angle of approximately 30 degrees to the vertical (Figure 8.75).
- The head, maxilla and mandible must be restrained using tape and sandbags or a frame.

The tongue should be pulled forward and moved out of the way by pushing and securing it against the mandible. The back of the head and neck should be supported with foam pads to avoid rotation. It is difficult to obtain a symmetrical view. If the mouth is not opened sufficiently, the coronoid processes will obscure the bullae. Asymmetrical views or views with the tongue superimposed on the bullae mimic middle ear disease. The endotracheal tube is usually removed for the exposure. The clinician must be prepared to reintubate and reposition the patient if the image is unsatisfactory.

- The X-ray beam is centred on the back of the mouth.

The open-mouth rostrocaudal view is used to examine and compare the tympanic bullae. Although it also provides a good image of the dens, which is visible between the two bullae, the degree of hyperflexion required to create the image is usually considered unsafe in animals with atlantoaxial instability and therefore discouraged. This view can also be used to assess for changes in the shape of the foramen magnum.

Rostral 10 degrees ventral–caudodorsal oblique view: bullae (cats)

- The cat is positioned in dorsal recumbency in a trough and the forelimbs are extended caudally. The head is flexed so that the base of the skull rests on the cassette and the hard palate is parallel with the X-ray beam and perpendicular to the table top. The nose is then tilted slightly towards the dorsal direction so that the hard palate forms an angle of 10 degrees with the vertical (Figure 8.76a).
- The X-ray beam is directed on the midline at the level of the angle of the mandibles. This 'nose-up' view is technically easier to obtain than the open-mouth rostrocaudal view.
- This modified view takes advantage of the comparatively large bullae in the cat, which project substantially below the skull base (Figure 8.76b).

The R10°V-CdDO view is used to assess the tympanic bullae in the cat.

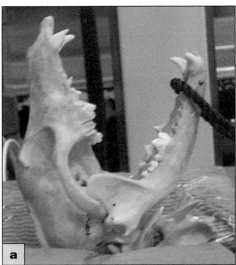
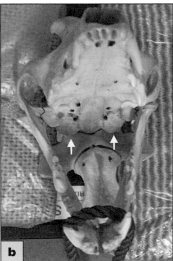
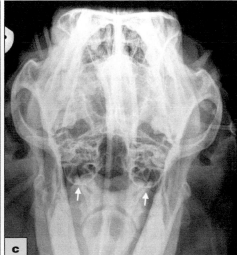

8.75 (a–b) Patient positioning for an open-mouth rostrocaudal view of the bullae (arrowed). The lower jaw is pulled out of the primary beam to avoid superimposition of the tongue, and the hard palate is tilted dorsally by 20–30 degrees. (c) The air-filled bullae (arrowed) are projected between the rami of the mandible.

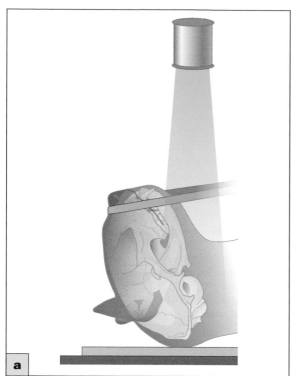

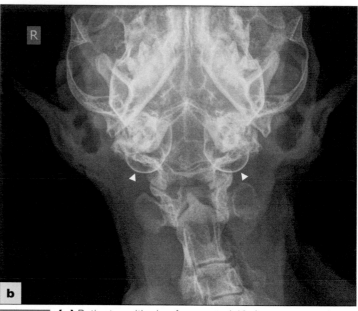

8.76 **(a)** Patient positioning for a rostral 10 degrees ventral–caudodorsal oblique (R10°V-CdDO) view of the bullae in a cat. The mouth is closed and the hard palate tilted 10 degrees towards the vertical. **(b)** The large bullae (arrowheads) are projected ventral to the skull base.

Specific approach to interpretation

Radiographic assessment is focused on determining whether:

- The tympanic bullae are filled with air or soft tissue
- The osseous bullae are intact or disrupted
- The changes are unilateral or bilateral
- There is nasopharyngeal involvement.

Common diseases

In most cases of ear disease, the pathology is unilateral and so comparison of the two sides (on symmetrical DV/rostrocaudal or comparable oblique lateral radiographs) is very useful for recognizing deviation from normal. On all radiographic views, the tympanic bullae are completely or at least partially superimposed on other structures such as the base of the tongue or the skull base, which complicates interpretation. It is important to note that bilateral sclerosis of the tympanic bullae can be present in normal older animals or may be the result of previous ear disease.

Otitis externa

Although external ear disease is usually assessed visually by otoscopy, radiography can be used to assess the extent and severity of the stenosis. Radiography is useful in unusual cases, such as atresia or avulsion of the external ear canal, as an assessment can be made of all the segments of the ear canal and compared with the opposite side. In cases of atresia, a segment of the external ear canal is absent. The vertical or horizontal ear canal can be affected. The intact segment terminates in a blind sac. With avulsion or traumatic separation of the external ear canal, there is a similar blind-ending external ear canal and the tympanic membrane cannot be visualized, but this tends to be more frequently associated with para-aural abscessation and middle ear disease.

Radiological features:

- The external ear canal is partially narrowed or completely occluded by thickening of the ear canal (hyperplasia) or accumulated discharge. Neoplastic masses of the external ear canal are indistinguishable from inflammatory changes.
- Mineralization of the ear canal is a bilaterally symmetrical finding in some older normal dogs, but when it is extensive and asymmetrical it is usually considered to be consistent with chronic otitis externa.
- In severe chronic otitis externa with marked proliferative hyperplasia, the ear canal may be expanded and resemble a mass lesion. Radiological assessment in these cases is usually limited to examination of the adjacent bulla, although it may be possible to establish from radiography if some part of the external ear canal is patent.
- With atresia of the vertical external ear canal, the air-filled external ear canal ends blindly and is separated from the bulla by soft tissue. Bulla changes are occasionally present.
- With traumatic avulsion of the external ear canal, the air-filled ear canal ends blindly and does not extend to the bulla. Para-aural soft tissue swelling and/or middle ear changes may be present.

Otitis media

Otitis media is most often associated with extension of otitis externa through the tympanic membrane. Radiographs of the bullae are primarily indicated for the assessment of animals with chronic otitis externa when the tympanum cannot be directly visualized, or when there is clinical suspicion of otitis media even if the tympanum appears to be intact. With severe otitis media there may be discomfort associated with opening the mouth if extensive para-aural changes are present. Radiographs should be obtained before flushing the ear. Caution should be exercised when assessing radiographs of bullae to avoid a false-positive diagnosis by misinterpreting soft tissue opacities overlying the bullae as originating from within the bullae.

Radiological features:

- Air within the bulla replaced by a soft tissue opacity (Figure 8.77).
- Sclerosis and thickening of the tympanic bulla wall as well as sclerosis and bony proliferation of the petrous temporal bone. Occasionally, there may be bony proliferation around the temporomandibular joint.
- Signs of otitis externa may be concurrent with otitis media.
- Lysis of the bony bulla wall and petrous temporal bone as well as para-aural soft tissue swelling may be present in chronic advanced disease. This indicates an aggressive process.
- Expansion (enlargement) of the diseased bulla (Figure 8.78) is an uncommon finding in middle ear disease. Thinning of the bulla wall due to bone atrophy may mimic bone lysis.
- Soft tissue mass dorsal to the soft palate due to nasopharyngeal polyps (cats).

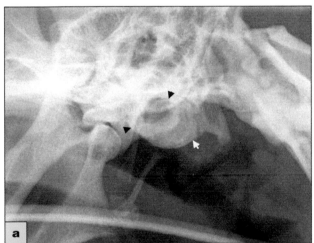

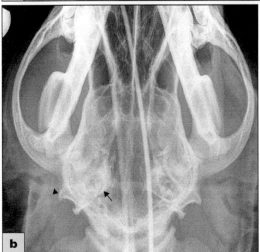

8.77 **(a)** Lateral oblique view of the right bulla and **(b)** DV view of the skull of a dog with otitis media. Air in the bulla has been replaced by a soft tissue/bone opacity consistent with otitis media (arrowed). The distal ear canal is mineralized (arrowheads).

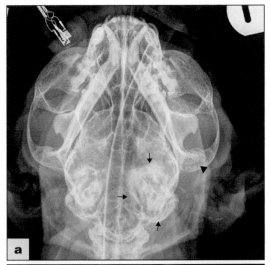

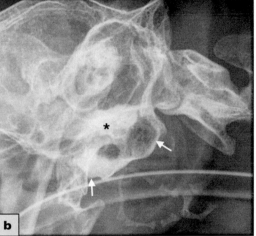

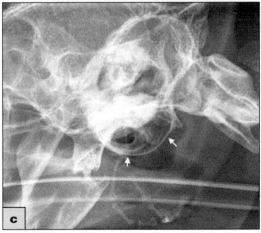

8.78 **(a)** DV and **(b)** left and **(c)** right lateral oblique views of the bullae of a cat with otitis media due to a polyp. (a) The left bulla is slightly enlarged and sclerotic (arrowed). A normal air-filled external ear canal cannot be recognized on the left side (arrowhead). (b) The left bulla is filled with a soft tissue opacity and is markedly sclerotic (arrowed). The dense petrous temporal bone lies dorsal to the bulla (*). (c) Normal right bulla (arrowed).

Osteolytic changes of the bulla or petrous temporal bone suggest an aggressive process associated either with infection or neoplasia; however, the radiological features are not specific for the underlying cause and, on occasion, infection may be accompanied by aggressive bone destruction and thus mistaken for neoplasia. Unstructured or disorganized new bone is not usually a feature of infection. Although lysis of the bulla wall may occur with otitis media, it is rare for it to extend to adjacent bones. Therefore, where this is identified, the more likely diagnosis is neoplasia.

Radiography is an insensitive technique for assessment of the presence of middle ear disease in the dog; reports suggest that between 25 and 40% of cases may be overlooked. A normal radiographic study, therefore, does not exclude otitis media. The identification of chronic, advanced or severe disease using radiography is usually possible. Recognition of increased opacity of the bulla in the dog is particularly difficult, even on DV views, despite the benefit of comparison with the opposite bulla when unilateral disease is suspected. Even slight rotation of the DV view may mimic pathology. Radiography is far more sensitive for the detection of middle ear disease in the cat and most cases can be identified.

Bilateral sclerosis of the bullae can be found in some normal aged animals, especially cats. The differential diagnoses for unilateral sclerosis and thickening of the bullae include nasopharyngeal polyps, neoplasia and, occasionally, craniomandibular osteopathy. Following ventral bulla osteotomy, the bulla wall may reform over time. Post-surgical complications include the development of fistulous tracts, osteomyelitis of the temporal and zygomatic temporal bones, and abscessation within the adjacent soft tissues.

When it is not possible to examine the tympanic membrane adequately by otoscopy, it can be assessed using radiography by infusing non-ionic water-soluble iodinated contrast medium (e.g. iohexol) into the external ear canal (canalography). A DV view of the skull should then be obtained. An intact tympanic membrane prevents contrast medium entering the tympanic bulla. The accumulation of contrast medium in the bulla confirms that the membrane is ruptured even if this is not evident on otoscopy. A false-negative result may occur if the flow of contrast medium is impeded by a thickened external ear canal wall or the aggregation of debris within the external ear canal. The presence of a ruptured tympanic membrane suggests otitis media.

Neoplasia

Malignant tumours of the ears and bullae are uncommon in the dog and cat (Figure 8.79) and tend to be locally invasive and destructive but rarely metastasize. Carcinomas (squamous cell carcinoma, ceruminous gland carcinoma) are most common. Tumours may arise from either the bullae or the external ear canals.

Radiological findings:

- Increased soft tissue opacity within the bulla and sclerosis or irregular thickening of the osseous bulla.
- In some cases, neoplastic processes lead to lysis of the osseous bulla and extend to the adjacent bony structures (base of the skull and the temporomandibular joint).
- Soft tissue tumours may extend into the adjacent structures, appearing as poorly marginated soft tissue masses, obliterating the ear canal and displacing fascial planes.

Distinguishing severe osteomyelitis (or complications arising from a previous bulla osteotomy) from

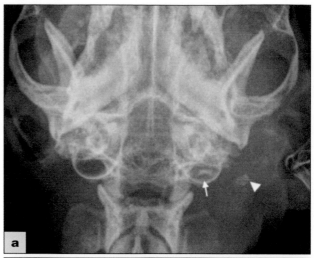

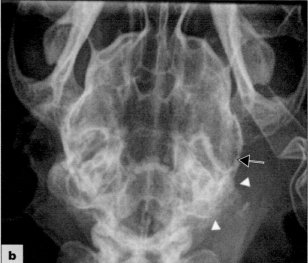

8.79 **(a)** Rostral 10 degrees ventral–caudodorsal oblique (R10°V-CdDO) and **(b)** DV views of the bullae of a cat with an aural tumour involving the left bulla. (a) The left tympanic bulla is of soft tissue opacity (arrowed). Note the extensive soft tissue swelling lateral to the bulla and displaced bone fragments (arrowhead). The air-filled external ear canal cannot be recognized. (b) On the DV view, the lateral aspect of the bulla appears disrupted (arrowheads) with displacement of the bone fragments laterally. Extensive lysis of the basicranium was also recognized on CT; however, these changes can only be suspected on radiography by the roughening and thinning of the lateral aspect of the cranial bones (arrowed).

neoplasia may be impossible in some cases as they can have a similar appearance. In extensive disease involving destruction of the bulla, the presence of disorganized or unstructured bone and lysis extending to the adjacent structures (temporomandibular joint and basicranium) makes a diagnosis of neoplasia more likely than osteomyelitis.

Nasopharyngeal polyps

In cats with signs of otitis media, in addition to obtaining views of the bullae, a lateral radiograph of the skull is useful to examine the nasopharynx for the presence of nasopharyngeal polyps. Feline nasopharyngeal polyps are benign fibrovascular growths that originate from the mucosa of the middle ear or Eustachian tube. Polyps may grow into the tympanic bulla, nasopharynx or ear canal.

Radiological appearance:

- Rounded intraluminal soft tissue mass filling the nasopharynx and displacing the soft palate ventrally (Figure 8.80).
- The rostral margin of the polyp may be indistinct but the caudal margin is defined by air.
- Soft tissue opacification of the ipsilateral bulla indicating concurrent signs of otitis media or a polyp within the bulla.
- Thickening of the tympanic bulla wall and increased soft tissue opacity within the bulla.
- The polyp may grow into the ear canal, leading to soft tissue obliteration of the ear canal with signs of otitis externa. Occasionally, nasopharyngeal polyps markedly enlarge, resulting in expansion and thinning of the affected bulla. This may give rise to an appearance of aggressive disease on radiography, which can be misinterpreted as a tumour.

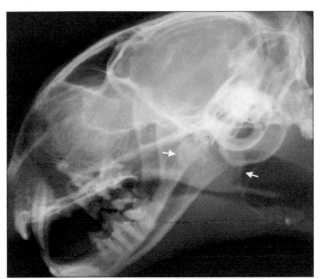

8.80 Lateral view of the pharynx of a cat with a nasopharyngeal polyp. An oval soft tissue mass (arrowed) lies dorsal to the soft palate and displaces it ventrally. Both the cranial and caudal borders are visible.

Otoliths

Otoliths appear as well defined, rounded or oval mineral opacities within the tympanic bulla and are sometimes associated with thickening of the bulla wall. Otoliths are probably formed due to mineralization of necrotic material or inflammatory polyps secondary to concurrent or previous episodes of otitis media. They may be an incidental finding.

Larynx and pharynx

Common indications

- Mass lesions involving the larynx and pharynx.
- Inspiratory dyspnoea, coughing, retching and gagging.
- Dysphagia.
- Swellings.
- Suspected foreign body injuries.

Radiographic views

- Lateral view (see Figure 8.1).
- DV view (usually of little value but may help when localizing foreign bodies).

Lateral view: pharynx

Positioning is as for lateral skull views. The mouth should be partially opened to reduce superimposition of dental structures and to better assess the air-filled oropharynx. The X-ray beam should be directed just caudal to the angle of the mandible. VD and DV views of the pharynx are of limited value due to superimposition of the skull and spine. The lateral view is used to assess for lesions of the oropharynx, nasopharynx, larynx, hyoid apparatus and retropharyngeal soft tissues.

Specific approach to interpretation

Radiographic assessment is focused on recognizing:

- Soft tissue masses
- Free gas in the fascial planes (penetrating foreign bodies)
- Displacement of the hyoid or larynx, indicating mass lesions
- Destruction of the hyoid.

Common diseases

Elongated and thickened soft palate

The soft palate normally extends to the tip of the epiglottis. Elongation of the soft palate is usually seen concurrently with thickening and narrowing or even occlusion of the nasopharynx (Figure 8.81). Thickening of the soft palate can be an artefact due to axial rotation of the head or may result from a primary inflammatory insult or neoplasia.

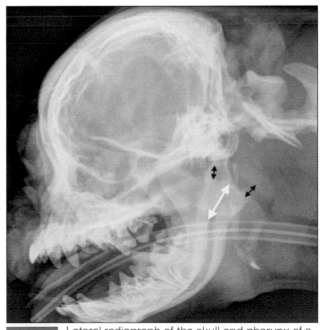

8.81 Lateral radiograph of the skull and pharynx of a brachycephalic dog. The soft palate is thickened and elongated (white arrow), the nasopharynx is narrowed (black arrows) and the thickened retropharyngeal tissues have displaced the pharynx ventrally. The caudal aspect of the soft palate extends beyond the tip of the epiglottis.

Pharyngeal and laryngeal foreign bodies

Foreign bodies can occur in both dogs and cats and may lead to acute or chronic pharyngeal and/or laryngeal disease.

- Pharyngeal stick injuries, bones, grass awns and fishhooks are commonly encountered foreign bodies.
- In acute injuries, there may be no radiographic changes if the foreign body is radiolucent.
- Cervical swelling due to haematomas or subcutaneous emphysema may be present with larger foreign bodies, such as sticks, as these are usually associated with some form of traumatic impalement.
- Animals with ingested foreign bodies, such as bones, usually present with acute signs of gagging or choking, although, surprisingly, they may also present chronically.

Radiological features:

- Acute injuries are associated with subcutaneous emphysema and swelling of the cervical soft tissues. In severe cases, haemorrhage and displacement of the larynx or cranial trachea may be present.
- Chronic injuries are associated with swelling and abscessation.
- Draining sinus tracts may be present and contain gas.
- Radiolucent retropharyngeal foreign bodies are hard to diagnose but may result in soft tissue swelling and bubbles of trapped gas (Figure 8.82). Geometric shapes may be present, suggestive of a foreign body. Particulate mineralized debris may be carried in by the penetrating foreign body and be recognized even if the foreign body itself is not. Foreign bodies may be visible if radiopaque or outlined by air.

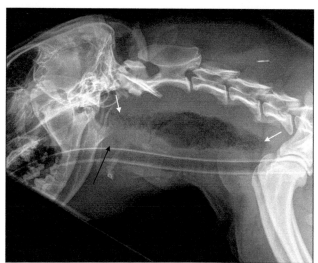

8.82 Lateral view of the pharynx of a dog with a retropharyngeal stick injury. A large retropharyngeal abscess extends from the pharynx to the level of the fifth cervical vertebra (white arrows). The abscess contains fluid and gas. The larynx and cervical trachea are displaced ventrally by the swelling and the nasopharynx is markedly narrowed (black arrow). Two large stick fragments were retrieved during surgery; however, they cannot be recognized on the radiograph.

If a discharging sinus is present, then sinography may be helpful in demonstrating the location of the foreign body. A probe or radiopaque marker should be used to identify the sinus and a non-ionic, water-soluble, iodine-containing contrast agent injected into the sinus tract. The tip of the catheter can be sutured into the sinus to prevent leakage of contrast medium. However, caution should be exercised when considering sinography. CT and MRI are considerably more useful for evaluating the presence of a foreign body as well as for assessing the location and extent of sinus tracts. Although these imaging modalities are more expensive, their use can reduce the likelihood that a revision surgery will be required. The identification of foreign bodies using sinography can be challenging as discharge and granulomatous tissue within the tract can mimic foreign bodies and confound the diagnosis.

Nasopharyngeal stenosis

Nasopharyngeal stenosis may be associated with reverse sneezing, retching, gagging or chronic rhinitis. The diagnosis may be apparent on a conventional lateral view (Figure 8.83), depending on the degree of stenosis, but the limitation of radiography is that the cross-sectional area of the stenosis cannot be demonstrated. Accurate positioning is required so that a comparison can be made if balloon dilation (bougienage) is used as a therapeutic option.

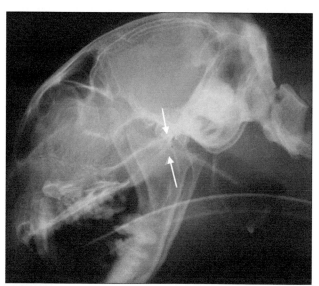

8.83 Nasopharyngeal stenosis. The junction between the posterior nares and the nasopharynx is kinked and narrowed (arrowed). Although contrast procedures can be used to demonstrate this abnormality, cross-sectional imaging is the technique of choice.

Radiological findings:

- The air-filled passage between the ventral nasal meatus and nasopharynx is narrowed or not visible.

Neoplasia

Pharyngeal tumours: Pharyngeal lesions are usually associated with soft tissue masses from adjacent structures displacing or invading the air space (caudal extension of nasal masses, oral or tonsillar squamous cell carcinoma or invasive adenocarcinoma of the salivary glands). Lymphoma can present as a primary nasopharyngeal mass and must be differentiated from a nasopharyngeal polyp.

Radiological features:

■ Soft tissue mass lesion filling defect within the nasopharynx or caudal pharynx (Figure 8.84).
■ Retropharyngeal swelling.
■ Displacement of the soft palate, hyoid or larynx.

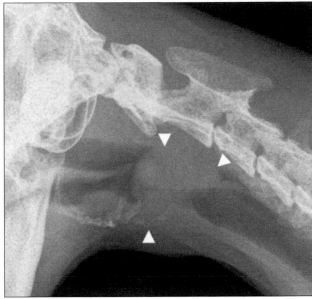

8.85 Lateral view of the pharynx of a cat with inspiratory dyspnoea due to a laryngeal mass (lymphoma). The larynx is markedly thickened by the concentric soft tissue mass (arrowheads). The pharynx is distended with air as a result of the obstruction caused by the laryngeal mass and respiratory effort. The cranial cervical trachea is also distended with air.

Radiological features:

■ General reduction in laryngeal air space.
■ Increase in opacity of the larynx due to soft tissue swelling.
■ Retropharyngeal lymph node enlargement causing displacement of the larynx and loss of the fascial plane fat.
■ Laryngeal obstruction may lead to signs of air-trapping in the thorax and stomach due to dyspnoea.

Thyroid tumours: Thyroid tumours, if large, appear as distinct, ventrally convex masses beneath C2–C4, causing pharyngeal compression and ventral displacement of the larynx and proximal trachea. Small lesions may not be recognized. If the tumour is associated with difficulties swallowing or regurgitation, a barium oesophagram can be used to assess for compression and displacement. Occasionally, invasion of the trachea and cervical vertebrae is recognized with large fixed thyroid masses. Cats with hyperthyroidism can present with a cranial cervical swelling. Radiography may demonstrate a mass caudal to the larynx. Chest radiographs, including the thoracic inlet, should be obtained as thyroid carcinoma can present with multiple masses, including lesions at the thoracic inlet and in the cranioventral mediastinum.

Salivary glands

There are four main paired salivary glands: the monostomatic and polystomatic sublingual salivary glands; the mandibular salivary glands; the zygomatic salivary glands; and the parotid salivary glands. The salivary glands are not visible on

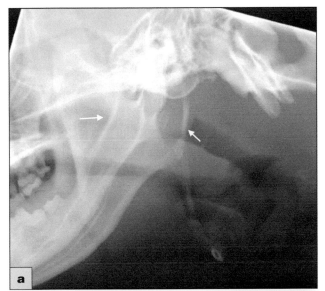

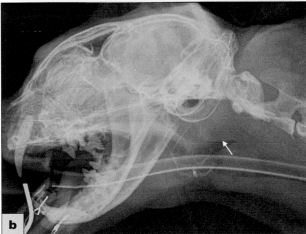

8.84 Lateral views of the pharynx of two cats with nasopharyngeal swellings. **(a)** A broad soft tissue mass fills the nasopharynx dorsal to the soft palate (arrowed). The mass does not displace the soft palate. The mass was confirmed as lymphoma but cannot be distinguished from a nasopharyngeal polyp based on radiographic appearance alone. **(b)** The broad-based soft tissue mass (arrowed) bulges into the caudal aspect of the pharynx, reducing the size of the normally air-filled space. The mass was confirmed as an extensive squamous cell carcinoma of the fauces, extending into the pharynx.

Laryngeal tumours: The most common canine laryngeal tumours are malignant epithelial tumours (e.g. carcinoma, squamous cell carcinoma, mast cell tumour) and rhabdomyoma. The most common laryngeal tumours in the cat are lymphosarcoma (Figure 8.85) and squamous cell carcinoma.

radiographs. Radiography is performed to rule out bone involvement, to assess the extent of the changes and to detect the presence of gas or radiopaque foreign bodies. A positive contrast study (sialography) is required to demonstrate that the salivary glands are intact. An abnormal sialogram, however, is non-specific and differentiation between pathology such as severe inflammation and neoplasia is usually not possible.

Common diseases

Sialoadenitis, salivary mucocele and sialoliths

Sialoadenitis is inflammation of the salivary glands. An underlying cause is not usually found. In severe cases, the changes may progress to necrosis and abscessation.

Salivary mucocele is the most commonly recognized clinical disease of the salivary gland. It is more common in the dog that than cat. A mucocele comprises an accumulation of saliva in the subcutaneous tissue and the consequent tissue reaction to the saliva. Trauma has been proposed as the cause of salivary mucocele. The sublingual salivary glands are most commonly associated with salivary gland mucocele.

Radiological features:

- Sialoadenitis (Figure 8.86) and salivary mucoceles result in soft tissue swellings ventral to the angle of the mandible and around the base of the ear.
- Sialography can be used to demonstrate the communication between the swellings and the salivary system and determine whether duct rupture is present (Figure 8.87).
- Sialoliths (Figure 8.88) appear as small, round or rod-shaped, radiopaque calculi within the salivary ducts. They are usually incidental findings.

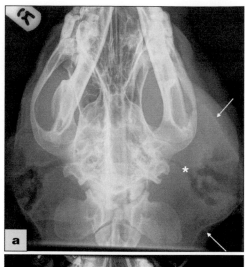
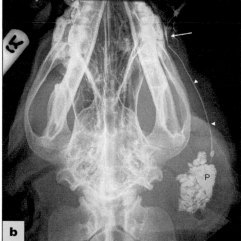

8.87 **(a)** VD survey radiograph and **(b)** sialogram of the skull of a dog with extensive cellulitis surrounding the left ear. (a) There is extensive swelling (arrowed) around the left external ear canal (*). (b) The parotid duct has been cannulated (arrowed) and the duct (arrowheads) has a normal thin, even appearance. The gland (P) is not disrupted and the contrast medium results in a normal 'cobble stone' appearance. The sialogram confirms that the cellulitis is not associated with the parotid gland.

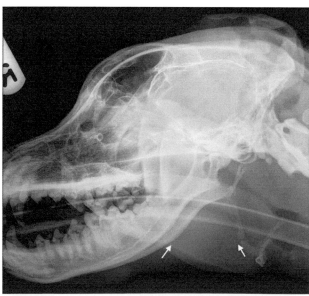

8.86 Lateral view of the skull of a dog with bilateral sialoadenitis. The radiographic changes are limited to soft tissue swelling caudoventral to the angle of the jaw (arrowed).

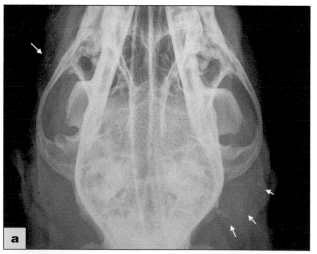

8.88 **(a)** VD radiograph of a dog with sialoliths. The sialoliths appear as small discrete mineralized bodies (arrowed) either singularly or in clusters. In this dog, they are bilateral. On the right, they are located close to the termination of the parotid duct of the buccal mucosa, opposite the fourth maxillary premolar, and on the left, they are located within the gland and proximal parotid duct. (continues) ▶

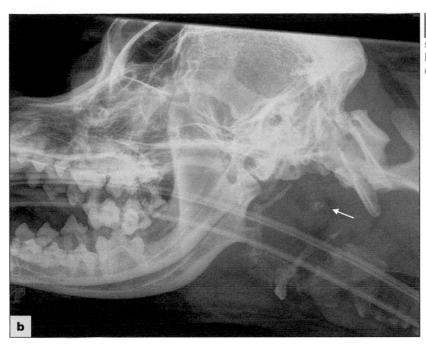

8.88 (continued) **(b)** Lateral radiograph of a dog with sialoliths. The sialoliths appear as small discrete mineralized bodies (arrowed) either singularly or in clusters.

Hyoid bones

Common indications
The indications for examination of the hyoid bones are similar to those for the larynx and pharynx (see earlier).

Radiographic views
The hyoid apparatus is best seen on a lateral view (see Figure 8.1) due to superimposition of other structures on the hyoid bones on the VD view. The animal may have to be extubated.

Specific approach to interpretation
The individual hyoid bones should be assessed carefully for displacement and fractures, as well as expansile and lytic lesions.

Common diseases

Trauma

- Trauma to the neck may cause fractures and luxation of the hyoid bones (Figure 8.89), resulting in perforation or laceration of the adjacent soft tissue structures.
- Irregular new bone production, bone lysis and/or periosteal reactions may be present in complicated trauma cases or infection of the soft tissues surrounding the hyoid apparatus (Figure 8.90). Open hyoid fractures can be complicated by osteomyelitis.

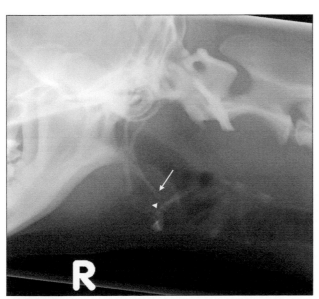

8.89 Lateral radiograph of the skull of a dog with hyoid bone trauma. There is a luxation between the right epihyoid and ceratohyoid bones. The distal epihyoid bone (arrowed) is displaced caudally relative to the ceratohyoid bone (arrowhead).

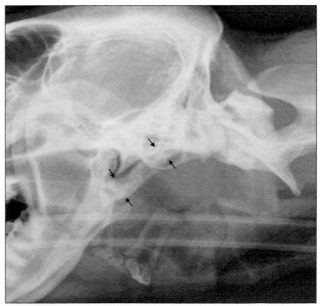

8.90 Lateral radiograph of the skull of a dog with chronic para-aural abscessation (left side) and hyoid bone changes. One of the stylohyoid bones (left) is markedly thickened (arrowed), mottled and sclerotic, representing chronic osteitis/periostitis. (Courtesy of Cambridge Veterinary School)

- Disarticulation of the hyoid from the basicranium may occur due to trauma or fracture.

Neoplasia

- Neoplasia is usually associated with destruction of the hyoid bones. Oral soft tissue masses invading the bone are the most likely cause.

References and further reading

Bischoff MG and Kneller SK (2004) Diagnostic imaging of the canine and feline ear. *Veterinary Clinics of North America: Small Animal Practice* **34**, 437–458

Coulsen A and Lewis N (2008) *An Atlas of Interpretative Anatomy of the Dog and Cat, 2nd edn.* Blackwell Publications, Oxford

Featherstone H and Llabres F (2003) Maxillary bone epithelial cyst in a dog. *Journal of Small Animal Practice* **44**, 541–545

Garosi LS, Dennis R and Schwarz T (2003) Review of diagnostic imaging of ear disease in the dog and cat. *Veterinary Radiology & Ultrasound* **44**, 137–146

Lamb CR, Richbell S and Mantis P (2003) Radiographic signs in cats with nasal disease. *Journal of Feline Medicine and Surgery* **5**, 227–235

Regodón S, Vivo JM, Franco A, Guillén MT and Robina A (1993) Craniofacial angle in dolicho-, meso- and brachycephalic dogs: radiological determination and application. *Annals of Anatomy* **175(4)**, 361–363

Schwarz T, Sullivan M and Hartung K (2000) Radiographic anatomy of the cribriform plate (lamina cribrosa) *Veterinary Radiology & Ultrasound* **41(3)**, 220–225

Schwarz T, Sullivan M and Hartung K (2000) Radiographic detection of defects of the nasal boundaries. *Veterinary Radiology & Ultrasound* **44**, 414–419

Tutt C (2006) *Small Animal Dentistry – A Manual of Techniques.* Blackwell Publications, Oxford

Verstraete FJM, Fiani N, Kass PH and Cox DP (2011) Clinicopathologic characterization of odontogenic tumors and focal fibrous hyperplasia in dogs: 152 cases (1995–2005). *Journal of the American Veterinary Medical Association* **238(4)**, 495–500

Verstraete FJM, Phillip PH and Terpak CH (1998) Diagnostic value of full mouth radiography in dogs. *American Journal of Veterinary Research* **59**, 686–691

Wykes PM (1991) Brachycephalic airway obstructive syndrome. *Problems in Veterinary Medicine* **3**, 188–197

Radiology of the vertebral column

9

Tobias Schwarz and Andrew Holloway

Radiographic assessment of the vertebral column is usually performed to investigate suspected disorders of the vertebral column and paravertebral soft tissues. As the spinal cord and nerves are not visible on survey radiographs, diagnostic conclusions are mainly drawn indirectly from its casing, the vertebral column. Therefore, it is not surprising that survey spinal radiography has a poor diagnostic yield in animals with neurological disease.

The challenges associated with radiography of the vertebral column include:

- Localization – accurate neurolocalization is required and should precede radiography to ensure that the correct spinal cord segments are imaged and to rule out multifocal disease
- Superimposition – paired structures (articular processes, pedicles) are superimposed on lateral views, and cardiovascular structures and the bowel are superimposed on the vertebral column on ventrodorsal (VD) views, creating multiple composite shadows which can mimic pathology
- Contrast – there is poor contrast of the paraspinal soft tissues and the soft tissues within the vertebral canal
- Bone loss – radiography is relatively insensitive for demonstrating bone loss. Considerable bone loss (30–50%) is required before changes are recognized on radiographs.

In most cases with suspected spinal disease, survey radiography is neither sufficient to make a specific and localized clinical diagnosis, nor sensitive enough to rule one out. Even for conditions of the vertebral column itself, such as fractures, radiography has been shown to have poor diagnostic sensitivity. A number of significant conditions that can be easily detected using radiography, such as discospondylitis, have a low clinical incidence. Other common diseases, such as spondylosis deformans, are clinically irrelevant.

Invasive contrast radiographic procedures (e.g. myelography) or non-invasive cross-sectional imaging modalities such as computed tomography (CT) and magnetic resonance imaging (MRI) are indicated for the majority of spinal disorders and have largely replaced radiography for the diagnosis of spinal disease in referral practice. Early diagnosis can be a significant advantage of cross-sectional imaging, but the availability and cost of these techniques remain disadvantages.

As long as the limitations of survey radiography are recognized, the technique remains valuable as a means to evaluate for conspicuous, and usually advanced, disease of the vertebrae, to assess vertebral alignment and bone density, and to monitor the changes associated with bone healing and remodelling. In addition, part of the vertebral column is usually included on thoracic, abdominal and pelvic radiographs, and it is important to be able to recognize significant vertebral changes. Radiographs of the vertebral column are also useful to screen for generalized or multifocal developmental, metabolic and neoplastic diseases. The vertebral column of many dogs with suspected orthopaedic problems (e.g. related to the shoulder or hip) and cats with suspected abdominal disease (e.g. megacolon or pain on renal palpation) are often imaged to rule out spinal cord disease as an alternative explanation of the clinical signs. However, this is of dubious value as the most common causes of spinal cord disorders cannot be diagnosed with survey radiography and the few conditions that can are relatively rare.

Indications

Common indications for survey radiography of the vertebral column include:

- Spinal pain:
  - Back pain, stiffness and pyrexia associated with draining sinus tracts of the flanks
  - Neck pain, in particular suspected atlantoaxial instability.
- Trauma with neurological deficits localized to the vertebral column
- Suspected congenital or developmental disease associated with spinal neurological signs in young animals or deformity of the vertebral column
- Paraparesis, hemiparesis or tetraparesis/tetraplegia
- Paraneoplastic syndromes associated with hypercalcaemia or hyperglobulinaemia.

In surgical patients radiography of the vertebral column is used for surgical planning and to obtain vertebral dimensions should implants be necessary, to evaluate the integrity and stability of surgical implants placed during spinal surgery and to assess the extent and location of changes at sites of previous surgical intervention.

Restraint and patient preparation

- Correct patient positioning is essential to produce radiographs of the vertebral column that are of diagnostic value. This is difficult to achieve in the conscious animal due to movement and muscle tension. Thus, in order to achieve accurate positioning with muscle relaxation, radiography of the vertebral column should almost always be performed under general anaesthesia.
- Justifiable exceptions are animals with suspected spinal trauma or instability (vertebral fractures, atlantoaxial subluxation) where the lack of muscular bracing can aggravate spinal cord injury during manipulation of the patient. However, the caveat is that in doing so, the already limited diagnostic yield of survey radiography of the vertebral column is drastically reduced. Handling should be kept to a minimum. Animals with suspected spinal trauma or instability can be secured on a rigid, radiolucent board to allow radiographs to be obtained without moving the animal further. Orthogonal views using a horizontal X-ray beam can also be obtained if radiation safety precautions are observed.
- Screening for generalized or multifocal conditions (osteopenia, multiple myeloma) often does not require perfect positioning.
- Immobilization for radiography of the vertebral column should be such that there is no risk of the patient falling or slipping from the X-ray table.
- The patient should be offered the opportunity to void (or an enema should be performed) as faecal material within the colon or a distended bladder complicates interpretation by creating multiple superimposed shadows.

Standard radiographic views

- For radiography of the vertebral column, the vertebrae need to be perfectly aligned with each other without axial rotation or sagging in the plane parallel to the supporting surface. To achieve this, it is often necessary to support the mid-cervical and mid-lumbar vertebral segments with a radiolucent positioning aid when obtaining lateral views. To limit axial rotation, the limbs should be supported and a radiolucent wedge can be placed under the sternum.
- Due to the divergence of the X-ray beam from the central ray, there is an increasing degree of geometric distortion towards the periphery of the image, leading to artificial lengthening of the peripheral vertebrae and narrowing of the intervertebral disc spaces. To minimize this artefact, radiographs are collimated only to include parts of the vertebral column, usually three or four

vertebrae for the cervical, thoracic and lumbar regions for both VD and lateral views, with some images centred on the border area between two regions.
- Lateral radiographs should be obtained initially, followed by VD views (Figure 9.1).
- When a lesion cannot be localized by the clinical or neurological examination, a radiographic examination of the entire vertebral column should be performed and should include at least 3–4 radiographs for cats and small dogs, and >6 radiographs in larger dogs.

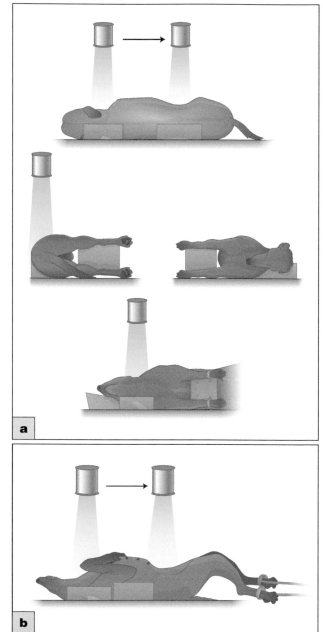

9.1 **(a)** Patient positioning for a lateral view of the vertebral column. The vertebral column is positioned parallel to the X-ray table and perpendicular to the X-ray beam by supporting the mid-cervical and mid-lumbar vertebral column using radiolucent positioning aids. This prevents the vertebral column from sagging in the sagittal plane. Supporting the skull, sternum and limbs limits rotation in the transverse plane. **(b)** Positioning for a VD view. The caudal cervical vertebral column and thorax are supported to prevent rotation.

Cervical vertebral column

Laterolateral view

- The sagittal plane of the head is maintained parallel to the X-ray table by supporting the muzzle with a foam wedge.
- The vertebral column is maintained parallel to the table with a foam support beneath the mid-cervical region. The alignment of the vertebral column is assessed using palpable anatomical landmarks such as the occipital protuberance and spinous processes of T1 to ensure that they are equidistant from the table.
- Depending on the conformation of the dog, further supports can be placed beneath the sternum and between the forelegs. The mid-lumbar region may also need to be supported.
- For the caudal cervical vertebral column, the forelimbs are retracted caudally using sandbags.
- Depending on the region of interest, the X-ray beam is centred on the:
  - Upper cervical vertebral column (C2–C3)
  - Lower cervical vertebral column (C5–C6)
  - Cranial thoracic vertebral column (T1–T8) (should be included in medium- to large-breed dogs with suspected cervical stenotic spondylomyelopathy as changes may also be evident within this segment).
- To evaluate specific areas, the beam is centred by palpating anatomical landmarks (e.g. for C1–C2 the wings of the atlas are palpated).
- To evaluate the caudal cervical vertebral column, exposure factors are increased due to the greater thickness of the soft tissues in this region.

Ventrodorsal view

- The thorax is supported using a radiolucent cradle and/or by foam supports.
- The mid-cervical vertebral column is supported by a foam pad.
- Overextension of the head often results in curvature of the vertebral column in the lateral plane. Supporting the nose in a neutral position limits this error.
- The cranial cervical intervertebral disc spaces tend to be aligned with the primary beam. The caudal spaces are at an angle to the primary beam. This can be overcome by rotating the tube head so that the beam is angled slightly from caudally to cranially.

Additional views

- Lateral oblique views of C1–C2 are used to demonstrate the dens.
- VD oblique views are used to demonstrate the intervertebral foramina.
- The open-mouth rostrocaudal view is described to evaluate the dens but should not be performed due to the risk of damage to the spinal cord. If evaluation of the dens is required, then a lateral oblique view should be obtained.
- Dynamic studies (extension, flexion and traction) are usually only performed following myelography (see later).

Thoracic vertebral column

Laterolateral view

- Alignment of the vertebral column is assessed by palpating anatomical landmarks (the spinous processes) to ensure they are parallel to the table. The sternum and cranial thoracic vertebral column may need to be elevated and supported by foam wedges.
- Depending on the region of interest, the X-ray beam is centred on the:
  - Cranial thoracic vertebral column (T1–T8)
  - Thoracolumbar junction (T13–L1).

Ventrodorsal view

- The animal is supported in a radiolucent trough or by foam wedges.
- Exposure factors must be increased to ensure adequate penetration, especially in deep-chested dogs.

Lumbar and lumbosacral vertebral column

Laterolateral view

- The mid-lumbar vertebral column should be supported using a small pad to avoid axial rotation and sagging.
- The hindlimbs should be parallel, with a pad placed between the limbs in large dogs.
- Palpation of the spinous (T13–L7/S1) and transverse processes provides landmarks to ensure that the long axis of the vertebral column and the transverse processes are parallel and perpendicular to the table, respectively.
- Depending on the region of interest, the X-ray beam is centred on the:
  - Thoracolumbar junction (T13–L1)
  - Mid-lumbar vertebral column (L3–L4)
  - Lumbosacral junction (L7–S1).

Ventrodorsal view

- Patient positioning is similar to that for a VD radiograph of the pelvis, although the centring points depend on the segments of interest.
- The hindlimbs are usually extended but can be flexed (neutral 'frog-legged' position) if necessary. Overextension of the hindlimbs leads to rotation and tilting of the vertebral column. If the back is not adequately supported with the legs in a neutral position, the vertebral column will curve to the left or right.

Additional views

- As the lumbosacral disc space and sacrum are not perpendicular to the X-ray beam, a true VD view of the lumbosacral disc space can only be obtained by angling the X-ray tube cranially (from a vertical position) by *approximately 30 degrees from the vertical.*
- Alternatively, pulling the hindlimbs cranially results in flexion of the lumbosacral junction and the disc space is then parallel to the table. This is called a flexed VD view.

Dynamic studies

Dynamic radiographic studies of the vertebral column in the dog are, in practice, limited to the cervical region.

- Flexed lateral views of the cranial cervical vertebral column are used to assess small-breed dogs (predominantly) with suspected atlantoaxial subluxation. The radiographs should only be obtained with the dog under general anaesthesia and the airway maintained by an endotracheal tube. Radiographs with the head moderately extended should be obtained initially, followed by radiography with the neck mildly flexed. If instability is not demonstrated, then additional radiographs can be obtained with the head in further flexion. Radiographs should not be obtained with the head in marked flexion to avoid the risk of further damage to the spinal cord.
- In cases with suspected cervical stenotic spondylomyelopathy, neutral and traction myelographic views can be used to demonstrate that compression of the spinal cord can be relieved by distraction. However, CT and MRI remain the preferred imaging techniques to evaluate the cervical spinal cord for changes associated with this condition.

Assessment of correct positioning

Cervicothoracic vertebral column

- The wings of the atlas should be superimposed.
- The transverse processes should be superimposed.
- The articular process joints should be parallel.
- The intervertebral discs should be of even thickness and regular shape.
- The rib heads should be superimposed.
- Anatomical features are symmetrical on the VD view.

Lumbosacral vertebral column

- The spinous processes should be superimposed on the mid-vertebral body on the VD view.
- The transverse processes should be superimposed on the lateral view.
- No axial rotation – the intervertebral disc spaces should be of even width and regular spacing.
- The wings of the ilia should be superimposed on views centred on the lumbosacral joint.
- Sacroiliac joints should be symmetrical on the VD view.

Radiographic exposure

- The radiographic technique is primarily directed at generating adequate penetration of the vertebral column, surrounding strong paravertebral musculature and soft tissues. The bone margins of the vertebrae should be well defined. Inappropriate exposure settings, film development or digital algorithms will influence the bone/soft tissue contrast and consequently the visibility of the bone margins. An intermediate to high kV (65–75 kV for a 30 kg dog) is required to achieve adequate penetration and a moderately high milliampere seconds (mAs) is needed to create sufficient film blackening (analogue film) or signal (digital film).
- To minimize the effect of scatter (generated by the thickness of the soft tissues and bone) a grid should be used. A Bucky grid positioned underneath the X-ray table allows cassettes to be changed without the need to reposition the patient. In addition, close collimation reduces the amount of scatter produced and improves contrast.
- Under general anaesthesia, relatively long exposure times can be used as little or no patient movement is expected.
- For radiography of the thoracic vertebral column, inducing temporary apnoea by hyperventilating the animal prior to exposure avoids movement artefacts.
- Fast film–screen combinations are used for most dogs weighing >10–15 kg. Detail film–screen combinations can be used for cats and small dogs.
- Computed and direct digital radiography are well suited for spinal radiography as they allow tissues with greatly different X-ray attenuation to be viewed using the same exposure factors. However, if inappropriate algorithms are used for processing raw data, the abrupt transition between cortical bone and soft tissue can create an artificial dark halo around the vertebrae on digital images.

Comparison with cross-sectional imaging

Radiography

- Allows alignment of the whole vertebral column to be easily assessed.
- Allows an overview of complex vertebral malformations.
- Allows routine reassessment of postoperative bone healing.
- Allows assessment of stability and integrity of implants.
- Low sensitivity and specificity.
- No information about the spinal cord or nerves without the use of contrast media.

Computed tomography

- Excellent for investigating trauma, vertebral malformations and developmental lesions, and intervertebral disc disease.
- Can be combined with myelography to improve information on spinal cord pathology.
- Provides a limited assessment of spinal cord changes (oedema, mass lesions, malacia (spinal cord necrosis), gliosis (scarring of the spinal cord) and atrophy) and peripheral nerves.

Magnetic resonance imaging

- Excellent soft tissue contrast, allowing detailed assessment of the spinal cord (MRI is the modality of choice in most cases of spinal cord disease).
- Allows assessment of the peripheral nerves and paraspinal soft tissues.
- Dynamic studies possible.   ▶

> ■ It can be difficult to obtain high quality, high resolution images of cats and small dogs using MRI. Artefacts from metal implants may compromise the diagnostic quality by obscuring the areas of interest. The radiofrequency coils used with some low-field systems may limit the assessment of the spinal cord in large- and giant-breed dogs.

Contrast studies

- ■ Myelography is a technique in which iodine-based contrast medium is injected into the subarachnoid space at either the cisternal or lumbar puncture sites for cerebrospinal fluid (CSF) collection (see Chapter 4).
- ■ The contrast-enhanced subarachnoid space outlines the spinal cord, allowing direct assessment of its shape and size (Figure 9.2).
- ■ Myelography requires practice in both performing the technique and interpreting the radiographs, and should not be performed by inexperienced clinicians. The technical procedure is therefore not discussed in this Manual. However, it is important to be familiar with the indications, principles of interpretation and contraindications for the procedure.
- ■ CSF should be collected and submitted as part of all myelographic studies, even if the presentation (e.g. intervertebral disc herniation) appears to be straightforward.
- ■ Other contrast procedures such as epidurography and discography are outdated and have been superseded by MRI and CT, which not only allow cross-sectional imaging but are considerably more sensitive and specific.

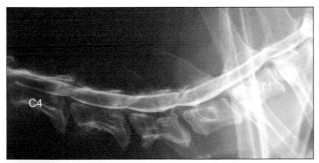

9.2 Lateral cervical myelogram of a German Shepherd Dog. The dorsal and ventral opaque columns of contrast medium in the subarachnoid space outline the margins of the spinal cord. The subarachnoid space is attenuated at the C4–C5, C5–C6, C6–C7 and T1–T2 intervertebral disc spaces. There is mild narrowing of the spinal cord at T1–T2. (Courtesy of L Jarrett)

Indications

The indications for myelography include:

- ■ To assess the site and extent of a lesion resulting in a transverse myelopathy (paresis/plegia/ataxia) as well as to determine an accurate neurolocalization
- ■ To determine the site and severity of spinal cord compression
- ■ To confirm the presence of diverticuli within the subarachnoid space, as suspected on CT or MRI.

Interpretation

The basic principles of interpretation of myelographic studies are:

- ■ Define the location of the lesion within the vertebral canal (Figure 9.3):
  - • Extradural
  - • Intradural–extramedullary
  - • Intramedullary.

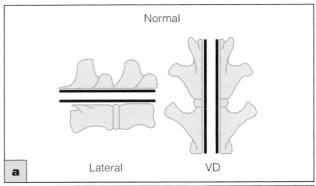

Normal

a | Lateral | VD

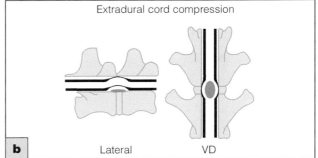

Extradural cord compression

b | Lateral | VD

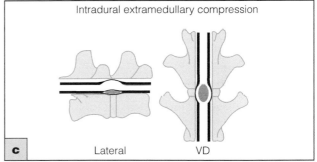

Intradural extramedullary compression

c | Lateral | VD

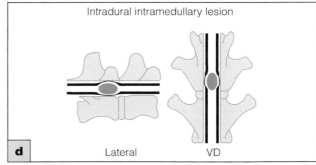

Intradural intramedullary lesion

d | Lateral | VD

9.3 Principles of myelographic interpretation. **(a)** Normal. **(b)** Ventral extradural compressive lesion (e.g. disc extrusion resulting in displacement or compression of the spinal cord on the lateral view and widening on the VD view). The subarachnoid space is narrowed on both views. **(c)** Intradural–extramedullary lesion (e.g. meningioma resulting in splitting of one of the contrast medium columns. This is best seen at the margins where pooling of contrast medium creates a 'golf-tee' sign). The cord is widened on the VD view. **(d)** Intramedullary lesion (e.g. spinal cord tumour). The spinal cord is widened and the subarachnoid space thinned on both views.

- Define the extent of a lesion and the relationship relative to the intervertebral disc space
- Provide an assessment of the severity and significance of a lesion
- Allow consideration of the nature of the lesion (i.e. intervertebral disc extrusion or protrusion, neoplastic mass or inflammatory process).

Complications

- There is an increased incidence of seizures following myelography, particularly in animals where a large volume of contrast medium is used with a cisternal puncture injection.
- Apnoea or death.
- Neurological status may worsen transiently following myelography. This may be more apparent in cases with cord swelling in which substantial pressure is required to inject the contrast medium beyond the affected area.
- Introduction of infection.
- Injection of contrast medium into the cord, resulting in a haematoma or myelomalacia.

Contraindications

- Multifocal neurological or brain disease.
- Inflammatory CSF sample.
- Unstable vertebral column.
- Infection at site of injection.
- Coagulopathy.
- Lower motor neuron disease.

Radiological interpretation

Normal anatomy

- Vertebrae are generally formed by three primary ossification centres (the vertebral body and the left and right halves of the vertebral arch). These can be identified on radiographs from birth. Secondary ossification centres develop later on for the vertebral processes and endplates.
- The atlas (C1) and axis (C2) vertebrae, in particular, have specific embryological and anatomical features.
  - The atlas has three centres of ossification: the vertebral body and the paired vertebral arches. There are no physes.
  - The axis has four centres of ossification: the dens, the body and the paired vertebral arches. A caudal physis is present.
- The cranial physes of the C3–L7 vertebrae close slightly earlier (5–6 months) than the caudal physes (9–10 months).
- The 'standard' anatomy of a vertebra consists of the body, the arch (lamina and paired pedicles) and paired articular processes, which articulate with the spinous process dorsally (Figure 9.4). Other processes are region-specific. From the second or third thoracic vertebra caudally, there are mammillary processes protruding dorsally from the transverse processes. Small accessory processes extend caudally from the pedicles of the mid-thoracic region caudally to the fifth or sixth

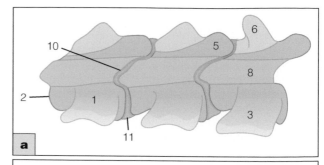

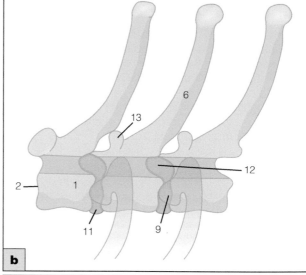

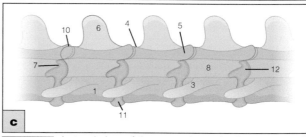

9.4 Lateral view of the normal vertebral structures of the **(a)** cervical, **(b)** thoracic and **(c)** lumbar vertebral column. 1 = vertebral body; 2 = endplate; 3 = transverse process; 4 = cranial articular process; 5 = caudal articular process; 6 = spinous process; 7 = accessory process; 8 = pedicle; 9 = rib head; 10 = articular process joint; 11 = intervertebral disc; 12 = intervertebral foramen; 13 = mammilary process.

lumbar vertebrae and contribute to the 'horsehead' shape of the intervertebral foramina. In the coccygeal region, small hemal processes extend ventrally to the coccygeal vertebrae. The cranial and caudal aspects of the vertebral canal of each vertebra are termed the cranial and caudal vertebral foramina, respectively.

- Dogs and cats normally have 7 cervical, 13 thoracic, 7 lumbar, 3 sacral and 6–23 coccygeal vertebrae (Figures 9.5 and 9.6). The vertebral body in the cat is more cylindrical than in the dog, and the arrangement of the vertebrae in the cat allows a greater degree of flexibility in the vertebral column. The sublumbar muscles in the cat are comparatively larger than in the dog and are most conspicuous on the VD view. The origin of the psoas minor muscle at the ventral vertebral margin visibly extends further cranially in the cat (T12) than in the dog (T13).

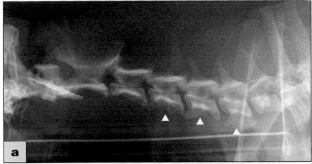

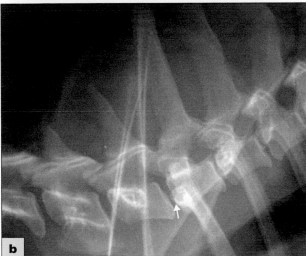

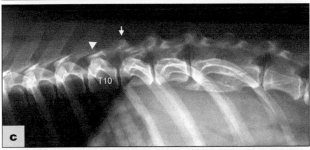

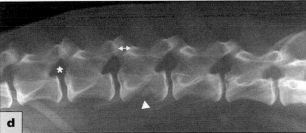

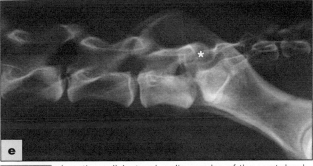

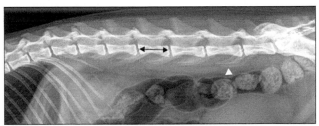

9.5 (continued) Lateral radiographs of the vertebral column of a skeletally mature dog.
(e) Lumbosacral vertebral column. Note that the larger, triangular, intervertebral disc space and indistinct articular joint space of L7–S1 (*) are normal features.

9.6 Lateral radiograph of the normal lumbar vertebral column in a cat. Note that the vertebral bodies of the lumbar vertebrae are elongated (arrowed) and that the forward projecting transverse processes have an elongated appearance (arrowhead).

9.5 Lateral radiographs of the vertebral column of a skeletally mature dog. **(a)** Cervical vertebral column. The C4–C6 vertebrae have large, ventrolaterally oriented, transverse processes (arrowheads). Note that the C2–C3 and C7–T1 intervertebral disc spaces are normally narrower than C4–C6. **(b)** Caudal cervical and cranial thoracic vertebral column. Superimposition of the head of the first rib on the C7–T1 intervertebral disc space may mimic intervertebral disc mineralization (arrowed).
(c) Caudal thoracic and cranial lumbar vertebral column. The diaphragmatic (T10) vertebra has dorsally oriented cranial (arrowed) and sagittally oriented caudal (arrowed) articular process joints. The T13 and L1 vertebrae are fused (block vertebra). **(d)** Lumbar vertebral column. Note the typical 'horsehead' shape of the intervertebral foramina (*) and articular process joint spaces (double arrow). The gradual narrowing of the caudal lumbar intervertebral disc spaces is due to geometric distortion. The ventral margin of L4 is indistinct due to hypaxial muscle attachments (arrowhead). (continues) ▶

- The vertebral canal is quite large at C1–C2, then narrows more caudally before enlarging in the regions of C6–T2 and L3–L6, to accommodate the cervical and lumbar intumescences of the spinal cord. The intervertebral disc spaces of C2–C3 and C7–T1 are often slightly narrower than other cervical disc spaces, whereas the L7–S1 intervertebral disc space is often slightly wider than other lumbar disc spaces.
- The area between two vertebrae can be divided into three spaces:
  - The intervertebral disc space is the space between the endplates of two adjacent vertebrae and contains the intervertebral disc supported dorsally and ventrally by longitudinal ligaments. The intervertebral disc consists of the central gelatinous nucleus pulposus and the peripheral annulus fibrosus, which is thinner dorsally than ventrally. The normal intervertebral disc is of soft tissue opacity on radiographs.
  - The intervertebral foraminal space is created by the superimposition of the paired intervertebral foramina, which consist of the opening between pedicles of neighbouring vertebral arches to allow passage of the spinal nerve and vessels. The shape differs between segments, but it is generally more distinct over the caudal aspect of the pedicle. The accessory process in the caudal thoracic and cranial lumbar vertebral column contributes to the typical 'horsehead' shape of the space in this region (Figure 9.7). In the cervical vertebral column, the foramina are angled obliquely and therefore a typical

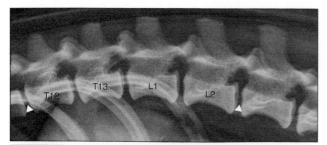

9.7 Lateral radiograph of the thoracolumbar vertebral column in a dog. The superimposition of the intervertebral foramina creates the typical 'horsehead' shape. The L1–L2 intervertebral disc space is most central on this view and thus appears largest. Towards the left of the image, the T12–T13 and T13–L1 intervertebral disc spaces appear gradually narrower, making assessment of the disc space width difficult. There is also faint mineralization of the nucleus pulposus at T11–T12 and L2–L3 (arrowheads).

'horsehead' is not recognized on a lateral view. The foramina in the cervical vertebral column can be seen without superimposition on lateral oblique views.

- The intervertebral articular joint space comprises the cartilage and synovium of both superimposed articular process joints. The articular process joints (also known as articular facet joints) are paired synovial (diarthroidal) joints allowing articulation of the vertebral arches of adjacent vertebrae. In the cervical and thoracic vertebral column, until T10 or T11, the joint is oriented in a dorsal plane and is mainly a sliding joint. From T11 to the caudal lumbar vertebral column, the joint space is oriented in a sagittal plane with caudally convex and cranially concave joint surfaces, allowing mainly horizontal movement and some vertical rotation. The cranial articular processes of T10 are often oriented in a dorsal plane, whereas the caudal processes are oriented in the sagittal plane. This feature is used to characterize T10 as the diaphragmatic vertebra. T11 is often the most cranial vertebra in which both the cranial and caudal articular process joints are oriented in a sagittal plane, and this is the most reliable feature to characterize it as the anticlinal vertebra (compared with other definitions). In the L6–L7 and L7–S1 joints, the orientation of the articular processes changes to a more dorsal plane, but they maintain the rounded surfaces. The diaphragmatic or anticlinal vertebra is used as a reference structure for lesion localization or surgical planning, in particular when the ribs cannot be used for this purpose.
- Generally, the spinous processes slope caudally up to and including the diaphragmatic vertebra. The spinous processes of the anticlinal vertebra and the vertebrae caudal to this slope cranially.
- The ventral margins of the L3–L4 vertebrae are often indistinct due to hypaxial muscle attachment.
- The cranial articular processes and vertebral arch of the S1 vertebra are often indistinct.

General approach

- The alignment of the vertebral canal should be assessed. It should be possible to trace the floor and roof of the canal smoothly across the intervertebral disc space without a step or change in angulation being evident. Although the vertebral canal widens between C6–T2 and L3–L6 to accommodate the cervical and lumbar intumescences of the spinal cord, this transition should be smooth. On VD views, the pedicles should be evenly spaced and parallel.
- Paired structures should be assessed for symmetry on VD views.
- The spinous processes should all be in a line. If the vertebral column is curved due to positioning or muscle spasm, the curvature of the line of the dorsal spinous processes should be smooth and gradual.
- The diameter of the vertebral canal is assessed between the dorsal aspect of the vertebral body and the ventral aspect of the lamina. The margin of the vertebral canal is not always clearly visible.
- The paravertebral tissues should be assessed for the presence of soft tissue swelling. This is best recognized ventral to the vertebral column, in the cervical region by displacement of the trachea, and in the lumbar region by changes in the fat opacity of the retroperitoneal space or the displacement of the kidneys and colon.
- The thickness and opacity of the cortical bone and trabeculation of the medulla should be assessed for changes in bone density and integrity. The periosteal surfaces should be assessed for reaction. In older cats, the trabecular pattern is often conspicuous and coarse.
- The intervertebral disc space should be of even width and similar in size to the adjacent disc spaces. The subchondral bone bordering the disc spaces should be intact. The opacity of the disc space should be the same as that of soft tissue.
- The shape and size of adjacent intervertebral foramina should be similar.

Röntgen signs

The vertebral column can be systematically assessed using Röntgen signs. Röntgen signs include geometric (location, size, shape, number, margination), opacity and functional signs. Radiographic changes are usually described using one or more Röntgen signs and an effort should be made to avoid relying on changes in opacity alone when evaluating spinal radiographs.

Location and alignment

- In the vertebral column, location refers in particular to the orientation and alignment of the vertebrae (Figure 9.8).
- Following trauma, displacement should be assessed by obtaining radiographs in two planes. Where instability is a concern, the orthogonal view should be obtained without moving the animal.
- In some congenital and developmental diseases, such as atlantoaxial subluxation or cervical stenotic spondylomyelopathy, dynamic views are necessary to demonstrate displacement.

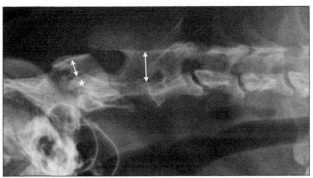

9.8 Röntgen signs: location and alignment. Lateral radiograph showing fused C2 and C3 block vertebrae in a cat. The odontoid process is enlarged, misshapen and oriented too dorsally (∗). The height of the vertebral canal at the level of the dens within C1 is considerably narrower than within C2 (double-headed arrows). These changes are likely to be clinically significant. Note the vestigial or narrowed intervertebral disc space between C2 and C3, and the change in shape of the cranial aspect of the C4 vertebral body to accommodate the angulation of the caudal endplate of the C2–C3 block vertebra. The diameter of the vertebral canal at C3–C4 is similar to that at C4–C5.

- Angulation or curvature of the vertebral column is usually due to vertebral malformation or instability but can also be due to muscle spasm or discomfort.
- Sacral fractures or sacroiliac subluxation are easily overlooked if lateral views are relied upon alone.

Size

- Enlargement of the vertebral canal (Figure 9.9) can occur with slowly growing proliferative tumours of the spinal cord, meninges or nerve roots. Meningiomas and peripheral nerve sheath tumours occur most frequently.
- Enlargement of the vertebra can be caused by osteoproliferative changes:
  - Benign lesions, including neoplasia (benign osteochondroma, a mushroom-like proliferation of displaced cartilage cells which subsequently ossify), benign new bone formation (spondylosis deformans or disseminated idiopathic skeletal hyperostosis) or callus formation and remodelling following fracture
  - Malignant neoplasia (usually primary bone tumour).
- Reduced vertebral length can be the result of:
  - Compression fractures (traumatic or pathological) (Figure 9.10)
  - Overriding fracture fragments (traumatic or pathological)
  - Congenital endocrinopathies (congenital hypothyroidism; Figure 9.11) and metabolic diseases (mucopolysaccharidosis)
  - Malformations such as a cleft vertebra or hemivertebra.
- The atlas (C1) is the vertebra most commonly reduced in length and size (hypoplasia). The vertebral body and arch of C1 are shortened and malformed, and the condition may be associated with malformation or absence of the occipital condyles and/or fusion of the atlas to the occipital bone (see Figure 9.12).

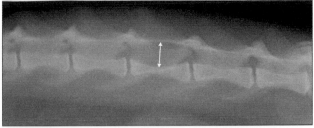

9.9 Röntgen sign: size. The vertebral canal within the L5 vertebral body is widened (double-headed arrow). The dorsal and ventral margins are expanded outwards and thinned. This represents a form of bone atrophy and remodelling typical of a slowly expanding mass. Final diagnosis: meningioma.

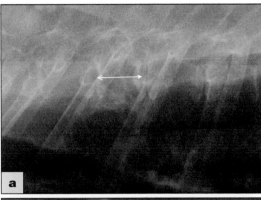

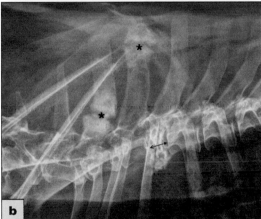

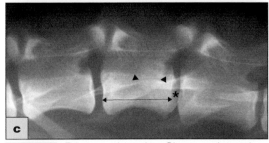

9.10 Röntgen sign: size. Shortened vertebra. **(a–b)** Lateral radiographs of the cranial thoracic spine of a dog with multiple myeloma. (a) The T3 vertebra is osteolytic and shortened (double-headed arrow) due to a compression fracture. There is an irregular periosteal reaction, suggesting that weakening of the vertebra was gradual, stimulating bone reaction. (b) At a later stage in the disease course, T3 has completely collapsed (double-headed arrow). Additional lesions and pathological fractures of the spinous processes are also present (∗). **(c)** Lateral radiograph of a dog with a traumatic L3 compression fracture. The L3 vertebra is shortened (double-headed arrow), sclerotic caudally (arrowheads) and the L3–L4 intervertebral disc space (∗) is reduced in size, consistent with a compression fracture and disc extrusion.

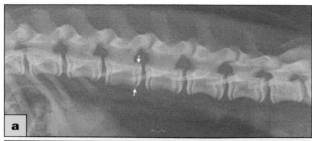

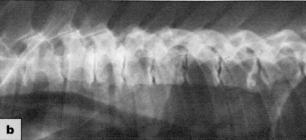

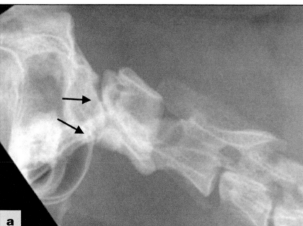

9.11 Röntgen sign: size. **(a)** Lateral view of the lumbar vertebral column of a 7-month-old dog with congenital hypothyroidism. Closure of the physes is delayed and the physes remain widened (arrowed). The vertebrae are reduced in length but the bone density is normal. **(b)** Lateral view of the thoracic vertebrae of a skeletally mature dog with congenital hypothyroidism, leading to epiphyseal dysplasia. The vertebrae are square and have irregular endplates.

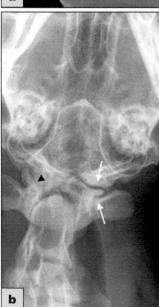

9.12 Röntgen sign: shape. Malformation of the occipitoatlantal articulation in a cat. **(a)** On the lateral view, the occipital condyles appear hypoplastic (arrowed). The anatomy of the atlas is generally normal except for a subtle change in the shape of the articular margin cranially. **(b)** On the VD view, the right occipital condyle is recognized to be normal in shape and size (arrowhead), whereas the left condyle is hypoplastic and flattened (arrowed) with adaptive remodelling of the cranial articular surface of the atlas.

- Due to the geometric distortion effect, there is artefactual gradual stretching of the vertebral silhouettes and narrowing of the intervertebral disc spaces towards the periphery of the image. Therefore, during assessment, vertebral and intervertebral disc space size must always be compared with both neighbouring vertebrae and discs, taking these gradual changes into account. A normal intervertebral disc space that is not located exactly in the centre of the image should be narrower than more centrally located disc spaces and wider than more peripherally located disc spaces. The gradual change in size of the vertebrae within each segment is normal.
- Reduced width or complete collapse of the intervertebral disc space is usually caused by intervertebral disc degeneration, with or without disc protrusion or extrusion, acute nucleus pulposus extrusion or trauma. Other causes of narrowing include congenital malformations (such as block vertebrae) and following fenestration of the intervertebral disc during spinal surgery. The intervertebral disc space may be widened (early) or narrowed (late) with discospondylitis. Narrowing of the intervertebral disc space is a more reliable finding of disc disease in younger rather than older animals as degeneration (which progresses with age) can lead to mild disc narrowing.
- The size of the normal articular process joint space can be altered:
  - Narrowed in intervertebral disc degeneration or following disc extrusion
  - Absent in vertebral luxation and subluxation and with abnormal orientation of facets (articular process joint tropism)
  - Widened in hypoplasia or aplasia of the articular processes or with neoplasia.
- The intervertebral foramen can be widened by an expansile mass. Peripheral nerve sheath tumours can result in this change, but soft tissue masses extending into the vertebral canal can occasionally lead to similar changes.

Shape

- There is marked normal variation in vertebral shape between the anatomical vertebral segments. The features of an individual vertebra are usually similar to those adjacent to it.
- Asymmetry may be an indication of disease or an incidental finding. The significance of asymmetry must be determined in combination with the other Röntgen signs.
- Vertebral anomalies and malformations may be clinically insignificant (e.g. block or transitional vertebrae).
- Remodelling of a vertebra, leading to a change in shape (Figure 9.12), is usually a feature of congenital or chronic and reactive disease rather than aggressive or acute disease.
- Lesions resulting in a change in vertebral shape originate due to processes within the vertebra itself or as a result of paravertebral soft tissues extending into the vertebra or vertebral canal (Figure 9.13).
- With congenital and developmental lesions resulting in narrowing of the vertebral canal

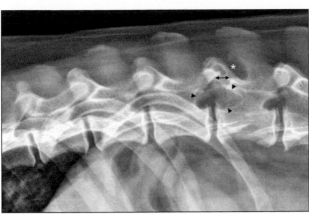

9.13 Röntgen sign: shape. Lateral radiograph of a dog with well demarcated osteolysis of the spinous process (*) and cranial articular processes of L2 (double-headed arrow), leading to an enlarged and abnormally shaped intervertebral foramen (arrowheads). The main differential diagnosis for this lesion would be a neoplastic process arising from the bone or paravertebral soft tissues.

(vertebral stenosis), the change in shape can be quite marked:

- Caudal cervical stenosis (cervical stenotic spondylomyelopathy) usually affects C4–C7. The cranial foramen of the vertebra is markedly smaller than the caudal foramen. The vertebral body is often malformed with a 'keel-shaped' appearance due to a defect in the cranial ventral border
- In lumbosacral stenosis, the change in shape of the vertebral canal is less marked compared with the caudal cervical region, but the associated malformation of L7–S1 is frequently complex if a transitional lumbosacral vertebra is present.
- With congenital lesions, although the bone has an abnormal shape, the cortical thickness and trabecular pattern are usually unchanged.
- Widening of the pedicles in congenital diseases, such as spina bifida, leads to focal widening of the vertebral canal, usually involving L7.
- Vertebral fractures result in a change in shape due to discontinuity of the cortices, changes in angulation of the vertebral elements and the displacement of fragments.
- The appearance of the cortical and trabecular bone of healed vertebral fractures is usually normal but remodelling can lead to a change in shape. Assessment should be focused on whether these changes encroach upon, or limit, the vertebral canal or intervertebral foramina.
- Significant post-surgical changes alter the shape and/or alignment of vertebrae due to:
  - Instability – recognized as subluxation, fracture of the articular process joints or proliferative new bone bridging the vertebral bodies or around the articular facets
  - The presence of a defect from a missing articular facet and lamina as a result of hemilaminectomy
  - The collapse of an intervertebral disc space as a result of fenestration.
- Deviations from the normally parallel intervertebral disc space shape can occur due to subluxation,

disc degeneration (Figure 9.14), discospondylitis, abnormalities of the endplates (such as Schmorl's node), osteochondritis dissecans (OCD) and fractures. A wedge-shaped disc space (narrower dorsally than ventrally) can suggest extrusion of intervertebral disc contents. However, it should be noted that the lumbosacral disc space normally has a slightly triangular shape.

- A change of shape in the dens, usually elongation and abnormal dorsal angulation, can be clinically significant.

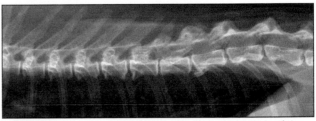

9.14 Röntgen sign: shape. Lateral radiograph of the thoracic vertebral column of a cat. Ventral bone spurs incompletely bridge several intervertebral disc spaces consistent with incidental spondylosis deformans. The intervertebral disc spaces are unequal in width, wedge-shaped with endplate sclerosis, with mineralization of the nuclei in some cases, indicative of intervertebral disc degeneration. Intervertebral disc disease in the cat is less common than in the dog. Where clinically significant, disease is usually chronic and progressive rather than due to acute extrusion. Radiographic changes such as these are of limited clinical significance.

Number
Whilst alteration in vertebral number may relate to reduced or increased deviation from the normal vertebral formula, a more important feature is whether the radiographic changes involve single (monostotic) or multiple (polyostotic) vertebrae (Figure 9.15). This, together with assessment of whether the vertebrae involved are contiguous or non-contiguous, has an important influence on the differential diagnoses that should be considered.

- Monostotic lesions are associated with primary neoplasia (less commonly, metastatic disease).
- Polyostotic lesions result from generalized neoplasia (multiple myeloma, lymphoma), metastases from pelvic neoplasia, haematogenous infection and soft tissue disease (neoplasia or infection extending into bone).
- Involvement of contiguous vertebrae occurs with metastasis from pelvic neoplasia, soft tissue neoplasia or infection extending to involve the vertebrae.
- Involvement of non-contiguous vertebrae ('skip lesions') is associated with haematogenous infection and metastatic neoplasia.

A reduction in the number of vertebrae rarely occurs in the cervical region, but is relatively common in the thoracic, lumbar and sacral vertebral regions in the dog and cat. This is usually caused by congenital malformations but some changes can be acquired. Recognizing these changes is important to determine anatomical landmarks in animals undergoing spinal surgery.

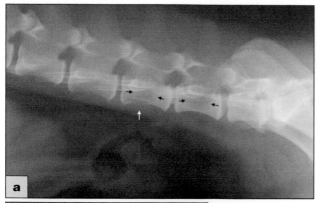

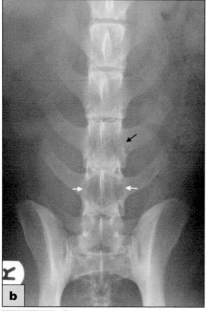

9.15 Röntgen sign: number. Lateral and VD views of the lumbosacral vertebral column of a dog with multiple myeloma. **(a)** Poorly circumscribed lysis of the L5 and L6 vertebral bodies is present (black arrows). The trabecular pattern is indistinct. An indistinct periosteal reaction borders the ventral margin of the L5 vertebral body. **(b)** The extent of the lysis of L5 (black arrow) and L6 (white arrows) is more evident on the VD view. Differentiating between monostotic and polyostotic lesions is an important feature to consider when evaluating radiographs of the vertebral column.

Opacity

Alterations in opacity primarily relate to an increase or decrease in bone substance.

Decreased bone opacity:

- This is due either to a decrease in bone substance (osteopenia) or to bone destruction (osteolysis).
- Radiography is relatively insensitive for determining reduced mineralization of the vertebral column. This is due to the limitations imposed by superimposition of structures as well as the ability of the film–screen combination or imaging plate to display attenuation of the X-ray beam.
- Generally, a decrease in bone density of 50% is required for reduced radiographic density of trabecular bone to be recognized. For cortical bone, a 25% decrease in bone density is required before changes are recognized on radiographs.

Osteopenia: This term is used to describe metabolic bone resorption, either regionally (disuse osteopenia) or generally due to calcium and phosphorus metabolism abnormalities. With osteopenia, the bone is normal but there is less of it. Diseases that should be considered in the dog and cat with generalized osteopenia include:

- Hyperparathyroidism (primary parathyroid, renal or nutritional) (Figure 9.16)
- Hypervitaminosis A (Figure 9.17) and hypovitaminosis D
- Mucopolysaccharidosis and hyperadrenocorticism (Figure 9.18).

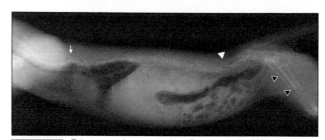

9.16 Röntgen sign: opacity. Osteopenia. Whole body radiograph of a 5-month-old cat with nutritional secondary hyperparathyroidism. There is marked generalized osteopenia, rendering the vertebral column poorly visible. Thoracic vertebral compression fractures have resulted in kyphosis (arrowed). There is caudal lumbar lordosis (white arrowhead) and the cortices of the femurs are thinned (black arrowheads).

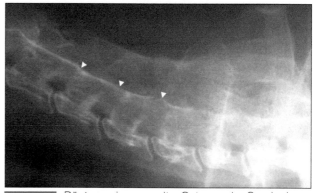

9.17 Röntgen sign: opacity. Osteopenia. Cervical vertebral column of a cat with hypervitaminosis A. There is a diffuse, smooth periosteal reaction bridging the dorsal aspect of the cervical vertebrae (arrowheads). There is also mild osteopenia of the vertebral bodies.

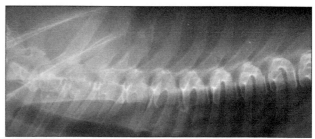

9.18 Röntgen sign: opacity. Osteopenia. Thoracic vertebral column of a dog with chronic hyperadrenocorticism. There is generalized osteopenia, making the vertebrae poorly distinct. The vertebral cortical margins stand out compared with the more demineralized medulla. Obesity also contributes to the low contrast in the image.

In many older cats a mild osteopenia is apparent, most likely related to reduced renal function. This is usually an incidental finding. In conditions such as extensive bridging spondylosis, the other parts of the vertebrae may be less mineralized, reflecting alteration in the parts of the bone responsible for load-bearing.

In the vertebral column, osteopenia is recognized on radiographs as:

- Generalized decreased bone opacity, leading to decreased contrast with the surrounding soft tissues
- Loss of fine trabecular bone pattern (only larger trabeculae remain visible)
- Thin but accentuated vertebral margin (the vertebrae appear 'framed')
- Secondary pathological fractures and spinal curvature deformity in advanced cases.

It can be difficult on radiographs to differentiate true osteopenia from loss of soft tissue/bone contrast due to technical factors such as large body thickness necessitating high kilovolt peak (kVp) settings, leading to increased scatter, underexposure or overexposure, or the selection of inappropriate reconstruction algorithms for digital images.

Osteolysis: This is the local or multifocal destruction of bone due to an active process (Figure 9.19). Aggressive soft tissue, bone and bone marrow neoplasia as well as aggressive fungal and bacterial infections can lead to osteolysis and eventually pathological vertebral fractures. Several radiographic features can be helpful:

- Osteolysis of a single vertebra not extending to others is typical for aggressive bone tumours (e.g. osteosarcoma). It is often associated with a very irregular periosteal reaction

- Osteolysis of adjacent vertebrae is seen more often with soft tissue neoplasia and infection. With infection, the associated periosteal reaction is typically more prominent than the osteolysis
- Osteolysis of multiple vertebrae (often as punched-out lesions) without an associated periosteal reaction is typical of bone marrow neoplasia (e.g. multiple myeloma and occasionally lymphoma).

Increased bone opacity: Increased bone opacity associated with the vertebral column includes changes involving the periosteum, cortical and trabecular bone, and periarticular and paravertebral new bone.

Sclerosis: This refers to an increase in bone opacity without alteration in the shape or size of the vertebra. It occurs as a consequence of Wolff's law, which states that bone adapts to the load under which it is placed. In areas of increased load, new bone is laid down on top of existing cortical and trabecular bone. In the vertebral column sclerosis is frequently observed in the vertebral endplates, associated with intervertebral disc degeneration, or bordering bone infection, and in articular processes with degenerative joint disease (Figure 9.20). Sclerosis is a feature of chronic disease.

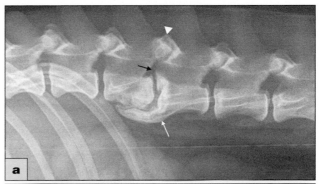

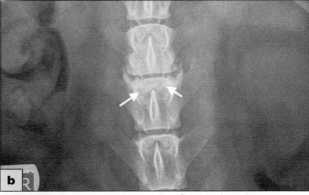

9.20 Röntgen sign: opacity. Osteosclerosis. **(a)** Lateral and **(b)** VD radiographs of the thoracolumbar vertebral column of a young dog with paraparesis. There is extensive remodelling associated with the L2–L3 vertebrae (white arrow). The intervertebral disc space is narrowed with marked sclerosis of the endplates bordering the disc space. A cleft is present within the cranial endplate of the L3 vertebra. The articular processes (arrowhead) appear irregular on the lateral view, but on the VD view they are normal in size. The intervertebral foramen is narrowed (black arrow). These changes are probably the consequence of trauma considering the collapsed disc space and the normal size of the vertebrae. Regardless of the cause, the changes indicate vertebral instability and adaptive changes to cope with the increased load. On MRI, the spinal cord was shown to be compressed by marked proliferation of protruding dorsal annulus.

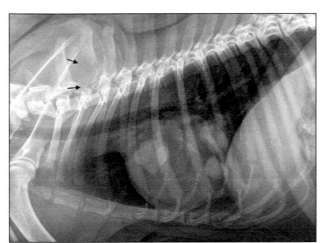

9.19 Röntgen sign: opacity. Osteolysis. Lateral radiograph of the thorax of a dog with neck pain. The purpose of radiography was to assess for pulmonary metastases. Note that an extensive lytic lesion has resulted in destruction of most of the spinous process and dorsal lamina of the second thoracic vertebra (arrowed). These changes are easily overlooked due to superimposition of the scapulae and emphasize the need to evaluate all parts of the image and the importance of not suspending the evaluation of the film when a conspicuous lesion, in this case multiple pulmonary metastases, is present.

Osteoproliferative disease: The extent of vertebral new bone may be marked or limited (Figure 9.21). Neoplasia (primary or soft tissue extending into the bone) can result in amorphous, poorly marginated and unstructured new bone. The changes associated with neoplasia are usually of a mixed pattern with both osteoproliferation and osteolysis. Inflammatory diseases involving the vertebrae are predominately osteoproductive; however, the periosteal reaction is more structured and may be florid. Cortical integrity is more likely to be preserved and the transition zone to normal bone is shorter.

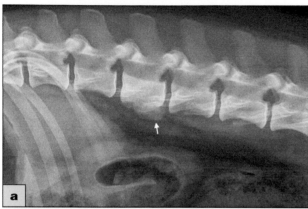

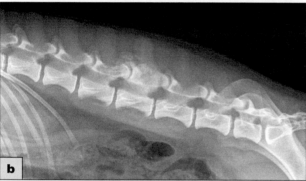

9.21 Röntgen sign: opacity. Osteoproliferation. **(a)** Lateral radiograph of the lumbar vertebral column of a dog with back pain due to vertebral osteomyelitis. A thick, smooth, periosteal reaction extends from the ventral border of the third lumbar vertebra (arrowed). The vertebral body overall is of increased opacity compared to adjacent vertebral bodies, due to the superimposition of florid, lateralized periosteal new bone. The changes were confirmed on MRI. Only a single vertebra was involved. **(b)** Lateral radiograph of the lumbar vertebral column of a dog with primary neoplasia of the L4 vertebra. The changes are predominantly productive involving the dorsal lamina of the vertebra. The location of the lesion and the amorphous new bone are indicative of a neoplastic process.

Periosteal reaction: Periosteal reactions are usually centred along the ventral and lateral aspects of the vertebral body (see Figure 9.21a). Location is an important feature. Changes in L3–L4 are most commonly associated with inflammatory diseases, whereas involvement of L5–L7, the sacrum, ilia and femora is often associated with local metastatic disease from aggressive neoplasms within the pelvis (carcinomas). The periosteal new bone associated with inflammation and infection is generally palisading and continuous. The appearance of new bone associated with neoplasia is variable and represented by unstructured periosteal new bone or amorphous tumoral new bone. In pelvic neoplasia that has metastasized to the caudal lumbar vertebral column, the periosteal reaction can appear aggressive, spiculated and interrupted. As periosteal reactions are commonly indistinct, the margins of the vertebrae should be examined with a bright light or high brightness monitor settings to avoid overlooking lesions.

Callus formation and remodelling: Healing vertebral fractures result in osseous callus formation and a local increase in radiographic opacity, followed by remodelling changes (Figure 9.22).

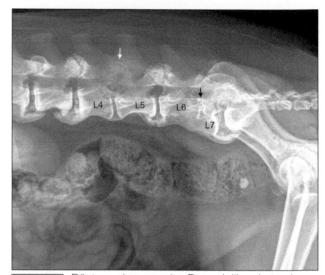

9.22 Röntgen sign: opacity. Remodelling. Lateral view of the lumbosacral vertebral column of a dog with remodelling changes following a displaced L7 fracture. The changes are chronic. The caudal aspect of the L7 vertebra is displaced ventrally. The displaced fragment has fused with the ventral aspect of the L6 vertebral body and the cranial aspect of the non-displaced L7 fragment (malunion). The intervertebral disc between L6 and L7 is still recognizable (black arrow). There is extensive remodelling and ventral spondylosis. The vertebral canal at the lumbosacral junction is irregularly widened. The changes associated with the L4–L5 vertebrae probably represent a congenital block vertebra rather than the result of trauma as the L4 vertebral body is shortened and the articular process joints are absent (white arrow).

Bone infarcts and islands: Focal areas of increased opacity in the vertebral bodies can occasionally be observed in the dog. These represent incidental bone islands or infarcts associated with an aggressive neoplastic lesion elsewhere in the body.

Osteopetrosis (myelofibrosis): Generalized increased bone opacity of the skeleton, including the vertebral column, can occasionally be observed in the cat (Figure 9.23) and, less commonly, in the dog. There is anecdotal evidence that this is associated with feline leukaemia virus (FeLV) or lymphoma in the cat. In the dog, osteopetrosis can be associated with pyruvate kinase deficiency. Other identified causes include chronic dietary calcium excess, hypervitaminosis D and myelosclerotic neoplasia.

Perivertebral new bone: New bone may be periarticular (articular process joints, osteophytosis) or associated with perivertebral ligaments and tendons (enthesiophytes).

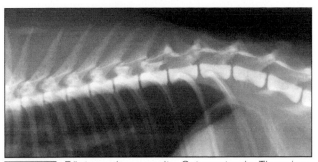

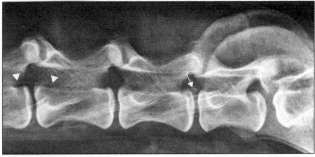

9.23 Röntgen sign: opacity. Osteopetrosis. There is a generalized, increased medullary opacity of the skeleton in this cat with lymphoma. This is particularly visible in the vertebral bodies.

9.25 Röntgen sign: opacity. Soft tissue mineralization. Lateral view of the lumbar vertebral column of a dog with ossification of the dura mater (dural ossification), outlining the spinal cord (automyelogram) (arrowheads). At L6–L7 mineralized disc material can be seen protruding into the vertebral canal and the dural sac is mildly deviated (arrowed). This does not provide sufficient information to determine whether a significant lesion is present.

Mineralization of soft tissues:

Nucleus pulposus mineralization: This is a hallmark feature of Hansen type I intervertebral disc degeneration (chondroid metaplasia). The appearance of the mineralization can be focal (involving the central zone of the nucleus alone), ring-like (involving the periphery of the nucleus) or involve the whole nucleus. It is not synonymous with, and does not indicate, intervertebral disc herniation. With Hansen type II degeneration (fibroid degeneration), disc mineralization occurs less frequently.

Intervertebral disc herniation: Herniation of intervertebral disc material into the vertebral canal can only be identified if the material is mineralized (chondroid degeneration) (Figure 9.24).

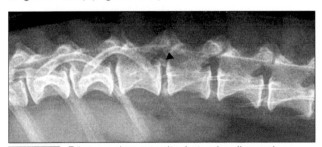

9.24 Röntgen sign: opacity. Lateral radiograph showing intervertebral disc degeneration and herniation in a chondrodystrophic dog. The L1–L2 intervertebral disc space is narrowed with mineralized disc material superimposed on the intervertebral foraminal space (arrowhead). These changes are consistent with a Hansen type I degeneration and disc extrusion. This finding is not sufficient to determine whether surgical intervention is justified as this material is not necessarily the clinically relevant lesion.

Dural ossification: The dura mater frequently ossifies (usually in plaques) in older large-breed dogs. This is an incidental degenerative process. Dural ossification is visible on radiographs (Figure 9.25) and, if deviated by extradural material, is suggestive of spinal cord compression (automyelogram). However, this is not a reliable method for diagnosing and localizing spinal cord compression.

Calcinosis circumscripta: This is an idiopathic condition with potential for malignancy, in which grape-like mineralization occurs in the vicinity of the synovial joints. Changes are most common around the cervical articular process joints.

Gas opacity:

Spinal vacuum phenomenon: Gas (mainly nitrogen) can accumulate in the clefts of a degenerated disc. The gas is resorbed from adjacent blood vessels. It occurs most commonly after stretching (e.g. lifting a heavy dog where its forelimbs and hindlimbs are suspended). The vacuum phenomenon is an indicator of disc degeneration but does not predict disc protrusion or extrusion.

Other causes: Other causes of gas accumulation, such as infection with gas-producing bacteria or following vertebral fracture, are extremely rare and not confined to the intervertebral disc.

Margination
The margins of the vertebrae may be altered due to the presence of lesions, which can result in:

- Expansile changes – usually neoplastic but occasionally inflammatory
- Periosteal reaction – reflecting either neoplastic or inflammatory processes. The location of the spinal segments in which the periosteal reaction is recognized is important
- Defects in the cortical margins of the body and endplates
- Fractures (Figure 9.26) – discontinuity of the cortical margins. In addition to the interruption of cortical integrity, the margins should be assessed for the presence of a periosteal reaction as this feature may be present with acute pathological fractures.

Function
The vertebral column allows a wide range of motion in different segments. If there is an insult leading to abnormal instability, secondary muscular bracing will reduce such motion to protect the spinal cord. To be able to diagnose the cause of instability on radiographs, hyperextension, flexion or traction may need to be applied (carefully) depending on the nature of the lesion. However, great care must be taken not to aggravate the clinical signs by doing so. Conditions in which dynamic assessment of the vertebral column might be indicated include:

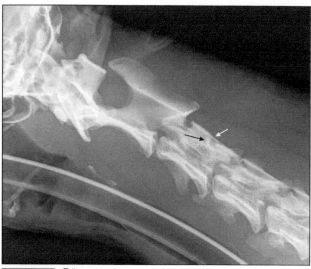

9.26 Röntgen sign: margination. Lateral radiograph of the cranial cervical vertebral column of a small-breed dog with a depression fracture of C3 following a bite to the neck from a larger dog. A discrete defect (white arrow) is present in the dorsal lamina of C3. The small cortical fragment (black arrow) is displaced ventrally and superimposed on the vertebral canal. Inadvertent axial rotation may have allowed the defect in the margin of the vertebral canal to be better visualized.

- Instability of the occipitoatlantal or atlantoaxial articulations
- Cervical spondylomyelopathy
- Cervical intervertebral disc protrusion
- Articular process joint pathology
- Lumbosacral intervertebral disc degeneration.

Common diseases

Specific spinal regions

Cervical vertebral column

Conditions that frequently affect the cervical vertebral column include:

- Instability of the occipitoatlantal or atlantoaxial articulations
- Articular process joint pathology (hypertrophy, malformation, malpositioning) resulting in stenosis
- Cervical stenotic spondylomyelopathy
- Intervertebral disc degeneration, protrusion and extrusion
- Neoplasia
- Infection
- Trauma.

Thoracic vertebral column

Conditions that frequently affect the thoracic vertebral column include:

- Vertebral malformation
- Cranial thoracic stenosis
- Intervertebral disc degeneration
- Neoplasia
- Infection
- Trauma.

Lumbar vertebral column

Conditions that frequently affect the lumbar vertebral column include:

- Vertebral malformation
- Intervertebral disc degeneration, protrusion and extrusion
- Articular process joint pathology
- Neoplasia
- Infection
- Trauma.

Sacral and coccygeal vertebral column

Conditions that frequently affect the sacral and coccygeal vertebral column include:

- Vertebral malformation
- Lumbosacral stenosis
- Intervertebral disc degeneration
- Neoplasia
- Infection
- Trauma.

Congenital malformations

Congenital malformations are very common, occurring in up to 25% of dogs. In many cases they are incidental and of no clinical significance; however, occasionally in cases of severe stenosis, they may be responsible for neurological signs (Figure 9.27).

Block vertebra

Block vertebrae (see Figures 9.8, 9.22 and 9.27) are usually caused by failure of somite segmentation. This results in osseous, partial or complete, fusion of two (or rarely more) adjacent vertebrae.

Radiological features:

- Fusion of the body, pedicles, laminae or spinal processes.
- Intervertebral disc space absent or vestigial. Articular process joint space between the two vertebrae may be absent or reduced in size.
- The length of the block vertebra is usually shorter than that of two normal vertebrae.
- Adjacent vertebrae adapt in shape to accommodate the abnormal angulation of the block vertebra.

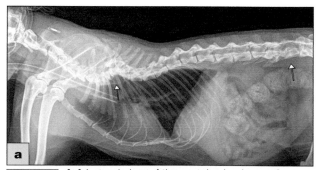

9.27 **(a)** Lateral view of the vertebral column of a young cat with multiple congenital malformations. There is marked kyphosis (dorsal angulation) of the thoracic vertebral column (arrowed). Radiography provides a global assessment of the changes; however, it is impossible to assess the nature and extent of the malformations with certainty. Accurate neurolocalization and cross-sectional imaging are required to establish whether the changes are of clinical significance and confirm any sites of stenosis (on MRI in this cat there was severe cord compression at T3–T4). The lumbosacral changes were not clinically significant. (continues) ▶

- The trabecular pattern and thickness of the cortical bone is normal.
- Block vertebrae do not usually cause clinical signs. In a minority of cases (typically associated with block vertebrae in the cervical region of the vertebral column), they may contribute to clinical signs due to:
  - Reduced vertebral or head mobility
  - Increased mobility and stress on neighbouring discs, which can lead to disc degeneration and/or ligamentous hypertrophy
  - Vertebral canal stenosis and spinal cord/nerve root compression due to excessive bone production.

Transitional vertebra

A transitional vertebra (Figure 9.28) is a congenital malformation resulting in a vertebra with the anatomical characteristics of another vertebral region. They occur

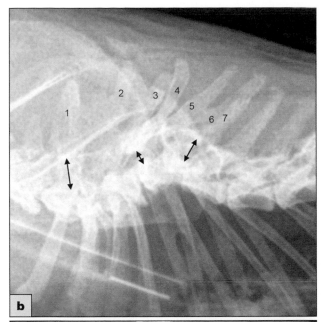

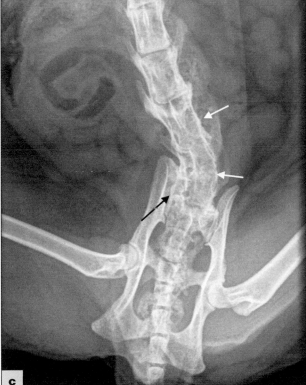

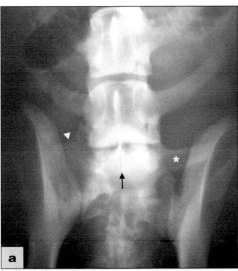

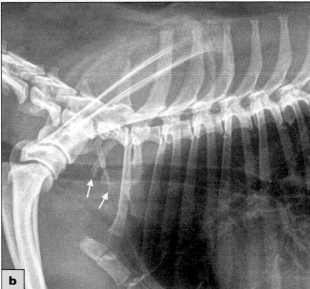

9.27 (continued) **(b)** Magnified lateral and **(c)** VD views of the vertebral column of a young cat with multiple congenital malformations. (b) The magnified view demonstrates narrowing of the vertebral canal at the level of T3–T4 (small double-headed arrow) compared to adjacent segments (large double-headed arrows). (c) Scoliosis (lateral deviation to the left) of the lumbar vertebral column (white arrows) and a transitional lumbosacral vertebra (black arrow) are evident. The malformations within both vertebral segments include block vertebrae, hemivertebrae, incomplete separation of the dorsal laminae and spinous processes and transitional vertebrae. Radiography provides a global assessment of the changes; however, it is impossible to assess the nature and extent of the malformations with certainty. Accurate neurolocalization and cross-sectional imaging are required to establish whether the changes are of clinical significance and confirm any sites of stenosis (on MRI in this cat there was severe cord compression at T3–T4). The lumbosacral changes were not clinically significant.

9.28 Transitional vertebrae. **(a)** VD view of the lumbosacral joint of a 5-month-old German Shepherd Dog. The transitional lumbosacral vertebra has a normal transverse process on the left (*) and an abnormal broad transverse process fused with the sacral wing on the right (arrowhead). The spinous process (arrowed) of the transitional vertebra is split (spina bifida). **(b)** Lateral view of the thorax of a dog. The transitional vertebra is located at C7. Note the elongated (rib-like), ventrally oriented transverse processes (arrowed).

at junctions between the regions. Further classification is based on which abnormal characteristics the vertebra has acquired. The changes may be unilateral or bilateral.

- Cervicalization – a thoracic vertebra with a missing rib.
- Thoracalization – a cervical or lumbar vertebra with a rib instead of a transverse process.
- Lumbarization – a thoracic or sacral vertebra with a transverse process instead of a rib or sacral wing.
- Sacralization – a lumbar or coccygeal vertebra with a sacral wing instead of a transverse process.

Radiological features:

- A comprehensive set of spinal radiographs, enabling a complete vertebral count, is required to accurately define the vertebrae which have gained or lost an anatomical feature (unilateral rib, transverse process). If this is not the case, the general term transitional vertebra is used to describe the vertebrae (i.e. transitional thoracolumbar or lumbosacral vertebra).
- Transitional vertebrae occur at the junction between vertebral segment regions.
- In most cases, the presence of a transitional vertebra is an incidental finding. Unilateral changes can lead to scoliosis and may promote lumbosacral disc degeneration. Previous claims that transitional lumbosacral vertebrae promote unilateral hip dysplasia have not been substantiated. However, transitional vertebrae do cause a number of practical problems:
  - Lumbosacral transitional vertebrae with unilateral changes prevent symmetrical positioning for VD radiographs of the hips and pelvis. This can lead to unjustified poor scoring in radiographic hip dysplasia screening
  - Unilateral or bilateral transitional vertebrae may lead to an error in anatomical localization when planning spinal surgery. For this reason, where surgical localization is based on rib palpation, it is essential to count the vertebrae of the relevant and neighbouring vertebral regions. Even where a diagnosis of intervertebral disc extrusion requiring surgical decompression has been reached by a preferred technique such as MRI, a VD radiograph provides a rapid, reliable means of demonstrating a transitional vertebra where there is uncertainty.

Hemivertebra

During embryogenesis the paired vertebral somites around the neural tube must separate into a cranial and a caudal segment to allow the spinal nerves to exit. The cranial segment then recombines with the caudal segment directly cranial to it. The process is known as metameric shift. Hemivertebrae represent anomalies of this orderly segmentation with displacement of the vertebral somites (hemi-metameric shift). The mismatch in the fusion pattern creates a wedge-shaped vertebra in either the sagittal or dorsal plane (Figure 9.29). It is very common in brachycephalic screw-tailed dogs such as Bulldogs, Pugs and Boston

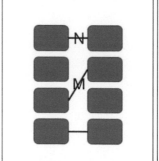
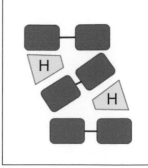

9.29 Hemivertebra formation. Normal, paired mesodermal segments (N) merge and form a cartilaginous precursor of a vertebral body. If a mismatch in the fusion pattern occurs, unmatched segments (M) form wedge-shaped hemivertebrae (H), resulting in vertebral curvature deformities.

Terriers. Hemivertebrae are often incidental, although anecdotal clinical signs are more likely to occur if the malformation is associated with lordosis.

Radiological features:

- Triangular or wedge-shaped vertebra on lateral or VD radiographs.
- Hemivertebrae can be associated with vertebral curvature deformations. Moderate to severe angulation of the vertebral column can result in scoliosis (lateral deviation of the vertebral column) (Figure 9.30) or kyphosis (dorsal deviation of the vertebral column) (Figure 9.31a) or a combination of both conditions.
- The bone is of normal appearance and mineralization.

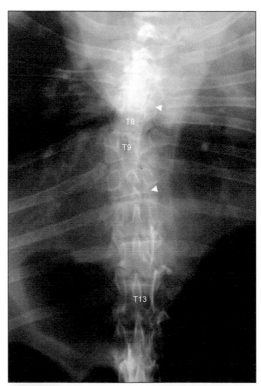

9.30 VD radiograph of a Bulldog showing scoliosis (arrowheads) and abnormal spacing of the ribs due to the formation of a hemivertebra at T8. These deformities are ubiquitous in brachycephalic breeds and only rarely cause clinical signs.

- Although usually incidental, marked vertebral canal stenosis is occasionally present resulting in neurological signs.
- The shape of adjacent vertebrae change to conform to the shape of the hemivertebra.
- The intervertebral discs are usually normal in shape.
- Osteophytes and osseous remodelling are not typically present. Instability is not a common feature of hemivertebrae, but in animals with neurological disease, cross-sectional imaging is essential to assess the significance of the changes.

Cleft vertebra

Cleft vertebra (also known as butterfly vertebra) occurs with persistence of the notochord or its sagittal cleavage. It results in a sagittal cleft through the vertebral body with funnel-shaped endplates. It is very common in brachycephalic screw-tailed dogs such as Bulldogs, Pugs and Boston Terriers.

Radiological features:

- On VD radiographs, the vertebra resembles the shape of a butterfly (Figure 9.31b).
- Reduced vertebral length (usually incidental).

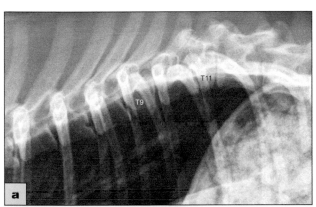

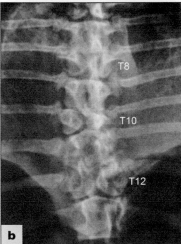

9.31 **(a)** Lateral radiograph of a Boston Terrier with thoracic hemivertebrae. The vertebral bodies of T9 and T11 are narrowed ventrally (triangular-shaped), resulting in kyphosis. These changes were incidental. Note also the central endplate defects in T5 and T7, consistent with incidental Schmorl's nodes. **(b)** Ventrodorsal radiograph of a brachycephalic dog with cleft or butterfly vertebrae at T8, T10 and T12. The bodies of these vertebrae are incompletely formed, giving them the shape of a butterfly.

Spina bifida

This is an incomplete fusion of the vertebral arch (see Figures 9.28 and 9.32) and may be associated with meningomyeloceles.

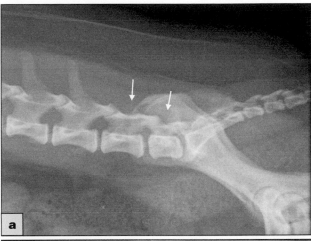

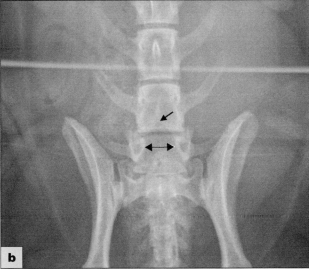

9.32 **(a)** Lateral and **(b)** VD views of the lumbosacral vertebral column of a dog with spina bifida. (a) The spinous process is hypoplastic in L6 and absent in L7 (arrowed). (b) The wide pedicles and absence of lamina and spinous process of L7 are noted on the VD view (double-headed arrow). The small cleft in the caudal lamina of L6 indicates a partial fusion defect (black arrow).

Radiological features:

- Changes are best identified on a VD radiograph.
- Variable appearance – the dorsal spinous processes may be absent or split (cleft).
- The vertebral arch (lamina) may be completely absent or incomplete.
- Spina bifida can affect one or several vertebrae. It is most commonly seen in the caudal lumbar (particularly L7) and sacral regions.
- Pedicles can be widened/laterally positioned.

Sacrococcygeal dysgenesis

This is a congenital anomaly in which the sacral and/or coccygeal vertebrae and spinal cord segments are absent. It is an autosomal dominant trait in Manx cats. The tail is usually absent. Sacrococcygeal dysgenesis (Figure 9.33) is often associated with other spinal cord anomalies. The clinical signs depend on the extent of the anomaly.

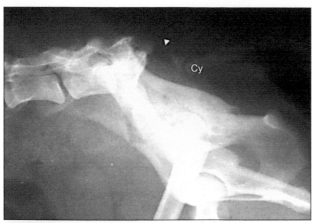

9.33 Sacrococcygeal dysgenesis in a Miniature Pinscher. The caudal part of the sacrum (arrowhead) and connection to the coccygeal vertebrae (Cy) are absent.

Radiological features:

■ Coccygeal and/or sacral vertebrae are absent.

Intervertebral disc disease

The term intervertebral disc disease encompasses degeneration, protrusion and extrusion. Degeneration of intervertebral discs is a common process in the dog and to a lesser degree in the cat. In chondrodystrophic dog breeds this condition is ubiquitous. Originally, two types of disc degeneration were described by (and named after) Hansen in the 1950s. More recently, a syndrome of acute disc extrusion of small volumes of largely non-degenerative disc material has been recognized which does not fit with the original Hansen classification. Progressive dehydration of the nucleus pulposus is the starting point for all forms of disc degeneration.

Intervertebral disc degeneration and herniation

Hansen type I disc degeneration:

■ Chondroid metaplasia of the dessicating nucleus pulposus leads to granular and often mineralized nuclear material.
■ High prevalence in chondrodystrophic dog breeds such as the Dachshund, Beagle, Cocker Spaniel and Pekingese.
■ Starts at a young age and is progressive.
■ Degenerate nucleus can extrude through a ruptured annulus into the vertebral canal.
■ If degenerative disc material is extruded, it usually results in acute spinal cord or nerve root compression, leading to extremity paralysis. Intermittent, progressive extrusion can also occur.

Hansen type II disc degeneration:

■ Fibrous metaplasia of the dessicating nucleus pulposus leads to fibrous nuclear material, which is not usually mineralized.
■ Prevalent in cats and non-chondrodystrophic dog breeds.
■ Starts in later stages of life and is progressive.
■ Partial annulus fibre tearing without complete rupture leads to bulging of the disc into the vertebral canal or intervertebral foramen. This is termed protrusion.
■ Slow onset, chronic condition which often starts with pain.

Acute non-degenerative disc extrusion:

■ This is a variation of type I disc degeneration and has also been termed low volume, high velocity disc extrusion or type III disc extrusion.
■ Acute rupture of the annulus by small, presumed high velocity, disc fragments propelled into the vertebral canal causes high impact spinal cord damage and extensive haemorrhage (contusion).
■ Disc material can also lacerate the dura mater and lead to a dural tear.

Radiological features:

■ Narrowed intervertebral disc space (Figures 9.34 and 9.35).
■ Narrowed articular process joint space.
■ Mineralization of an intervertebral disc.
■ Gas within the intervertebral disc (spinal vacuum phenomenon).
■ Sclerotic endplates.

Intervertebral disc extrusion

Intervertebral disc degeneration is a common phenomenon which *per se* does not cause clinical signs. Only some degenerated discs protrude or extrude into the vertebral canal and cause spinal cord or nerve root compression with clinical signs. Survey radiography is insensitive for the diagnosis of spinal cord compression except when:

■ The protruding or extruded material is mineralized and visible within the vertebral canal
■ The dura mater is ossified and visibly deviated inward by disc material (automyelogram).

However, even under these circumstances survey radiography is unreliable to localize, lateralize and assess the degree of spinal cord compression. Many

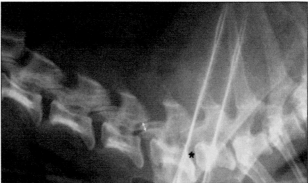

9.34 Lateral radiograph of the caudal cervical vertebral column of a Toy Poodle with acute neurological signs. The C6–C7 intervertebral disc space is narrowed and wedge-shaped, indicating disc degeneration (*) and probable extrusion. The osteophyte extending from the caudoventral border of C6 is indicative of chronic instability. Although the survey radiographs support the presumptive diagnosis of intervertebral disc herniation, cross-sectional imaging (preferably) or myelography is required to confirm and lateralize the lesion. The C5–C6 articular process joints are widened (double-headed arrow).

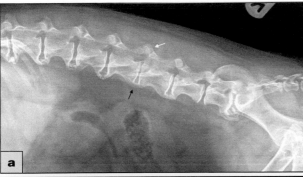

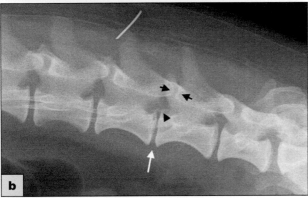

9.35 Lateral lumbar spinal radiographs of two Dachshunds with signs of hindlimb paresis.
(a) Multiple degenerative changes including narrowing of the L4–L5 (black arrow), L5–L6 and lumbosacral intervertebral disc spaces are visible. The L4–L5 facet joint is also narrowed (white arrow). It is not possible to determine which of the changes is most significant on survey radiographs alone. **(b)** The L5–L6 intervertebral disc space (white arrow) is the only one which is narrowed and is accompanied by narrowing of the facet joint (black arrows) and intervertebral foramen (arrowhead). A small amount of granular mineralized material lies within the ventral vertebral canal, dorsal to the intervertebral disc space. It is likely that the herniated degenerated disc material is responsible for the clinical signs but this and the lateralization, extent and degree of cord compression must be confirmed by myelography or cross-sectional imaging. The linear metal structure is a hypodermic needle placed to facilitate identification of the correct disc space at surgery.

dogs have multiple disc protrusions or extrusions, of which only some may be mineralized. The mineralized lesion visible on radiographs is not necessarily the clinically relevant lesion. Thus, survey radiography alone is not an appropriate method to diagnose spinal cord compression by intervertebral disc protrusion or extrusion.

Protrusion and extrusion of the intervertebral discs occurs most frequently between T9 and T13 in the dog. This is attributed to the lack of an intercapital ligament, which connects both rib heads on the floor of the vertebral canal and provides additional protection for the spinal cord in these vertebrae. However, mid-thoracic intervertebral disc protrusions do occur, particularly in German Shepherd Dogs, and should be considered.

Radiological features:

- Mineralized material, if present, is recognized superimposed on the intervertebral foramen on lateral views.
- The location of the material immediately dorsal to the intervertebral disc space is an important

feature of disc extrusion; although with extrusion of a large volume of disc, mineralized material may distribute extensively both cranially and caudally to the disc space.
- Oblique views of the caudal vertebral endplates, superimposition of the head of the ribs (thoracic vertebral column) and superimposition of the accessory processes or tips of the transverse processes (lumbar vertebral column) may mimic herniated intervertebral disc material. Accurate positioning is the most important step to differentiate artefacts from genuine extrusion.
- Mineralized material that has herniated laterally can be recognized superimposed on the intervertebral foramen on oblique views of the cervical vertebral column or VD views of the thoracolumbar vertebral column.

Fibrocartilaginous embolism

Fibrocartilaginous embolism involves acute spinal vascular occlusion by material transported from the nucleus pulposus. The mechanism is unclear, but it is possibly associated with intervertebral disc degeneration. It is an acute onset asymmetrical neuropathy, which is non-painful and non-progressive after 24 hours.

Radiological features

- Usually normal appearance of the vertebral column at the site of neurolocalization.
- Can be associated with non-specific slight narrowing of the intervertebral disc space.

Schmorl's node

This is occasionally recognized in the dog, particularly chondrodystrophic breeds. It consists of a defect in the central osseous vertebral endplate, allowing protrusion of disc material into the vertebral body. It is an incidental finding.

Radiological features

- Concave vertebral endplates (see Figure 9.31a).

Vertebral canal stenosis

Stenosis may be focal or segmental, affecting one to several adjacent vertebrae, or generalized, affecting the entire vertebral column. The stenosis may be absolute, where the narrowed osseous spinal canal results in attenuation of the spinal cord, or relative, where the vertebral canal is reduced in diameter compared with normal animals and there is the potential for cord attenuation secondary to soft tissue changes, vertebral instability or bony proliferation. Vertebral canal stenosis can be caused by:

- Any proliferative process (neoplasia, discospondylitis, disc protrusion, ligamentous hypertrophy and synovial proliferation)
- Osseous processes (articular process joint malformation, vertebral malformation, fractures, luxation and excessive callus formation).

Only mineralized or osseous forms of stenosis are visible on survey radiography. Myelography or cross-sectional imaging is required to demonstrate vertebral canal stenosis fully. There are several specific forms of vertebral canal stenosis, including:

- Malalignment due to occipitoatlantal malformation, cervical stenotic spondylomyelopathy and lumbosacral stenosis
- Malformation of the vertebrae and vertebral canal
- Articular process hypertrophy/malformation (involving the mid-cervical vertebral column in Bassett Hounds and other large- and giant-breed dogs as a component of cervical stenotic spondylomyelopathy)
- Disc-associated stenosis where disc degeneration (usually type II) with annulus protrusion results in acquired stenosis in animals with a pre-existing relative osseous stenosis
- Developmental stenosis due to hypothyroidism, mucopolysaccharidosis, multiple cartilaginous exostoses or osteochondrosis
- Occasionally hemivertebrae and transitional vertebrae
- Post-healing remodelling.

Cervical stenotic spondylomyelopathy

Cervical stenotic spondylomyelopathy (also known as Wobbler syndrome) (Figure 9.36) is a developmental abnormality in young or middle-aged predominantly large-breed dogs, where a combination of factors including disc protrusion, vertebral subluxation and malformation, articular process joint enlargement, and compensatory ligamentous hypertrophy result in sequential compression of the cervical spinal cord at the level of the intervertebral disc spaces. Several subtypes exist:

- C2–C4 vertebral canal stenosis in Bassett Hounds due to disc protrusion, malformation of the lamina and dorsal ligament hypertrophy
- Dorsal and ventral C3–C7 vertebral canal stenosis in young Great Danes and C5–C7 in young or middle-aged Dobermanns due to disc protrusion, dorsal and yellow ligament hypertrophy, and vertebral malformation and malarticulation of C7 and to a lesser degree C6. These vertebrae are wedge-shaped (lack of normal cranioventral

margin) with dorsal rotation or displacement of the cranial aspect of the vertebral body. The vertebral canal is funnel-shaped
- Dorsolateral C4–C7 vertebral canal stenosis in older Great Danes due to malformation of the articular process joints
- T2–T5 vertebral canal stenosis. Usually large-breed dogs with the conformation typical of Mastiffs (stenosis is usually dorsolateral) or Dobermanns (dorsoventral stenosis). Cross-sectional imaging is required to demonstrate stenosis.

In many cases, radiographic signs are only suggestive of disease and MRI is needed for complete characterization of the condition.

Radiological features:

- The radiographic features are those of caudal cervical vertebral malformation, instability and stenosis together with secondary degenerative changes.
- Vertebral body malformation leads to malalignment of adjacent vertebrae. The dorsocranial aspect of C7 and occasionally C5–C6 rotate dorsally, narrowing the vertebral canal.
- Narrowing of the vertebral canal (vertebral canal stenosis). The height of the vertebral canal cranially (cranial vertebral foramen) is reduced compared with caudally (caudal vertebral foramen). This condition usually involves the caudal cervical vertebrae (C5–C7). Consequently, the vertebral canal has a funnel-shape. These changes must be distinguished from normal mild narrowing of the cranial vertebral foramen.
- Malformation and/or osseous hypertrophy of the articular process joints may be seen on both lateral and VD views.
- Intervertebral disc space narrowing or collapse and decreased size of the intervertebral foramina.
- Remodelling changes (sclerosis of the endplates, remodelling of vertebral bodies and ventral spondylosis).

Lumbosacral stenosis

With lumbosacral stenosis, the clinical signs are typical of cauda equina compression and include:

- Pelvic limb weakness and lower motor neuron signs relating to the bladder, tail and anus
- Pain on movement of the tail or compression of the lumbosacral junction
- Hindlimb lameness.

Lumbosacral stenosis is caused by:

- Congenital anomalies (stenosis; Figure 9.37) including stenotic lumbosacral joints in some German Shepherd Dogs
- Developmental abnormalities such as lumbosacral osteochondritis dissecans. This is a relatively rare developmental disease seen in German Shepherd Dogs and Belgian Shepherd Dogs associated with incomplete ossification of the dorsal aspect of the S1 endplate or, less commonly, the caudal endplate of L7 (Figure 9.38). Displaced cartilage

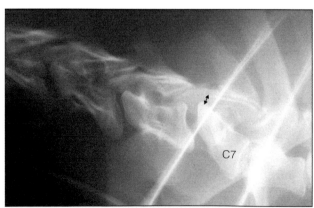

9.36 Lateral radiograph of the caudal cervical vertebral column of a young Dobermann with cervical stenotic spondylomyelopathy (Wobbler syndrome). The C7 vertebra is wedge-shaped and rotated in a clockwise direction and the cranial vertebral foramen is markedly narrowed (double-headed arrow). These changes result in marked vertebral canal stenosis.

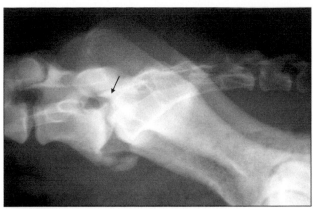

9.37 Lateral radiograph showing lumbosacral disc degeneration in a large-breed dog. The endplates are sclerotic and the dorsal lamina (arrowed) and vertebral body of S1 are subluxated ventrally in relation to L7, contributing to the vertebral canal stenosis.

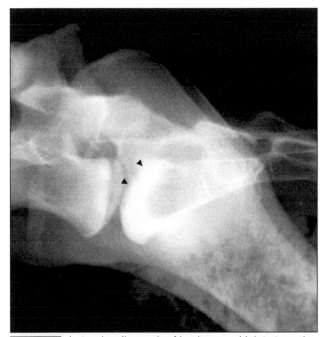

9.38 Lateral radiograph of lumbosacral joint stenosis in a 3-year-old German Shepherd Dog with sacral osteochondrosis. The cranial endplate of S1 is not ossified dorsally (arrowheads), resulting in a flattened appearance. Small mineralized fragments are superimposed on the vertebral canal.

- fragments can compress the cauda equina and cause clinical signs
- Intervertebral disc disease
- Malalignment and instability
- Masses
- Infection
- Fractures.

Radiological features:

- In osteochondritis dissecans, the cranial endplate of S1 or, less commonly, the caudal endplate of L7, is abnormal with an osseous defect of the dorsal endplate margin. A mineralized displaced fragment(s) may be present bordering the defect or superimposed on the vertebral canal. These changes may be obscured by florid degenerative changes.

- In congenital stenosis, the sacrum may be subluxated (ventrally) relative to L7. Angulation of the sacrum relative to the L7 vertebra may be abnormal. Stenosis of the vertebral canal within the L7 vertebra and at the lumbosacral junction may be associated with a transitional lumbosacral vertebra. Radiographs only demonstrate the extent of the osseous changes; cross-sectional imaging is required to demonstrate the full extent of all changes.
- In degenerative lumbosacral stenosis, the intervertebral disc space may be narrowed or collapsed with sclerosis of the endplates. Perivertebral degenerative changes (ventral and lateral spondylosis and facet hypertrophy) are often florid.
- In discospondylitis, there is destruction of the vertebral endplates, and initial disc space widening followed by disc space narrowing or collapse. Rarely, subluxation or fracture of articular facet joints may be present.

Occipitoatlantal and atlantoaxial articulation abnormalities

Incomplete ossification of the atlas: The atlas vertebra is created by a complex ossification process. In the dog, incomplete atlas ossification leading to atlanto-axial instability or atlanto-occipital overlap has been reported (Figure 9.39).

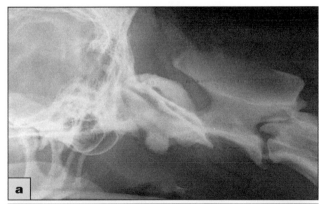

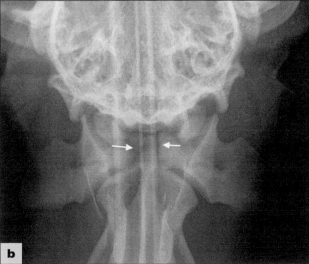

9.39 **(a)** Lateral and **(b)** VD radiographs of a young dog with incomplete ossification of the atlas. The changes cannot be assessed on the lateral view, but on the VD view the arches of the atlas are not fused (arrowed), allowing direct visualization of the odontoid process.

Atlantoaxial subluxation: This usually occurs in small-breed (toy) dogs but large dog breeds are occasionally affected. Clinical signs include neck pain, low head carriage and varying degrees of ataxia and tetraparesis. The most important consideration is that the clinical signs, even in cases with congenital disease, may only be demonstrated later in life, often following minor trauma. Atlantoaxial instability should not be discounted based on age.

Radiological features:

- The cranial aspect of the spinous process of C2 is displaced relative to the dorsal arch of C1 (Figure 9.40). The displacement is usually in the order of a few millimetres.
- Instability may not be evident on a neutral lateral survey radiograph. Subsequent radiographs following incremental flexion of the neck may be needed to demonstrate instability. Care must be taken that in demonstrating instability clinical signs are not exacerbated.
- An abnormally shaped or absent odontoid process of the axis (dens) may be recognized. The dens may be shortened.
- Trauma may result in fracture of the dens.

Abnormalities of the odontoid process of the axis vertebra: The axis vertebra bears the odontoid process, which acts as a pivot for the rotation of the atlas vertebra. It is held in position by several ligaments.

Radiological features:

- Dens aplasia or hypoplasia. The odontoid process may be absent (Figure 9.41) or incompletely formed, leading to atlantoaxial instability and spinal cord compression.
- Dorsal dens angulation. The odontoid process may be abnormally shaped with dorsal angulation, leading to spinal cord compression.
- Odontoid ligament rupture, leading to abnormal mobility of the odontoid process (atlantoaxial instability) and spinal cord compression.
- Avulsion of the cranial tip of the odontoid process. This is a secondary ossification centre, which can avulse due to trauma or underlying osteochondritis dissecans.

A lateral oblique radiograph (rotated head and atlas) is best for visualization of the odontoid process. This view allows the odontoid process to be projected free from the rotated wings of the atlas.

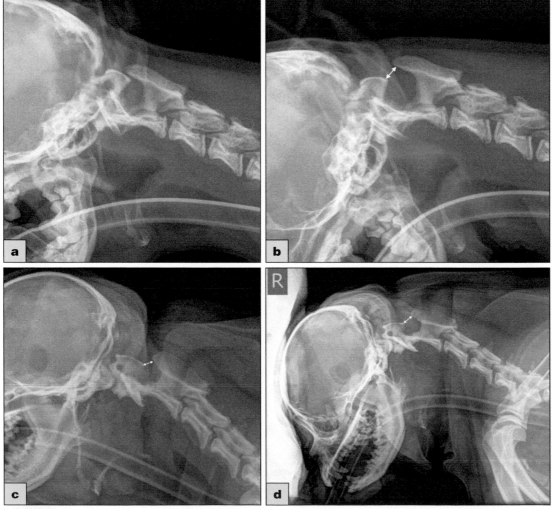

9.40 (a, c) Neutral and (b, d) moderately flexed lateral radiographs of the cranial cervical vertebral column of two dogs with atlantoaxial instability. Instability results in widening of the space between the dorsal arch of C1 and the dorsal arch of C2 during flexion (double-headed arrow). The instability is more marked in (b) than in (d).

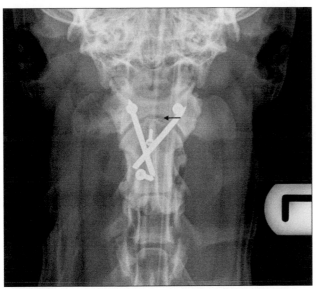

9.41 VD radiograph of a skeletally mature Miniature Schnauzer with atlantoaxial instability due to agenesis of the dens. Note the absence of a normal odontoid process (arrowed). The instability has been stabilized using crossed pins, screws and bone cement.

Vertebral fractures

Radiography has poor sensitivity for the detection of vertebral fractures. A fracture of the spinous or transverse processes is often readily visible, whereas vertebral body and arch fractures are often compression fractures, leading to vertebral shortening and mild alterations in shape. Healed fractures often lead to the formation of block vertebrae. When correlating radiographic and clinical findings, it is important to remember that the degree of vertebral displacement does not always correlate well with the severity of neurological dysfunction. Significant displacement during a traumatic incident, leading to severe spinal cord injury, may not be evident at the time of radiography when fracture fragments are partially or completely reduced by the effect of muscle contraction and pain.

For the assessment of stability of vertebral fractures, a three-compartment module has been developed:

- The dorsal compartment comprises the articular processes, laminae, pedicles, spinous processes and supporting soft tissue structures
- The middle compartment includes the dorsal longitudinal ligament, the dorsal aspect of the annulus fibrosus of the intervertebral disc and the dorsal part of the vertebral body
- The ventral compartment contains the rest of the vertebral body, the lateral and ventral annulus fibrosus, the nucleus pulposus and the ventral longitudinal ligament.

If more than one compartment is affected by a fracture, then it is deemed unstable. Great care should be taken to avoid additional spinal cord injury during positioning for radiography and surgery. General anaesthesia results in muscle relaxation, which may allow further displacement of the unstable spinal column.

The lateral view is the most useful, but both lateral and VD views are required to document all abnormalities. Careful review of two orthogonal views of the vertebral column may allow the nature of the injury (i.e. overextension/flexion, rotation, avulsion or compression) to be determined. Knowledge of the mechanism of injury is useful for predicting the degree of resultant instability and selecting a method of fixation. Occasionally, stress radiography may help to further delineate the nature of the injury; however, stress images are usually not necessary when two orthogonal views have been obtained and should generally be avoided because manipulation of the vertebral column increases the risk of further vertebral displacement. Myelography is usually not indicated unless a mass effect has not been documented by plain radiography and the neurological status of the animal would warrant surgery if one were present. The presence of bone lysis or production in animals with an acute onset of pain, paresis or paralysis usually indicates a pre-existing pathological condition (neoplasia). The thoracolumbar region is most commonly affected in dogs, whereas the sacrococcygeal region is most commonly affected in cats. The entire vertebral column should be imaged as a precaution.

Radiological features:

- Vertebral body fractures may be transverse or oblique with disruption of the dorsal or ventral cortex or endplate (Figures 9.42 and 9.43). Due to the support of the paravertebral muscles and flexibility of the vertebral column, the degree of displacement may be difficult to detect despite significant cord injury. Examination for malalignment of the spinous processes on VD radiographs is useful to evaluate for subtle displacement.
- Subluxation may be associated with fractures of the articular processes. Careful assessment of the alignment of the vertebral canal is necessary to identify the changes.
- Marked displacement of fragments indicates severe cord damage, usually transection.
- Physeal separation may be seen in immature animals (usually <1 year old).
- Compression fractures can be recognized by:
  - Shortened vertebra
  - Angulation of the vertebral column
  - Increased bone density due to compression and overlap of the trabeculae.

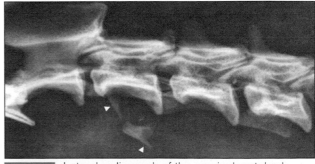

9.42 Lateral radiograph of the cervical vertebral column of a Fox Terrier that had been attacked by another dog. The transverse processes of C3 are fractured and displaced (arrowheads). However, it remains difficult to assess whether fractures of the vertebral bodies or arches are present.

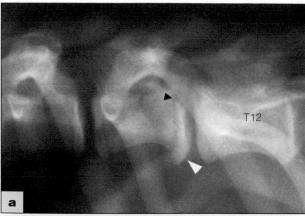

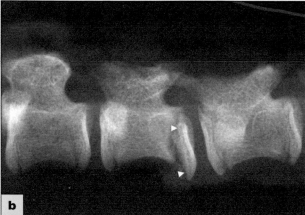

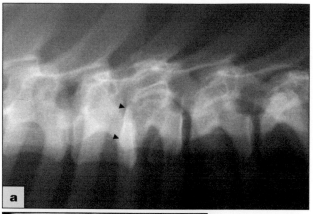

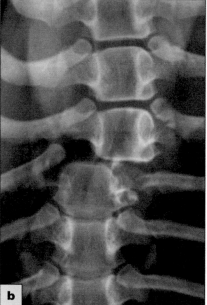

9.43 Lateral radiographs of the caudal thoracic vertebral column of a dog involved in a car accident. **(a)** The caudal endplate of T11 is minimally displaced. It is barely visible: the dorsal (black arrowhead) and ventral (white arrowhead) margins of the ventrally displaced endplate are shown. **(b)** Radiograph taken at post-mortem. The endplate fracture is clearly visible (arrowheads). Muscular bracing often prevents fracture displacement *in vivo*, making radiographic assessment difficult.

- Neural arch fractures are difficult to assess on survey radiographs unless accompanied by dorsal displacement of fracture fragments.
- A narrowed or collapsed intervertebral disc space may indicate traumatic disc herniation.
- Soft tissue swelling (haemorrhage, retroperitoneal organ damage) may be recognized ventral to the vertebral column. In addition, the radiographs should be assessed for signs of pulmonary haemorrhage, rib fractures and fractures of the appendicular skeleton.
- Pathological fractures:
  - Decreased bone density, indicating neoplasia, osteopenia or infection, should be assessed
  - Periosteal reactions, indicating a pre-existing bone disease, should be assessed
  - Lack of sharp margins of fracture fragments due to previous bone lysis.
- Care must be taken to ensure that multiple fractures are not overlooked.

Vertebral luxation and subluxation

Complete vertebral luxation usually leads to severing of the spinal cord with catastrophic consequences (Figure 9.44). In the coccygeal vertebrae, tail fractures and luxations are usually treatable with amputation.

9.44 **(a)** Lateral view of the thoracic vertebral column of a dog involved in a car accident. The T5 and T6 vertebrae overlap (arrowheads), indicating vertebral luxation. **(b)** DV radiograph taken at post-mortem showing complete T5–T6 intervertebral and right vertebrocostal joint luxation, as well as a fracture of T6, causing complete transection of the spinal cord.

Although difficult to acquire in a vertebral trauma patient, two orthogonal views are essential to assess a vertebral luxation.

- Atlanto-occipital overlap has been reported in small-breed dogs, where the arch of the atlas protrudes into an enlarged foramen magnum and compresses the cerebellar vermis, contributing to the clinical signs of Chiari malformation.
- Atlantoaxial instability is caused by insufficient anchoring of the odontoid process of the axis to the floor of the axis, resulting in spinal cord hyperextension and compression.
- Subluxation of the C5–C6 articular processes has been reported in two Poodles, caused by dog fight injuries, and was recognized on VD radiographs (Basinger *et al.*, 1986).
- Trauma can cause rupture of the intervertebral ligaments and result in abnormal flexion or extension, leading to spinal cord compression. In cervical spondylomyelopathy, cervical subluxation is part of the complex pathophysiology of this condition.

- Lumbosacral degenerative disc disease is often associated with a degree of vertebral subluxation, which contributes to cauda equina compression.

Degenerative conditions

Spondylosis deformans: This is a degenerative disease with osteophyte/enthesiophyte formation along the ventral or lateral endplate margin, bridging the intervertebral space. As with any osteophytosis, it is believed to be associated with joint instability. It is ubiquitous in the dog and cat and progressive with age. Despite recognition of this condition in the dog since the 1930s, there is to date no scientific publication that convincingly documents any clinical relevance.

Radiological features:

- Consists of bridging ventral or lateral new bone formation at the endplates, often with a trabecular bone pattern.
- Osseous fragments can be disconnected from the vertebra.

The main relevance of spondylosis deformans is to differentiate it from other forms of pathology. In particular, lateral spondylosis on a lateral radiograph can mimic discal mineralization or other forms of bony proliferation.

Osteoarthritis of the articular process joints: The significance of proliferative changes associated with articular process joints is uncertain (Figure 9.45). Pain and reduced range of motion or stiffness may result, but are not necessarily associated with neurological signs. In the cervical vertebral column, arthrosis, osteophytosis and hypertrophy of the articular process joints is associated with lateralized (bilateral) osseous stenosis (Figure 9.46).

Disseminated idiopathic skeletal hyperostosis: This is an idiopathic condition with extensive new bone formation along the entire ventral and lateral margins of several vertebrae, bridging the intervertebral disc spaces and eventually leading to block vertebra formation. The condition is very common in Boxers (Figure 9.47) and Great Danes, and rarely causes any clinical signs apart from a stiff gait.

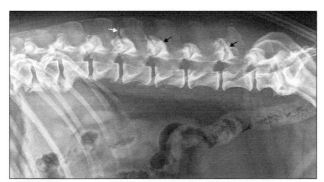

9.45 Lateral view of the lumbar vertebral column of a dog showing extensive degenerative changes. Florid new bone surrounds the articular processes (black arrows) and between the lamina and base of the spinous processes of adjacent vertebrae (white arrow). The changes, although dramatic, are often of limited significance other than reduced flexibility of the vertebral column.

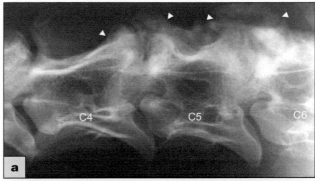

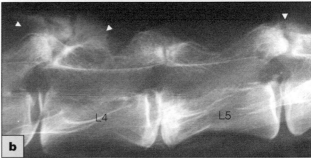

9.46 Lateral radiographs of **(a)** the cervical and **(b)** the lumbar vertebral column in a Great Dane. (a) The C4–C5 and C5–C6 articular process joints are misshapen and surrounded by massive osteophytosis (arrowheads). These changes can arise as a result of osteochondrosis and lead to stenosis of the cervical vertebral canal as part of the cervical stenotic spondylomyelopathy. (b) The lumbar articular process joints at L3–L4, L4–L5 and L5–L6 (arrowheads) are also affected.

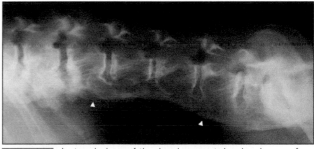

9.47 Lateral view of the lumbar vertebral column of a skeletally mature Boxer with continuous bone formation (arrowheads) along the ventral aspect of the lumbar vertebral bodies (disseminated idiopathic skeletal hyperostosis), leading to vertebral body enlargement, abnormal shape and fusion. Despite its dramatic appearance, this was an incidental finding.

Recent studies have shown that block vertebra formation in dogs creates increased stress on the intervertebral disc spaces of adjacent vertebral segments, which can lead to intervertebral disc protrusion (adjacent segment syndrome) (Ortega *et al.*, 2012).

Radiological features:

- Smooth continuous ventral and lateral new bone formation along the thoracic, lumbar and sacral vertebral column.

Vertebral periosteal reactions

Periosteal reactions can occur secondary to neoplastic or inflammatory conditions. The degree of irregularity reflects the aggressiveness of the lesion. The most common causes include:

- Primary or metastatic vertebral or soft tissue neoplasia. Pelvic (prostatic, cystic, urethral) carcinomas are associated with an irregular periosteal reaction along L6 to S3
- Aggressive discospondylitis or spondylitis, in particular with fungal, mycobacterial and protozoal disease
- Hypervitaminosis A, particularly in the cervical vertebrae of cats.

Articular process joint malformation

Malformation of the articular processes is relatively common in the dog and usually occurs without any clinical consequences as they are located lateral to the vertebral canal (Figure 9.48). Malformation must be dramatic to encroach upon the spinal canal.

- Articular process joint tropism is a term used to describe bilateral asymmetry of the articular process joint orientation. This is most commonly seen in the caudal lumbar vertebral column of German Shepherd Dogs and is thought to promote degenerative joint disease and abnormal loading of the vertebral column. The asymmetry in the articular process joint can be recognized on VD radiographs.

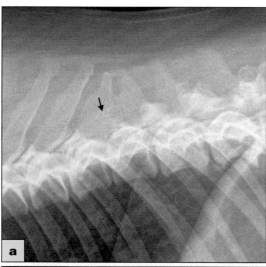
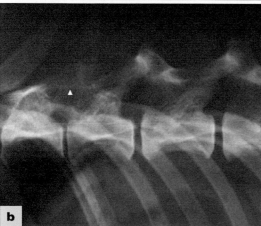

9.48 Lateral radiographs showing the absence of the articular process joints in two dogs. **(a)** Mid-thoracic block vertebra without articular processes (arrowed). **(b)** Absence of articular process joints at T10–T11 (arrowhead). This was an incidental finding. Note also the narrowing of the intervertebral disc space at T10–T11, indicating disc degeneration.

- Aplasia or marked hypoplasia of an articular process can lead to compensatory hypertrophy of the opposing articular process, joint instability and dorsal spinal cord compression. In most cases, such changes are mild and non-compressive.
- Malformation, osteochondrosis, trauma and infection of the articular process joint can all lead to end-stage degenerative joint disease with osteophyte formation. On radiography, this often manifests as exuberant irregular new bone formation around the articular process joints with lack of a normal joint space.

Vertebral curvature deformations

Abnormal alignment of the vertebral column is occasionally seen in the dog and cat. It is often incidental, but can become clinically significant if the spinal cord is compressed.

Scoliosis: This is abnormal lateral deviation of the vertebral column. Common causes include:

- Hemivertebra
- Transitional vertebra
- Vertebral luxation
- Vertebral malunion fracture
- Unilateral chronic muscular spasm or fibrosing changes.

Kyphosis: This is abnormal dorsal deviation of the vertebral column. Common causes include:

- Hemivertebra
- Vertebral luxation
- Vertebral malunion fracture
- Muscular, spinal or abdominal pain.

Lordosis: This is abnormal ventral deviation of the vertebral column. Common causes include:

- Hemivertebra
- Vertebral luxation
- Vertebral malunion fracture
- Brainstem injury (opisthotonus) for cervical lordosis
- Muscle spasm or fibrotic changes.

Inflammatory bone disease

Spondylitis: Spondylitis or osteomyelitis of the vertebral body occurs secondary to foreign bodies, penetrating wounds, paravertebral infections and haematogenous infection (due to conditions, such as portosystemic shunts, that reduce the normal immune response). The majority of cases with spondylitis involve the thoracolumbar vertebral column with signs referable to the hindlimbs. Common signs include pain, stiffness and reluctance to rise. The cervical vertebral column is only occasionally involved and clinical signs include neck pain and low head carriage. Single or multiple draining sinuses may be present. Neurological signs are only present when there is cord compression following extension of inflammatory disease into the vertebral canal, resulting in empyema (infection of the epidural space) or dural involvement.

Radiological features:

- Focal (monostotic) or segmental (multiple adjacent vertebrae) involvement. Determining the site of involvement can be helpful in reaching a diagnosis. Involvement of the L2–L5 vertebrae is highly suggestive of a migrating foreign body (Figure 9.49).

■ Soft tissue swelling:
- In the cervical region may lead to ventral or lateral displacement of the trachea or larynx
- In the sublumbar region recognized as a soft tissue opacity or mass with displacement of the kidneys or colon.

■ Periosteal changes with paravertebral infections are recognized early in the course of the disease, whereas with haematogenous spondylitis they tend to appear later. The periosteal reaction can be ventral or lateralized. The ventral cortices may become indistinct.

■ The trabecular pattern in the medulla is usually unaltered with paravertebral infections, except in chronic disease or if the vertebral body is penetrated by a foreign body. With haematogenous or atypical infections (fungal), the vertebral changes are variable and can have a lytic, productive or mixed appearance. Biopsy may be necessary to distinguish vertebral infection from a neoplastic lesion in some cases.

■ Chronic remodelling may result in bridging ventral spondylosis.

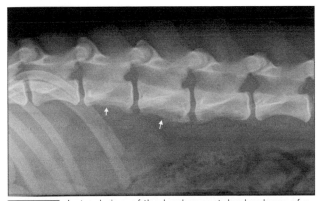

9.49 Lateral view of the lumbar vertebral column of a dog with spondylitis involving L2 and L3. The periosteal reaction (arrowed) is palisading and continuous along the ventral aspect of the vertebral bodies. The pattern is typically associated with a migrating foreign body.

Discospondylitis: Infection of the intervertebral disc occurs secondary to haematogenous dissemination of septic emboli or paravertebral infection associated with penetrating wounds or migrating foreign bodies. Bacteraemia can be secondary to urinary tract infection, bacterial endocarditis, immunecompromise and spinal surgery. Clinical signs include spinal pain, stiffness, pyrexia and systemic disease. Neurological deficits are not present unless there is empyema or instability due to disc herniation or fractures. Multiple sites of discospondylitis may be present with haematogenous infection or in immunocompromised animals. Involvement of non-contiguous vertebrae tends to support a diagnosis of haematogenous involvement.

Radiological features:

■ Cervical involvement is uncommon whereas thoracolumbar involvement is more frequently seen.

■ Widening of the intervertebral disc space occurs initially, progressing to disc space collapse (Figure 9.50).

■ Endplate destruction (Figure 9.51). The vertebral bodies appear shortened and sequestra may form within the vertebral endplates.

■ Sclerosis of the vertebral endplates bordering areas of subchondral destruction.

■ Although discospondylitis can affect dogs of any age, in the immature animal before the growth plates have closed, the lesions may be centred on the vertebral physis. The physis may be widened

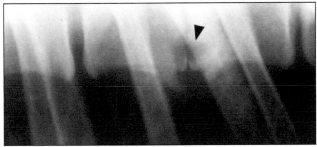

9.50 Magnified lateral view of the T7–T8 intervertebral disc space of an Irish Setter with early-stage discospondylitis. Note the disc space collapse and irregular osteolysis in both endplates (arrowhead).

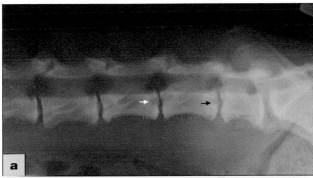
a

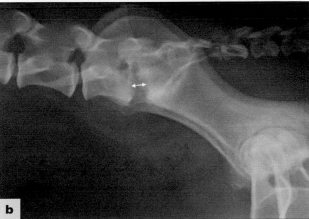
b

9.51 Lateral radiographs of the lumbosacral vertebral column of two dogs with discospondylitis.
(a) There is destruction of the cranial and caudal endplates and subchondral bone bordering the L5–L6 (white arrow) and L6–L7 (black arrow) intervertebral disc spaces. Destruction of the cranial endplates at these sites is subtle. The predominant feature is bone lysis; sclerosis is limited.
(b) The destruction of the endplates and subchondral bone at the L7–S1 intervertebral disc space is more marked than in (a), resulting in widening of the intervertebral disc space (double-headed arrow). The L7 and S1 vertebrae are shortened, the vertebral endplates are irregular and the disc space has collapsed.

and bordered by irregular bone on either side. The physis may subluxate.

- Instability may lead to subluxation/luxation if the articular processes are involved.
- Changes are centred on the intervertebral disc until late in the course of the disease. A periosteal reaction with discospondylitis is a feature of advanced disease.
- Progression and remodelling can lead to bony ankylosis of one or more vertebrae.

Neoplasia

Primary vertebral tumours: Osteosarcomas and chondrosarcomas are the most common primary vertebral tumours. Large dogs are more frequently affected. They usually result in monostotic lesions. Haemopoietic neoplasia, of which multiple myeloma is the most common but which also includes lymphoma, results in polyostotic lesions. Clinical signs may be slow to develop but progression is rapid when they do arise. Pain is often a significant feature of spinal tumours and is frequently evident before neurological deficits are recognized. This alone justifies survey radiography (Figures 9.52 to 9.54), ruling out the need for cross-sectional imaging (if the clinical assessment and neurolocalization are accurate).

Radiological features:

- Single vertebra is usually involved.
- Centred on the vertebral body, arches and lamina (less common). Lesion is not centred on the intervertebral disc space. The lesion does not cross the intervertebral disc space, but occasionally in advanced cases adjacent vertebrae are involved by extension.
- A paravertebral soft tissue mass may be evident but this is uncommon.

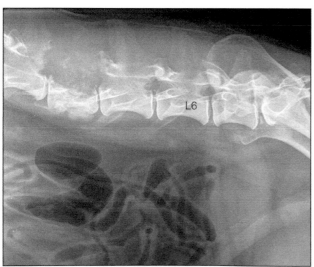

9.52 Lateral view of the lumbar vertebral column of a dog with an extensive primary vertebral tumour involving L4. Extensive destruction of the spinous process, lamina, and cranial and caudal articular processes and vertebral body predominates, but new bone is also present along the ventral margin of the vertebral body. The lesion is unusual as, although it clearly arises from one vertebra, it extends to involve the lamina and articular processes of the adjacent vertebrae. This probably reflects the advanced changes.

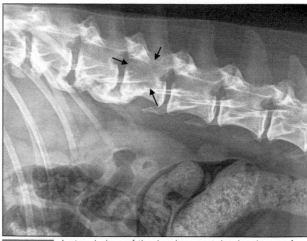

9.53 Lateral view of the lumbar vertebral column of a dog with a primary vertebral tumour involving L3. The lesion is large and predominately lytic (arrowed). Despite this, the lesion is easily overlooked if the clinician is distracted by the extensive degenerative changes (ventral spondylosis and periarticular osteophytes).

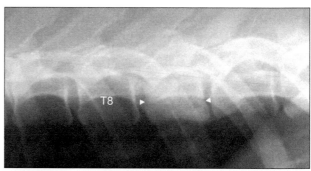

9.54 Lateral view of the caudal thoracic vertebrae of a dog with vertebral neoplasia of T9 (arrowheads). The only radiographic finding was mild sclerosis of the T9 vertebral body.

- The appearance is variable – predominantly destructive/lytic or mixed pattern.
- Destruction most commonly involves the dorsal and ventral cortices and endplates.
- Pathological fractures may occur.
- There may be collapse of the intervertebral disc space and subluxation.

Multiple myeloma:

Radiological features:

- Polyostotic lesions are usually evident (see Figure 9.15). Rarely, solitary lesions (solitary plasmacytoma) may occur, usually in the cat.
- Variably sized lytic foci are present. They are usually small and punctuate (3–5 mm) but appear larger when confluent.
- The vertebral column, pelvis, sternum and ribs are all often involved.
- Unaffected bone has a normal appearance.
- Pathological fractures often appear as compression fractures.

Metastatic neoplasia:

- One or more vertebrae may be involved. Contiguous vertebrae may be affected in animals with pelvic neoplasia.

- 'Skip' lesions may be present with other haematogenous metastatic neoplasia.
- Metastatic neoplasia may appear as a periosteal reaction along the ventral aspect of the caudal lumbar vertebrae from pelvic tumours (in particular, prostatic carcinomas and transitional cell carcinomas). The periosteal reaction may involve the sacrum and ilium.
- Any part of the vertebra may be involved (Figures 9.55 and 9.56).
- A soft tissue component is uncommon.
- Local lymphadenopathy may be present (sublumbar lymph nodes in metastatic neoplasia from the pelvis).

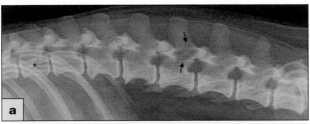

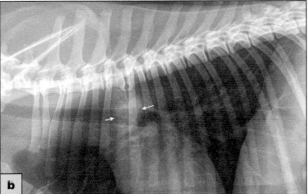

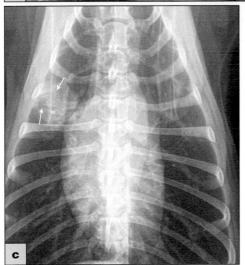

9.55 **(a)** Lateral view of the lumbar vertebral column and **(b)** lateral and **(c)** VD views of the thorax of a dog with vertebral metastasis. (a) The dorsal lamina of the fourth lumbar vertebra is disrupted (arrowed). The margin of the area of lysis is ragged and poorly circumscribed. On MRI, the medulla of the T13 vertebral body was also seen to be completely replaced by the tumour. This change cannot be appreciated on the radiograph (*) due to superimposition of the ribs and the insensitivity of radiographs in demonstrating bone lysis. (b–c) Careful evaluation of the thorax reveals an expansile, destructive lesion of the proximal third of the right fourth rib (arrowed) and pathological fracture of the rib.

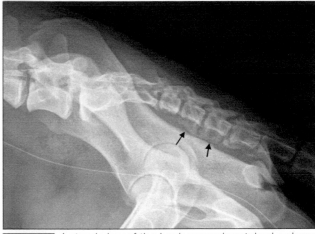

9.56 Lateral view of the lumbosacral vertebral column of a male dog with urethral neoplasia. Thick, palisading new bone (arrowed) is present along the ventral margin of multiple coccygeal vertebrae. The change is consistent with metastatic disease.

Soft tissue neoplasia invading bone: Soft tissue tumours invading the vertebral column are uncommon but primary mesenchymal tumours (injection site sarcoma in the cat) or retroperitoneal tumours may produce radiographic changes.

- Soft tissue tumours invading the vertebral column usually involve several adjacent vertebrae.
- Paravertebral soft tissue masses may be quite large but are difficult to distinguish from paravertebral muscles.
- A periosteal reaction may be present along the ventral or lateral aspect of one or more vertebral bodies.
- Masses are often first recognized if normal symmetry is lost (e.g. due to destruction of the transverse processes).
- Lysis of the spinous processes may be present with soft tissue sarcomas (injection site sarcomas) (Figure 9.57) involving the cranial thorax in the cat.

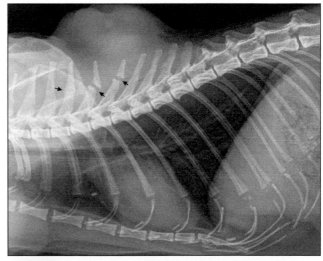

9.57 Lateral view of the thorax of a cat with a large soft tissue sarcoma between the scapulae. Infiltration of the mass into the dorsal spinous processes has resulted in pathological fractures of the mid-portion of the T4 and T5 dorsal spinal processes (arrowed). A mild periosteal reaction borders the fracture site (including T3).

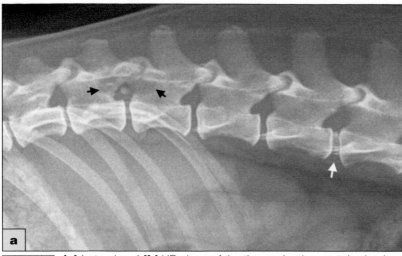
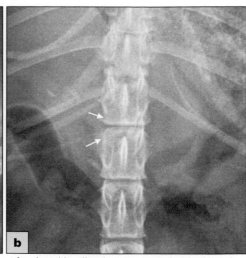

9.58 **(a)** Lateral and **(b)** VD views of the thoracolumbar vertebral column of a dog. Hemilaminectomy and spinal cord decompression for intervertebral disc extrusion had previously been performed. Neurological signs recurred 1 year later. (a) The missing articular process is difficult to recognize on the lateral view but the borders (black arrows) of the laminectomy are visible. The nucleus of the intervertebral disc at L3–L4 is mineralized (white arrow). (b) On the VD view, the missing process joint is appreciated better (white arrows). There does not appear to be any indication of instability as a result of the previous surgery.

Tumours of the nerve roots, cord and meninges:
Survey radiographic changes are often unremarkable. In rare cases with slow tumour growth, expansion results in bone (pressure) atrophy.

Radiological features:

- Enlargement of the vertebral canal and intervertebral foramina.
- Thinning of the vertebral body or lamina.

Post-surgical changes: Significant post-surgical changes can alter the shape and/or alignment of the vertebrae and include:

- Instability, recognized as subluxation, fracture of the articular process joints or proliferative new bone bridging the vertebral bodies or around the articular facets (see Figure 9.9)
- The presence of a defect from a missing articular process and lamina as a result of hemilaminectomy (Figure 9.58)
- Collapse of an intervertebral disc space as a result of fenestration.

References and further reading

Baines EA, Grandage J, Herrtage ME and Baines SJ (2009) Radiographic definition of the anticlinal vertebra in the dog. *Veterinary Radiology and Ultrasound* **50(1)**, 69–73
Basinger RR, Bjorling De and Chambers JN (1986) Cervical spinal luxation in two dogs with entrapment of the cranial articular process of C6 over the caudal articular process of C5. *Journal of the American Veterinary Medical Association* **217**, 862–864
Davis J (2006) Spine – intervertebral disc disease and 'Wobbler syndrome'. In: *BSAVA Manual of Canine and Feline Musculoskeletal Imaging*, ed. FJ Barr and RM Kirberger, pp. 247–256. BSAVA Publications, Gloucester
Kirberger RM (2006) Spine – general. In: *BSAVA Manual of Canine and Feline Musculoskeletal Imaging*, ed. FJ Barr and RM Kirberger, pp. 220–232. BSAVA Publications, Gloucester
Lang J (2006) Spine – lumbosacral region and cauda equina syndrome. In: *BSAVA Manual of Canine and Feline Musculoskeletal Imaging*, ed. FJ Barr and RM Kirberger, pp. 257–271. BSAVA Publications, Gloucester
Llabres-Diaz F, Petite A, Saunders J and Schwarz T (2008) The thoracic boundaries. In: *BSAVA Manual of Canine and Feline Thoracic Imaging*, ed. T Schwarz and V Johnson, pp. 340–376. BSAVA Publications, Gloucester
McConnell JF (2012) Imaging of neurological emergencies. In: *Small Animal Neurological Emergencies*, ed. S Platt and L Garosi, pp. 83–120. Manson Publishing, London
McEvoy FJ (2006) Spine – conditions not related to intervertebral disc disease. In: *BSAVA Manual of Canine and Feline Musculoskeletal Imaging*, ed. FJ Barr and RM Kirberger, pp. 233–246. BSAVA Publications, Gloucester
Ortega M, Goncalves R, Haley A, Wessmann A and Penderis J (2012) Spondylosis deformans and diffuse idiopathic skeletal hyperostosis (DISH) resulting in adjacent segment disease. *Veterinary Radiology and Ultrasound* **53(2)**, 128–134

Index